COUNSELOR
PREPARATION

COUNSELOR PREPARATION

Programs, Faculty, Trends

11th Edition

Thomas W. Clawson
The National Board for Certified Counselors

Donna A. Henderson
Wake Forest University

Wendi K. Schweiger
The National Board for Certified Counselors

with

Daniel R. Collins
The National Board for Certified Counselors

Brunner-Routledge

New York and Hove

Published in 2004 by
Brunner-Routledge
29 West 35th Street
New York, NY 10001
www.brunner-routledge.com

Published in Great Britain by
Brunner-Routledge
27 Church Road
Hove, East Sussex
BN3 2FA
www.brunner-routledge.co.uk

Brunner-Routledge is an imprint of the Taylor & Francis Group
Printed in the United States of America on acid-free paper.

10 9 8 7 6 5 4 3 2 1

Library of Congress Cataloging-in-Publication Data is available from the Library of Congress.
ISBN 0-415-93553-9 (hb)

Contents

PART B: COUNSELOR PREPARATION PROGRAM STRUCTURE

PART C: COUNSELOR PREPARATION PROGRAMS

Preface

This book is the work of current, past, and future counselor educators. Our perspective is, therefore, to make available data that will be relevant as a resource while continuing the tradition of what we in the profession fondly call the "Hollis and Wantz Directory."

Begun in 1970, *Counselor Preparation* has been the only longitudinal record of our counselor education programs. As our profession has more clearly defined itself, the number of programs has become smaller and better delineated. This shrinking of "counselor preparation" programs is a result of professional concerns as well as four distinct changes in selection by the authors.

First, and very significant, the Council for the Accreditation of Counseling and Related Educational Programs (CACREP) standards have been the most influential voluntary training ideas introduced to professional counseling. As CACREP standards have become the flagship determination of a professional counseling program, many institutions have been influenced to abandon programs that would never be accredited. So, as programs become more stringent and are subjected to outside review, fewer remain.

Second, the authors of *Counselor Preparation* began in the 9th edition to eliminate educational institutions that were not counselor preparation. The history of counselor education shows us that many early programs were part of, or housed in, schools of psychology, social work, or family studies. Counseling developed standards and moved toward professionalization starting in the 1960s; these early changes provided us with reason to eliminate a great number of listed programs, but it is not correct to assume that counselor education programs have diminished greatly. What has changed the most is our willingness to label a program counselor education.

A third factor that has affected the numbers of programs listed was the 9th edition elimination of training institutes that were not degree granting. Training institutes provide service for the mental health professions but are not academically accredited. All programs listed in this book are part of a regionally accredited institution of higher education.

Fourth, the response rate from institutions is remarkably low. The authors delayed this edition because counselor education programs were slow in returning surveys or simply ignored requests. We find this astounding, considering the widespread use of *Counselor Preparation* and the free advertising provided by program descriptions. We do understand that there are many pressing needs within institutions that can move our survey to the bottom of the pile. We also may be seeing an economic trend. Because counselor education is in a very healthy era in terms of enrollment and job opportunities, free advertising of a program is not necessarily beneficial. When applications outnumber admission spaces, programs may not be looking for any more publicity. We would like to suggest that, even when applications are high, having more students explore a broader range of institutions can only lead to more diversity of student populations and to better selection possibilities.

The authors are indebted to so many people for the time and energy they contributed to the first online Counselor Preparation Survey. This data will be saved and re-sent to institutions for the next, updated 12th edition. We hope to include more programs and promise to begin international reporting of counseling programs.

Some data from this book will appear on the NBCC Website, www.nbcc.org.

Thomas W. Clawson, Ed.D., NCC, LPC
Executive Director, National Board for Certified Counselors, Inc.®

Donna A. Henderson, Ph.D., NCC, LPC
Associate Professor, Department of Counseling, Wake Forest University

Wendi K. Schweiger, M.S./Ed.S., NCC, LPC
Research Associate/Counselor-in-Residence
National Board for Certified Counselors, Inc.®

A Tribute to Joe Hollis

This serial approach to reviewing counselor preparation programs remains unique to our profession. Joseph W. Hollis, Ed.D., NCC, began this collection in the late 1960s in an effort to document what counselor education was doing, who was involved in the preparation, and where programs were located. As counseling became more professional, the need for *Counselor Preparation* as a resource grew steadily. Soon the early editions of the book became known for the two authors, Joe Hollis and Richard Wantz. The book today is often referred to as the Hollis and Wantz directory, even though Dr. Richard Wantz of Wright State University has not been a coauthor for a decade. Dr. Wantz's long-term contribution to this series has greatly added to our archives.

This is the first preface of *Counselor Preparation* that does not have the personal hand of Joe Hollis shining through. Joe passed away in November of 2002 while data collection was still in progress. Joe's death is a sad event with a meaningful history to be told. We will talk about Joe Hollis on later pages. Now we would like to look at the age of our profession: the developmental age.

In 2002, the American Counseling Association marked its 50th anniversary. Many of the original leaders in our field are still leading, but many have passed away. In counselor education, we are experiencing a time of many retirements and deaths of the stalwarts of our profession. This is occurring partly because counselor education found its most dominant rise in the mid-1960s. Many young professors created the first syllabi, engineered the first schedules, and politicked master's degree programs through university senates. These pioneering professors began to retire in the past decade in great numbers. They are remembered on plaques, in scholarships, and in their written work. Moreover, they are responsible for several generations of youthful professionals who have made a mark on American society. We salute Joe Hollis with this book; we salute our hundreds of other mentors as well for their dedication and for nurturing a new profession.

TO JOSEPH W. HOLLIS

Joe was born in Waverly, Missouri, where he graduated from high school and attended the University of Missouri-Kansas, receiving his first degree in 1948. Joe then went on to the University of Colorado, receiving his doctorate. Joe also served our country while in the United States Army during World War II.

He came to Muncie, Indiana, in 1954, teaching Psychology at Ball State University. This is where he also served as Chairman of the Department of Counseling Psychology and Guidance Services. Dr. Hollis spent 30 years of his life dedicated to his students and colleagues, retiring in 1984.

In 1965, Dr. Hollis published his first major publication and another in 1969, building an interest in publishing. Dr. Hollis was author of more than ten books and was the author of articles and chapters in many publications. Joe started a publishing company in the garage of his home, and this is where he founded Accelerated Development Publishing Company. (Excerpted from the Joseph W. Hollis memorial program.)

I have had two major experiences with Joe Hollis that have taught me how much he knew and how respected he was. Joe hired me to teach for Ball State University's Overseas Counselor Education Program in 1981. It was a turning point in my career and in my life. Later, as executive director of NBCC, I called him to express concern for the continuation of *Counselor Preparation*. NBCC teamed with Joe to continue the 9th and 10th editions of *Counselor Preparation*.

My insider memories of working for and with Joe are many. I suppose my most significant memory is helping edit two editions of *Counselor Preparation*. Both editions were primarily written by Joe—and by that I mean handwritten. I still have a huge pile of paper constituting the bulk of the 10th edition in Joe's handwriting. He didn't like computers.

Possibly the most telling story about Joe Hollis and his work is the lasting impression he made. I am currently coauthoring *Counselor Preparation* with Donna Henderson and Wendi Schweiger. Even though we are the new authors, we still call it, file it, and remember it as the "Hollis Book."

Also known as the Hollis and Wantz directory, this title was not one that Brunner-Routledge of the Taylor & Francis Group wanted to see disappear.

I was always glad to get a chance to sit with Joe and talk about the profession. He knew something about practically everybody in counselor education and either published or tried to contract every author in our field. I can close my eyes and see him in his stunning green sport coat, with the biggest smile possible, telling a student what books and ideas were hot. In his mid-70s he said to me, "I'm not ready to retire, but I just love my wife and want to spend more time with her. Tom, I hope you have as fulfilling a career as I have had." Joe wished us all his success and gave so many of us opportunities to shine.

In the 2003 issue of *Counseling Today*, Dawn Pennington, Editor-in-Chief, created a tribute to Joe Hollis. The following is her edited article that has captured so much of Joe's essence.

Publisher, Editor, Counseling
'Hero' Hollis Passes Away at Age 80

By Dawn A. Pennington, Managing Editor, Counseling Today

Joseph W. Hollis, a counselor educator who not only was extensively published since 1965, but was also instrumental in assisting many of his students to become published as well, died on Nov. 23, 2002. He was 80.

In addition to dedicating three decades of his life to educating the next generations of counselors, Dr. Hollis, along with his students, actively participated in the advancement of the counseling profession. He was one of the founders of the Counselors Association for Humanistic Education and Development, which is celebrating its 50th anniversary this year, and he also served as its president in 1975–76.

In addition to his involvement in the American Counseling Association, "He was very instrumental in getting C-AHEAD started," says Don C. Locke, adding, "He was also very active in state and regional organizations." Dr. Locke received his doctorate from Ball State University when Hollis chaired the Counseling Psychology doctoral program.

"As co-founder of C-AHEAD, he was very much involved in reconstituting it," Richard Wantz said. "It was a dying organization— he was encouraged to look at revamping it and giving it some life." Wantz was an early collaborator with Hollis, editing *Counselor Preparation*.

C-AHEAD continues to honor Dr. Hollis and his first wife, with its Joe and Lucille Hollis Publications Award, established in 1985 for

Dr. Hollis and his late first wife. This award recognizes leadership and expertise in the publishing arena and has been given to 18 individuals to date who have made a significant impact in humanistically oriented publications.

The annual ACA convention was a place where Dr. Hollis always made a grand appearance. "He would always have an exhibit booth for Accelerated Development," Locke said, noting that his second wife, Marcy, was also a regular attendee. He was also a presence in the Association for Counselor Education and Supervision (ACES).

His passion for counseling was paralleled by a passion for publishing. Not only was he the founder and editor of C-AHEAD's newsletter, *Infochange*, but he also founded the Accelerated Development Publishing Company during the 1970s. The latter venture enabled Dr. Hollis to provide a number of counselors with the opportunity to become published for the first time. "He was an inspiration to many in the publishing world as editor of Accelerated Development," said Richard Wantz, associate professor at Wright State University in Ohio.

Accelerated Development, which was initially headquartered in Dr. Hollis' garage, was eventually moved to a house he purchased, in which he also rented space to graduate students. "He was a person who wasn't afraid to try something different," Wantz said.

"It may sound strange, since I only met Joe face-to-face on a few occasions, but he had a monumental impact on my life and my professional career," said Howard Rosenthal, a professor and program coordinator of human services at St. Louis Community College. "In fact, he literally changed the course of my life for the better."

Rosenthal credited Hollis as the inspiration for his successful venture into publishing books. After giving numerous lectures on suicide prevention, "Everybody kept saying, 'Where's your book?' Of course, I hadn't written one," he said. "Since I was working on another book with a rather famous agent, I told her about my idea to write a suicide prevention text. She said the idea was a 'downer,' and she refused to look at it. She also never sold my other book!"

That was 1998, and that is also when he contacted Dr. Hollis, noting that he'd seen his name on a catalog. "Joe was a straight shooter. [He] wrote me back and said, 'Look, you either have something or you don't. Send me three pages.'"

"I sent Joe the three pages," he continued. "He said 'you have something,' and he gave me a contract on my first book." Rosenthal noted that Dr. Hollis always corresponded directly with himself and others through handwritten notes and never through assistants or public relations departments.

Dr. Hollis's own publishing career dated back to 1965, when he published the first of his ten books, in addition to a number of articles and chapters in other publications. Eventually, Accelerated Development became a subsidiary of the Taylor & Francis Group. "I suspect he had an entrepreneurial spirit," Locke said.

Accelerated Development focused on publications that would benefit counselor educators, according to Wantz. He collaborated with Dr. Hollis for 25 years on such publications, contributing to several of the 10 editions of "Counselor Preparation" manuals that Dr. Hollis later authored with the National Board for Certified Counselors.

"I suspect that publication has been cited by more counseling students in research papers than any other publication in history," Locke said, noting that Hollis first began writing and researching these books in the 1970s, updating the series every three years thereafter.

Dr. Hollis was the 1997 recipient of ACA's Extended Research Award. "One thing I learned from Joe was his emphasis on research and publication of one's writings as criteria for [becoming] a good professional," Locke said, noting that, "Joe encouraged [us as students and new counselors] and made it clear that was what he wanted."

The NBCC held a special interest for Dr. Hollis, who believed firmly in counselor licensure. "I also remember the time he let his NBCC certificate lapse—a braver man than I—so he could take the exam and make certain the test prep materials truly worked," Rosenthal said. "Fortunately, they did. Joe only sold a product [i.e., book or tape] if he really believed in it."

Something else he believed in was in the accreditation of graduate counseling programs. "Ball State was one of the first universities to apply to the Council for Accreditation of Counseling and Related Educational Programs [CACREP]," Wantz said. "I don't know if they would have gone for that if Joe wasn't involved."

Later, according to Wantz, Ball State's counseling psychology program would go up for accreditation. "It was turned down initially, but Joe felt they had a strong program," he said. The program later became accredited.

Dr. Hollis's list of accomplishments as a publisher, editor, writer and educator wouldn't be complete without the term "mentor."

"Joe was my major counseling professor at Ball State University in Muncie, Indiana, back in the late '60s," said Jim White, director of elementary/secondary services with ACT, Inc., East Region. "His specialty was careers, and his instruction took for me . . . as a career focus has been a part of all my life work to date."

"He was a very open professor who invited us to take chances and think 'out of the box,'" White continued. "In later years, I saw Joe at conferences where we were both exhibiting. He was always so welcoming and always seemed to remember who you were, even after 20-plus years! He was indeed a special man who made a major impact on the lives of so many."

Don C. Locke, a counselor educator at the North Carolina State University in Raleigh, as well as the director of the doctoral program at its Asheville Graduate Center, also got his start in publishing under Dr. Hollis' wing. But before that, he was a student of Dr. Hollis.

"[Dr. Hollis] was instrumental to my getting a contract for my first book, 'Psychological Techniques for Teachers,'" Locke said. "He was also instrumental in getting me into the doctoral program [at Ball State University, where Dr. Hollis was the director of its doctoral program]—he encouraged me and sponsored me."

"Joe was a career counselor type, always a very supportive and super-nice man," Locke continued. Wantz added that Dr. Hollis was a "vocational expert" and that he was often hired by federal courts to share his expertise during court hearings.

"He was very much a believer in the counseling model and the right of counselors to exist," Wantz said.

The counseling model, for Dr. Hollis, also included serving as a role model to his students, whether it meant taking them on the road with him to conferences, having lunch with them or inviting them into his home for classes.

"He was the kind of person who did a great deal at the university level, then on the professional level," Locke said, noting that it was a natural progression for Dr. Hollis to subsequently invite students to accompany him in his many endeavors.

"He was very giving to his students and included them in presentations, conferences and seminars [that would benefit them]," Wantz said, noting that Dr. Hollis also in this manner exposed his students to the professional groups in which he was so active. He was invited by Dr. Hollis to attend ACA's convention in Atlantic City when he was a student.

"It was also not uncommon for students to be invited to The Flamingo in Muncie," he continued. "He and his wife ate out every day, and to be invited to dine with them was a wonderful personal touch."

This personal touch helped the professional impact to become even more profound.

Locke recalled a professional issues class that he attended on Tuesday afternoon in Dr. Hollis's home. "I think it was Joe who really gave me the foundation and encouraged my interest in professional issues," he said, noting how inspired he became, learning about items of critical interest to aspiring counseling professionals during these seminars.

"In his home, he had a library where he held classes—which is not typical of most faculty members," Wantz said.

Locke recalled a class on learning-oriented reactive simulation, where, "You were placed in situations that you would face in your profession [through role play]," he said.

Wantz noted that Dr. Hollis even enlisted the campus police to bring an even higher element of reality to the role play, much to the surprise of his students.

Not only did Dr. Hollis leave an impression on the counseling students he mentored, but he also made a mark on the president's house at Ball State University. According to Wantz, Dr. Hollis was head of a committee that worked on the design of the nine-story building, and it came to be known affectionately as the "Hollis Hilton."

His writers recall him fondly as well.

"Joe gave me my start in the publishing business, and I will never forget it," Rosenthal said, noting that he dedicated his most recently published book to Dr. Hollis as well as to his late father. "Life is strange. Several minutes after [learning of Dr. Hollis's death] the UPS truck dropped off a shipment of my new book, the 'Human Services Dictionary.' It was like a sign. The book was an arduous project that I started on with Joe's blessing many years ago. I feel a deep sadness knowing I won't be able to send Joe a copy."

Rosenthal's recent inscription to Dr. Hollis reads, "Many people live their entire lives and never have the good fortune to meet an individual with the vision and integrity that is radiated by Dr. Joseph Hollis. Therefore, I consider myself to be a very lucky person."

When Rosenthal first learned that Dr. Hollis had passed away, he noted, "My wife said, 'You lost a mentor,' and I said, 'Yes, I did.'"

"They say there really aren't any more heroes nowadays, but that just isn't true," he added.

— —

Good mentors are hard to give up. In the end, the great mentors leave us with knowledge (and wanting more), pleasurable memories (always there to recall), and confidence (that we've absorbed so freely). Losing them is difficult, yet they leave us with great gifts to pass on.

Thomas W. Clawson, Ed.D., NCC, LPC
Executive Director
National Board for Certified Counselors, Inc.®

Acknowledgments

The authors thank the National Board for Certified Counselors, Inc., and Affiliates (NBCC) for their continued support of this important series. NBCC bears the cost of all data collection, programming, clerical assistance in the manuscript phase, and communication costs. We thank the NBCC directors for their continued efforts to present this book as a service to the counseling profession.

Hundreds of counseling professionals helped gather data for the individual counseling programs listed in this book. We are deeply indebted to each of them for the time spent on our extensive survey.

Members of the NBCC staff who were involved in this project were many. Of special importance is Dan Collins who fashioned the new data collection form to a computer-based tool, compiled data with the programming he pioneered, and then went on to offer numerous helpful advances for our data. Dan Paredes at NBCC was a lifesaver when the final deadline loomed. He saved countless hours from our days with his work on this edition. Mary Frazier, in usual form, typed all of Tom Clawson's contributions with a sharp editing eye.

Brunner-Routledge, a division of the Taylor & Francis Group publishers, provided editorial service, business direction, marketing, and, most of all, encouragement. Emily Epstein shepherded us from beginning to end.

CACREP executive director, Dr. Carol Bobby, and her staff, Jenny Gunderman and Nan Bayster, were very helpful in providing up-to-date accredited program listings as well as CACREP subject editing. The CACREP board gave permission for use of the CACREP service mark appearing throughout the book. To them we are indebted.

Part A

Purpose and Design

## Chapter 1

The Profession

This volume contains descriptions of educational programs that prepare counselors at the opening of the 21st century. The extent and focus of those programs has altered as counseling has evolved into its current form. Therefore, we will begin with a look at the beginnings of the profession.

MILESTONES IN THE HISTORY OF COUNSELING

The roots of the counseling profession were planted as the 20th century began. In 1908, Frank Parsons founded the Boston Vocational Bureau, a place designed to help young people find jobs. Jesse Davis was the first person to set up a guidance program in public schools in 1907, and Clifford Beers advocated for better facilities and treatment for the mentally ill in his 1908 book, *A Mind That Found Itself*. The development of tests for military recruits during both world wars also contributed to the need for counselors. Other people who influenced this fledgling profession were William Fainey Harpers, Lightner Witmer, Morris S. Viteles, Alfred Binet, G. Stanley Hall, and even Sigmund Freud during his visit to the United States.

To become a discipline or body of knowledge, the counseling movement needed to meet specific criteria.

1 *Specific body of knowledge with recognized training programs.* To be considered a profession, a body of knowledge must be accumulated in the area. One indication of this being accomplished was that by 1964 the U.S. Department of Health, Education, and Welfare listed 327 institutions of counselor preparation.

2 *Professional organization of peers.* The professional organization of peers in counseling began with the National Vocational Guidance Association in 1913 and in 1914 with the National Association of Deans of Women, which was later named the National Association of Women Deans and Counselors. Over 20 professional associations have evolved as the specialties in the profession have increased.

3 *Accreditation of training programs.* Established standards and supervision help ensure the quality of training programs. The largest accreditation body for counseling programs is the Council for Accreditation of Counseling and Related Educational Programs (CACREP).

4 *Supervised clinical training.* In addition to extensive classroom instruction, clinical training under the supervision of qualified professional practitioners is required in the education of counselors. The amount of clinical experience is measured in clock hours, with the required number steadily increasing throughout the years.

5 *Certification of practitioners.* Certification refers to the process of gaining certification from a professional organization. The credential affirms that a board of professionals in an area of specialization has reviewed the qualifications of a person and found the individual well qualified. The National Board for Certified Counselors (NBCC) is the largest organization that certifies counselors.

6 *Legal recognition and licensure.* The legal recognition of counselors in private practice has occurred with state and federal laws and acts. Currently 47 states have enacted licensure laws for counselors. A license law stipulates those who can call themselves counselors and what functions they can perform. Therefore, state licensure establishes qualification standards and limits of practice.

MAJOR STEPS TO BECOMING A PROFESSIONAL COUNSELOR

To enter the profession of counseling, a person must complete several activities.

1 Graduating with a baccalaureate degree.

2 Applying to a graduate degree program in counseling. (The selection of the program may depend on program location, desired specialty area, whether the program is accredited, credentials of the faculty, and other things.)

3 Being accepted and enrolling in a counselor preparation program.

4 Completing the academic coursework. (The number of academic hours varies with the kind of program and with the institution. The minimum is generally 48 or more graduate-level academic semester hours, which may include hours for practicum and internship.)

5 Completing a practicum. (The number of clock hours required varies with the program.)

6 Completing a supervised clinical internship. (The number of clock hours required, the type of setting, and the amount of supervision varies from program to program.)

7 Graduating from the counselor preparation program with the equivalent of a master's degree or higher.

8 Applying to the state board and obtaining state licensure.

9 Applying to the national certification board and obtaining certification.

CREDENTIALING OF COUNSELORS AS PRACTITIONERS

A person is eligible for credentialing only after completing a program of study; however, the program requirements or length may determine how quickly some credentials can be obtained. Students would be well advised to carefully consider the program(s) being researched and what opportunities are provided to explore their skills, expectations, and interests during any program of study. Students should gain as much information as possible about potential credentialing opportunities from each program they are considering, review each one, and compare among programs to identify a challenging professional environment and personal growth experience for them as students and future counseling professionals.

State Licensure

Obtaining state licensure means meeting state board requirements that are determined by each state. It is important for candidates to consider the state or states where they might want to practice. Requirements can also vary within any state, depending on the setting in which one would like to practice and the area of practice chosen. For example, requirements for licensure often differ for mental health counselors, marriage and family counselors/therapists, school counselors, rehabilitation counselors, and student affairs practice professionals. The differences can include the amount of academic semester hours required, the type and amount of clinical experience required, and the type and amount of supervised clinical practice hours. For the basic information and the most recent regulations, contact the state board within the state in which you are interested in practicing. Contact information for each state board (as of March 2003) is listed below.

State Boards for State Counselor Licensure/Certification

Alabama   *Law passed 1979.* Dr. Walter Cox, Executive Officer, Alabama Board of Examiners in Counseling, 950 22nd Street North,

Suite 670, Birmingham, AL 35203; (205) 458-8717/1-800-822-3307; e-mail: cox7267@aol.com

Alaska *Law passed 1998.* Ms. Carol Whelan, Board of Professional Counselors, Division of Occupational Licensing, P.O. Box 110806, Juneau, AK 99811-0806; (907) 465-2551; FAX: (907) 465-2974; Website: www.commerce.state.ak.us/occ

Arizona *Law passed 1988.* Ms. Debra Rinaldo, Executive Director, Arizona Board of Behavioral Health Examiners, 1400 West Washington, Room 350, Phoenix, AZ 85007; (602) 542-1882; FAX: (604) 542-1830; e-mail: behavioral_health@pop.state.az.us ; Website: aspin.asu.edu/~azbbhe

Arkansas *Law passed 1979.* Dr. Ann K. Thomas, Executive Director, Arkansas Board of Examiners in Counseling, P.O. Box 70, Magnolia, AR 71754-0070; (870) 901-7055; FAX: (870) 234-1842; e-mail: arboec@sbcglobal.net ; Website: www.state.ar.us/abec

California Dean Porter, Executive Director, CA Registry of Professional Counselors & Paraprofessionals, 2555 East Chapman Avenue, Suite 201, Fullerton, CA 92831; (714) 284-8857; FAX: (714) 871-5132; Website: www.california-registry.org

The CA Registry is a voluntary registry for professionals and paraprofessionals in that state. The only state credential available for counselors is the Marriage, Family, and Child Therapist. NCCs/ LPCs moving to California can contact the relevant board here: Marriage, Family, Child Therapist, Board of Behavioral Sciences, 400 R Street, Suite 3150, Sacramento, CA 95814-6240; (916) 445-4933; FAX: (916) 323-0707; e-mail: BBSWebMaster@bbs.ca.gov; Website: www.bbs.ca.gov

Colorado *Law passed 1988.* Mr. Gene Merrdink, Administrative Assistant, State Board of Licensed Professional Counselor Examiners, 1560 Broadway, Suite 1370, Denver, CO 80202; (303) 894-7766; FAX: (303) 894-7790; e-mail: joan.seggerman@state.co.us; Website: www.dora.state.co.us/registrations/men.htm

Connecticut *Law passed 1997.* Ms. Lawanda Scott, Professional Counselor Licensure, Department of Public Health, 410 Capitol Avenue—MS # 12APP, P.O. Box 340308, Hartford, CT 06134-0308; (860) 509-7561; FAX: (860) 509-8457; Website: www.dph.tate.ct.us

Delaware *Law passed 1987.* Ms. Gayle Franzelino, Administrative Assistant, Board of Professional Counselors of Mental Health, 861 Silver Lake Boulevard, Cannon Building—Suite 203, Dover, DE 19904; (302) 739-4522; FAX: (302) 739-2711

District of Columbia *Law passed 1992.* Ms. Graphelia Ramseur, Administrator, D.C. Board of Professional Counseling, Department of Health, 825 N. Capital Street NE, 2nd Floor, Washington, DC 20002; (202) 442-4775/(202) 442-9200; FAX: (202) 442-9431

Florida *Law passed 1981, revised 1987.* Ms. Carole Timin, Regulatory Specialist, Board of Clinical Social Work, Marriage and Family Therapy, and Mental Health Counseling, 4052 Bald Cypress Way, Bin # C0-8, Tallahassee, FL 32399-3250; (850) 245-4444 ext. 3434; e-mail: carol_timin@doh.state.fl.us ; Website: www.doh.state.fl.us/mqu

Georgia *Law passed 1984.* Mr. Ken Smith, Composite Board of Professional Counselors, Social Workers, and Marriage & Family Therapists, Examining Boards Division, 237 Coliseum Drive, Macon, GA 31217; (478) 207-1670; FAX: (478) 207-1676

Guam *Law passed 1989.* Ms. Teofila P. Cruz, Licensing Administrator, Department of Public Health & Social Services, The Guam Board of Allied Health Examiners, P.O. Box 2816, Agana, GU 96910; (671) 734-7295/(671) 735-7399; FAX: (671) 734-2066

Hawaii There is no licensure law in Hawaii at this time.

Idaho *Law passed 1982.* Ms. Janice Wiedrick, Board Secretary, Idaho State Counselor Licensing Board, Bureau of Occupational Licenses, Owyhee Plaza, 1109 Main Street, Suite 220, Boise, ID 83702-5642; (208) 334-3233; FAX: (208) 334-3945; e-mail: jwiedric@ibol.state.id.us

Illinois *Law passed 1992.* Ms. Cheryl Foxx, Board Liaison, Illinois Department of Professional Regulations, 320 West Washington Street, 3rd Floor, Springfield, IL 62786; (217) 782-8556; FAX: (217) 782-7645

Indiana *Law passed 1997.* Mr. Wade A. Lowhorn, Director, IN Social Work, Marriage & Family Therapist & Mental Health Counselor Board, Health Professions Bureau, 402 W. Washington Street, Room 041, Indianapolis, IN 46204; (317) 234-2064; FAX: (317) 233-4236; e-mail: hpb5@hpb.state.in.us ; Website: www.in.gov/hpb

Iowa *Law passed 1991.* Ms. Judith Manning, Board Administrator, Iowa Board of Behavioral Science Examiners, IA Department of Public Health, Lucas State Office Building, 4th Floor, Des Moines, IA 50319; (515) 281-4413; FAX: (515) 281-3121

Kansas *Certification Law passed 1987.* Legislature law passed 1996 and 1999. Ms. Pat Martin, Behavioral Sciences Regulatory Board, 712 S. Kansas Avenue, Topeka, KS 66603-3817; (785) 296-3240; FAX: (785) 296-3112; e-mail: lvawter@ink.org ; Website: www.ink.org/public/bsrb

Kentucky *Law passed 1996, revised in 2000.* Ms. Judy Jennings, Board Administrator, Division of Occupations and Professions, P.O. Box 1360, Frankfort, KY 40602; (502) 564-3296, ext. 226; FAX:

(502) 564-4818; e-mail: judy.jennings@mail.state.ky.us; Website: www.state.ky.us/agencies/finance/occupations

Louisiana *Law passed 1987*. Ms. Lin Falcon, Administrative Assistant, Licensed Professional Counselors, Board of Examiners, 8631 Summa Avenue, Suite A, Baton Rouge, LA 70809; (225) 765-2515; FAX: (225) 765-2514

Maine *Law passed 1989*. Ms. Ann Head, Executive Director, Maine Board of Counseling Professionals Licensure, State House Station, #35, Augusta, ME 04333; (207) 624-8603; FAX: (207) 624-8637

Maryland *Law passed 1985*. Ms. Aileen Taylor, Administrator, State of Maryland, MD Department of Health & Mental Hygiene, Board of Professional Counselors and Therapists, Metro Executive Center, 3rd Floor, 4201 Patterson Avenue, Baltimore, MD 21215-2299; (410) 764-4732; FAX: (410) 764-5987

Massachusetts *Law passed 1987*. Ms. Jodi Bornstein, Administrative Assistant, Board Allied Mental Health & Human Services Professions, 239 Caiseway Street, 5th Floor, Boston, MA 02114; (877) 773-7462; FAX: (617) 727-2366; e-mail: jodi.b.bornstein@state.ma.us

Michigan *Law passed 1988*. Ms. Patty Marsh, Processor, Michigan Board of Counseling, The Office of Health Services, P.O. Box 30670, Lansing, MI 48909; (517) 335-0918; FAX: (517) 373-2179

Minnesota *Law passed 2003*. Further information not available at time of publication. Check NBCC Website.

Mississippi *Law passed 1985*. Ms. Ann Cox, Mississippi State Board of Examiners for Licensed Professional Counselors, 319 S. Main Street, Yazoo City, MS 39194; (888) 860-7001; Website: www.lpc.state.ms.us

Missouri *Law passed 1985*. Ms. Loree Kessler, Executive Director, Division of Professional Registration, Committee for Professional Counselors, 3605 Missouri Boulevard, P.O. Box 1335, Jefferson City, MO 65102; (573) 751-0018; FAX: (573) 526-3489; e-mail: couns@mail.state.mo.us; Website: www.ecodev.state.mo.us/pr/counselr

Montana *Law passed 1985*. Ms. Mary C. Hainlin, Program Manager, Board of Social Work Examiners & Professional Counselors, Department of Commerce, Professional & Occupational Licensing Division, 301 South Park, 4th Floor, P.O. Box 200513, Helena, MT 59620-0513; (406) 841-2369; FAX: (406) 841-2309; e-mail: compolswp@state.mt.us; Website: www.discovermontana.com/dli/bsd/index.htm

Nebraska *Law passed 1986*. Mr. Chris Childs, Credentialing Coordinator, Nebraska Board of Examiners in Mental Health Practice,

P.O. Box 94986, Lincoln, NE 68509-9486; (402) 471-2117; FAX: (402) 471-3577

Nevada   There is no licensure law in Nevada at this time.

New Hampshire   *Certification law passed 1992, licensure law passed 1998.* Ms. Peggy Lynch, New Hampshire Board of Mental Health Practice, 49 Donovan Street, Concord, NH 03301; (603) 271-6762; e-mail: plynch@dhhs.state.nh.us

New Jersey   *Law passed 1993.* Mr. Dennis Gonzalez, Executive Director, New Jersey Division of Consumer Affairs, State Board of Marriage & Family Therapy Examiners, Professional Counselor Examiners Committee, P.O. Box 45007, Newark, NJ 07101; (973) 504-6415; FAX: (973) 648-3536

New Mexico   *Law passed 1993.* Ms. Eva Baca, New Mexico Therapy Practice Board, Regulation & Licensing Department, 2055 Pacheco Street, Suite 300, P.O. Box 25101, Santa Fe, NM 87505; (505) 476-7102; FAX: (505) 476-7148

New York   *Law passed 2002.* New York State Board for Mental Health Practitioners, New York State Education Department, 89 Washington Avenue, Second Floor, Albany, NY 12234-1000; (518) 474-3817; e-mail: mhpbd@mail.nysed.gov; Website: www.op.nysed.gov

North Carolina   *Registry law passed 1983, licensure law passed 1993.* Ms. Vanessa Pantoja, Board Administrator, North Carolina Board of Licensed Professional Counselors, P.O. Box 1369, Garner, NC 27529-1369; (919) 661-0820; FAX: (919) 779-5642; Website: www.NCBLPC.org

North Dakota   *Law passed 1989.* Ms. Marge Ellefson, Executive Secretary, North Dakota Board of Counselor Examiners, 2112 10th Avenue SE, Mandan, ND 58554; (701) 667-5969; FAX: (701) 667-5969; e-mail: ndbce@btigate.com; Website: sendit.nodak.edu/NDBCE

Ohio   *Law passed 1984.* Ms. Beth Farnsworth, Executive Director, Counselor & Social Worker Board, 77 South High Street, 16th Floor, Columbus, OH 43266; (614) 466-0912; FAX: (614) 728-7790

Oklahoma   *Law passed 1985.* Mr. Mike Blazi, Administrator, Licensed Professional Counselors Advisory Board, Oklahoma State Department of Health, 1000 NE 10th Street, Oklahoma City, OK 73117-1299; (405) 271-6030; FAX: (405) 271-1918

Oregon   *Law passed 1989.* Ms. Julia M. Cooley, Board Administrator, Oregon Board of Licensed Professional Counselors & Therapists, 3218 Pringle Road, SE #160, Salem, OR 97302-6312; (503) 378-5499; e-mail: lpc.lmft@state.or.us; Website: www.oblpct.state.or.us

Pennsylvania   *Law passed 1998.* Ms. Sandra Matter, Board Administrator, State Board of Social Workers, Marriage and Family Therapists, and Professional Counselors, P.O. Box 2649, Harrisburg, PA

17105; (717) 783-2454; FAX: (717) 787-7769; e-mail: socialwo@pados.state.pa.us

Rhode Island *Law passed 1987.* Ms. Donna Dickerman, Administrative Officer, RI Board of Mental Health Counselors and Marriage and Family Division of Professional Regulation, 3 Capitol Hill, Room 104, Providence, RI 02908-5097; (401) 222-2827 ext. 106; FAX: (401) 222-1272; e-mail: donnad@doh.state.ri.us

South Carolina *Law passed 1985, revised law enacted 1998.* Ms. Kitty Cox, Administrator, South Carolina Department of Labor Licensing Regulations, Division Professional & Occupational Licensing, Box 11329, Columbia, SC 29211-1329; (803) 896-4658; FAX: (803) 896-4719; Website: www.llr.sc.edu/pol

South Dakota *Law passed 1990.* Ms. Joyce Vos, Executive Secretary, South Dakota Board of Counselor Examiners, 307 S. Menlo Avenue, Sioux Falls, SD 57104; (605) 331-2927; FAX: (605) 331-2043

Tennessee *Law passed 1984.* Ms. Sherry Owens, Board Administrator, TN State Board of Professional Counselors, Marital & Family Therapists & Clinical Pastoral Therapists, 1st Floor, Cordell Hull Building, 425 5th Ave. North, Nashville, TN 37247-1010; (615) 532-3202/(888) 310-4650; FAX: (615) 532-5164; Website: www.state.tn.us/health

Texas *Law passed 1981.* Mr. Stephen Mills, Executive Director, Texas State Board of Examiners for Professional Counselors, 1100 West 49th Street, Austin, TX 78756-3183; (512) 834-6658; FAX: (512) 834-6789; Website: www.tdh.state.tx.us/hcqs/plc/lpc.htm

Utah *Law passed 1994.* Mr. Dan S. Jones, Bureau Manager, Department of Occupational Professional Licensing, 160 E 300 S, Box 146741, Salt Lake City, UT 84114-6741; (801) 530-6720; FAX: (801) 530-6511; e-mail: dsjones@utah.gov; Website: www.commerce.state.ut.us/web/commerce/dopl/dopl1.htm

Vermont *Law passed 1988.* Ms. Dianne LaFaille, Staff Assistant, Secretary of State's Office, Board of Allied Mental Health Practitioners, Redstone Building, 26 Terrace Street, Drawer 09, Montpelier, VT 05609-1106; (802) 828-2390; FAX: (802) 828-2465; e-mail: dlafaill@sec.state.vt.us; Website: www.sec.state.vt.us

Virginia *Law passed 1976.* Ms. Evelyn Brown, Executive Director, Virginia Board of Professional Counselors, Department of Health Professionals, 6606 West Broad Street, 4th Floor, Richmond, VA 23230; (804) 662-9912

Washington *Law passed 1987.* Ms. Sandy Lewis, Department of Health, Counselor Programs, 310 Israel Road SE, Tumwater, WA 98504-7850; (360) 236-4700; FAX: (360) 236-4981; e-mail: sandy.lewis@doh.wa.gov; Website: doh.wa.gov

West Virginia   *Law passed 1986.* Ms. Jean Ann Johnson, Executive Director, West Virginia Board of Examiners in Counseling, Marshall University Graduate College, P.O. Box 129, Ona, WV 25545; (800) 520-3852; FAX: (304) 767-3062; e-mail: counselingboard@msn.com; Website: www.state.wv.us/wvbec

Wisconsin   *Law passed 1992.* Dr. Kimberly Nania, Bureau Director, Wisconsin Department of Regulation Licensing, P.O. Box 8935, Madison, WI 53708; (608) 266-0145; FAX: (608) 267-0644; Website: badger.state.wi.us/agencies/drl/Regulation/html

Wyoming   *Law passed 1987.* Ms. Veronica Skoranski, Acting Executive Director, Mental Health Professions Licensure Board, First Bank Plaza, 2020 Carey Avenue, Suite 201, Cheyenne, WY 82002; (307) 777-7788; FAX: (307) 777-6005

Certification

In general, practitioners who are more highly credentialed are better respected among their peers, clients, and among others with whom they work. Certification is also an excellent source of professionalism and professional representation to the general public. Credentials may be provided from at least three different sources.

The National Board for Certified Counselors

Obtaining certification from a nationally recognized certification board is a very important way for professionals to know that they are well qualified and current in their skills and practices. It is also perhaps the most important way to communicate to potential and current clients and other members of the community that the counselor is well trained and a qualified member of a nationally recognized professional organization. The most widely recognized certification board for counselors is the National Board for Certified Counselors (NBCC) with approximately 35,000 certified counselors. To become certified by the NBCC, a counselor must present evidence of specifically required graduate-level academic and clinical experience and pass one or more specifically required examinations. If a counselor's program of study is being completed in a CACREP (Council for Accreditation for Counseling and Related Educational Programs) accredited program, the student may take the test early (last term of the program), provided the counseling program participates in the graduate student application process.

An individual who has obtained the National Counselor Certification (NCC) credential has the responsibility to keep current with training and education. NBCC requires that 100 continuing education hours (CEUs) be obtained every five years from NBCC-approved programs. The approved training program must provide a certificate of satisfactory completion with the specific number of CEUs indicated.

Some counselors practice in more than one area of specialization. As a result, they may need to be certified in more than one area. The NBCC currently offers certifications in General Practice Counseling, Clinical Mental Health Counseling, School Counseling, and Addictions Counseling. For other specializations, certifications are offered from other certification boards with the result being that counselors may hold certifications from two or more certification boards to match their areas of practice.

Academic Degree

Another important type of credential is an academic degree including the individual's major area of specialization. The minimum academic degree for counselors is the master's degree. The major area of study or specialization is an important and visible part of one's academic credentials. This area of specialization should be congruent with one's area of practice. For example, an M.A. in counseling with a major or track in school counseling would be more appropriate and relevant to be used in schools than in a community setting. Generally speaking, the more advanced the degree (i.e., a Ph.D. as compared to an M.A.), the stronger the credentials. However, the reputation of the academic department and college or university as well as accreditation of programs from such organizations as CACREP are also significant to one's academic credentials.

Credentials and Membership in Area of Practice

Counselors should expect to become active members in one or more relevant professional organizations. This involvement assists in allowing the professional counselor to keep abreast of important professional issues and avenues of research. It also allows the professional the ability to network within the profession and area of specialization. Professional organizations often issue certification to qualified members in various areas of specialization, and organizations may also recognize qualified members through membership classification.

Continuing Education Units

Continuing education (CEs) designate credit for participating in an educational opportunity as a means of updating and developing the skills of professionals. Most counseling licenses and certifications require a certain number of CEs in order to renew or update that license or certification. CE programs or courses vary in duration of time based on the topic and the sponsor of the program.

To offer a program that results in CEs, the offering agency (sponsor) must have each program approved by the credentialing and/or licensing board for which the CEs are being offered as relevant. Each certification body has the right to determine how many CEs a particular program is worth.

SUMMARY

These descriptions provide an overview of the development, growth, and maintenance of the counseling profession. As counseling has expanded, preparation programs have responded by offering specialized studies for training people to offer mental health care to a wide range of clients. Coursework now occurs at the graduate level and includes clinical experiences that are supervised by a well-qualified professional in a clinical setting with clients.

The increase in counseling has also stimulated the establishment of state boards to regulate practice. Accreditation organizations have been founded to inspect and accredit education programs. National certification organizations, such as the National Board for Certified Counselors (NBCC), have offered credentials to both general practice and specialty counselors. The profession continues to expand, self-regulate, and provide learning opportunities in various settings and formats. This volume presents a study of the state of counselor education training programs in 2003.

## Chapter 2

Research Design
and Data Source

The ten preceding editions of *Counselor Preparation* formed the outline for the research design and data sources of this edition. Over the years, additions and deletions to the survey have created a very different look. Following in this chapter is a sample of the most recent survey form.

DATA COLLECTION PROCEDURE

Institutions having master's and doctoral degrees designated as counseling were invited in late spring 2002 to complete the online or paper version of the data collection form (Table 2.1). As in the past, many additions and deletions as well as formating changes were made. Care was taken to include only programs that profess the education of counselors and counselor educators.

Follow-up e-mails and letters were sent regularly to ensure the most complete listing possible. After five months of data collection, forms were again solicited at the conference of the Association for Counselor Education and Supervision (ACES). In March 2003, each responding program was contacted for final verification and changes.

Of note in this edition is our new system of banking data for future use. NBCC completed the online form with all previously collected data and merged or added all new data. Those data will now be available for all succeeding editions.

Listings of counselor education program institutions were derived from three sources. NBCC maintains a listing of counseling programs for business purposes, including testing and certification of counselors. Merged lists from the Council for Accreditation of Counseling and Related Educational Programs (CACREP) and Chi Sigma Iota (CSI) counseling honorary society, as well as university Websites, are regularly used by NBCC for updating this list.

When an institution of higher education houses counseling programs in more than one department, they are treated as separate programs. Every effort has been and will be made to include all counselor preparation units. New and unlisted programs are encouraged to take part in future surveys.

Table 2.1. Data Collection Form

nbcc ™
national board for certified counselors, inc. and affiliates

COUNSELOR PREPARATION 2002–2003: PROGRAMS, PERSONNEL, TRENDS

Programs include master's, specialist, and doctoral degrees with majors in community, mental health, school, college, student affairs (counseling emphasis, developmental emphasis, administrative emphasis), addictions, career, gerontological, marriage and family, pastoral, rehabilitation, counselor education, and other counseling specialties.

Please enter the data for your institution, save this document with your data, and e-mail it as an attachment to CounselorPreparation@nbcc.org.

A. Administrative Unit	
Name of Administrator	
Administrator's Title	
Department	
College/University	
Address	
City	
State	
Zip plus 4	
Country	
Department's Telephone Number	
Department's Fax Number	
Department's E-mail Address	
Dean's Name and College Location	
Department's Website Address	
☐ College or University Holds Regional Accreditation	

Ethnicity of instructors—mark all that apply

☐ African-American

☐ Asian-American

☐ Caucasian

☐ Hispanic

☐ Native American

☐ Pacific Islander

☐ Multiracial (a descendent of more than one of the above)

Other

Uniqueness of Department and/or Counseling Program

State the uniqueness of the department, faculty, students, and programs. This may communicate an academic climate to potential students.	
Research interests and current projects of faculty members:	

☐ **Please check here if you or your institution will order Counselor Preparation 11th Ed., at the reduced rated offered survey participants**

This is necessary so we can confirm and authenticate the data submitted.

E-mail address of the individual who supplied data	

If different from above, enter the Name and Telephone Number of the Individual Who Supplied Data

Name

Telephone

Today's Date | Select   **2002**

B. Faculty

Directions: Please list the counselor preparation faculty, highest academic degree for each, percentage of time assigned to the programs, academic rank, administrative title, and whether or not the person is state and national credentialed (e.g., LPC, NCC) and each e-mail address. Leave none of the applicable sections blank.

First Name	MI	Last Name	Highest Degree	Academic Rank	<21%	22–40	41–60	61–80	>81%	LPC	NCC	Other	E-mail
				Select	☐	☐	☐	☐	☐	☐	☐	☐	
				Select	☐	☐	☐	☐	☐	☐	☐	☐	
				Select	☐	☐	☐	☐	☐	☐	☐	☐	
				Select	☐	☐	☐	☐	☐	☐	☐	☐	
				Select	☐	☐	☐	☐	☐	☐	☐	☐	
				Select	☐	☐	☐	☐	☐	☐	☐	☐	
				Select	☐	☐	☐	☐	☐	☐	☐	☐	
				Select	☐	☐	☐	☐	☐	☐	☐	☐	
				Select	☐	☐	☐	☐	☐	☐	☐	☐	
				Select	☐	☐	☐	☐	☐	☐	☐	☐	
				Select	☐	☐	☐	☐	☐	☐	☐	☐	
				Select	☐	☐	☐	☐	☐	☐	☐	☐	
				Select	☐	☐	☐	☐	☐	☐	☐	☐	
				Select	☐	☐	☐	☐	☐	☐	☐	☐	
				Select	☐	☐	☐	☐	☐	☐	☐	☐	
				Select	☐	☐	☐	☐	☐	☐	☐	☐	
				Select	☐	☐	☐	☐	☐	☐	☐	☐	
				Select	☐	☐	☐	☐	☐	☐	☐	☐	
				Select	☐	☐	☐	☐	☐	☐	☐	☐	
				Select	☐	☐	☐	☐	☐	☐	☐	☐	
				Select								☐	

Percent of teaching staff in professional counseling practice: %

C. Program Information for Master's or Specialist Degree Programs

Directions: List only programs with graduate degree. For each master's (e.g., MA, MS, MEd) or specialist (e.g., EdS, CAGS) degree program you offer in a counseling area, please supply the information requested. Leave blank any data not applicable to programs.

Degree Awarded	Type of Counseling/Therapy											
	Community	Mental Health	School	College	Student Affairs	Addictions	Career	Geronto-logical	Marriage & Family	Other	Pastoral	Rehab
(e.g., MA, MS, MEd)	☐	☐	☐	☐	☐	☐	☐	☐	☐	☐	☐	☐
(e.g., EdS, CAGS)	☐	☐	☐	☐	☐	☐	☐	☐	☐	☐	☐	☐
Number of Students												
Admitted Yearly												
Graduated Yearly												
Females (enrolled)												
Males (enrolled)												

Ethnicity of students—click all that apply

☐ African-American
☐ Asian-American
☐ Caucasian
☐ Hispanic
☐ Native American
☐ Pacific Islander
☐ Multiracial (a descendent of more than one of the above)

Other

Admission Requirements: For each master's (e.g., MA, MS, MEd) or specialist (e.g., EdS, CAGS) degree program

For Test (Specify score)	Community	Mental Health	School	College	Student Affairs	Addictions	Career	Geronto-logical	Marriage & Family	Other	Pastoral	Rehab
GRE: Total												
Verbal												
Quantitative												
Analytical												
MAT												
Undergrad GPA												
Work Experience # Years Required												
Letters Recommen-dation # Required												
Personal Interview Required	☐	☐	☐	☐	☐	☐	☐	☐	☐	☐	☐	☐

☐ **Institutional Financial Aid Available**

Graduation Requirements—For Master's Degrees

Master's Degrees	Community	Mental Health	School	College	Student Affairs	Addictions	Career	Gerontological	Marriage & Family	Other	Pastoral	Rehab
# Semester Hours												
or Quarter Hours												
# Practicum Clock Hours												
# Internship Clock Hours												
Thesis Required	☐	☐	☐	☐	☐	☐	☐	☐	☐	☐	☐	☐
Comprehensive Exam	☐	☐	☐	☐	☐	☐	☐	☐	☐	☐	☐	☐
CPCE Used	☐	☐	☐	☐	☐	☐	☐	☐	☐	☐	☐	☐
Oral Comprehensive	☐	☐	☐	☐	☐	☐	☐	☐	☐	☐	☐	☐
Portfolio	☐	☐	☐	☐	☐	☐	☐	☐	☐	☐	☐	☐

Graduation Requirements—For Specialist Degrees

Specialist Degrees	Community	Mental Health	School	College	Student Affairs	Addictions	Career	Gerontological	Marriage & Family	Other	Pastoral	Rehab
# Semester Hours												
or Quarter Hours												
# Practicum Clock Hours												
# Internship Clock Hours												
Thesis Required	☐	☐	☐	☐	☐	☐	☐	☐	☐	☐	☐	☐
Comprehensive Exam	☐	☐	☐	☐	☐	☐	☐	☐	☐	☐	☐	☐
CPCE Used	☐	☐	☐	☐	☐	☐	☐	☐	☐	☐	☐	☐
Oral Comprehensive	☐	☐	☐	☐	☐	☐	☐	☐	☐	☐	☐	☐
Portfolio	☐	☐	☐	☐	☐	☐	☐	☐	☐	☐	☐	☐

Placement of Graduates: For Each Master's (e.g., MA, MS, MEd) or Specialist (e.g., EdS, CAGS) Degree Program

First Year after Graduation—Estimate percentage; Each column with an entry must total 100%

	Community Mental Health	School	College	Student Affairs	Addictions	Career	Geronto-logical	Marriage & Family	Other	Pastoral	Rehab
Advanced Graduate Programs	%	%	%	%	%	%	%	%	%	%	%
Managed Care (HMO, HMP, PPO, EAP)	%	%	%	%	%	%	%	%	%	%	%
Private Practice—Solo/Group	%	%	%	%	%	%	%	%	%	%	%
Agency Practice	%	%	%	%	%	%	%	%	%	%	%
Other	%	%	%	%	%	%	%	%	%	%	%
Other Setting											
School Counseling											
Elementary	%	%	%	%	%	%	%	%	%	%	%
Middle	%	%	%	%	%	%	%	%	%	%	%
Secondary	%	%	%	%	%	%	%	%	%	%	%
Higher Education/ Student Affairs	%	%	%	%	%	%	%	%	%	%	%
Total of Above	100%	100%	100%	100%	100%	100%	100%	100%	100%	100%	100%

D. Program Information for Doctoral Degree Programs

Directions: For each doctoral degree program you offer in a counseling area, please supply the information requested. Leave blank any columns or data not applicable to programs.

Degree Awarded	Community Mental Health	School	College	Student Affairs	Addictions	Career	Geronto-logical	Marriage & Family	Other	Pastoral	Rehab	Counselor Education
Education	☐	☐	☐	☐	☐	☐	☐	☐	☐	☐	☐	☐
Ed.D.	☐	☐	☐	☐	☐	☐	☐	☐	☐	☐	☐	☐
Ph.D.	☐	☐	☐	☐	☐	☐	☐	☐	☐	☐	☐	☐
D.Reh.	☐	☐	☐	☐	☐	☐	☐	☐	☐	☐	☐	☐
D.Min.	☐	☐	☐	☐	☐	☐	☐	☐	☐	☐	☐	☐
Other (specify)												
Number of Students												
Admitted Yearly												
Graduated Yearly												
Females (enrolled)												
Males (enrolled)												

Ethnicity of students—click all that apply

- ☐ African-American
- ☐ Asian-American
- ☐ Caucasian
- ☐ Hispanic
- ☐ Native American
- ☐ Pacific Islander
- ☐ Multiracial (a descendent of more than one of the above)

Other

Admission Requirements for Doctoral Programs

For Test (Specify score)	Community	Mental Health	School	College	Student Affairs	Addictions	Career	Geronto-logical	Marriage & Family	Other	Pastoral	Rehab	Counselor Education
GRE:													
Total													
Verbal													
Quantitative													
Analytical													
MAT													
Master's Required	☐	☐	☐	☐	☐	☐	☐	☐	☐	☐	☐	☐	☐
Graduate GPA Required													
Work Experience # Years Required													
Letters Recommen-dation # Required													
Personal Interview Required	☐	☐	☐	☐	☐	☐	☐	☐	☐	☐	☐	☐	☐

Graduation Requirements—For Doctoral Degrees

Doctoral Degrees	Community	Mental Health	School	College	Student Affairs	Addictions	Career	Gerontological	Marriage & Family	Other	Pastoral	Rehab	Counselor Education
# Semester Hours													
or Quarter Hours													
# Practicum clock hours													
# Internship clock hours													
Dissertation required	☐	☐	☐	☐	☐	☐	☐	☐	☐	☐	☐	☐	☐
Comprehensive Exam	☐	☐	☐	☐	☐	☐	☐	☐	☐	☐	☐	☐	☐
CPCE Used	☐	☐	☐	☐	☐	☐	☐	☐	☐	☐	☐	☐	☐
Oral Comprehensive	☐	☐	☐	☐	☐	☐	☐	☐	☐	☐	☐	☐	☐
Portfolio	☐	☐	☐	☐	☐	☐	☐	☐	☐	☐	☐	☐	☐

Placement of Graduates: For Each Doctoral Degree Program

First Year After Graduation—Estimate percentage; each column with an entry must total 100%)

	Community	Mental Health	School	College	Student Affairs	Addictions	Career	Geronto-logical	Marriage & Family	Other	Pastoral	Rehab	Counselor Education
Advanced Graduate Programs	%	%	%	%	%	%	%	%	%	%	%	%	%
Managed Care (HMO, HMP, PPO, EAP)	%	%	%	%	%	%	%	%	%	%	%	%	%
Private Practice—Solo/Group	%	%	%	%	%	%	%	%	%	%	%	%	%
Agency Practice	%	%	%	%	%	%	%	%	%	%	%	%	%
Other	%	%	%	%	%	%	%	%	%	%	%	%	
Other Setting													
School Counseling													
Elementary	%	%	%	%	%	%	%	%	%	%	%	%	%
Middle	%	%	%	%	%	%	%	%	%	%	%	%	%
Secondary	%	%	%	%	%	%	%	%	%	%	%	%	%
Higher Education/Student Affairs	%	%	%	%	%	%	%	%	%	%	%	%	%
Total of Above	100%	100%	100%	100%	100%	100%	100%	100%	100%	100%	100%	100%	100%

For All Degrees and Programs

Contact Person for the Program

	Master's	Specialist	Doctoral
Community			
Mental Health			
School			
College			
Student Affairs			
Addictions			
Career			
Gerontological			
Marriage & Family			
Other			
Pastoral			
Rehab			
Counselor Education			

E. Courses To Be Added and/or Dropped

Directions: Please check areas where you anticipate a course will be added or dropped within the next three years.

Area in which course is applicable	Drop	Add
Abuse of Individual	☐	☐
Addictions	☐	☐
Adventure Counseling	☐	☐
Advocacy	☐	☐
Career/Life Planning	☐	☐
Computer and Related Technology	☐	☐
Consultation	☐	☐
Crisis / Violence Counseling	☐	☐
Diversity	☐	☐
Experiential Component	☐	☐
Forensic Counseling	☐	☐
Gender Studies	☐	☐
Gerontological Counseling	☐	☐
Grief Counseling	☐	☐
Group Work	☐	☐
Human Sexuality	☐	☐
Intelligence Testing	☐	☐
Internet Use	☐	☐
Legal / Ethical Issues	☐	☐
Life Coaching	☐	☐
Marriage and Family Counseling	☐	☐
Play Therapy	☐	☐
Projective Assessment	☐	☐
Psychodiagnosis	☐	☐
Psychopharmacology	☐	☐
Rehabilitation	☐	☐
Research Methods	☐	☐
School Counseling	☐	☐
Social Justice	☐	☐
Special Needs Populations	☐	☐
Sports Counseling	☐	☐
Supervision	☐	☐
Teaching	☐	☐
Teaming and Collaboration	☐	☐
Technology	☐	☐
Testing, Appraisal, Assessment	☐	☐
Theory Component	☐	☐
Wellness	☐	☐
Other (Specify)	☐	☐

F. Program Changes

Directions: Please check areas where you anticipate a program change, increase or decrease, within the next three years.

Anticipated Change	Decrease	Increase
Admission Requirements	☐	☐
Course Offerings—Approximate Number	☐	☐
Clinical Supervision	☐	☐
Diversity Recruiting of Faculty	☐	☐
Diversity Recruiting of Students	☐	☐
Faculty FTE	☐	☐
Financial Aid	☐	☐
Graduation Requirements	☐	☐
National Accreditation (e.g., CACREP, CORE)	☐	☐
Number of Degree Majors	☐	☐
Number of Distance Education Courses	☐	☐
Number of Off-Campus Courses	☐	☐
Number of On-Line Courses	☐	☐
Other (Specify)	☐	☐

G. Related Graduate Programs

Directions: Please check other programs on your campus that prepare mental health workers.

☐ Clinical Social Workers	
☐ Marriage and Family Therapists	
☐ Psychologists	
☐ Arts Therapists	
☐ Psychiatric Nurses	
☐ Psychiatrists	
☐ Organizational Behaviorists	
☐ Communications	
☐ International Studies	
☐ Other (Specify)	

H. Institutional Specialized Accreditation

Directions: Please indicate your plans regarding program accreditation during 2002, 2003, and 2004.

Accrediting Body	Program	Now Have Accreditation	Plan to Drop Accreditation (year)	Applying for Accreditation
CACREP	College Counseling			
	Community Counseling			
	Community Counseling/Career Counseling			
	Community Counseling/Gerontological Counseling			
	Counselor Education and Supervision			
	Marriage and Family Counseling			
	Mental Health Counseling			
	School Counseling			
	Student Affairs / Counseling Emphasis			
	Student Affairs / Professional Practice Emphasis			
CORE	Rehabilitation Counseling			
AAPC	Pastoral Counseling			

Counselor Preparation
Program Structure

## Chapter 3

Academics

Professional counselors have received a graduate degree at the master's, specialist, or doctoral level. Students are awarded those degrees by completing counselor preparations programs that have a sequence of curricular and clinical experiences. Clinical experiences include the supervised practice of counseling skills. That practice may occur in a clinic or laboratory housed in a college or university. Students may also be placed in community, school, or other settings. Academic experiences are related to the curriculum. These include the expected course work, examinations, culminating project, thesis, or dissertation, and other professional activities such as teaching, assisting in a classroom, or working on scholarly projects with the faculty and/or a mentor. Counselor education faculty members provide and supervise these academic experiences. Therefore, the qualifications, interests, and interpersonal styles of the faculty significantly contribute to the quality of the program. The information that follows introduces some ways to compare faculty contributions across different programs and departments.

PROGRAM ADMINISTRATION

Counselor education programs generally exist within an academic unit that is located in an educational institution, college, or university. The academic unit may offer other programs such as psychology, teacher education, human services programs, or other types of studies.

The accreditation(s) that have been granted to the academic unit and the institution of higher education indicate that the administrative unit meets or exceeds the standards set by the accreditation body. People who graduate from a program in which the administrative unit holds accreditation may have been exposed to a more comprehensive prospective with broader opportunities. Some career options may also be determined on whether the person's degree comes from an accredited program in an accredited institution.

Other possible benefits of accreditation include resources, equipment, and personnel that are allocated based on the prestige of the program within the university, community, or profession. Accredited programs may receive higher recognition and greater funding that leads to strengthened educational experiences for students.

PROGRAM ACCREDITATION

Accreditation of preparation programs in the United States is a voluntary process, and the accreditation bodies are independent from the federal and state governments. In most cases, the professional association initially established the related accreditation body. Each accreditation body establishes criteria to be met by the program before accreditation. If a department offers more than one program, each program must be evaluated separately for accreditation. Thus, a department may have some programs that are accredited and others that are not. Accreditation is generally for a specific time (usually two to five years) and must be reevaluated for continuation of accreditation each time the accreditation period expires.

Obtaining accreditation requires several steps. An important part is the self-evaluation by the department's faculty and staff, for which each accreditation body has specific guidelines. Once the self-evaluation is completed, and faculty and staff believe they meet the criteria, they ask the accreditation body to make their evaluation. Often a team of professionals makes a campus visit and performs an on-site evaluation. That report is then sent to the accreditation body and is revised and approved by the relevant board. From the time the department starts the process until the board approval is often two or more years. Obligations on the part of the program wishing to be accredited include (a) preparation of a self-study report, (b) application fees, (c) visitation fees, (d) membership fees, and (e) a separate evaluation of each program. Advantages of program accreditation include (a) providing assurance that the program meets high professional standards, (b) ensuring periodic review of the program, (c) assuring applicants that the program meets high standards, (d) offering graduates of the program advantages (i.e., quicker access to licensure) related to having graduated from an accredited program, and (e) providing a source of pride for faculty, students, and the college or university as they contribute to or become involved in a nationally recognized program.

Accreditation Bodies

The following are three accrediting bodies for counseling programs.

American Association of Pastoral Counselors (AAPC)

The American Association of Pastoral Counselors was "founded in 1963 as an organization which certifies pastoral counselors, accredits pastoral counseling centers, and approves training programs" (www.aapc.org). Membership is open to individuals in seven categories. Pastoral counseling programs can be accredited as training programs, service centers, or both. Currently there are 37 training programs accredited by AAPC listed on the AAPC Website.

Contact information for the AAPC:

American Association of Pastoral Counselors
950A Lee Highway
Fairfax, VA 22031-2303
Phone: (703) 385-6967
FAX: (703) 352-7725
E-mail: info@aapc.org
Website: www.aapc.org

Council for Accreditation of Counseling and Related Educational Programs (CACREP)

The Council for Accreditation of Counseling and Related Education Programs (CACREP) is an independent council created by the American Counseling Association (ACA) and its divisions to develop, implement, and maintain standards of preparation for the counseling profession's degree programs. Its purpose is to work with institutions offering graduate-level programs in counseling and related educational fields so that they might achieve and maintain accreditation status. As an accrediting agency for the counseling profession, CACREP's scope includes master's level programs in Career Counseling; College Counseling; Community Counseling; Marital, Couple and Family Counseling/Therapy; Mental Health Counseling; School Counseling; Student Affairs; and doctoral programs in Counselor Education and Supervision. CACREP is recognized as a specialized accrediting agency by the Council for Higher Education Accreditation (CHEA). Table 3.1 lists the number of programs accredited in the United States as of April 2003.

Currently, 47 states, the District of Columbia, Guam, and Puerto Rico offer state-level credentialing or licensure for counselors. Currently, 35 states and the District of Columbia accept the National Counselor Exam (NCE) administered by the National Board for Certified Counselors, Inc. and Affiliates (NBCC). Students in CACREP accredited programs are eligible to

Table 3.1. Number of CACREP-Accredited U.S. Programs and Their Classification

Kind of Program	Number of Programs
Community counseling	129
Mental health counseling	29
School counseling	150
College counseling	2
Student affairs	1
Student affairs practice in higher education/ college counseling emphasis	33
Student affairs practice in higher education/ professional practice emphasis	11
Career counseling	6
Marital, couple, and family counseling/therapy	26
Gerontological counseling	2

take the NCE exam during the final term of their program when their program elects to participate in this graduate student application process for the National Certified Counselor (NCC) credential. In addition, students who graduate from CACREP-accredited programs are not required to complete the two years of post-master's experience required of graduates of programs not accredited by CACREP in order to become credentialed by NBCC.

Contact information for the CACREP:

Council for Accreditation of Counseling and Related Educational Programs
5999 Stevenson Avenue
Alexandria, VA 22304-3302
Phone: (703) 823-9800, ext. 301
FAX: (703) 823-1581
E-mail: cacrep@aol.com

Each table in this edition was checked against the accreditation list issued by CACREP.

Council on Rehabilitation Education (CORE)

Accreditation of Rehabilitation Counselor Education (RCE) programs by CORE promotes the "effective delivery of rehabilitation services to individuals with disabilities" by fostering "continuing review and improvement of master's degree–level RCE programs." The CORE's accreditation process promotes "program self-improvement rather than outside censure" (www.core-rehab.org). CORE is accredited by the Council on Higher Education Accreditation and is a member of the Association of Specialized and

Professional Accreditors. Currently, there are 93 CORE-accredited master's-level rehabilitation programs listed on the CORE Website.

Contact information for the CORE organization:

Council on Rehabilitation Education, Inc.
1835 Rohlwing Road, Suite E
Rolling Meadows, IL 60008
(850) 878-4966
FAX: (850) 878-3183
E-mail: dclink@wans.net

DEGREES HELD BY FACULTY

The total number of faculty members reported from the responding programs was 1611. As can be seen from Table 3.2, Faculty Rank and Degree, the majority of those hold terminal degrees, Ph.D. or Ed.D. Further faculty information specific to each program can be found in Parts D and E in this book. Table 3.2 also provides a summary of the academic rank of the faculty members. The rank held may not reflect many specifics about a department or about an individual faculty member. Rank may be related to the amount of time a faculty member has been teaching at an institution of higher education. Rank may also indicate the academic or scholarly contributions made by the faculty member such as professional publications, research, or teaching achievements.

CREDENTIALS HELD BY FACULTY

Credentials other than rank and degree provide another measure of faculty qualifications and commitment to the profession. Chapter 1 contains an outline of the process of obtaining a credential. Maintaining the credential usually requires continuing education as well as periodic checks by the state licensing board and the certifying body. A summary of credentials

Table 3.2. Faculty Rank and Degree

Academic Rank	Degree		
	Ph.D.	Ed.D.	Other
Full Professor	293	115	5
Associate	282	81	11
Assistant	335	58	25
Adjunct	78	14	54
Instructor	50	10	43
Lecturer	24	7	18

Table 3.3. Summary of NCCs and LPCs Held by the Faculty

Number Reported	Credential
543	LPC—Licensed Professional Counselor
561	NCC—National Certified Counselor

reported for faculty members from responses to the data collection form appears in Table 3.3.

The National Board for Certified Counselors, Inc. (NBCC)

NBCC is the largest credentialing body for counselors. Its purpose and scope are as follows:

> The National Board for Certified Counselors, Inc. (NBCC), an independent not-for-profit credentialing body, was incorporated in 1982 to establish and monitor a national certification system, to identify for professionals and the public those counselors who have voluntarily sought and obtained certification, and to maintain a register of those counselors. This process grants recognition to counselors who have met predetermined NBCC standards in their training, experience, and performance on the National Counselor Examination for Licensure and Certification (NCE), the most portable test in counseling. NBCC represents more than 35,000 National Certified Counselors (NCCs) as of June 2003, and forty-four states and the District of Columbia have adopted NBCC licensure examinations as part of their statutory credentialing process. (Both the NCE and the National Clinical Mental Health Examination are NBCC licensure examinations.)
>
> NBCC was initially created as an independent, not-for-profit 501(c)(6) corporation by the American Counseling Association (ACA). NBCC is now an independent credentialing body with close ties to ACA. While ACA concentrates on professional development, including publications, workshops and government relations in the counseling field, NBCC focuses on promoting quality counseling through certification and setting national practice standards.
>
> Since October 1985, NBCC has been accredited by the National Commission for Certifying Agencies (NCCA). NCCA is an independent national regulatory organization that monitors the credentialing processes of its member agencies. Accreditation by the commission represents the foremost organizational recognition in national certification.

Requirements for the NCC are as follows. Applicants must:

- Hold a master's degree with a major study in counseling from a regionally accredited university and have a minimum of 48 semester or 72 quarter hours of graduate-level coursework, with at least one course in each of the following areas: Human Growth and Development, Social and Cultural Foundations, Helping Relationships, Group Work, Career and Lifestyle Development, Appraisal, Research and Program Evaluation, and Professional Orientation and Ethics. NBCC defines a major study in counseling as one in which more than half (but no less than 24 semester hours or quarter equivalent) of the degree credits reflect the required coursework.

- Document two academic terms of supervised field experience in a counseling setting. Applicants have only one academic term of field experience: they may substitute one additional year of post-master's supervised experience (1,500 extra hours of activities directly related to counseling and 50 extra hours of face-to-face supervision) beyond the required two years of post-master's supervised experience.
- Document two years of post-master's counseling experience with 3,000 client contact hours and 100 hours of face-to-face supervision.
- Provide two professional endorsements, one of which must be from a recent supervisor.
- Pass the National Counselor Examination for Licensure and Certification (NCE). (www.nbcc.org)

Of the 1,611 faculty members listed, 550 were reported as holding NCC credentials, which represents 34% percent of the total.

Chi Sigma Iota

Faculty and students and others may align with Chi Sigma Iota, the International Counseling Academic and Professional Honor Society, which was established in 1985. The goals of this society focus on providing recognition for outstanding academic achievement or outstanding service within the counseling profession and on linking students, educators, practitioners, and administrators in various counseling settings. With the aim of both personal and professional development for its members, Chi Sigma Iota is committed to upholding high standards. The purposes of the group as noted in Article I (1.3) of the by-laws are:

> To promote scholarship, research, professionalism, and excellence in counseling, and to recognize high attainment in the pursuit of academic and clinical excellence in the field of counseling. (Chi Sigma Iota, 1994)

Those goals are met primarily through the activities of the local chapters as well as through the support of the headquarters staff and officers. Since its inception, Chi Sigma Iota as an organization and many of its members have assumed leadership roles in the profession.

Chi Sigma Iota has a chapter at 239 colleges and universities. Note that only one Chi Sigma Iota chapter exists in each institution; therefore, if two or more counseling programs are offered, only one chapter will be listed for that campus. More information can be found at www.csi-net.org.

FACULTY TIME DEVOTED TO COUNSELOR PREPARATION

Graduate or advanced graduate courses require faculty time devoted to consulting, supervising, and teaching. The amount of available time varies from counseling program to program. One possible way to compute this variable is to compare the assigned faculty time to the number of students in the program. The ratio, student per faculty full-time equivalency (Stu/Fac FTE), is an indicator of faculty availability. The data included in Part D, Data on Each Department, could be used to perform this computation. The number of students admitted to all counselor preparation programs or the number of students graduating can be totaled. Next, compute the total time reported for all faculty and divide the sum by the number of faculty members. That will provide a rough estimate of student per faculty full-time equivalency.

Another way to review faculty time available is reviewing the percentage of time devoted to counselor preparation programs as reported for this study. The data collection form asked respondents to indicate one of five percentage groupings: 0–21%, 22–40%, 41–60%, 61–80%, 81–100%. Of the 1,606 responses to this question, more than half (52%) indicated faculty time devoted to counselor preparation amounted to 81–100%. Those percentages are reported in Table 3.4.

DEGREES OFFERED

Students in counselor preparation programs may be pursuing a master's degree, an educational specialist's degree, or a doctoral degree. Entry-level programs with fifth or sixth year programs are more common. For this edition, 484 entry-level programs, 78 specialist programs, and 70 doctoral-level programs responded. Chapter 4 contains summary information about

Table 3.4. Percentage of Faculty Time Devoted to Counselor Preparation Programs

0–21%	23%
22–40%	9%
41–60%	10%
61–80%	6%
81–100%	52%
Total responses	1,606
No responses	40

entry-level programs and Part E of this book has particulars for each specialty area program. Chapter 5 includes information about doctoral-level study in counselor education. At each level, programs determine criteria for the admission and graduation of students. All programs determine the minimum number of academic courses to be completed and the clinical experience that is to be included in the preparation program.

CLINICAL EXPERIENCE DURING TRAINING

The clinical experience in counselor preparation programs often occurs in two parts, a practicum and an internship. The practicum may happen early in a program and internship may come later in the sequence of training. Both components require direct supervision by a qualified supervisor with both group and individual formats for supervision. The number of clock hours required for practicum and internship vary from program to program. CACREP standards list practicum as a 100-hour experience and internship as a 600-hour requirement. The site for clinical experiences depends on the location of the college or university and the community resources. The goal of most programs is to provide an in-depth experience at a site that has working conditions similar to the student's career goals. The next two chapters contain descriptions of counselor education programs that help students move toward those goals.

REFERENCES

American Association of Pastoral Counselors. (2003). About pastoral counseling. Retrieved April 28, 2003, from http://www.aapc.org/about.htm

Chi Sigma Iota. (1994). Bylaws. Retrieved April 28, 2003, from www.csi-net.org

The Council for Accreditation of Counseling and Related Educational Programs. (2003, April). Directory of accredited programs. Alexandria, VA: CACREP.

Council on Rehabilitation Education (2003). CORE: Council on rehabilitation education. Retrieved April 28, 2003, from http://www.core-rehab.org/

Hollis, J. W. & Dodson, T. A. (1999). *Counselor preparation* (10th ed.). Philadelphia: Accelerated Development.

National Board for Certified Counselors. (2003). Retrieved April 28, 2003, from www.nbcc.org.

Counselor Preparation Programs

## Chapter 4

Entry-Level Counselor Preparation Programs

Professional counselors pursue a master's degree program with specialty study in an identified area. Most often students in counselor preparation programs focus on the core areas of human growth and development, assessment, group work, counseling theories and skills, career development, research and program evaluation, professional identity, and social and cultural diversity. Besides these foundation courses, students not only take courses specific to their specialty area of counseling but they also participate in their supervised clinical experiences appropriate to their intended areas of practice. CACREP standards for the scope of this type of academic and clinical experience can be reviewed at the organization's web address: www.counseling.org/cacrep.

PROGRAMS OFFERED AND ACCREDITATION

Information was collected from 484 programs that responded to the data reporting form. Programs indicated if the counseling areas of community, mental health, school, college, student affairs, addictions, career, gerontological, marriage and family, and other specialty types were offered in their institution. According to these data, the specialty areas of community with 117 programs and school counseling with 171 programs were by far the most commonly identified. Those two programs constituted 59.5% of all programs offered by those responding. The other specialty areas that were offered, in descending order of frequency, include mental health, marriage and family, student affairs, other, college, career, addictions, and gerontological counseling. Table 4.1 provides information about the number of departments and accredited programs offering entry-level programs.

Table 4.I. Number of Departments Responding and Number of Accredited Programs in Entry Level Counselor Preparation

	Community	Mental Health	School	College	Student Affairs	Addictions	Career	Geron- tological	Marriage & Family	Other
NPR	117	54	171	15	40	7	8	3	44	25
CP	129	29	150	2	45 (all)	–	6	2	26	–
APR	80	20	98	2	36 (all)	–	3	1	14	–

APR: Accredited programs responding; CP: CACREP programs accredited; NPR: Number of programs responding.

ADMISSIONS AND GRADUATES

The greatest number of counseling students enroll and graduate from the programs of community counseling and school counseling. Table 4.2 contains the average number of students admitted yearly and the average number of students graduated annually for the counseling preparation programs that reported this information.

ADMISSION REQUIREMENTS

Counselor preparation programs require a variety of information before admitting students. Standardized tests such as the Graduate Record Examination (GRE) and the Miller Analogies Test (MAT) are used by some programs as a part of their admission requirements. Of the programs that responded to this query, 266 reported requiring the GRE and 109 reported requiring the MAT. Programs also reported the average grade point average (GPA) of students admitted. Across all responding programs that average amounts to a 2.85 GPA. Table 4.3 details how many specialty programs require the standardized test and the average reported GPA of students admitted.

Some programs ask applicants to have completed some work experience, submit recommendation letters, or participate in an interview. Of those programs who responded, 58 required work experience, 374 asked for letters of recommendation, and 275 held interviews for applicants to their programs. Information specific to specialty area programs can be found in Table 4.4.

Table 4.2. Number of Students Admitted and Number of Students Graduated Yearly in Entry-Level Counseling Programs

Programs	Number of Programs Responding	Average Admitted Yearly	Average Graduated Yearly
Community	107	26	21
Mental Health	49	22	14
School	157	22	18
College	12	7	5
Student Affairs	37	12	10
Addictions	5	10	8
Career	5	8	7
Gerontological	3	7	5
Marriage & Family	34	17	14
Other	19	14	9

Table 4.3. Admission Requirements to Entry-Level Counseling Programs

Programs	NPR	GRE	MAT	NPR	Average GPA
Community	117	62	31	98	2.87
Mental Health	56	37	10	46	2.92
School	171	97	44	142	2.86
College	15	8	2	13	2.81
Student Affairs	41	23	4	32	2.80
Addictions	7	4	2	3	2.83
Career	9	3	1	6	2.8
Gerontological	3	2	1	3	3.0
Marriage & Family	46	22	16	31	2.85
Other	30	8	12	22	2.74

GRE: Graduate Record Examination; MAT: Miller Analogies Test; NPR: Number of programs responding.
Note: Entries under GRE and MAT columns reflect the number of programs that reported that they use either of these as an admission requirement.

CLINICAL EXPERIENCES REQUIRED

Counselor preparation programs reported supervised practicum and internship clock hours that must be completed before graduation. These programs may vary these hours according to the specialty area being pursued. According to CACREP standards, practicum in entry-level programs includes 100 clock hours with 40 or more of those hours in direct service. Practicum also involves group supervision of 1.5 hours per week and individual supervision of 1 hour per week. CACREP standards outline the clock hours of internship as a minimum of 600 hours with 240 or more of those involving direct service. Information provided on the data collection form indicated

Table 4.4. Other Admission Requirements to Entry-Level Counseling Programs

Programs	Number of Programs Responding	Working Experience	Recommen-dation Letters	Interviews
Community	117	8	107	72
Mental Health	56	8	49	32
School	171	18	147	108
College	15	0	9	11
Student Affairs	41	11	31	21
Addictions	7	0	6	2
Career	9	0	7	3
Gerontological	3	0	3	1
Marriage & Family	46	6	33	25
Other	30	0	14	16

Note: Entries under Work Experience, Recommendation Letters, and Interviews columns indicate the number of programs that replied that indicated positively that they required these for admission.

Table 4.5. Graduation Requirements for Master's Degrees in Counseling: Clinical Hours Required

Programs	NPR	Practicum Hours	NPR	Internship Hours
Community	106	118	105	583
Mental Health	46	200	43	721
School	156	131	140	562
College	14	110	13	540
Student Affairs	31	121	36	537
Addictions	5	200	5	600
Career	3	133	3	600
Gerontological	1	100	3	433
Marriage & Family	31	192	28	621
Other	13	176	12	641

NPR: Number of programs responding.
Note: Entries under Practicum Hours and Internship Hours are average numbers for all programs that responded to these items.

an average of 148 practicum hours and 560 internship hours being required in the programs that responded. Table 4.5 contains information related to required practicum and internship hours.

GRADUATION REQUIREMENTS

One standard requirement for graduation from a counselor preparation program is the successful completion of coursework. The average number of graduate hours required for the 431 programs that responded to this portion of the data collection form was 50.8 semester hours. Those who reported quarter hours averaged at 69.83. Further information is contained in Table 4.6.

Table 4.6. Graduation Requirements for Master's Degrees in Counseling: Academic Course Hours Required

Programs	Number of Programs Responding	Semester Hours	Quarter Hours
Community	109	51	74
Mental Health	50	58	82
School	166	50	61
College	14	49	72
Student Affairs	39	46	—
Addictions	5	49	—
Career	5	51	—
Gerontological	3	50	—
Marriage & Family	35	58	82
Other	17	46	48

Note: Entries under Semester Hours and Quarter Hours are average numbers for all programs that responded to these items.

Table 4.7. Graduation Requirements for Master's Degrees in Counseling: Other Requirements

Programs	Number of Programs Responding	Thesis	Comprehensive Exam	Oral Exam	Portfolio
Community	85	5	69	12	26
Mental Health	38	5	31	9	7
School	124	7	100	17	47
College	11	0	8	1	3
Student Affairs	17	3	2	2	7
Addictions	2	1	1	1	0
Career	3	0	1	1	0
Gerontological	2	0	0	0	2
Marriage & Family	17	0	3	6	9
Other	11	4	7	4	2

Note: Entries under Thesis, Comprehensive Exam, Oral Exam, and Portfolio reflect the number of programs that indicated that these were part of their graduation requirements.

Programs may have other exit requirements. Examples of some other graduation requirements are a thesis, comprehensive examination, oral examination, or portfolio. Programs may ask students for one or more of these projects. According to the data collected, 25 responding programs require a thesis, 222 have a comprehensive examination, 53 have oral examinations, and 103 include portfolios as part of their graduation requirements. The numbers of the 310 programs that answered this portion of the data collection form as mandating one or more of those projects are tabulated in Table 4.7.

Some students may choose to pursue an Educational Specialist degree or a Certificate of Advanced Graduate Study in counseling. The academic hours and clinical hours required by those responding programs are outlined in Table 4.8. As noted below the table, interpreting the information is difficult because of the variations in reporting. Graduates of the 78 specialist programs that responded must complete a thesis (10), comprehensive examination (51), oral examination (13), and/or a portfolio (22). That information is summarized in Table 4.9.

JOB SETTINGS AFTER GRADUATION

Our study indicates the majority of graduates from counselor preparation programs find employment in settings related to their specialty areas the first year after completing their programs. According to information reported on the data collection form, 67% of community counseling graduates and 67% of mental health counseling graduates find employment in agencies after graduation; 87% of school counselors are hired in schools,

Table 4.8. Graduation Requirements for Specialist Degrees in Counseling: Academic and Clinical Hours

Academic Hours		Clinical Hours			
Semester Hours	NPR	Practicum Hours	NPR	Intern Hours	NPR
10–20	4	0–100	28	0–100	0
21–30	47	101–200	9	101–200	3
31–40	0	201–300	6	201–300	12
41–50	8	301–400	2	301–400	2
51–60	11	401–500	1	401–500	1
61–70	10	501–600	1	501–600	44
71–80	18	over 600	0	over 600	6
81–90	1				

NPR: Number of programs responding.
Note: It is possible that some of the programs responding answered this item as an addition to requirements for their master's degrees, which may account for the programs with low requirements in semester hours, practicum hours, or internship hours. All specialist programs were collapsed to get the data above rather than separating them by type of program.

and 40% of college counselors work in higher education/student affairs. The majority of graduates in addictions, gerontological, and marriage and family also work in agencies. More details regarding percentages of graduates and their job settings the first year after completing entry-level programs can be found in Table 4.10. Some graduates choose to pursue an advanced degree after finishing the entry-level program. The next chapter contains information about doctoral-level preparation programs.

SUMMARY

The information reported for entry-level counselor preparation programs has been further summarized in Tables 4.11 and 4.12.

Table 4.9. Graduation Requirements for Specialist Degrees in Counseling: Other Requirements

Number of Programs Responding	Thesis Exam	Comprehensive Exam	Oral	Portfolio
78	10	51	13	22

Note: All specialist programs were collapsed to get the data above rather than separating them out by type of program.

Table 4.10. Job Settings in First Year After Completing Entry-Level Programs

Job Placement After Graduation	Number of Programs Responding	Percent of Graduates
Community		
Advanced graduate programs	70	13.42%
Managed care	60	10.03%
Private practice	64	9.20%
Agency practice	92	67.65%
Elementary schools	8	10.21%
Middle schools	36	2.67%
Secondary schools	35	2.94%
Higher education/student affairs	37	2.35%
Mental Health		
Advanced graduate programs	39	14.87%
Managed care	32	16.34%
Private practice	34	10.44%
Agency practice	42	67.79%
Elementary schools	1	21%
Middle schools	9	0
Secondary schools	8	0
Higher education/student affairs	10	0.5%
School		
Advanced graduate programs	91	9.09%
Managed care	54	0.04%
Private practice	44	0.27%
Agency practice	61	5.41%
Elementary schools	41	29.30%
Middle schools	130	28.77%
Secondary schools	133	29.29%
Higher education/student affairs	106	36.11%
College		
Advanced graduate programs	11	9.09%
Managed care	11	5.45%
Private practice	7	1.43%
Agency practice	7	5.24%
Elementary schools	1	30.7%
Middle schools	2	0%
Secondary schools	3	10.23%
Higher education/student affairs	5	40.6%
Student Affairs		
Advanced graduate programs	28	16.43%
Managed care	18	0.56%
Private practice	18	0
Agency practice	19	2.21%
Elementary schools	2	47.5%
Middle schools	16	0
Secondary schools	15	0.67%
Higher education/student affairs	19	21.26%

Addictions

Advanced graduate programs	3	8.33%
Managed care	3	33.33%
Private practice	2	10%
Agency practice	5	62%
Elementary schools	0	—
Middle schools	1	0
Secondary schools	1	0
Higher education/student affairs	1	0

Career

Advanced graduate programs	3	18.33%
Managed care	3	3.33%
Private practice	3	3.33%
Agency practice	3	16.67%
Elementary schools	0	—
Middle schools	2	0
Secondary schools	2	2.5%
Higher education/student affairs	3	16.67%

Gerontological

Advanced graduate programs	1	5%
Managed care	1	15%
Private practice	1	5%
Agency practice	2	52.5%
Elementary sSchools	1	5%
Middle schools	0	—
Secondary schools	0	—
Higher education/student affairs	0	—

Marriage & Family

Advanced graduate programs	28	16.03%
Managed care	19	16.05%
Private practice	26	16.19%
Agency practice	30	60.13%
Elementary schools	1	0
Middle schools	7	0.86%
Secondary schools	6	0.86%
Higher education/student affairs	5	0%

Other

Advanced graduate programs	9	26.88%
Managed care	3	3.33%
Private practice	4	13.75%
Agency practice	9	45%
Elementary schools	2	5%
Middle schools	4	18.75%
Secondary schools	4	25%
Higher education/student affairs	6	50.83%

Notes: Numbers do not add up to 100%. This is because averages were only taken of programs that responded for each item, and this was not consistent. In addition, not all programs entered their data so that it would equal 100% as a total. Also, 0 is listed as a response if the program entered this as a response. It is not assumed that no response equals a response of 0.

Table 4.11. Entry-Level Program Summary: Admission Requirements

	Average No. Admitted	Average No. Graduated	Require GRE	Require MAT	Average GPA	Require Experience	Require Letters	Require Interviews
Community	26	21	62	31	2.87	8	107	72
Mental Health	22	14	37	10	2.92	8	49	32
School	22	18	97	44	2.86	18	147	108
College	7	5	8	2	2.81	0	9	11
Student Affairs	12	10	23	4	2.80	11	31	21
Addictions	10	8	4	2	2.83	0	6	2
Career	8	7	3	1	2.80	0	7	3
Gerontological	7	5	2	1	3.00	0	3	1
Marriage & Family	17	14	22	16	2.85	6	33	25
Other	14	9	8	12	2.74	0	14	16

GRE = Graduate Record Examination; MAT: Miller Analogies Test.
Note: Please use caution in comparisons. Recall from the tables earlier in this chapter that the number of programs responding to these questions on the Data Collection Form varied considerably. Refer to the information in Part E of this book for information specific to each specialty program.

Table 4.12. Entry-Level Program Summary: Graduation Requirements

	Semester Hours	Quarter Hours	Practicum Hours	Internship Hours	Thesis	Comp	Oral	Portfolio
Community	51	74	118	583	5	69	12	26
Mental Health	58	82	200	721	5	31	9	7
School	50	61	131	562	7	100	17	47
College	49	72	110	540	0	8	1	3
Student Affairs	46	—	121	537	3	2	2	7
Addictions	49	—	200	600	1	1	1	0
Career	51	—	133	600	0	1	1	0
Gerontological	50	—	100	433	0	0	0	2
Marriage & Family	58	82	192	621	0	3	6	9
Other	46	48	176	641	4	7	4	2

Note: Please use caution in comparisons. Recall from the tables earlier in this chapter that the number of programs responding to these questions on the data collection form varied considerably. Refer to the information in Part E of this book for information specific to each specialty program.

## Chapter 5

Doctoral-Level Counselor Preparation Programs

Professional counselors may also choose to pursue a doctoral degree program. Those programs build upon the foundations of the entry-level program. CACREP accredits doctoral-level counselor education and supervision programs. CACREP standards for the scope of type of academic and clinical experience can be reviewed at the web address: www.counseling.org/cacrep

PROGRAMS OFFERED AND ACCREDITATION

Information was collected from 70 programs that responded to the data reporting form. Programs indicated if the counseling areas of community, mental health, school, college, student affairs, addictions, career, gerontological, marriage and family, counselor education, and other specialty types were offered at their institution. According to these data, the specialty areas of counselor education with 38 programs was the most commonly identified. Counselor education programs constituted 54.2% of all doctoral programs offered. The other areas, in descending order of frequency, include school, other, community, mental health, student affairs, marriage and family, addictions, and careers. No doctoral programs in college or gerontological counseling were reported. Table 5.1 provides information about the doctoral level number of departments and accredited programs.

Table 5.1. Number of Departments Responding and Number of Accredited Programs in Doctoral-Level Preparation Programs

Departments Responding	70
Community	5
Mental Health	4
School	9
College	0
Student Affairs	3
Addictions	1
Career	1
Gerontological	0
Marriage & Family	2
Counselor Education	38
Other	7
Accreditation Information: CACREP Programs	
Counselor Education and Supervision	45
Accredited Programs Responding	
Counselor Education	30

ADMISSIONS AND GRADUATES

Doctoral-level programs enroll and graduate fewer students than entry-level programs. The average number admitted yearly ranges from one to nine students. The average number of students who graduate from doctoral-level programs ranges from one to six annually. Table 5.2 contains the average number of students admitted and graduated annually for counseling preparation programs that reported this information.

Table 5.2. Number of Students Admitted and Graduated Yearly in Doctoral-Level Programs

Programs	Number of Programs Responding	Average Admitted Yearly	Average Graduated Yearly
Community	7	4	3
Mental Health	3	6	6
School	6	7	6
College	1	5	5
Student Affairs	3	3	1
Addictions	1	1	1
Career	1	1	—
Gerontological	0	—	—
Marriage & Family	2	2	2
Counselor Education	28	9	6

ADMISSION REQUIREMENTS

Doctoral-level counselor preparation programs require a variety of information before admitting students. Standardized tests such as the Graduate Record Examination (GRE) and the Miller Analogies Test (MAT) are used by some programs as a part of their admission requirements. Of the 70 programs that responded to this query, 52 require the GRE and 8 require the MAT. Programs also reported the average grade point average (GPA) of students admitted. Across all programs that average is a 3.31 GPA. Table 5.3 details how many specialty programs require the standardized test and the average GPA of students admitted.

Some programs ask that applicants have work experience, submit recommendation letters, or participate in an interview. Doctoral-level programs may also require students seeking admission to have completed a master's degree. Again, 70 programs answered the data collection form regarding these admission requirements. Of those programs, 24 reported requiring work experience, 64 required letters of recommendation, and 59 held interviews for applicants to their programs. Sixty-one programs reported requiring a master's degree as a portion of the admission criteria. Information specific to specialty area programs can be found in Table 5.4.

CLINICAL EXPERIENCES REQUIRED

Doctoral-level counselor preparation programs reported supervised practicum and internship clock hours that must be completed before graduation. These programs may vary the hours according to the specialty area being pursued. Information provided on the data collection form indicated

Table 5.3. Admission Requirements to Doctoral-Level Programs

Programs	NPR	GRE	MAT	NPR	Average GPA	Master's Required
Community	5	5	1	4	3.28	5
Mental Health	4	2	1	3	3.27	2
School	9	8	0	7	3.26	9
College	0	—	—	0	—	—
Student Affairs	3	3	0	3	3.17	3
Addictions	1	1	0	1	3.50	1
Career	1	1	0	1	3.60	0
Gerontological	0	—	—	0	—	—
Marriage & Family	2	2	0	2	3.40	2
Counselor Education	38	25	4	9	3.22	33
Other	8	5	2	5	3.09	6

GRE: Graduate Record Examination; MAT: Miller Analogies Test; NPR: Number of programs responding.
Note: Entries under GRE and MAT columns reflect the number of programs that reported they use either of these as an admission requirement.

Table 5.4. Other Admission Requirements

Programs	Number of Programs Responding	Work Experience	Recommen- dation Letters	Interviews
Community	5	2	5	5
Mental Health	4	0	2	2
School	9	5	9	8
College	0	—	—	—
Student Affairs	3	1	3	2
Addictions	1	1	1	1
Career	1	0	1	1
Gerontological	0	—	—	—
Marriage & Family	2	0	2	2
Counselor Education	38	14	35	34
Other	8	1	6	4

Note: Entries under Work Experience, Recommendation Letters, and Interviews columns are the number of programs that indicated positively that they required these for admission.

an average of 236 practicum hours and 791 internship hours being required in the 46 programs that responded. Table 5.5 contains information related to required practicum and internship hours.

GRADUATION REQUIREMENTS

A standard requirement for graduation from a doctoral-level counselor prepa- ration program is the successful completion of coursework. The average number of graduate hours required for the doctoral-level programs that re-

Table 5.5. Clinical Hours Required for Doctoral Degree

Programs	NPR	Practicum Hours	NPR	Internship Hours
Community	4	150	5	520
Mental Health	2	138	3	1,267
School	4	500	9	656
College	0	—	0	—
Student Affairs	2	140	3	453
Addictions	0	—	1	600
Career	1	100	1	600
Gerontological	0	—	0	—
Marriage & Family	1	100	2	900
Counselor Education	27	261	34	668
Other	5	500	5	1,460

NPR: Number of Programs Responding.
Note: Entries under Practicum Hours and Internship Hours are average numbers for all programs that responded to these items.

Table 5.6. Academic Hours Required for Doctoral Degree

Programs	Number of Programs Responding	Semester Hours	Quarter Hours
Community	5	81	—
Mental Health	3	99	—
School	9	86	—
College	0	—	—
Student Affairs	3	105	—
Addictions	1	100	—
Career	1	82	—
Gerontological	0	—	—
Marriage & Family	2	101	—
Counselor Education	33	86	—
Other	5	92	120

Note: Entries under Semester Hours and Quarter Hours are average numbers for all programs that responded to these items.

sponded to this portion of the data collection form was 85 semester hours. One program reported 120 quarter hours needed for graduation. Further information is contained in Table 5.6.

Programs may have other exit requirements. Examples of some other graduation requirements are a thesis or dissertation, comprehensive examination, oral examination, or portfolio. Programs may ask students for one or more of these projects. According to the data collected from 70 programs, 64 reported requiring a thesis or dissertation, 49 reported having a comprehensive examination, 41 have oral examinations, and 7 include portfolios as part of their graduation requirements. The number of specialty programs that answered this portion of the data collection form concerning one or more of those projects are tabulated in Table 5.7.

JOB SETTINGS AFTER GRADUATION

The job settings of graduates in the first year after completing the doctoral-level counselor education program mirror many of those of entry-level practitioners. According to information reported on the data collection form, 54% of community counseling graduates and 40% of mental health counseling graduates find employment in agencies after graduation; 72.8% of school counselors are hired in schools. The majority of graduates in addictions counseling and marriage and family counseling also work in agencies. More details regarding percentages of graduates and their job settings the first year after completing doctoral-level programs can be found in Table 5.8.

Table 5.7. Other Graduation Requirements for Doctoral Degree

Programs	Number of Programs Responding	Thesis/ Dissertation	Compre- hensive Exam	Oral Exam	Portfolio
Community	5	4	5	4	0
Mental Health	4	3	3	2	0
School	9	9	1	6	1
College	0	—	—	—	—
Student Affairs	3	2	2	1	0
Addictions	1	1	1	1	0
Career	1	1	1	0	0
Gerontological	0	—	—	—	—
Marriage & Family	2	2	2	1	0
Counselor Education	38	35	30	22	3
Other	7	7	4	4	3

Note: Entries under Thesis, Comprehensive Exam, Oral Exam, and Portfolio reflect the number of programs that responded positively that these were part of their graduation requirements.

Table 5.8. Job Settings of Graduates in First Year After Completing Doctoral-Level Programs

Job Placement After Graduation	Number of Programs Responding	Percentage of Graduates
Community		
Advanced graduate programs	2	10.5%
Managed care	3	14%
Private practice	4	28.75%
Agency practice	5	54%
Elementary schools	2	13.5%
Middle schools	1	5%
Secondary schools	1	15%
Higher education/student affairs	1	20%
Mental Health		
Advanced graduate programs	0	—
Managed care	0	—
Private practice	0	—
Agency practice	1	40%
Elementary schools	1	20%
Middle schools	0	—
Secondary schools	0	—
Higher education/student affairs	0	—

School

Advanced graduate programs	2	10.5%
Managed care	1	0
Private practice	3	10%
Agency practice	2	40%
Elementary schools	1	20%
Middle schools	5	25.8%
Secondary schools	4	27%
Higher education/student affairs	5	43.6%

College
No programs responding

Student Affairs

Advanced graduate programs	3	6.67%
Managed care	2	0
Private practice	2	5%
Agency practice	2	0
Elementary schools	2	17.5%
Middle schools	2	0
Secondary schools	2	0
Higher education/student affairs	2	0

Addictions

Advanced graduate programs	1	20%
Managed care	0	—
Private practice	1	20%
Agency practice	2	65%
Elementary schools	0	—
Middle schools	0	—
Secondary schools	0	—
Higher education/student affairs	0	—

Career
No programs responded

Gerontological
No programs responded

Marriage & Family

Advanced graduate programs	1	2%
Managed care	1	5%
Private practice	1	5%
Agency practice	2	90%
Elementary schools	1	8%
Middle schools	0	—
Secondary schools	0	--
Higher education/student affairs	0	—

(*Continued*)

Table 5.8. Continued

Job Placement After Graduation	Number of Programs Responding	Percentage of Graduates
Counselor Education		
Advanced graduate programs	19	26.84%
Managed care	15	5.73%
Private practice	24	17.79%
Agency practice	19	20.88%
Elementary schools	11	19.7%
Middle schools	12	4.5%
Secondary schools	12	3.58%
Higher education/student affairs	14	6%
Other		
Advanced graduate programs	3	0
Managed care	5	20.2%
Private practice	6	16.83%
Agency practice	5	30.8%
Elementary schools	4	7.75%
Middle schools	3	0
Secondary schools	3	0
Higher education/student affairs	3	1.67

Note: Numbers do not add up to 100%. This is because averages were only taken of programs that responded for each item, and this was not consistent. In addition, not all programs entered their data so that it would equal 100% as a total. Also, 0 is listed as a response if the program entered this as a response. It is not assumed that no response equals a response of 0.

Chapter 6

Pastoral and Rehabilitation Programs

Two other specialty area programs, pastoral and rehabilitation counseling, responded to our study. An organization that sets standards for pastoral counselor training is the American Association of Pastoral Counselors. The Council on Rehabilitation Education (CORE) accredits programs in rehabilitation counseling. The Council's recommendations for programs can be accessed at www.core-rehab.org.

PROGRAMS OFFERED AND ACCREDITATION

Information was collected from five entry-level and one doctoral pastoral counseling program. Twenty-eight entry-level and one doctoral-level rehabilitation counseling program responded. Table 6.1 provides information about the number of departments and accredited entry-level programs.

ADMISSIONS AND GRADUATES

Entry-level programs in pastoral counseling enroll an average of 8 students each year and have an average of 6 graduates annually. The one doctoral-level pastoral counseling program that responded admits 12 students yearly and graduates 8. The 25 entry-level rehabilitation counseling programs that answered the study average 17 students admitted each year with 11 graduating on an annual basis. Two doctoral-level rehabilitation counseling programs admit and graduate an average of three students annually. See Table 6.2 for the number of students admitted and graduating annually.

Table 6.1. Number of Departments Responding and Number of Accredited Programs in Pastoral and Rehabilitation Programs

Department and Program Data
Entry-Level Departments Responding
    Pastoral   5
    Rehabilitation   28
Doctoral-Level Departments Responding
    Pastoral   1
    Rehabilitation   2

Accreditation Information
AAPC Programs   37
CORE Programs   93
(from www.core-rehab.org/states/index.html)

Accredited Programs Responding
    Pastoral   —
    Rehabilitation   23

Departments Planning to Apply for Accreditation Within Next Three Years
    AAPC   —
    CORE   4

ADMISSION REQUIREMENTS

As with other counselor preparation programs, pastoral and rehabilitation programs have requirements for admission. Students are required to have GRE scores in two of the five pastoral entry-level programs. Fifteen of the 28 entry-level rehabilitation programs reported requiring the GRE, as do 2 of the doctoral-level rehabilitation programs. Programs also reported the average grade point average (GPA) of students admitted. Table 6.3 details how many specialty programs require the standardized test; the average

Table 6.2. Number of Students Admitted and Graduated Yearly in Pastoral and Rehabilitation Programs

Programs	Number of Programs Responding	Average Admitted Yearly	Average Graduated Yearly
Entry Level			
Pastoral	4	8	6
Rehabilitation	25	17	11
Doctoral Level			
Pastoral	1	12	8
Rehabilitation	2	3	3

Note: Entry-level program information is a combination of master's and specialist degrees.

Table 6.3. Admission Requirements to Pastoral and Rehabilitation Programs

Programs	NPR	GRE	MAT	NPR	Average GPA
Entry Level					
Pastoral	5	2	0	2	2.75
Rehabilitation	28	15	7	23	2.88
Doctoral Level					
Pastoral	1	0	0	0	—
Rehabilitation	2	2	0	2	3.25

GPA: Grade point average; GRE: Graduate Record Examination; MAT: Miller Analogies Test; NPR: Number of programs responding.
Note: Entry-level program information is a combination of master's and specialist degrees. Entries under GRE and MAT columns reflect the number of programs that reported that they use either of these as an admission requirement.

GPA of students admitted provides more details on those admission standards.

Some programs ask applicants to have completed some work experience, to submit recommendation letters, or participate in an interview. Table 6.4 details how pastoral and rehabilitation programs answered the data collection form regarding these admission requirements.

CLINICAL EXPERIENCES REQUIRED

Pastoral and rehabilitation counseling preparation programs reported supervised practicum and internship clock hours that must be completed before graduation. Information provided on the data collection form indicated

Table 6.4. Other Admission Requirements to Pastoral and Rehabilitation Programs

Programs	Number of Programs Responding	Work Experience	Recommendation Letters	Interviews
Entry Level				
Pastoral	4	0	3	2
Rehabilitation	27	2	23	21
Doctoral Level				
Pastoral	1	1	1	1
Rehabilitation	2	1	2	2

Note: Entry-level program information is a combination of master's and specialist degrees. Entries under Work Experience, Recommendation Letters, and Interviews columns reflect the number of programs that reported that they use these as admission requirements.

Table 6.5. Clinical Hours Required for Pastoral and Rehabilitation Programs

Programs	NPR	Practicum Hours	NPR	Intern Hours
Entry Level				
Pastoral	2	100	3	333
Rehabilitation	26	143	28	598
Doctoral Level Programs				
Pastoral	0	—	1	1,500
Rehabilitation	2	1,080	1	2,000

NPR: Number of programs responding.
Note: Entry-level program information is a combination of master's and specialist degrees. Entries under Practicum Hours and Internship Hours are average numbers for all programs that responded to these items.

an average of 100 practicum hours and 333 internship hours are required in the pastoral counseling entry-level programs, with 1,500 internship hours at the doctoral level. Rehabilitation counseling programs that responded averaged 143 practicum hours and 598 internship hours at the entry level and 1,080 practicum hours and 2,000 internship hours at the doctoral level. Table 6.5 contains information related to required practicum and internship hours.

GRADUATION REQUIREMENTS

These programs vary in the number of graduate hours required for graduation. The average number of graduate hours required for the three entry-level pastoral counseling programs that responded to this portion of the data collection form was 67 semester hours and 60 hours for the doctoral level. Thirty-two rehabilitation counseling programs average 51 semester hours for an entry-level program, and three doctoral level programs require 103 semester hours or 145 quarter hours. This information is shown in Table 6.6.

Table 6.6. Acacemic Hours Required for Pastoral and Rehabilitation Programs

Programs	Number of Responding	Semester Hours	Quarter Hours
Entry Level			
Pastoral	3	67	—
Rehabilitation	32	51	—
Doctoral Level Programs			
Pastoral	1	60	—
Rehabilitation	3	103	145

Note: Entry-level program information is a combination of master's and specialist degrees. Entries under Semester Hours and Quarter Hours are average numbers for all programs that responded to these items.

These programs may have other exit requirements. Examples of some other graduation requirements are a thesis, comprehensive examination, oral examination, or portfolio. Programs may ask students for one or more of these projects. Information from the pastoral and rehabilitation programs that answered this portion of the data collection form are shown in Table 6.7.

Table 6.7. Other Requirements for Graduation for Pastoral and Rehabilitation Programs

Programs	Number of Programs Responding	Thesis	Comprehensive Exam	Oral Exam	Portfolio
Entry Level					
Pastoral	5	2	0	2	2
Rehabilitation	28	6	20	4	3
Doctoral Level					
Pastoral	1	1	1	0	0
Rehabilitation	1	1	0	1	0

Note: Entry-level program information is a combination of master's and specialist degrees. Entries under Thesis, Comprehensive Exam, Oral Exam, and Portfolio reflect the number of programs that responded positively that these were part of their graduation requirements.

Chapter 7

Expectations: Anticipated Changes in Trends

Several programs that responded to the data collection form provided information about changes that were anticipated for the next three years. Those alterations involved the addition or deletion of specific courses, accreditation status, and other modifications. The following provides summaries of those plans.

COURSES

The continually expanding body of knowledge from which best practices in counseling emerge necessitates a responsive curriculum. Therefore, many programs reported plans to alter some courses. Of the 101 programs that responded to this section of the Data Collection Form, they listed the most common courses for being added to the curriculum as addictions, play therapy, crisis/violence counseling, supervision, and marriage and family counseling. Respondents indicated very few courses being dropped, with only four reports of career and marriage and family courses to be omitted. Table 7.1 provides a tally of responses.

ACCREDITATION STATUS OF PROGRAMS

As noted in earlier chapters, counselor preparation programs may seek accreditation. Receiving that status indicates the program adheres to standards set by the accrediting body. Table 7.2 shows that school counseling

Table 7.1. Academic Areas in Which Departments Anticipate Adding or Dropping One or More Courses Within the Next Three Years

Academic Areas	Add	Drop
Abuse of Individual	7	1
Addictions	20	1
Adventure Counseling	4	1
Advocacy	8	0
Career/Life Planning	4	4
Computer and Related Technology	5	0
Consultation	14	3
Crisis/Violence Counseling	18	1
Diversity	11	0
Experiential Component	5	0
Forensic Counseling	4	0
Gender Studies	5	0
Gerontological Counseling	9	0
Grief Counseling	11	1
Group Work	4	0
Human Sexuality	6	1
Intelligence Testing	0	1
Internet Use	5	0
Legal/Ethical Issues	12	1
Life Coaching	2	0
Marriage and Family Counseling	15	4
Play Therapy	20	2
Projective Assessment	0	0
Psychodiagnosis	6	1
Psychopharmacology	8	2
Rehabilitation	2	1
Research Methods	3	1
School Counseling	8	2
Social Justice	6	0
Special Needs Populations	6	0
Sports Counseling	2	0
Supervision	15	2
Teaching	2	0
Teaming and Collaboration	3	0
Technology	3	1
Testing, Appraisal, Assessment	3	0
Theory Component	3	1
Wellness	6	3
Other	0	0
Total	265	35
Number of Departments Responding	N = 101	

and community counseling programs have the majority of accredited programs that responded to this survey. Information on other specialty areas that are accredited, plan to seek accreditation, or intend to drop accreditation is contained in that table also.

Table 7.2. Accreditation Status of Programs

Accreditation Body	Program	Now Have	Applying For	Plan to Drop
CACREP	College Counseling	2	—	—
	Community Counseling	80	12	—
	Career Counseling	3	2	—
	Gerontological Counseling	1	—	—
	Counselor Education and Supervision	30	4	—
	Marital, Couple, and Family Counseling/Therapy	14	8	—
	Mental Health Counseling	20	6	—
	School Counseling	98	27	1
	Student Affairs/College Counseling Emphasis	24	4	—
	Student Affairs/Professional Practice Emphasis	11	4	—
CORE	Rehabilitation Counseling	23	3	—
AAPC	Pastoral Counseling	—	—	—
Total		284	70	1
Number of Programs Responding			N = 141	

PROGRAM CHANGES ANTICIPATED

As well as changes in the curriculum, counselor preparation programs may anticipate making other modification to refine their offerings. The programs that answered this portion of the data collection form indicated much increased effort in diversity recruiting of both faculty and students. The other changes noted most often were seeking accreditation and providing more distance education and online courses. Table 7.3 summarizes these responses.

OTHER MENTAL HEALTH PROGRAMS

Several counselor education respondents provided information relative to related programs on their campus. Most often those related programs were psychology and social work. Further descriptions of the frequencies that related programs were reported appears in Table 7.4.

TRENDS

Earlier editions of *Counselor Preparation* have compared data across years. We have reported the responses to the survey without interpretation. However, readily apparent in this and other editions is the dynamic nature of the profession. Many counselor education preparation programs are being strengthened, many are revising to meet the changing needs of the practi-

Table 7.3. Program Changes Anticipated by Departments Within Next Three Years

Anticipated Program Changes	Increase	Decrease
Admission requirements	21	—
Course offerings—approximate number	38	2
Clinical supervision	21	—
Diversity recruiting of faculty	70	—
Diversity recruiting of students	75	—
Faculty full-time equivalency	32	6
Financial aid	21	—
Graduation requirements	13	—
National accreditation (e.g., CACREP)	45	—
Number of degree majors	22	4
Number of distance education courses	44	2
Number of off-campus courses	35	2
Number of online courses	40	1
Other	—	—
Totals	477	17
Number of Programs Responding	N = 143	

tioner, more are incorporating technology into delivery systems, and more are populated with faculty who hold well-respected credentials. For the ongoing growth and development of the profession and the mental health needs of those counselors serve, we hope these will be challenges on which we continue to build.

Table 7.4. Availability of Other Mental Health Program(s) at Same College or University Where Counselor Preparation Program Offered

Mental Health Program Offered on Campus	Number of Programs Responding
Clinical social workers	46
Marriage and family therapists	20
Psychologists	80
Arts therapists	9
Psychiatric nurses	23
Psychiatrists	16
Organizational behaviorists	16
Communications	29
International Studies	17
Other	19

Part D

Data on Each
Department

Keys for Part D: Data on Each Department

M – Master's degree (i.e. M.A., M.S., M.Ed.)

S – Specialist degree (i.e. Ed.S., C.A.G.S.)

D – Doctoral degree (i.e. Ph.D., Ed.D.)

R – Required

NP – Not Provided

CPCE – Counselor Preparation Comprehensive Exam

Full Prof. – Full Professor

Assoc. – Associate Professor

Assist. – Assistant Professor

ACS – Approved Clinical Supervisor

CAC – Certified Alcoholism (Addictions) Counselor

CADC – Certified Alcohol and Dependency Counselor

CADAC – Certified Alcohol and Drug Abuse Counselor

CCDC – Certified Clinical Dependence Counselor

CCMHC – Certified Clinical Mental Health Counselor

CLPC – Clinical Licensed Professional Counselor

CRC – Certified Rehabilitation Counselor

CSC – Certified School Counselor

LCDC – Licensed Clinical Dependence Counselor

LCP – Licensed Counseling Professional

LCPC – Licensed Clinical Professional Counselor

LMFC – Licensed Marriage and Family Counselor

LMHC – Licensed Mental Health Counselor

LMHP – Licensed Mental Health Professional

LPC – Licensed Professional Counselor

LPCC – Licensed Professional Clinical Counselor

LSAC – Licensed Substance Abuse Counselor

MAC – Master Addictions Counselor

MFCC – Marriage, Family, Child Counselor

NCC – National Certified Counselor

NCCC – National Certified Career Counselor

NCGC – National Certified Gerontological Counselor

NCSC – National Certified School Counselor

PCC – Professional Clinical Counselor

RCC – Registered Clinical Counselor

RPCC – Registered Professional Career Counselor

AAMFT – American Association of Marriage and Family Therapy

AAPC – American Association of Pastoral Counselors

ABPP – American Board of Professional Psychology

ACSW – Academy of Certified Social Workers

ASCH – American Society of Clinical Hypnotherapy

BCD – Board Certified Diplomat in Clinical Social Work

CCAS – Certified Clinical Addictions Specialist

CGP – Certified Group Psychotherapist

CMFT – Certified Marriage and Family Therapist

CORE – Council on Rehabilitation Education

CSP – Certified School Psychologist

CSW – Clinical Social Worker

CVE – Certified Vocational Evaluator

DCSW – Doctorate of Clinical Social Work

HSPP – Health Service Provider in Psychology

LCSW – Licensed Clinical Social Worker

LMFT – Licensed Marriage and Family Therapist

LP – Licensed Psychologist

LPE – Licensed Psychological Evaluator

MCC – Master Certified Coach

MHSP – Mental Health Service Provider

NCSP – National Certified School Psychologist

RPT – Registered Play Therapist

RPT-S – Registered Play Therapist - Supervisor

RN – Registered Nurse

AL: Auburn University

2084 Haley Center
Auburn, AL 36849-6222
United States

Dean Francis Kochan, Dean College of Education, 3084 Haley Center, Auburn University, Auburn, AL 36849
Administrator Holly Stadler, Professor
Department Department of Counseling & Counseling Psychology
(334) 844-5160, fax (334) 844-2860, ccp@auburn.edu,
www.auburn.edu/academics/education/ccp

Key See key for Data on Each Department (this section) on page 79.

Program

Accreditation Regional Accreditation, **CACREP:** Community Counseling, **CACREP:** Counselor Education and Supervision, **CACREP:** School Counseling

CACREP

Uniqueness The department and faculty are committed to preparing professional counselors to work with a diverse clientele in schools and communities. The mission statement for the department and objectives for individual programs can be found on the departmental webpage www.auburn.edu/academics/education/ccp

Degrees
- Community Counseling: M.
- School Counseling: M.
- Other: PhD, D.
- Counselor Education: EdD, PhD.

Contact
- Community Counseling: M = Irene Houston.
- School Counseling: M = Debra Cobia.
- Other: D = NP.
- Counselor Education: D = Jamie Carney.

Admission and Graduation Data

Admission
Requirements
- Community Counseling(M): GPA 3.00; GRE 1000; GRE V 400; GRE Q 400; GRE A 0.
- School Counseling(M): GPA 3.00; GRE 1000; GRE V 400; GRE Q 400; GRE A 0.
- Other(D): NP.
- Counselor Education(D): GRE 1000; GRE V 400; GRE Q 400.

Enrollment
- Community Counseling(M): 15-20 Admitted yearly; 15-20 Graduated yearly; 22 Female; 5 Male.
- School Counseling(M): 5-10 Admitted yearly; 5-10 Graduated yearly; 8 Female; 2 Male.
- Other(D): 5 Admitted yearly; 5 Graduated yearly; 25 Female; 5 Male.
- Counselor Education(D): 1-2 Admitted yearly; 3-6 Graduated yearly; 12 Female; 1 Male.

Diversity
- African-American; Asian-American; Caucasian; Other.

Graduation
Requirements
- Community Counseling(M): 48 Class hours; 100 Practicum hours; 600 Internship hours; Comprehensive exam; CPCE; Oral exam; Portfolio.
- School Counseling(M): 48-51 Class hours; 100 Practicum hours; 600 Internship hours; Comprehensive exam; CPCE; Oral exam; Portfolio.
- Other(D): NP.
- Counselor Education(D): 50 Post-master's Class hours; 100 Practicum hours; 600 Internship hours; Oral exam; Dissertation; Portfolio.

Postgraduation activity: Advanced education and employment setting percentages.

- Community Counseling(M): 5 Advanced education; 90 Agency practice; 5 Other.
- School Counseling(M): NP.
- Other(D):
- Counselor Education(D): 80 Advanced education; 5 Agency practice; 5 Middle school; 5 Secondary school; 5 Student affairs.

Planned Program Modifications

Courses
Drop
- NP.
Add
- NP.

Other
Decrease
- NP.
Increase
- Faculty FTE.

Related Programs Marriage and Family Therapists
Psychology

Faculty

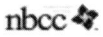 Percent of faculty reported with NCC certification: 33%.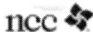

Percent in professional counseling practice: 66%.

Research interests Faculty biographical information and research interests can be found on the Counseling
and Counseling Psychology webpage

Diversity   • African-American; Caucasian; Other.

Name, Degree, Rank, State/National Credentials, % time devoted to program, email
• Buckhalt, Joseph A; Ph.D.; Full Prof.; <21%; *buckhja@auburn.edu*
• Carney, Jamie; Ph.D.; Assoc.; NCC; >81%; *carneyjs@auburn.edu*
• Cobia, Debra C; Ed.D.; Full Prof.; LPC, NCC; >81%; *cobiadc@mail.auburn.edu*
• Houston, Irene; Ph.D.; Assist.; LPC; >81%; *houstis@auburn.edu*
• Liddle, Becky; Ph.D.; Assoc.; <21%; *liddlbj@auburn.edu*
• Middleton, Renee A; Ph.D.; Assoc.; 22-40%; *middlre@auburn.edu*
• Pipes, Randolph B; Ph.D.; Full Prof.; <21%; *pipearb@auburn.edu*
• Stadler, Holly A; Ph.D; Full Prof.; <21%; *stadlha@auburn.edu*
• Suh, Suhyun; Ph.D.; Assist.; NCC; >81%; *suhyusu@auburn.edu*

Has CHI SIGMA IOTA (International Counseling Society) chapter.

AL: The University of Alabama

Box 870231
Tuscaloosa, AL 35487-0231
USA

Dean   John P. Dolly — College of Education
Administrator   S. Allen Wilcoxon, Ed.D., Program Chair
                       Department   Educational Studies in Psychology, Research Methodology, and Counseling
                                       (205) 348-7579, fax (205) 348-7584, awilcoxo@bamaed.ua.edu,
                                       counselored.ua.edu

Key   See key for Data on Each Department (this section) on page 79.

Program
Accreditation   Regional Accreditation, **CACREP:** Community Counseling, **CACREP:** Counselor Education
                   and Supervision, **CACREP:** School Counseling, **CORE:** Rehabilitation Counseling

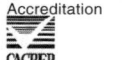

Uniqueness   This program offers some distance learning via interactive technology (no on-line curriculum),
                   though the majority of course work is completed in a traditional on-campus format.

Degrees   • Community Counseling: M, S.
                   • School Counseling: M, S.
                   • Rehabilitation Counseling: M, S.
                   • Counselor Education: PhD.

Contact   • Community Counseling: M, S = S. Allen Wilcoxon, Ed.D..
                   • School Counseling: M, S = Karla D. Carmichael, Ph.D..
                   • Rehabilitation Counseling: M, S = Jamie F. Satcher, Ph.D..
                   • Counselor Education: D = S. Allen Wilcoxon, Ed.D..

Admission and Graduation Data
Admission
Requirements   • Community Counseling(M): GPA 3.00; GRE 1000(V+Q); MAT 50.
                   • Community Counseling(S): GPA 3.00; GRE 1000(V+Q); MAT 50.
                   • School Counseling(M): GPA 3.00; GRE 1000(V+Q); MAT 50.
                   • School Counseling(S): GPA 3.00; GRE 1000(V+Q); MAT 50.
                   • Rehabilitation Counseling(M): GPA 3.00; GRE 1000(V+Q); MAT 50.
                   • Rehabilitation Counseling(S): GPA 3.00; GRE 1000(V+Q); MAT 50.
                   • Counselor Education(D): Masters and GPA 3.00; GRE 1000(V+Q); MAT 50; 1 Year work
                     experience.

Enrollment   • Community Counseling(M & S): 14 Admitted yearly; 9 Graduated yearly; 28 Female;
                     8 Male.
                   • School Counseling(M & S): 6 Admitted yearly; 3 Graduated yearly; 11 Female.
                   • Rehabilitation Counseling(M & S): 14 Admitted yearly; 12 Graduated yearly; 17 Female;
                     6 Male.
                   • Counselor Education(D): 9 Admitted yearly; 4 Graduated yearly; 13 Female; 6 Male.

Diversity   • African-American; Asian-American; Caucasian; Hispanic; Multiracial.

Graduation
Requirements   • Community Counseling(M): 60 Class hours; 100 Practicum hours; 600 Internship hours;
                     Comprehensive exam; Portfolio.
                   • Community Counseling(S): 30 Class hours; 300 Internship hours; Portfolio.
                   • School Counseling(M): 48 Class hours; 100 Practicum hours; 600 Internship hours;
                     Comprehensive exam; Portfolio.
                   • School Counseling(S): 30 Class hours; 300 Internship hours; Portfolio.
                   • Rehabilitation Counseling(M): 48 Class hours; 100 Practicum hours; 600 Internship hours;
                     Comprehensive exam; Portfolio.
                   • Rehabilitation Counseling(S): 30 Class hours; 300 Internship hours; Portfolio.
                   • Counselor Education(D): 72 Class hours; 300 Practicum hours; 600 Internship hours;
                     Comprehensive exam; Dissertation.

Postgraduation activity: Advanced education and employment setting percentages.
                   • Community Counseling(M & S): 25 Advanced education; 5 Managed care; 5 Private
                     practice; 70 Agency practice.
                   • School Counseling(M & S): 15 Advanced education; 40 Elementary school; 10 Middle
                     school; 35 Secondary school.
                   • Rehabilitation Counseling(M & S): 5 Advanced education; 10 Managed care; 85 Agency
                     practice.
                   • Counselor Education(D): 5 Managed care; 25 Private practice; 25 Agency practice; 15
                     Secondary school; 10 Student affairs; 20 Other.

Planned Program Modifications

Courses	Drop	Add
	• NP.	• Psychopharmocology.

Other	Decrease	Increase
	• Number of Distance Education Courses	• NP.
	• Number of Off-Campus Courses.	

Related Programs Clinical Social Workers
Marriage and Family Therapists
Psychology
Organizational Behaviorists
Communications

Faculty

nbcc ❧.   Percent of faculty reported with NCC certification: 50%.   ncc ❧

Percent in professional counseling practice: 50%.

Research interests Faculty research interests include counselor development, counselor supervision, ethical/legal aspects of counseling, play therapy, marriage/family counseling.

Diversity   • Caucasian; Multiracial.

Name, Degree, Rank, State/National Credentials, % time devoted to program, email
- Burnham, Joy S; PhD; Assist.; LPC, NCC; >81%; *jburnham@bamaed.ua.edu*
- Carmichael, Karla D; PhD; Assoc.; LPC, NCC, National Registered Play Therapist; >81%; *kcarmich@bamaed.ua.edu*
- Dunn, Patrick L; PhD; Assist.; CRC; >81%; *pdunn@bamaed.ua.edu*
- Satcher, Jamie F; EdD; Full Prof.; CRC; >81%; *jsatcher@bamaed.ua.edu*
- Stephens, Barry N; PhD; Adjunct; LPC, CRC; >81%; *bstephen@bamaed.ua.edu*
- Wilcoxon, S. Allen; EdD; Full Prof.; LPC, NCC, LMFT; >81%; *awilcoxo@bamaed.ua.edu*

Has CHI SIGMA IOTA (International Counseling Society) chapter.

AL: Troy State University

10 McCartha Hall
Troy, AL 36081
USA
Dean   Dr. Donna Jacobs
Administrator   Dr. Dianne Gossett, Dept. Chair
Department   Psychology, Counseling and Foundations of Education
(334) 670-3350, fax (334) 670-3291, dgossett@troyst.edu,
eddean@troyst.edu

Key   See key for Data on Each Department (this section) on page 79.

Program
Accreditation   Regional Accreditation; **CORE:** Rehabilitation Counseling

Uniqueness

Degrees   • Community Counseling: M.
• School Counseling: M.
• Rehabilitation Counseling: M.

Contact   • Community Counseling: M = Jeane Wright.
• School Counseling: M = Dianne Gossett.
• Rehabilitation Counseling: M = Linda Williams.

Admission and Graduation Data
Admission
Requirements   • Community Counseling(M): GPA 2.50; GRE 850; MAT 33; Interview.
• School Counseling(M): GPA 2.50; GRE 850; MAT 33; Interview.
• Rehabilitation Counseling(M): GPA 2.50; GRE 850; MAT 33; Interview.

Enrollment   • Community Counseling(M): 40 Admitted yearly; 45 Graduated yearly.
• School Counseling(M): 15 Admitted yearly; 5 Graduated yearly.
• Rehabilitation Counseling(M): 5 Admitted yearly.

Diversity   • African-American; Caucasian; Hispanic; Multiracial.

Graduation
Requirements   • Community Counseling(M): 48 Class hours; 100 Practicum hours; 600 Internship hours;
Comprehensive exam.
• School Counseling(M): 48 Class hours; 100 Practicum hours; 600 Internship hours;
Comprehensive exam.
• Rehabilitation Counseling(M): 48 Class hours; 100 Practicum hours; 600 Internship hours;
Comprehensive exam.

Postgraduation activity: Advanced education and employment setting percentages.
• Community Counseling(M): NP.
• School Counseling(M): NP.
• Rehabilitation Counseling(M): NP.

Planned Program Modifications
Courses   Drop   Add
• NP.   • NP.

Other   Decrease   Increase
• NP.   • National Accreditation
• Number of Degree Majors
• Number of Distance Education Courses.

Related Programs

Faculty

nbcc ❧   Percent of faculty reported with NCC certification: 60%.   ncc ❧

Percent in professional counseling practice: NP.

Research interests

Diversity   • African-American; Caucasian.

Name, Degree, Rank, State/National Credentials, % time devoted to program, email
• Gossett, Dianne; EdD; LPC, NCC; 61-80%; *dgossett@troyst.edu*
• Wright, Jeanne; PhD; LPC, NCC; >81%; *jwright@troyst.edu*

- Williams, Linda S; PhD; LPC, CRC; >81%; *lindaw@troyst.edu*
- Ritter, Sandra; PhD; NCC; >81%; *shritter@troyst.edu*
- Warren, Fernelle; PhD; <21%; *fwarren@troyst.edu*

Has CHI SIGMA IOTA (International Counseling Society) chapter.

AL: University of Montevallo

Station 6380
Montevallo, AL 35115
USA
Dean   Beth Counce, Interim Dean, College of Education
Administrator   Lee Doebler, Professor, Chair
                    Department   Counseling, Leadership, and Foundations
                                    (205) 665-6380, fax (205) 665-6349, doebler@montevallo.edu,
                                    www.montevallo.edu

Key   See key for Data on Each Department (this section) on page 79.

Program
   Accreditation   Regional Accreditation

   Uniqueness   Program tracks in community counseling, marriage and family counseling, and school
                    counseling allow students to meet academic requirements for licensure and certification in a
                    hands-on, student centered environment.

   Degrees   • Community Counseling: M.
                    • School Counseling: M.
                    • Marriage and Family Counseling: M.

   Contact   • Community Counseling: M = Debbie Grant.
                    • School Counseling: M = Charlotte Daughhetee.
                    • Marriage and Family Counseling: M = Stephanie G. Puleo.

Admission and Graduation Data
Admission
   Requirements   • Community Counseling(M): GPA 2.50; GRE 850; MAT 35; Interview.
                    • School Counseling(M): GPA 2.50; GRE 850; MAT 35; Interview.
                    • Marriage and Family Counseling(M): GPA 2.50; GRE 850; MAT 35; Interview.

   Enrollment   • Community Counseling(M): 20 Admitted yearly; 18 Graduated yearly; 35 Female; 5 Male.
                    • School Counseling(M): 10 Admitted yearly; 9 Graduated yearly; 15 Female; 1 Male.
                    • Marriage and Family Counseling(M): 10 Admitted yearly; 9 Graduated yearly; 20 Female; 4
                      Male.

   Diversity   • African-American; Caucasian; Hispanic; Multiracial; Other.

Graduation
   Requirements   • Community Counseling(M): 48 Class hours; 100 Practicum hours; 600 Internship hours;
                      Comprehensive exam; CPCE; Portfolio.
                    • School Counseling(M): 48 Class hours; 100 Practicum hours; 600 Internship hours;
                      Comprehensive exam; CPCE; Portfolio.
                    • Marriage and Family Counseling(M): 60 Class hours; 100 Practicum hours; 900 Internship
                      hours; CPCE; Portfolio.

   Postgraduation activity: Advanced education and employment setting percentages.
                    • Community Counseling(M): 2 Advanced education; 3 Private practice; 87 Agency practice;
                      3 Other.
                    • School Counseling(M): 2 Advanced education; 30 Elementary school; 34 Middle school; 34
                      Secondary school.
                    • Marriage and Family Counseling(M): NP.

Planned Program Modifications
   Courses   Drop   Add
                    • NP.   • Marriage and Family Counseling.

   Other   Decrease   Increase
                    • NP.   • Course Offerings
                                               • National Accreditation.

Related Programs

Faculty

   nbcc ❖   Percent of faculty reported with NCC certification: 20%.   ncc ❖

   Percent in professional counseling practice: 40%.

   Research interests counselor preparation and professional development

Diversity   •   Caucasian.

Name, Degree, Rank, State/National Credentials, % time devoted to program, email
- Doebler, Lee K; PhD; Full Prof.; 22-40%; *doebler.montevallo.edu*
- Puleo, Stephanie G; PhD; Assoc.; NCC, LMFT; >81%; *puleos@montevallo.edu*
- Thrower, Elizabeth E; PhD; Assoc.; 41-60%; *throwe@montevallo.edu*
- Grant, Debbie D; PhD; Assist.; >81%; *grantdd@montevallo.edu*
- Daughhetee, Charlotte; PhD; Assist.; LPC, LMFT; >81%; *daughh@montevallo.edu*

Has CHI SIGMA IOTA (International Counseling Society) chapter.

AL: University of North Alabama

UNA Box 5107
Florence, AL 35632-0001
USA
Dean   Fred Hattabaugh, College of Education
Administrator   J. Paul Baird, Associate Professor and Coordinator
                    Department   Counselor Education Program
                                    (256) 765-4667, fax (256) 765-4159, pbaird@unanov.una.edu, www.una.edu

Key   See key for Data on Each Department (this section) on page 79.

Program
Accreditation   Regional Accreditation

Uniqueness   Strong emphasis on counseling skills development. Program provides practical support for
                 students/graduates seeking to qualify for licensure by administering Counselor Preparation
                 Comprehensive Examination and National Counselor Examination.

Degrees   • Community Counseling: M.
                 • School Counseling: M.

Contact   • Community Counseling: M = J. Paul Baird.
                 • School Counseling: M = J. Paul Baird.

Admission and Graduation Data
Admission
Requirements   • Community Counseling(M): GPA 3.00; GRE 900; GRE V 450; GRE Q 450; MAT 40;
                   Interview.
                 • School Counseling(M): GPA 3.00; GRE 900; GRE V 450; GRE Q 450; MAT 40; Interview.

Enrollment   • Community Counseling(M): 15 Admitted yearly; 12 Graduated yearly; 33 Female; 7 Male.
                 • School Counseling(M): 15 Admitted yearly; 12 Graduated yearly; 5 Male.

Diversity   • African-American; Asian-American; Caucasian; Native American; Multiracial.

Graduation
Requirements   • Community Counseling(M): 48 Class hours; 100 Practicum hours; 600 Internship hours;
                   Comprehensive exam; CPCE.
                 • School Counseling(M): 48 Class hours; 100 Practicum hours; 600 Internship hours;
                   Comprehensive exam; CPCE.

Postgraduation activity: Advanced education and employment setting percentages.
                 • Community Counseling(M): 30 Managed care; 20 Private practice; 35 Agency practice; 5
                   Secondary school; 5 Student affairs.
                 • School Counseling(M): 5 Advanced education; 40 Elementary school; 20 Middle school; 35
                   Secondary school.

Planned Program Modifications
Courses   Drop   Add
                 • NP.   • NP.

Other   Decrease   Increase
                 • NP.   • NP.

Related Programs

Faculty

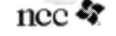   Percent of faculty reported with NCC certification: 67%.

Percent in professional counseling practice: NP.

Research interests Counselor supervision, the role of leisure activities in career development,
                   academic success and failure among college students, advanced empathy skills,
                   the use of popular music and movies in counselor training.

Diversity   • Caucasian.

Name, Degree, Rank, State/National Credentials, % time devoted to program, email
• Baird, J. Paul; PhD; Assoc.; LPC, NCC; >81%; *pbaird@unanov.una.edu*
• Loew, Sandra A; PhD; Assist.; LPC, NCC; >81%; *sloew@unanov.una.edu*
• Pearson, Quinn M; PhD; Assoc.; LPC; >81%; *qpearson@unanov.una.edu*

Has CHI SIGMA IOTA (International Counseling Society) chapter.

AL: University of South Alabama

	UCOM 3700, College of Education
	Mobile, AL 36688-0002
	USA
Dean	Dr. George Uhlig, UCOM 3614
Administrator	Dr. Joseph G. Law, Jr., Program Coordinator, Counseling and Psychometry
	Department Behavioral Studies and Educational Technology
	(251) 380-2861, fax (251) 380-2713, jlaw@usouthal.edu,
	www.southalabama.edu/coe/bset

Key See key for Data on Each Department (this section) on page 79.

Program

Accreditation   Regional Accreditation

Uniqueness   All instructors have doctoral degrees and are active in community service. One professor is president of the state counseling association, another is active on the boards of several human service agencies.

Degrees
- Community Counseling: M.
- School Counseling: M, S.
- Other: M.
- Rehabilitation Counseling: M.

Contact
- Community Counseling: M = Dr. Joseph G. Law, Jr.
- School Counseling: M = Dr. Jean Clark.; S = NP.
- Other: M = Dr. Joe Law for psychometry.
- Rehabilitation Counseling: M = Dr. Joseph G. Law, Jr.

Admission and Graduation Data

Admission

Requirements
- Community Counseling(M): GPA 3.00.
- School Counseling(M): GPA 3.00.
- School Counseling(S): GPA 3.00.
- Other(M): GPA 3.00.
- Rehabilitation Counseling(M): GPA 3.00.

Enrollment
- Community Counseling(M): 23 Admitted yearly; 10 Graduated yearly.
- School Counseling(M & S): 16 Admitted yearly; 9 Graduated yearly.
- Other(M): 12 Admitted yearly; 8 Graduated yearly.
- Rehabilitation Counseling(M): 12 Admitted yearly; 8 Graduated yearly.

Diversity
- Caucasian; Native American; Multiracial.

Graduation

Requirements
- Community Counseling(M): 48 Class hours; 100 Practicum hours; 600 Internship hours; Comprehensive exam.
- School Counseling(M): 39 Class hours; 100 Practicum hours; 300 Internship hours; Comprehensive exam.
- School Counseling(S):
- Other(M): 39 Class hours; 300 Internship hours; Comprehensive exam.
- Rehabilitation Counseling(M): 54 Class hours; 100 Practicum hours; 600 Internship hours; Comprehensive exam.

Postgraduation activity: Advanced education and employment setting percentages.
- Community Counseling(M): NP.
- School Counseling(M & S).
- Other(M): NP.
- Rehabilitation Counseling(M): NP.

Planned Program Modifications

Courses	Drop	Add
	• NP.	• Human Sexuality
		• Supervision.

Other	Decrease	Increase
	• NP.	• Admission Requirements
		• Number of Distance Education Courses
		• Number of On-Line Courses.

Related Programs Psychology
Psychiatric Nurses

Faculty

nbcc   Percent of faculty reported with NCC certification: 80%.   ncc

Percent in professional counseling practice: 60%.

Research interests   Active research is carried out on counseling folks with PTSD, ADHD, learning disabilities and other disorders. One faculty member has published research on the practice of body piercing and another is norming an adult personality test.

Diversity   •   Caucasian; Native American; Multiracial.

Name, Degree, Rank, State/National Credentials, % time devoted to program, email
- Law, Joseph G; EdD; Full Prof.; LPC, NCC, Lic.Psychologist; >81%; *jlaw@usouthal.edu*
- Guest, Charles L; PhD; Assoc.; LPC, NCC; >81%; *cguest@usouthal.edu*
- McIntosh, Irene; PhD; Assoc.; NCC; >81%; *imcintos@usouthal.edu*
- Clark, Jean; PhD; Assoc.; <21%; *jclark@usouthal.edu*
- Millner, Vaughn; PhD; Assist.; LPC, NCC; 41-60%; *vmillner@usouthal.edu*

Has CHI SIGMA IOTA (International Counseling Society) chapter.

AR: University of Arkansas at Little Rock

	2801 S. University Avenue Little Rock, AR 72204 USA
Dean	Angela Sewall, EdD, College of Education
Administrator	Larry R. Dickerson, PhD, Graduate Program Coordinator
	Department Counseling, Adult and Rehabilitation Education (501) 569-3428, fax (501) 569-3547, lrdickerson@ualr.edu, www.teletrain.com/ualr

Key   See key for Data on Each Department (this section) on page 79.

Program

Accreditation   Regional Accreditation, **CORE:** Rehabilitation Counseling

Uniqueness   The 54-semester hour Master of Arts in Rehabilitation Counseling program is completely online and utilizes the latest in asynchronous videostreaming and chromakey technology to create a learning environment comparable to the on-campus class experience.

Degrees   • Rehabilitation Counseling: M.

Contact   • Rehabilitation Counseling: M = Larry R. Dickerson, PhD.

Admission and Graduation Data

Admission

Requirements   • Rehabilitation Counseling(M): GPA 2.75; Interview.

Enrollment   • Rehabilitation Counseling(M): 138 Admitted yearly; 15 Graduated yearly; 97 Female; 41 Male.

Diversity   • African-American; Asian-American; Caucasian; Hispanic; Native American; Multiracial.

Graduation

Requirements   • Rehabilitation Counseling(M): 54 Class hours; 100 Practicum hours; 600 Internship hours.

Postgraduation activity: Advanced education and employment setting percentages.
• Rehabilitation Counseling(M): 10 Advanced education; 10 Private practice; 80 Agency practice.

Planned Program Modifications

Courses	Drop	Add
	• NP.	• Rehabilitation • Wellness.

Other	Decrease	Increase
	• NP.	• Admission Requirements • Course Offerings • Diversity Recruiting of Faculty • Faculty FTE • Financial Aid • Number of Degree Majors • Number of Distance Education Courses • Number of On-Line Courses.

Related Programs Clinical Social Workers
Other

Faculty

 Percent of faculty reported with NCC certification: 22%.

Percent in professional counseling practice: 56%.

Research interests The technology and psychology of Distance Learning; Increasing accessibility of educational materials for persons with disabilities; Techniques for improving collection and utilization of Program Evaluation data.

Diversity   • African-American; Caucasian; Hispanic.

Name, Degree, Rank, State/National Credentials, % time devoted to program, email
• Dickerson, Larry R; PhD; Full Prof.; CRC, Licensed Psychologist; >81%; *lrdickerson@ualr.edu*
• Garner, William E; RhD; Assoc.; LPC, NCC, CRC, CDMS; >81%; *wegarner@ualr.edu*
• Cochran, William A; PhD; Assist.; Licensed Psychologist; 22-40%; *wacjct@comcast.net*
• Harris, Dawn F; EdD; Assist.; LPC, NCC, Licensed Psychologist; <21%; *dfharris60@aol.com*

- Ortega, Raymond; EdD; Assist.; CRC; <21%; *rorte@earthlink.net*
- Wolffe, Karen; PhD; Assist.; <21%; *75254.2250@compuserve.com*
- Croston, Yvonne M; MS; Instructor; <21%; *ymcroston@ualr.edu*
- Hope, Robert C; MS; Instructor; CRC; <21%; *rchope@ualr.edu*
- Smith, Thomas E; EdD; Full Prof.; <21%; *tesmith1@ualr.edu*

AZ: Arizona State University

Payne 302, Mc-0611
Tempe, AZ 85287-0611
USA
Dean   Eugene Garcia, Payne 104
Administrator   Elsie Moore, Division Director
           Department   Psychology in Education
                     (480) 965-3384, fax (480) 965-0300, dpe@asu.edu,
                     http://coe.asu.edu/psyched

Key   See key for Data on Each Department (this section) on page 79.

Program

Accreditation   Regional Accreditation, **CACREP:** Community Counseling

Uniqueness   Nationally ranked master's program in counseling and doctoral program in counseling psychology. Programs focus on multicultural counseling competence.

Degrees
- Community Counseling: M.
- School Counseling: M.
- Other: M.

Contact
- Community Counseling: M = Terence Tracey.
- School Counseling: M = Andrea Dixon Rayle.
- Other: M = NP.

Admission and Graduation Data

Admission

Requirements
- Community Counseling(M): GPA no minima; GRE R; GRE V no minima; GRE Q no minima; GRE A no minima; MAT yes.
- School Counseling(M): GRE R; MAT yes.
- Other(M): NP.

Enrollment
- Community Counseling(M): 50 Admitted yearly; 45 Graduated yearly; 105 Female; 38 Male.
- School Counseling(M): 15 Admitted yearly.
- Other(M): NP.

Diversity
- African-American; Asian-American; Caucasian; Hispanic; Native American; Pacific Islander; Multiracial.

Graduation

Requirements
- Community Counseling(M): 60 Class hours; 100 Practicum hours; 600 Internship hours; Comprehensive exam; CPCE.
- School Counseling(M): 60 Class hours; 100 Practicum hours; 600 Internship hours; Comprehensive exam; CPCE.
- Other(M): NP.

Postgraduation activity: Advanced education and employment setting percentages.
- Community Counseling(M): 15 Advanced education; 25 Managed care; 10 Private practice; 40 Agency practice; 10 Other.
- School Counseling(M): 10 Elementary school; 20 Middle school; 40 Secondary school; 20 Other.
- Other(M): NP.

Planned Program Modifications

Courses	Drop		Add
	• NP.	• NP.	
Other	Decrease		Increase
	• NP.	• NP.	

Related Programs

Faculty

     Percent of faculty reported with NCC certification: **100**%.   ncc

Percent in professional counseling practice: 90%.

Research interests	Multicultural counseling competence assessment and training, ethnic identity, acculturation, school and mental health evaluation, test interpretation, counseling process and outcome, supervision, vocational assessment and development, wellness, mattering and meaning-in-life issues, psychological interventions over the internet, at-risk populations, optimal development, genetic counseling, school counseling, substance abuse, and counselor development.
Diversity	• African-American; Asian-American; Caucasian; Hispanic; Native American.

Name, Degree, Rank, State/National Credentials, % time devoted to program, email
- Arciniega, G. M; PhD; Assoc.; LPC, NCC; 41-60%; *m.arciniega@asu.edu*
- Arredondo, Patricia; PhD; Assoc.; NCC; 41-60%; *empower@asu.edu*
- Claiborn, Charles D; PhD; Full Prof.; NCC, psychol.; 41-60%; *claiborn@asu.edu*
- Glidden-Tracey, Cynthia E; PhD; Assist.; NCC, psychol; 41-60%; *cglidden@asu.edu*
- Homer, Judith; PhD; Assoc.; NCC, psychol; 41-60%; *jhomer@asu.edu*
- Hood, Stafford; PhD; Assoc.; NCC; 41-60%; *stafford.hood@asu.edu*
- Horan, John J; PhD; Full Prof.; NCC, psychol; 41-60%; *horan@asu.edu*
- Kerr, Barbara; PhD; Full Prof.; NCC, psychol; 41-60%; *bkerr@asu.edu*
- Kinnier, Richard T; PhD; Full Prof.; NCC, psychol; 41-60%; *kinnier@asu.edu*
- McWhirter, J. J; PhD; Full Prof.; NCC, psychol; 41-60%; *mcwhirter@asu.edu*
- Robinson Kurpius, Sharon; PhD; Full Prof.; NCC, psychol; 41-60%; *sharon.kurpius@asu.edu*
- Tracey, Terence J; PhD; Full Prof.; NCC, psychol; 41-60%; *ttracey@asu.edu*
- Rayle, Andrea Dixon; PhD; Assist.; NCC; 22-40%; *andrea_dixon.rayle@asu.edu*

AZ: University of Phoenix

4605 East Elwood Street
Phoenix, AZ 85040
USA

Dean   Patrick Romine, Ph.D.
Administrator   Patrick Romine, Ph.D., Dean
                     Department   College of Social andnd Behavioral Sciences
                                     (480) 557-1074, patrick@phoenix.edu

Key   See key for Data on Each Department (this section) on page 79.

Program
Accreditation   Regional Accreditation, **CACREP:** Community Counseling

CACREP

Uniqueness   This is a program for working adults. Courses are at night and on weekends.

Degrees   • Marriage and Family Counseling: M.

Contact   • Marriage and Family Counseling: M = Paul Hagenburger, M.A..

Admission and Graduation Data
Admission
Requirements   • Marriage and Family Counseling(M): GPA 2.50; 2 Years work experience; Interview.

Enrollment   • Marriage and Family Counseling(M): 40 Admitted yearly; 35 Graduated yearly; 110
                   Female; 70 Male.

Diversity   • African-American; Asian-American; Caucasian; Hispanic; Multiracial.

Graduation
Requirements   • Marriage and Family Counseling(M): 54 Class hours; 300 Practicum hours; Portfolio.

Postgraduation activity: Advanced education and employment setting percentages.
                 • Marriage and Family Counseling(M): 25 Advanced education; 20 Managed care; 15 Private
                   practice; 40 Agency practice.

Planned Program Modifications
Courses   Drop   Add
                 • NP.   • NP.

Other   Decrease   Increase
                 • NP.   • Clinical Supervision
                                                   • National Accreditation.

Related Programs Marriage and Family Therapists

Faculty

nbcc   Percent of faculty reported with NCC certification: 0%.   **ncc**

Percent in professional counseling practice: 98%.

Research interests

Diversity   • NP.

Name, Degree, Rank, State/National Credentials, % time devoted to program, email
• Bessel, Jennifer; PhD; Adjunct; <21%; *jlbessel@peoplec.com*
• Billingsly, Galy; PhD; Adjunct; Psychologist; <21%; *dr-gayle@con.net*
• Burns, Kathy; MA; Adjunct; MFT; 41-60%; *kathyburns@cox.net*
• Burt, Barbara; MA; Adjunct; MFT; 22-40%; *bjburt@myexcel.com*
• Buttler, Catherine; MA; Adjunct; 22-40%; *cmbutler@cox.net*
• Gimber, Pilar; MA; Adjunct; MFT; 22-40%; *PilarGimber@yahoo.com*
• Dickinson, Page; MA; Adjunct; MFT; 22-40%; *PEDolphin@aol.com*
• Fisher, Steve; PsyD; Adjunct; Psy.; 22-40%; *stevefisher@earthlink.net*
• Fox, Erik; PhD; Adjunct; Psy; 41-60%; *erikfox@san.rr.com*
• Fox, Patrica; MA; Adjunct; 22-40%; *pattifx@pacbell.net*
• Gazaway, Betty; PsyD; Adjunct; MFT; 41-60%; *bgazaway@san.rr.com*
• George, Patricia; MA; Adjunct; MFT; 22-40%; *mswpat@cox.net*
• Gold, Jerry; PhD; Adjunct; Psy; 41-60%; *gold.jerry@scrippshealth.org*
• Hagenburger, Paul; MA; Full Prof.; MFT; 61-80%; *hagenburger@cox.net*

- Hannibal, Barbara; MA; Adjunct; MFT; 22-40%; *bhannibal@juno.com*
- Lunceford, Lynn; MA; Adjunct; MFT; 61-80%; *lunceford@email.unphx.edu*
- Morrison, Carrie; PhD; Adjunct; MFT; 41-60%; *Doc2Too@aol.com*
- Pascale, Lucile; PhD; Adjunct; Psy; 41-60%; *lpascale@alliant.edu*
- Pruitt, Beverly; MA; Adjunct; MFT; 41-60%; *bpruitt@san.rr.com*
- Simonet, Christopher; PhD; Adjunct; Psy; 41-60%; *chrissimonet@hotmail.com*
- Tedeschi, Gary; PhD; Adjunct; Psy; 41-60%; *gtedeschi@ucsd.edu*

Has CHI SIGMA IOTA (International Counseling Society) chapter.

CA: California Lutheran University

	60 W. Olsen Road
	Thousand Oaks, CA 91360-2787
	United States

Dean

Administrator Gail Uellendahl, Ph.D., Director of Counseling & Guidance Program
Department   School of Education
(805) 493-3420, uellenda@clunet.edu

Key   See key for Data on Each Department (this section) on page 79.

Program

Accreditation   Regional Accreditation

Uniqueness   Highly qualified, professionally active, student-centered faculty. Practitioner oriented programs grounded in theory and supported by research. Small classes provide individualized attention and effective teaching practices.

Degrees   • School Counseling: M.
• Student Affairs: M.

Contact   • School Counseling: M = NP.
• Student Affairs: M = NP.

Admission and Graduation Data

Admission

Requirements   • School Counseling(M): GPA 3.00; GRE 900; Interview.
• Student Affairs(M): GPA 3.00; GRE 900; Interview.

Enrollment   • School Counseling(M): NP.
• Student Affairs(M): NP.

Diversity   • African-American; Asian-American; Caucasian; Hispanic; Native American; Pacific Islander; Multiracial.

Graduation

Requirements   • School Counseling(M): 48 Class hours; 100 Practicum hours; 600 Internship hours; Comprehensive exam; Portfolio.
• Student Affairs(M): 38 Class hours; 150 Practicum hours; 150 Internship hours.

Postgraduation activity: Advanced education and employment setting percentages.
• School Counseling(M): 98 Advanced education; 10 Elementary school; 25 Middle school; 65 Secondary school.
• Student Affairs(M): 80 Advanced education; 100 Other.

Planned Program Modifications

Courses   Drop   Add
• NP.   • NP.

Other   Decrease   Increase
• NP.   • NP.

Related Programs Marriage and Family Therapists

Faculty

nbcc ❖   Percent of faculty reported with NCC certification: 0%.   ncc ❖

Percent in professional counseling practice: 65%.

Research interests School counselors use of assessment, resiliency in students, outcomes of elementary school counseling.

Diversity   • African-American; Asian-American; Caucasian; Hispanic.

Name, Degree, Rank, State/National Credentials, % time devoted to program, email
• Atkinson, Jan; M; Adjunct; <21%;
• Espalin, Charles; EdD; Adjunct; <21%;
• Holder, Linda; Adjunct; PPS; <21%;
• Jew, Cynthia; PhD; Assoc.; >81%;
• Greaves, Kathy; Other; Adjunct; <21%;
• Gorbach, Karen; PhD; Adjunct; <21%;
• Holmboe, David; Other; Adjunct; PPS; <21%;

- Haber, Pauline; Other; Adjunct; PPS; <21%;
- Konantz, James; Other; Adjunct; PPS; <21%;
- Lingens, Hans; EdD; 41-60%;
- Meyers, Cheryl; Other; Adjunct; PPS; <21%;
- Murray-Ward, Mildred; PhD; Assoc.; 41-60%;
- Roth, Richard; Other; Adjunct; <21%; *uellenda@clunet.edu*
- Sheldon, Susan; PhD; Adjunct; <21%;
- Uellendahl, Gail; PhD; Assoc.; >81%;
- Wallace, Valerie; Other; Adjunct; PPS; <21%;
- Wolenik, Rita; EdD; Assist.; PPS; >81%;

CA: California State University-Fresno

5005 N. Maple Avenue, M/S Ed 3
Fresno, CA 93741-8025
United States

Dean Paul Shaker, Kremen School of Ed & Human Development
Administrator Ronald Kiyuna, Chairperson
Department Department of Counseling, Special Ed, & Rehabilitation
(559) 278-0340, fax (559) 278-0045, ronaldK@csufresno.edu,
http://education.csufresno.edu/departments/cse/counsped.html

Key See key for Data on Each Department (this section) on page 79.

Program
Accreditation Regional Accreditation, **CACREP:** Marriage and Family Counseling, **CORE:** Rehabilitation
Counseling

CACREP

Uniqueness Our Counselor Education Programs are noted for their strong emphasis on scholarship and
pratical application.

Degrees
• School Counseling: M.
• Marriage and Family Counseling: M.
• Rehabilitation Counseling: M.
• Student Affairs: M.

Contact
• School Counseling: M = Sarah Lam.
• Marriage and Family Counseling: M = Sari H. Dworkin.
• Rehabilitation Counseling: M = Charles Arokiasamy.
• Student Affairs: M = Sarah Lam.

Admission and Graduation Data
Admission
Requirements
• School Counseling(M): GPA 2.75; Interview.
• Marriage and Family Counseling(M): GPA 2.75; Interview.
• Rehabilitation Counseling(M): GPA 2.75.
• Student Affairs(M): GPA 2.75.

Enrollment
• School Counseling(M): 30 Admitted yearly; 20 Graduated yearly.
• Marriage and Family Counseling(M): 40 Admitted yearly; 30 Graduated yearly.
• Rehabilitation Counseling(M): 15 Admitted yearly; 10 Graduated yearly.
• Student Affairs(M): 20 Admitted yearly; 14 Graduated yearly.

Diversity
• African-American; Asian-American; Caucasian; Hispanic; Native American; Pacific
Islander; Multiracial.

Graduation
Requirements
• School Counseling(M): 48 Class hours; 600 Practicum hours.
• Marriage and Family Counseling(M): 60 Class hours; 80 Practicum hours; 600 Internship
hours.
• Rehabilitation Counseling(M): 60 Class hours.
• Student Affairs(M): NP.

Postgraduation activity: Advanced education and employment setting percentages.
• School Counseling(M): 10 Elementary school; 20 Middle school; 70 Secondary school.
• Marriage and Family Counseling(M): 10 Advanced education; 10 Managed care; 20 Private
practice; 50 Agency practice; 10 Other.
• Rehabilitation Counseling(M): 30 Private practice; 70 Agency practice.
• Student Affairs(M): 100 Other.

Planned Program Modifications
Courses	Drop	Add
	• NP.	• Psychopharmocology.

Other	Increase	Increase
	• NP.	• NP.

Related Programs

Faculty

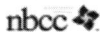 Percent of faculty reported with NCC certification: 40%.

Percent in professional counseling practice: 33%.

Research interests   Dr. Sari H. Dworkin—lesbian, gay, bisexual research and interests; Dr. Ronald Kiyuna—
                       Social Justice, Trauma; Dr. Charles Arokiasamy—Rehab theory, policy, TBI, Substance
                       Abuse; Dr. Chris Lucey—social justice, adolescent depression, suicide; Dr. Claire Sham-
                       Choy—Acadmic & Career self-efficacy; trust in minority/majority student/teacher,
                       counselor dyads; Dr. Diane Gehart—Post Modern Family Therapy Process & Outcome; Dr.
                       Sarah Lam—English Proficiency and Performance of non-native speaker counseling
                       students; Dr. Juan Garcia—Hispanic Institute of Transcultural Psychotherapy; Dr. Dan
                       Smith—Use of Internet in teaching counseling skills, transition from school to agency/
                       private practice counseling

Diversity   • African-American; Asian-American; Caucasian; Hispanic; Other.

Name, Degree, Rank, State/National Credentials, % time devoted to program, email
• Arokiasamy, Charles; PhD; Full Prof.; NCC; >81%; *charles@csufresno.edu*
• Dworkin, Sari H; PhD; Full Prof.; NCC, LMFT, Psych; >81%; *sarid@csufresno.edu*
• Garcia, Juan C; PhD; Full Prof.; LMFT; >81%; *juang@csufresno.com*
• Gehart-Brooks, Diane; PhD; Assist.; LPC, Texas; >81%; *dianeb@csufresno.edu*
• Kiyuna, Ronald S; EdD; Full Prof.; LMFT, Psych; >81%; *ronaldc@scufresno.edu*
• Lucey, Christopher F; PhD; Assist.; LPC, NCC, LMFT; >81%; *clucey@csufresno.edu*
• Smith, Dan H; EdD; Full Prof.; LMFT; >81%; *dans@csufresno.edu*
• Lam, Sarah; EdD; Assist.; LMFT; >81%; *renees@csufresno.edu*
• Degeneffe, Charles; PhD; Assist.; NCC;
• Sham-Choy, Claire; EdD; Assist.; >81%;

Has CHI SIGMA IOTA (International Counseling Society) chapter.

CA: Chapman University

Orange, CA, United States
92866
Dean
Administrator   John Snodgrass, Registar
Department   Transcript Services
(714) 997-6584 or (714) 744-7885, fax (714) 744-7984,
www.chapman.edu

Key   See key for Data on Each Department (this section) on page 79.

Program
Accreditation

Uniqueness   All instructors that I had at the Tucson satellite campus were full-time working professionals.

Degrees   •

Contact   •

Admission and Graduation Data
Admission
Requirements   •

Enrollment   •

Diversity   •   NP.

Graduation
Requirements   •

Postgraduation activity: Advanced education and employment setting percentages.
•

Planned Program Modifications
Courses   Drop   Add
• NP.   • NP.

Other   Decrease   Increase
• NP.   • NP.

Related Programs

Faculty

nbcc   Percent of faculty reported with NCC certification: 0%.   ncc

Percent in professional counseling practice: NP.

Research interests One instructor was President of the Arizona Counselors Association. Another instructor does research with marriage and family issues. Another instructor is doing work with horses in her therapy.

Diversity   •   Caucasian.

Name, Degree, Rank, State/National Credentials, % time devoted to program, email

CA: San Diego State University

3590 Camino del Rio North
San Diego, CA 92108
United States
Dean Lionel Meno, College of Education
Administrator Fred R. McFarlane, Professor and Chairperson
Department Department of Adm, Rehab & Post-Secondary Education
(619) 594-6406, fax (619) 594-4208, fmcfarla@mail.sdsu.edu,
http://www.interwork.sdsu.edu

Key See key for Data on Each Department (this section) on page 79.

Program
Accreditation CORE: Rehabilitation Counseling

Uniqueness Focus on rehabilitation counseling, diversity; specializations in mental health, certificate in
rehabilitation administration. Extensive use of distance education. Over 40% persons with
disabilities and diverse ethnic backgrounds.

Degrees • Rehabilitation Counseling: M.

Contact • Rehabilitation Counseling: M = Fred McFarlane.

Admission and Graduation Data
Admission
Requirements • Rehabilitation Counseling(M): GPA 2.75; GRE 950; Interview.

Enrollment • Rehabilitation Counseling(M): 25 Admitted yearly; 12 Graduated yearly.

Diversity • NP.

Graduation
Requirements • Rehabilitation Counseling(M): 60 Class hours; 9 Practicum hours; 600 Internship hours.

Postgraduation activity: Advanced education and employment setting percentages.
• Rehabilitation Counseling(M): 5 Advanced education; 10 Managed care; 25 Private
practice; 25 Agency practice; 5 Student affairs; 20 Other.

Planned Program Modifications
Courses	Drop		Add
	• NP.	• NP.	

Other	Decrease		Increase
	• NP.	• NP.	

Related Programs NP.

Faculty

nbcc Percent of faculty reported with NCC certification: 0%. ncc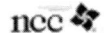

Percent in professional counseling practice: NP.

Research interests Professional development; distance education;assistive technology; deafness employment;
mental health; employment; working with diverse groups.

Diversity • African-American; Asian-American; Caucasian; Hispanic; Native American; Pacific
Islander.

Name, Degree, Rank, State/National Credentials, % time devoted to program, email
• Atkins, Bobbie J; PhD; *batkins@mail.sdsu.edu*
• Jacobs, Ron; PhD; *rjacobs@mail.sdsu.edu*
• McFarlane, Fred R; PhD; *fmfarla@mail.sdsu.edu*
• Sax, Caren; EdD; *csax@mail.sdsu.edu*
• Olney, Marj; PhD; *olney@interwork.sdsu.edu*

CA: San Jose University

One Washington Square
San Jose, CA 95192-0076
United States
Dean   Susan Meyers, 101 Sweeney Hall
Administrator   Xiaolu Hu, Chair
            Department   Department of Counseling Education
                        (408) 924-3668, fax (408) 924-4137, edco@email.sjsu.edu,
                        http://sweeneyhall.sjsu.edu/eld/coed/index.html

Key   See key for Data on Each Department (this section) on page 79.

Program

Accreditation   NP.

Uniqueness   NP.

Degrees
- School Counseling: M.
- Career Counseling: M.
- College Counseling: M.
- Student Affairs: M.

Contact
- School Counseling: M = NP.
- Career Counseling: M = NP.
- College Counseling: M = NP.
- Student Affairs: M = NP.

Admission and Graduation Data

Admission

Requirements
- School Counseling(M): NP.
- Career Counseling(M): NP.
- College Counseling(M): NP.
- Student Affairs(M): NP.

Enrollment
- School Counseling(M): 60 Admitted yearly; 50 Graduated yearly.
- Career Counseling(M): NP.
- College Counseling(M): NP.
- Student Affairs(M): 30 Admitted yearly; 20 Graduated yearly.

Diversity
- NP.

Graduation

Requirements
- School Counseling(M): 48 Class hours; 600 Internship hours; Comprehensive exam; Thesis.
- Career Counseling(M): NP.
- College Counseling(M): NP.
- Student Affairs(M): 48 Class hours; 400 Internship hours; Thesis.

Postgraduation activity: Advanced education and employment setting percentages.
- School Counseling(M): 60 Advanced education; 15 Elementary school; 15 Middle school; 30 Secondary school; 40 Other.
- Career Counseling(M): NP.
- College Counseling(M): 20 Advanced education.
- Student Affairs(M): 20 Advanced education.

Planned Program Modifications

Courses	Drop	Add
	• NP.	• NP.

Other	Decrease	Increase
	• NP.	• Admission Requirements
		• Clinical Supervision
		• Diversity Recruiting of Faculty
		• Diversity Recruiting of Students
		• Faculty FTE
		• Number of Distance Education Courses
		• Number of Off-Campus Courses
		• Number of On-Line Courses.

Related Programs NP.

Faculty

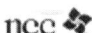 nbcc Percent of faculty reported with NCC certification: 10%. ncc

Percent in professional counseling practice: NP.

Research interests NP.

Diversity • African-American; Asian-American; Caucasian; Native American; Pacific Islander; Multiracial.

Name, Degree, Rank, State/National Credentials, % time devoted to program, email
• Hughey, Andrew R; PhD; Full Prof.; >81%;
• Aptica, Lewis; PhD; Full Prof.; >81%;
• Oliver, Lisa; PhD; Assist.; >81%;
• Hu, Xiaolu; PhD; Full Prof.; NCC; >81%;
• Kelley, Gene; PhD; Assoc.; >81%;
• Saterfield, Harry; PhD; Assoc.; 61-80%;
• Berta, Steve; MA; Lecturer; PPSC; <21%;
• Bender, Donna; MA; Lecturer; 61-80%;
• Sheen, Marion; PhD; Lecturer; >81%;
• Ogimachi, Shawn; MA; Lecturer; 41-60%;

CA: School of Education, La Sierra University

Riverside, CA 92515
USA
Dean   Norman Powell, School of Education
Administrator   Lennard A. Jorgensen, Chair
        Department   School Psychology and Counseling
                (909) 785-2267, fax (909) 785-2205, ljorgens@lasierra.edu

Key   See key for Data on Each Department (this section) on page 79.

Program
Accreditation   NP.

Uniqueness   Our program is small, thus very personal. While we are a private Christian university, we accept all religious affiliations. Currently we have Protestants, Catholics, Hindu, and Muslim students (Very Multicultural).

Degrees   • School Counseling: M, S.

Contact   • School Counseling: M, S = Lennard A. Jorgensen.

Admission and Graduation Data
Admission
Requirements   • School Counseling(M): GPA 3.0; GRE 1000; GRE V 500; GRE Q 500; GRE A 500; Interview.
              • School Counseling(S): GPA 3.0; GRE 1000; GRE V 500; GRE Q 500; GRE A 500; Interview.

Enrollment   • School Counseling(M & S): 20 Admitted yearly; 10 Graduated yearly; 5 Male.

Diversity   • African-American; Asian-American; Caucasian; Hispanic; Multiracial.

Graduation
Requirements   • School Counseling(M): 450 Practicum hours; Comprehensive exam; Portfolio.
              • School Counseling(S): 500 Practicum hours; 1200 Internship hours; Comprehensive exam; Portfolio.

Postgraduation activity: Advanced education and employment setting percentages.
              • School Counseling(M & S): 33.3 Elementary school; 33.3 Middle school; 33.3 Secondary school.

Planned Program Modifications
Courses	Drop		Add
	• NP.		• Abuse of Individual.

Other	Decrease		Increase
	• NP.		• NP.

Related Programs

Faculty

   Percent of faculty reported with NCC certification: 33%.   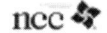

Percent in professional counseling practice: NP.

Research interests Social policy, psychopathology, mental retardation, human sexuality, and technology used to teach counseling

Diversity   • Asian-American; Caucasian; Multiracial.

Name, Degree, Rank, State/National Credentials, % time devoted to program, email
• Ji, Chang-ho; PhD; Assoc.; statistics; 22-40%; *cji@lasierra.edu*
• Clarke-Pine, Dora; PhD; Assoc.; >81%; *dclarke@lasierra.edu*
• Jorgensen, Lennard A; PhD; Assoc.; NCC, school counseling/psychology/licensed clinical psyhologist; >81%; *ljorgens@lasierra.edu*

CA: University of San Diego, School of Education

5998 ALcala Park
San Diego, CA 92110-2492
US
Dean   Dean Paula Cordeiro, School of Education
Administrator Lonnie Rowell, Program Director
                   Department   Counseling Program(
                                   619) 260-7441, fax (619) 260-6826, lrowell@sandiego.edu,
                                   http://www.acusd.edu/soe/programs/counselng/

Key   See key for Data on Each Department (this section) on page 79.

Program
  Accreditation

    Uniqueness   M.A. in Counseling with specializations in school, college and career. Program offers study
                   abroad classes arranged around international counseling conference. San Diego provides
                   multicultural opportunities at internship sites. Students get involved in local, state and
                   national professional associations.

    Degrees   • School Counseling: M.
                   • Career Counseling: M.
                   • Other: M.

    Contact   • School Counseling: M = Lonnie Rowell.
                   • Career Counseling: M = Susan Zgliczynski.
                   • Other: M = Ken Gonzalez - College.

Admission and Graduation Data
Admission
    Requirements   • School Counseling(M): GPA 2.75; 1 Year work experience; Interview.
                   • Career Counseling(M): GPA 2.75; 1 Year work experience; Interview.
                   • Other(M): GPA 2.75; 1 Year work experience; Interview.

    Enrollment   • School Counseling(M): 25 Admitted yearly; 25 Graduated yearly; 10 Male.
                   • Career Counseling(M): 15 Admitted yearly; 10 Graduated yearly; 16 Female; 2 Male.
                   • Other(M): 15 Admitted yearly; 12 Graduated yearly; 15 Female; 5 Male.

    Diversity   • African-American; Asian-American; Caucasian; Hispanic; Native American; Pacific
                   Islander; Multiracial.

Graduation
    Requirements   • School Counseling(M): 48 Class hours; 100 Practicum hours; 600 Internship hours;
                   Comprehensive exam.
                   • Career Counseling(M): 48 Class hours; 100 Practicum hours; 600 Internship hours;
                   Comprehensive exam.
                   • Other(M): 48 Class hours; 100 Practicum hours; 600 Internship hours; Comprehensive
                   exam.

  Postgraduation activity: Advanced education and employment setting percentages.
                   • School Counseling(M): 10 Agency practice; 25 Elementary school; 25 Middle school; 40
                   Secondary school.
                   • Career Counseling(M): 10 Advanced education; 10 Private practice; 20 Agency practice;
                   30 Student affairs; 30 Business Other.
                   • Other(M): 10 Advanced education; 20 Agency practice; 70 Student affairs.

Planned Program Modifications

Courses	Drop	Add
	• NP.	• Advocacy
		• Consultation
		• Supervision.

Other	Decrease	Increase
	• Faculty FTE	• Course Offerings
	• Number of Degree Majors.	• Clinical Supervision
		• National Accreditation
		• Number of On-Line Courses.

Related Programs Marriage and Family Therapists
                   Communications
                   International Studies

Faculty

nbcc ❧   Percent of faculty reported with NCC certification: 25%.   ncc ❧

Percent in professional counseling practice: NP.

Research interests Research interests of faculty include school violence prevention, success of first generation college students, multicultural assessment issues, global cultural competence and use of online learning in preparing counselors.

Diversity   •   African-American; Asian-American; Caucasian; Hispanic; Multiracial.

Name, Degree, Rank, State/National Credentials, % time devoted to program, email
• Rowell, Lonnie L; PhD; Assoc.; >81%;
• Johnson, Ronn; PhD; Assoc.; >81%;
• Zgliczynski, Susan M; PhD; Assoc.; NCC, RPCC - CA; >81%;
• Gonzalez, Kenneth; PhD; Assist.; >81%;

Has CHI SIGMA IOTA (International Counseling Society) chapter.

CO: Adams State College

208 Edgemont Blvd.
Alamosa, CO 81102
USA

Dean   Dr. Don Basse, School of Education and Graduate Studies
Administrator Susan Varhely, PhD, LPC, Program Coordinator
                  Department   Psychology & Counselor Education
                  (719) 587-7626, fax (719) 587-8421, ascpsych@adams.edu,
                  http://counselored.adams.edu

Key   See key for Data on Each Department (this section) on page 79.

Program

Accreditation   Regional Accreditation, **CACREP:** Community Counseling, **CACREP:** School Counseling

Uniqueness   A hands-on, involved faculty. Unique distance program with full-time faculty teaching most of the courses.

Degrees   • Community Counseling: M.
              • School Counseling: M.

Contact   • Community Counseling: M = Dr. Susan Varhely.
              • School Counseling: M = Dr. Susan Varhely.

Admission and Graduation Data

Admission
Requirements • Community Counseling(M): GPA 2.75; GRE 1250; GRE V NA; GRE Q NA; GRE A NA; MAT 37.
              • School Counseling(M): GPA 2.75; GRE 1250; GRE V NA; GRE Q NA; GRE A NA; MAT 37.

Enrollment   • Community Counseling(M): 60 Admitted yearly; 58 Graduated yearly; 58 Female; 24 Male.
              • School Counseling(M): 60 Admitted yearly; 58 Graduated yearly; 7 Male.

Diversity   • African-American; Asian-American; Caucasian; Hispanic; Native American; Pacific Islander; Multiracial.

Graduation
Requirements • Community Counseling(M): 60 Class hours; 100 Practicum hours; 600 Internship hours; Comprehensive exam.
              • School Counseling(M): 60 Class hours; 100 Practicum hours; 600 Internship hours; Comprehensive exam.

Postgraduation activity: Advanced education and employment setting percentages.
              • Community Counseling(M): 66 Agency practice; 5 Elementary school; 5 Middle school; 10 Secondary school; 10 Other.
              • School Counseling(M): NP.

Planned Program Modifications

Courses   Drop   Add
                    • NP.   • Crisis/Violence Counseling.

Other   Decrease   Increase
                    • NP.   • Diversity Recruiting of Faculty
                                                   • Diversity Recruiting of Students
                                                   • Number of Distance Education Courses
                                                   • Number of Off-Campus Courses
                                                   • Number of On-Line Courses.

Related Programs

Faculty

nbcc   Percent of faculty reported with NCC certification: 50%.   ncc

Percent in professional counseling practice: 33%.

Research interests Outcome research, trauma, play therapy, spirituality, counselor education issues.

Diversity   • Caucasian; Hispanic.

Name, Degree, Rank, State/National Credentials, % time devoted to program, email
- Calhoun, Ken A; PhD; Assist.; LPC, NCC; >81%; *kacalhou@adams.edu*
- Filer, Rex D; PhD; Full Prof.; LPC, Licensed Counseling Psychologist; >81%; *rdfiler@adams.edu*
- Manzanares, Mark G; ABD; Assist.; >81%; *mgmanzan@adams.edu*
- McCartney, Teri J; PhD; Assoc.; LPC, NCC; >81%; *tjmccart@adams.edu*
- O'Halloran, Theresa M; PhD; Assoc.; LPC, NCC; >81%; *tmohallo@adams.edu*
- Varhely, Susan C; PhD; Full Prof.; LPC; >81%; *scvarhel@adams.edu*

Has CHI SIGMA IOTA (International Counseling Society) chapter.

CO: Denver Seminary

	P.O. Box 100,000 Denver, CO 80250-0100 USA
Dean	Dr. Randy MacFarland
Administrator	Dr. James R. Beck, Counseling Division Chair
	Department Counseling Division
	(303) 762-6954, fax (303) 762-6976, Jim.Beck@DenverSeminary.edu, www.denverseminary.edu

Key   See key for Data on Each Department (this section) on page 79.

Program

Accreditation	Regional Accreditation, **CACREP:** Community Counseling

CACREP

Uniqueness	The seminary context in which this program is located gives students an opportunity to integrate their professional counseling skills with Christianity.

Degrees	• Community Counseling: M. • Marriage and Family Counseling: DMin. • Other: M. • Pastoral Counseling: M.

Contact	• Community Counseling: M = James R. Beck. • Marriage and Family Counseling: D = NP. • Other: M = NP. • Pastoral Counseling: M = NP.

Admission and Graduation Data

Admission

Requirements	• Community Counseling(M): GPA 3.00. • Marriage and Family Counseling(D): NP. • Other(M): GPA 2.50. • Pastoral Counseling(M): GPA 2.50.

Enrollment	• Community Counseling(M): 75 Admitted yearly; 50 Graduated yearly; 60% Female; 40% Male. • Marriage and Family Counseling(D): NP. • Other(M): 15 Admitted yearly; 10 Graduated yearly; 60% Female; 40% Male. • Pastoral Counseling(M): 10 Admitted yearly; 5 Graduated yearly; 100% Male.

Diversity	• African-American; Asian-American; Caucasian; Hispanic; Native American; Multiracial.

Graduation

Requirements	• Community Counseling(M): 62 Class hours; 125 Practicum hours; 600 Internship hours. • Marriage and Family Counseling(D): NP. • Other(M): 62 Class hours; 400 Internship hours; Comprehensive exam. • Pastoral Counseling(M): 92 Class hours; 400 Internship hours; Oral exam.

Postgraduation activity: Advanced education and employment setting percentages.
- Community Counseling(M): 50 Private practice; 40 Agency practice; 5 Other.
- Marriage and Family Counseling(D):
- Other(M): 50 Private practice; 50 Other.
- Pastoral Counseling(M): 5 Advanced education; 95 Other.

Planned Program Modifications

Courses	Drop	Add
	• NP.	• NP.

Other	Decrease	Increase
	• NP.	• Faculty FTE • Financial Aid • Number of Degree Majors • Number of Distance Education Courses.

Related Programs

Faculty

 Percent of faculty reported with NCC certification: 40%.   ncc ❖

Percent in professional counseling practice: 80%.

Research interests Victim assistance; cross-cultural issues in supervision; brief therapy; personality theory and the Christian Scriptures.

Diversity   • Caucasian; Hispanic; Native American.

Name, Degree, Rank, State/National Credentials, % time devoted to program, email
* Beck, James R; PhD; Full Prof.; NCC, Psychologist; >81%; *jim.beck@denverseminary.edu*
* Winfrey, Joan; PhD; Full Prof.; psychologist; >81%; *Joan.Winfrey@denverseminary.edu*
* Cappa, Steve; PsyD; Assist.; >81%; *Steve.Cappa@denverseminary.edu*
* Suarez, Elisabeth; PhD; Assist.; LPC, NCC; >81%; *elisabeth.suarez@denverseminary.edu*
* McCormack, Janet; MDiv; Instructor; Board Certified Chaplain; 61-80%; *janMcCormack@denverseminary.edu*

CO: University of Colorado at Colorado Springs

Dean
Administrator

PO Box 7150   1420 Austin Bluffs Pkwy
Colorado Springs, CO
Dean David Nelson
Beverly Snyder, Department Chair
Department   Counseling and Leadership
(719) 262-4120, fax (719) 262-4110, bevsnyder@uccs.edu,
uccs.edu/Academics

Key   See key for Data on Each Department (this section) on page 79.

Program
Accreditation   Regional Accreditation, **CACREP:** Community Counseling, **CACREP:** School Counseling

CACREP

Uniqueness   Strong emphasis on personal growth through three 2 hour labs taken each of the first three
semesters. Opportunity to specialize in Play therapy, Hypnotherapy, Experiential Education or
Reality Therapy/Choice Theory. Transpersonal approaches to counselor development.
Program also offers a master's degree in Leadership in Counseling.

Degrees
- Community Counseling: M.
- School Counseling: M.
- Student Affairs: M.
- Other: M.

Contact
- Community Counseling: M = Beverly Snyder.
- School Counseling: M = Donna Kelsch.
- Student Affairs: M = Beverly Snyder.
- Other: M = David Fenell.

Admission and Graduation Data
Admission
Requirements
- Community Counseling(M): GPA 2.50; 3 Years work experience; Interview.
- School Counseling(M): GPA 2.75; Interview.
- Student Affairs(M): GPA 2.75; Interview.
- Other(M): GPA 2.75; Interview.

Enrollment
- Community Counseling(M): 20 Admitted yearly; 15 Graduated yearly; 10 Female; 5 Male.
- School Counseling(M): 40 Admitted yearly; 35 Graduated yearly; 10 Male.
- Student Affairs(M): 5 Admitted yearly; 5 Graduated yearly; 3 Female; 2 Male.
- Other(M): 20 Admitted yearly; 20 Graduated yearly.

Diversity
- African-American; Asian-American; Caucasian; Hispanic; Native American; Pacific
Islander; Multiracial.

Graduation
Requirements
- Community Counseling(M): 49 Class hours; 100 Practicum hours; 600 Internship hours;
Comprehensive exam; Portfolio.
- School Counseling(M): 49 Class hours; 100 Practicum hours; 600 Internship hours;
Comprehensive exam; Portfolio.
- Student Affairs(M): 49 Class hours; 100 Practicum hours; 600 Internship hours;
Comprehensive exam; Portfolio.
- Other(M): 40 Class hours.

Postgraduation activity: Advanced education and employment setting percentages.
- Community Counseling(M): NP.
- School Counseling(M): NP.
- Student Affairs(M): NP.
- Other(M): NP.

Planned Program Modifications
Courses   Drop   Add
- NP.   - NP.

Other   Decrease   Increase
- NP.   - NP.

Related Programs Psychology
Psychiatric Nurses
Communications

Faculty

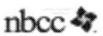 Percent of faculty reported with NCC certification: **100**%.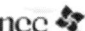

Percent in professional counseling practice: NP.

Research interests Retention of college students, particularly diverse populations.School counseling: Standards based comprehensive developmental approach.Marriage and family issues. Sexual harassment among school children.Bullying and conflict resolution.

Diversity • African-American; Caucasian; Hispanic.

Name, Degree, Rank, State/National Credentials, % time devoted to program, email
• Snyder, Beverly A; EdD; Assoc.; LPC, NCC, lmhc; >81%; *bsnyder@uccs.edu*
• Fenell, David; PhD; Full Prof.; NCC, Psych; >81%; *fenelld@soc.mil*
• Kelsch, Donna; EdD; Assist.; LPC, NCC, Schl Psych; >81%; *dkelsch@uccs.edu*
• Williams, Rhonda; EdD; Assist.; LPC, NCC; >81%; *rwilliam@!uccs.edu*

Has CHI SIGMA IOTA (International Counseling Society) chapter.

CO: University of Colorado at Denver

CB 106, PO Box 173364
Denver, CO 80217-3364
USA
Dean   Lynn Rhodes
Administrator   Marsha Wiggins Frame, Associate Professor and Chair
                      Department   Counseling Psychology & Counselor Education
                                      (303) 556-8367, fax (303) 556-4479, Jane_Lipscomb@ceo.cudenver.edu,
                                      http://soe.cudenver.edu

Key   See key for Data on Each Department (this section) on page 79.

Program
    Accreditation   Regional Accreditation, **CACREP:** Community Counseling, **CACREP:** Marriage and Family
                     Counseling, **CACREP:** School Counseling

    Uniqueness   We have a strong focus on multiculturalism and diversity. We have a highly diverse faculty.

    Degrees   • Community Counseling: M.
                     • School Counseling: M.
                     • Career Counseling: M.
                     • Marriage and Family Counseling: M.

    Contact   • Community Counseling: M = Andrew Helwig.
                     • School Counseling: M = Joseph Lasky.
                     • Career Counseling: M = Andrew Helwig.
                     • Marriage and Family Counseling: M = Marsha Wiggins Frame.

Admission and Graduation Data
Admission
    Requirements   • Community Counseling(M): GPA 2.75; GRE 900; MAT 40; Interview.
                     • School Counseling(M): GPA 2.75; GRE 900; MAT 40; Interview.
                     • Career Counseling(M): GPA 2.75; GRE 900; MAT 40; Interview.
                     • Marriage and Family Counseling(M): GPA 2.75; GRE 900; MAT 40; Interview.

    Enrollment   • Community Counseling(M): 25 Admitted yearly; 25 Graduated yearly; 160 Female;
                       40 Male.
                     • School Counseling(M): 45 Admitted yearly; 40 Graduated yearly.
                     • Career Counseling(M): 5 Admitted yearly.
                     • Marriage and Family Counseling(M): 50 Admitted yearly; 40 Graduated yearly.

    Diversity   • African-American; Asian-American; Caucasian; Hispanic; Native American; Multiracial.

Graduation
    Requirements   • Community Counseling(M): 60 Class hours; 150 Practicum hours; 600 Internship hours;
                       Comprehensive exam.
                     • School Counseling(M): 60 Class hours; 150 Practicum hours; 600 Internship hours;
                       Comprehensive exam.
                     • Career Counseling(M): 60 Class hours; 150 Practicum hours; 600 Internship hours; CPCE;
                       Oral exam.
                     • Marriage and Family Counseling(M): 63 Class hours; 150 Practicum hours; 600 Internship
                       hours.

    Postgraduation activity: Advanced education and employment setting percentages.
                     • Community Counseling(M): NP.
                     • School Counseling(M): NP.
                     • Career Counseling(M): NP.
                     • Marriage and Family Counseling(M): NP.

Planned Program Modifications
    Courses   Drop   Add
                     • NP.   • NP.

    Other   Decrease   Increase
                     • NP.   • Diversity Recruiting of Faculty
                                                              • Diversity Recruiting of Students
                                                              • Number of Distance Education Courses
                                                              • Number of On-Line Courses.

Related Programs Communications

Faculty

nbcc Percent of faculty reported with NCC certification: 40%. ncc

Percent in professional counseling practice: 10%.

Research interests Many faculty are involved in research regarding culture and diversity. One is interested in spirituality and counseling. Another focuses on career development.

Diversity • African-American; Caucasian; Hispanic; Native American.

Name, Degree, Rank, State/National Credentials, % time devoted to program, email
- Byers, Steven R; PhD; Assist.; >81%; *Steve_Byers@ceo.cudenver.edu*
- Helwig, Andrew A; PhD; Full Prof.; LPC, NCC; >81%; *Andrew_Helwig@ceo.cudenver.edu*
- Frame, Marsha Wiggins; PhD; Assoc.; LPC, NCC, LMFT; >81%; *mframe@ceo.cudenver.edu*
- Estrada, Diane; PhD; Assist.; NCC, LMFT; >81%; *Diane_Estrada@ceo.cudenver.edu*
- Rutter, Philip A; PhD; Assist.; Licensed Psychologist; >81%; *Phil_Rutter@ceo.cudenver.edu*
- Williams, Carmen Braun; PhD; Assoc.; Licensed Psychologist; >81%; *carmen_williams@ceo.cudenver.edu*
- Harding, Susan S; PhD; Instructor; LPC, Licensed Psychologist; >81%; *susan_harding@ceo.cudenver.edu*
- Lasky, Joseph F; EdD; Assist.; LPC; 41-60%; *Joe_Lasky@ceo.cudenver.edu*
- Larsen, Patricia A; PsyD; Instructor; Licensed Psychologist; >81%; *Pat_Larsen@ceo.cudenver.edu*
- Goalstone, Janet; PhD; Instructor; LPC, NCC; 22-40%; *Janet_Goalstone@ceo.cudenver.edu*

Has CHI SIGMA IOTA (International Counseling Society) chapter.

CO: University of Northern Colorado

McKee 248; Box 131
Greeley, CO 80639
USA

Dean   Eugene Sheehan; College of Education
Administrator Tracy Baldo, Professor and Coordinator of Counselor Education Programs
                  Department   Professional Psychology
                                 (970) 351-2731, fax (970) 351-2625, tammy.alexander@unco.edu,
                                 www.unco.edu/coe/ppsy

Key   See key for Data on Each Department (this section) on page 79.

Program

Accreditation   Regional Accreditation, **CACREP:** Community Counseling, **CACREP:** Counselor Education
                  and Supervision, **CACREP:** Marriage and Family Counseling, **CACREP:** School Counseling

Uniqueness   Our programs have a strong clinical focus. Our graduates leave as strong clinicians. The
                  faculty and students form collegial professional relationships.

Degrees   • Community Counseling: M.
                  • School Counseling: M.
                  • Marriage and Family Counseling: M.
                  • Counselor Education: PhD.

Contact   • Community Counseling: M = Basilia Softas-Nall.
                  • School Counseling: M = Linda Black.
                  • Marriage and Family Counseling: M = William Walsh.
                  • Counselor Education: D = Tracy Baldo.

Admission and Graduation Data

Admission

Requirements   • Community Counseling(M): GPA 3.00; Interview.
                  • School Counseling(M): GPA 3.00; Interview.
                  • Marriage and Family Counseling(M): GPA 3.00; Interview.
                  • Counselor Education(D): Masters and GPA 3.25; GRE 1000; GRE V 500; GRE Q 500;
                    GRE W 3.5.

Enrollment   • Community Counseling(M): 50 Admitted yearly; 48 Graduated yearly; 38 Female; 12 Male.
                  • School Counseling(M): 25 Admitted yearly; 22 Graduated yearly; 17 Female; 8 Male.
                  • Marriage and Family Counseling(M): 25 Admitted yearly; 23 Graduated yearly; 17 Female;
                    8 Male.
                  • Counselor Education(D): 6 Admitted yearly; 6 Graduated yearly; 13 Female; 5 Male.

Diversity   • African-American; Asian-American; Caucasian; Hispanic; Native American; Pacific
                    Islander; Multiracial.

Graduation

Requirements   • Community Counseling(M): 60 Class hours; 340 Practicum hours; 600 Internship hours;
                    Comprehensive exam.
                  • School Counseling(M): 57 Class hours; 340 Practicum hours; 600 Internship hours;
                    Comprehensive exam.
                  • Marriage and Family Counseling(M): 66 Class hours; 468 Practicum hours; 600 Internship
                    hours.
                  • Counselor Education(D): 89 Class hours; 1270+ Practicum hours; 1200 Internship hours;
                    Comprehensive exam; Oral exam; Dissertation.

Postgraduation activity: Advanced education and employment setting percentages.
                  • Community Counseling(M): 20 Advanced education; 10 Managed care; 15 Private practice;
                    50 Agency practice; 5 Other.
                  • School Counseling(M): 15 Advanced education; 15 Elementary school; 30 Middle school;
                    40 Secondary school.
                  • Marriage and Family Counseling(M): 25 Advanced education; 10 Managed care; 20 Private
                    practice; 45 Agency practice.
                  • Counselor Education(D): 30 Private practice; 70 Other.

Planned Program Modifications

Courses   Drop   Add
                  • NP.   • Career/Life Planning
                                               • Consultation
                                               • Crisis/Violence Counseling.

Other   Decrease   Increase
                         • NP.   • Diversity Recruiting of Faculty
                                                           • Diversity Recruiting of Students
                                                           • Number of Off-Campus Courses.

Related Programs Psychology
                   Other

Faculty

nbcc 💠   Percent of faculty reported with NCC certification: 43%.   ncc 💠

Percent in professional counseling practice: 40%.

Research interests White Privilege; Counselor Education and Supervision; Women's issues; Adolescent
                  issues

Diversity   • Caucasian; Hispanic; Native American.

Name, Degree, Rank, State/National Credentials, % time devoted to program, email
• Athanasiou, Michelle; PhD; Assoc.; <21%; *michelle.athanasiou@unco.edu*
• Baldo, Tracy; PhD; Full Prof.; LPC, NCC; >81%; *tracy.baldo@unco.edu*
• Bardos, Achilles; PhD; Full Prof.; <21%; *achilles.bardos@unco.edu*
• Black, Linda; EdD; Assist.; LPC, NCC; >81%; *linda.black@unco.edu*
• Copeland, Ellis; PhD; Full Prof.; <21%; *ellis.copeland@unco.edu*
• D'Amato, Rik; PhD; Full Prof.; <21%; *rik.damato@unco.edu*
• Gonzalez, David; PhD; Full Prof.; <21%; *david.gonzalez@unco.edu*
• Crepeau-Hobson, Franci; PhD; Assist.; <21%; *franci.crepeau-hobson@unco.edu*
• Johnson, Brian; PhD; Assoc.; 22-40%; *brian.johnson@unco.edu*
• Magnuson, Sandy; EdD; Assoc.; LPC, NCC; >81%; *sandy.magnuson@unco.edu*
• O'Halloran, Sean; PhD; Full Prof.; 22-40%; *sian.ohalloran@hotmail.com*
• Shaw, Sarah; EdD; Full Prof.; NCC; >81%; *sarah.shaw@unco.edu*
• Softas-Nall, Basilia; PhD; Full Prof.; NCC; >81%; *basilia.softas-nall@unco.edu*
• Walsh, William; PhD; Full Prof.; NCC; >81%; *william.walsh@unco.edu*

Has CHI SIGMA IOTA (International Counseling Society) chapter.

CO: University of Phoenix

5475 Tech Center Drive
Colorado Springs, CO 80919
Dean   Patrick Romine, located in Phoenix, Az.
Administrator Linda Roan, College Campus Chair
Department   Health and Human Services
(719) 599-5282, fax (719) 599-7973, John.West@phoenix.edu,
Patrick.Romine@phoenix.edu

Key   See key for Data on Each Department (this section) on page 79.

Program
Accreditation   Regional Accreditation

Uniqueness   The schedule and academic climate are designed for the adult learner. Full-time students
attend class one night a week, accompanied by a flexible study group session each week.

Degrees   • Community Counseling: M.
• School Counseling: M.

Contact   • Community Counseling: M = John West.
• School Counseling: M = John West.

Admission and Graduation Data
Admission
Requirements   • Community Counseling(M): GPA 2.50; 3 Years work experience; Interview.
• School Counseling(M): GPA 2.50; 3 Years work experience; Interview.

Enrollment   • Community Counseling(M): 30 Admitted yearly; 30 Female; 15 Male.
• School Counseling(M): NP.

Diversity   • African-American; Asian-American; Caucasian; Hispanic; Native American; Multiracial.

Graduation
Requirements   • Community Counseling(M): 51 Class hours; 100 Practicum hours; 600 Internship hours;
Portfolio.
• School Counseling(M): 49 Class hours; 600 Internship hours; Portfolio.

Postgraduation activity: Advanced education and employment setting percentages.
• Community Counseling(M): NP.
• School Counseling(M): NP.

Planned Program Modifications
Courses   Drop   Add
• NP.   • NP.

Other   Decrease   Increase
• NP.   • Diversity Recruiting of Faculty
• Diversity Recruiting of Students
• National Accreditation.

Related Programs Organizational Beaviorists

Faculty

nbcc ❖   Percent of faculty reported with NCC certification: 0%.   ncc ❖

Percent in professional counseling practice: 100%.

Research interests Mediation; Teenage violence; Addictions(various populations); Child abuse

Diversity   • Caucasian; Hispanic; Multiracial.

Name, Degree, Rank, State/National Credentials, % time devoted to program, email
• Duffin, Dennis; D; Instructor; 41-60%; *dduffin@email.uophx.edu*
• Wood, Meredith; M; Instructor; LPC, also holds second masters and certification in school psychology;
<21%; *mwoods@email.uophx.edu*
• Jones, Terry; D; Instructor; licensed psychiatrist; <21%; *tjones@email.uophx.edu*
• Sellers, Mark; M; Instructor; LPC, also holds masters of school psycology; <21%;
msellers@email.uophx.edu

CT: Saint Joseph College

	1678 Asylum Avenue
	West Hartford, CT 06117
Dean	Dr. Clark Hendley
Administrator	Richard W. Halstead, Ph.D., Chair
	Department Counselor Education
	(860) 231-5333, fax (860) 231-5774, rhalstead@sjc.edu,
	www.sjc.edu/counseloreducation

Key   See key for Data on Each Department (this section) on page 79.

Program

Accreditation   Regional Accreditation

Uniqueness   The Counselor Education Department offers degrees in Community Counseling and a degree in School Counseling where students may, if they choose to, specialize in tracks in child welfare or pastoral counseling. All programs within the masters degree offer education and training based on a competency based outcome model.

Degrees
- Community Counseling: M.
- School Counseling: M.

Contact
- Community Counseling: M = Richard W. Halstead, Ph.D.
- School Counseling: M = NP.

Admission and Graduation Data

Admission

Requirements
- Community Counseling(M): MAT R; Interview.
- School Counseling (M): Interviews.

Enrollment
- Community Counseling(M): 24 Admitted yearly; 18 Graduated yearly; 90 Female; 10 Male.
- School Counseling (M): NP.

Diversity
- African-American; Asian-American; Caucasian; Hispanic; Multiracial.

Graduation

Requirements
- Community Counseling(M): 48 Class hours; 100 Practicum hours; 600 Internship hours; Comprehensive exam; Portfolio.
- School Counseling (M): 48 Class hours.

Postgraduation activity: Advanced education and employment setting percentages.
- Community Counseling(M): 10 Managed care; 5 Private practice; 84 Agency practice.
- School Counseling (M): NP.

Planned Program Modifications

Courses	Drop	Add
	• NP.	

Other	Decrease	Increase
	• NP.	• Diversity Recruiting of Students.

Related Programs Marriage and Family Therapists

Faculty

nbcc ❧   Percent of faculty reported with NCC certification: 12%.   ncc ❧

Percent in professional counseling practice: NP.

Research interests Mulitcultural counseling and supervision, spiritual care in counseling, spiritual assessment, schema focused assessment of client core issues in counseling and clinical supervision

Diversity
- African-American; Caucasian.

Name, Degree, Rank, State/National Credentials, % time devoted to program, email
- Halstead, Richard; PhD; Assoc.; LPC, NCC; >81%; *rhalstead@sjc.edu*
- Durham, Judie; PhD; Assist.; LPC; >81%; *jdurham@sjc.edu*
- Topper, Charlie; EdD; Assoc.; LPC; >81%; *ctopper@sjc.edu*
- Totah, Norma; MSW; Instructor; MSW; 22-40%;
- Emswiler, Jim; MA; Instructor; LPC; 22-40%;
- Kennedy, Stan; PhD; Instructor; 22-40%;
- Berne, Pat; PhD; Instructor; Psych.; 22-40%;
- Savory, Lou; PhD; Instructor; Psych; 22-40%;

DC: The George Washington University

2134 G Street, N.W.
Washington, DC 20052
United States

Dean   Mary Hatwood Futrell, Graduate School of Education and Human Development
Administrator Pat Schwallie-Giddis, Ph.D., Director of Graduate Programs in Counseling
                   Department   Department of Counseling, Human & Organizational Studies
                                 (202) 994-0829, fax (202) 994-6642, gsehdapp@gwu.edu,
                                 gsehd.gwu.edu~chaos

Key   See key for Data on Each Department (this section) on page 79.

Program

Accreditation   Regional Accreditation, **CACREP:** Community Counseling, **CACREP:** School Counseling,
                 CORE: Rehabilitation Counseling, **CACREP:** Counselor Education and Supervision

CACREP

Uniqueness   Diversity of field placements in DC area, reputation in cross cultural counseling, close
              student faculty relationships, diverse student body. Certificate in Culturally and Linguistically
              Diverse Persons.

Degrees   • Community Counseling: M.
           • School Counseling: M.
           • Other: S.
           • Rehabilitation Counseling: M.
           • Counselor Education: EdD, PhD.

Contact   • Community Counseling: M = Chris D. Erickson, Ph.D..
           • School Counseling: M = Pat Schwallie-Giddis, Ph.D..
           • Other: S = Pat Schwallie-Giddis, Ph.D..
           • Rehabilitation Counseling: M = Jorge Garcia, Rh.D..
           • Counselor Education: D = Richard Lanthier, Ph.D..

Admission and Graduation Data

Admission

Requirements   • Community Counseling(M): GPA 3.00; GRE 1000; GRE V 500; GRE Q 500; GRE A 500;
                  MAT 50%; Interview.
                • School Counseling(M): GPA 3.00; GRE 1000; GRE V 500; GRE Q 500; GRE A 500; MAT
                  50%; Interview.
                • Other(S):
                • Rehabilitation Counseling(M): GPA 3.00; GRE 1000; GRE V 500; GRE Q 500; GRE A 500;
                  MAT 50%; Interview.
                • Counselor Education(D): Masters and GPA 3.50; GRE 1000; GRE V 500; GRE Q 500;
                  GRE A 500; 2 Years work experience.

Enrollment   • Community Counseling(M): 15 Admitted yearly; 10 Graduated yearly; 12 Female; 3 Male.
              • School Counseling(M): 15 Admitted yearly; 10 Graduated yearly; 12 Female; 3 Male.
              • Other(S).
              • Rehabilitation Counseling(M): 10 Admitted yearly; 10 Graduated yearly; 7 Female; 3 Male.
              • Counselor Education(D): 10 Admitted yearly; 40 Female; 10 Male.

Diversity   • African-American; Asian-American; Caucasian; Hispanic; Native American; Pacific
               Islander; Multiracial; Other.

Graduation

Requirements   • Community Counseling(M): 48 Class hours; 100 Practicum hours; 600 Internship hours.
                • School Counseling(M): 48 Class hours; 100 Practicum hours; 600 Internship hours.
                • Other(S): 36 Class hours; 100 Practicum hours; 300 Internship hours; Comprehensive
                  exam.
                • Rehabilitation Counseling(M): 48 Class hours; 100 Practicum hours; 600 Internship hours.
                • Counselor Education(D): 69 Class hours; 300 Practicum hours; 600 Internship hours;
                  Comprehensive exam; Oral exam; Dissertation.

Postgraduation activity: Advanced education and employment setting percentages.
                • Community Counseling(M): 20 Advanced education; 4 Managed care; 10 Private practice;
                  33 Agency practice; 33 Other.
                • School Counseling(M): 10 Advanced education; 33 Elementary school; 10 Middle school;
                  27 Secondary school.
                • Other(S).
                • Rehabilitation Counseling(M): 20 Advanced education; 40 Agency practice; 40 Other.
                • Counselor Education(D): 40 Advanced education; 60 Other.

Planned Program Modifications

Courses	<u>Drop</u>	<u>Add</u>
	• NP.	• NP.

Other	<u>Decrease</u>	<u>Increase</u>
	• NP.	• Diversity Recruiting of Faculty
		• Diversity Recruiting of Students
		• Number of Distance Education Courses
		• Number of On-Line Courses.

Related Programs Psychology
Arts Therapists
Psychiatric Nurses
Psychiatrists
Organizational Beaviorists
International Studies

Faculty

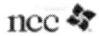

Percent of faculty reported with NCC certification: 64%.

Percent in professional counseling practice: 20%.

Research interests Diversity research.

Diversity   • Caucasian; Hispanic.

Name, Degree, Rank, State/National Credentials, % time devoted to program, email
• Erickson, Chris D; PhD; Assist.; NCC; >81%; *cerick@gwu.edu*
• Dew, Donald; EdD; Full Prof.; NCC, CORE; <21%; *Dondew@gwu.edu*
• Garcia, Jorge G; RhD; Assoc.; LPC, NCC, CORE; 61-80%; *Garcia@gwu.edu*
• Heddesheimer, Janet; PhD; Full Prof.; NCC; <21%; *Heddesh@gwu.edu*
• Hoare, Carol; EdD; Full Prof.; 41-60%; *Choare@gwu.edu*
• Hergenrather, Kenneth C; PhD; Assist.; NCC, CORE; >81%; *hergenkc@gwu.edu*
• Lanthier, Richard; PhD; Assist.; 41-60%; *lanthier@gwu.edu*
• Linkowski, Don C; PhD; Full Prof.; LPC, NCC, CORE; 61-80%; *Dcl@gwu.edu*
• Marotta, Sylvia A; PhD; Assoc.; LPC, Psych; 41-60%; *syl@gwu.edu*
• McGuire-Kuletz, Maureen; EdD; Assist.; NCC; 41-60%; *mkuletz@gwu.edu*
• Termaat, Mercedes; PhD; Assist.; LPC, RAT; >81%; *mtermaat@gwu.edu*

Has CHI SIGMA IOTA (International Counseling Society) chapter.

DE: University of Delaware

261 Student Center
Newark, DE 19716
United States

Dean   Daniel Rich
Administrator John. B. Bishop, Associate Professor
                  Department   Department of Individual and Family Studies
                                (302) 831-8107, fax (302) 8312148, John.Bishop@udel.edu,
                                http://www.udel.edu/ifst/

Key   See key for Data on Each Department (this section) on page 79.

Program

Accreditation   Regional Accreditation

Uniqueness   Either major requires two years of full-time study, excluding summer sessions. Strong
                 emphasis on supervised practice. Faculty are also professionals in Student Life Division.

Degrees   • College Counseling: M.
                 • Student Affairs: M.

Contact   • College Counseling: M = John Bishop.
                 • Student Affairs: M = John Bishop.

Admission and Graduation Data

Admission

Requirements   • College Counseling(M): GPA 2.50; GRE 1050; Interview.
                 • Student Affairs(M): GPA 2.50; GRE 1050; Interview.

Enrollment   • College Counseling(M): 6 Admitted yearly; 6 Graduated yearly; 10 Female; 2 Male.
                 • Student Affairs(M): 6 Admitted yearly; 6 Graduated yearly; 8 Female; 4 Male.

Diversity   • African-American; Caucasian; Multiracial.

Graduation

Requirements   • College Counseling(M): 48 Class hours; 210 Practicum hours; 420 Internship hours;
                   Comprehensive exam.
                 • Student Affairs(M): 48 Class hours; 210 Practicum hours; 420 Internship hours.

Postgraduation activity: Advanced education and employment setting percentages.
                 • College Counseling(M): 10 Advanced education; 90 Other.
                 • Student Affairs(M): 10 Advanced education; 90 Other.

Planned Program Modifications

Courses   Drop   Add
                 • NP.   • Group Work.

Other   Decrease   Increase
                 • NP.   • Course Offerings
                                                  • Diversity Recruiting of Faculty
                                                  • Diversity Recruiting of Students
                                                  • Faculty FTE.

Related Programs PsychologyPsychiatric Nurses

Faculty

nbcc ❧   Percent of faculty reported with NCC certification: 0%.   ncc ❧

Percent in professional counseling practice: NP.

Research interests College student culture; student development; counseling in higher education

Diversity   • African-American; Asian-American; Caucasian.

Name, Degree, Rank, State/National Credentials, % time devoted to program, email
• Bauer, Karen W; PhD; Assist.; <21%; *KBauer@udel.edu*
• Beale, Charles L; EdD; Assist.; 22-40%; *Beale.Charles@udel.edu*
• Bishop, John B; PhD; Assoc.; 41-60%; *John.Bishop@udel.edu*
• Brooks, Timothy F; EdD; Assist.; <21%; *Timothy.Brooks@udel.edu*
• Hollingsworth, Merris A; PhD; Assist.; 22-40%; *Merris.Hollingsworth@udel.edu*
• Prime, Marilyn S; EdD; <21%; *MPrime@udel.edu*
• Lewis, Jonathan D; PhD; Assist.; 22-40%; *Jonathan.Lewis@udel.edu*

- Sharf, Richard S; PhD; Assoc.; 22-40%; *Richard.Sharf@udel.edu*
- Sharkey, Stuart J; MEd; Assist.; 22-40%; *Stuart.Sharkey@udel.edu*
- Yamada, Vivian A; PsyD; Assist.; 22-40%; *Vivian.Yamada@udel.edu*
- Brunelle, John P; PhD; Assist.; 22-40%; *brunelle@udel.edu*
- Fleming, Mark C; PhD; Assist.; 22-40%; *mfleming@udel.edu*

FL: Carlos Albizu University

2173 N.W. 99th Avenue
Miami, FL 33172-2209
USA

Dean   N/A
Administrator Diana Barroso, M.S., LMHC, Director of Master's Programs
             Department   Master's Programs
                       (305) 593-1223, fax (305) 702-7806,
                       http://www.albizu.edu

Key   See key for Data on Each Department (this section) on page 79.

Program

Accreditation   Regional Accreditation

Uniqueness   Carlos Albizu University is committed to training culturally sensitive professionals in the mental health field.

Degrees   • Mental Health Counseling: M.
             • School Counseling: M.
             • Marriage and Family Counseling: M.

Contact   • Mental Health Counseling: M = Diana Barroso, M.S., LMHC.
             • School Counseling: M = Diana Barroso, M.S., LMHC.
             • Marriage and Family Counseling: M = Diana Barroso, M.S., LMHC.

Admission and Graduation Data

Admission
Requirements • Mental Health Counseling(M): GPA 3.00; Interview.
             • School Counseling(M): GPA 3.00; Interview.
             • Marriage and Family Counseling(M): GPA 3.00; Interview.

Enrollment   • Mental Health Counseling(M): 38 Admitted yearly; 7 Graduated yearly; 39 Female; 19 Male.
             • School Counseling(M): 11 Admitted yearly; 11 Graduated yearly; 20 Female; 1 Male.
             • Marriage and Family Counseling(M): 13 Admitted yearly; 11 Graduated yearly; 23 Female; 8 Male.

Diversity   • African-American; Asian-American; Caucasian; Hispanic; Multiracial.

Graduation
Requirements • Mental Health Counseling(M): 61 Class hours; 1000 Practicum hours; Comprehensive exam.
             • School Counseling(M): 49 Class hours; 240 Practicum hours; Comprehensive exam.
             • Marriage and Family Counseling(M): 52 Class hours; 300 Practicum hours; Comprehensive exam.

Postgraduation activity: Advanced education and employment setting percentages.
             • Mental Health Counseling(M): NP.
             • School Counseling(M): NP.
             • Marriage and Family Counseling(M): NP.

Planned Program Modifications

Courses   Drop   Add
             • NP.   • NP.

Other   Decrease   Increase
             • NP.   • NP.

Related Programs Marriage and Family Therapists
             Psychology

Faculty

nbcc ❖   Percent of faculty reported with NCC certification: 5%.   ncc ❖

         Percent in professional counseling practice: 95%.

Research interests Cross cultural and minority issues, psychotherapy outcomes, women's issues, history of ethnicity, anxiety sensitivity in the elderly, treatment of juvenile deliquents, systems family therapy, gay and lesbian issues, addictive behaviors, psychopathology, domestic violence, psychopharmacology, and play therapy.

Diversity   • African-American; Asian-American; Caucasian; Hispanic; Multiracial.

Name, Degree, Rank, State/National Credentials, % time devoted to program, email
- Abraham, Kondoor; PsyD; Adjunct; LPC; <21%;
- Barron, Irma; MS; Adjunct; LMHC; <21%; *sobecats@aol.com*
- Bravo, Irene; PhD; Adjunct; <21%; *ibravo@albizu.edu*
- Clark, Carol; PhD; Adjunct; LMHC; 41-60%; *carollclark@worldnet.att.net*
- Diaz, Tania; PsyD; Adjunct; <21%; *tdiaz@tui.edu*
- Domingo, Lamberto; PsyD; Adjunct; LMHC; <21%; *lsdomingo@aol.com*
- Finch, Teresa; PsyD; Adjunct; <21%;
- Garcia, Manolo; PsyD; Adjunct; <21%;
- Gonzalez, Maria; MS; Adjunct; LMFT; 22-40%; *casy007@netside.net*
- Haber, Karen; PsyD; Adjunct; 22-40%;
- Insua-Auais, Mayte; PsyD; Adjunct; NCC; 41-60%; *mayte_insua@uhc.com*
- Reznik, Eric; PsyD; Adjunct; <21%;
- Santana, Niurka; PhD; Adjunct; 22-40%; *nikkisantana@hotmail.com*
- Stephenson, Edward; PhD; Adjunct; 22-40%;
- Valiente, David; PhD; Adjunct; <21%;
- Valiente, Marilyn; PhD; Adjunct; LMHC; <21%;
- Simon, Matthew; PsyD; Adjunct; LMHC; <21%; *mdspsyd@netzero.net*
- Orta, Luis; PhD; Adjunct; <21%
- Barroso, Diana; MS; Assoc.; LMHC; >81%; *dbarroso@albizu.edu*
- Sydnor, Denise; PsyD; Assoc.; >81%; *dsydnor@albizu.edu*

FL: Florida Atlantic University

College of Education
Boca Raton, FL 33431-0991
USA
Dean Greg Aloia, Ph.D. College of Education
Administrator Dr. Alex Miranda, PhD, Chair
Department Department of Counselor Education
(561) 297-3602, fax (561) 297-2309, cnslred@fau.edu,
www.coe.fau.edu/counsel

Key See key for Data on Each Department (this section) on page 79.

Program
Accreditation Applied for CORE: Rehabilitation Counseling

Uniqueness Department emphasis is upon connecting research knowledge based on "best of practice" with the development of student competencies in their counseling specialization area. A community counseling clinic is maintained in the department where students receive live supervision in counseling practice. Courses are offered in several formats including traditional weekly evening courses, saturday courses and modular intensive courses to meet varying needs of students. Department also maintains a counseling resource library and computer/internet access for students. The department is actively involved with several international projects with counseling organizations and schools including Europe, Africa, Asia, and Latin America.

Degrees
• Mental Health Counseling: M, S.
• School Counseling: M, S.
• Marriage and Family Counseling: S.
• Rehabilitation Counseling: M.

Contact
• Mental Health Counseling: M, S = Dr. Alex Miranda.
• School Counseling: M, S = Dr. Greg Brigman.
• Marriage and Family Counseling: S = Dr. Alex Miranda.
• Rehabilitation Counseling: M = Dr. Larry Kontosh.

Admission and Graduation Data
Admission
Requirements
• Mental Health Counseling(M): GPA ~3.00; GRE ~1000; Interview.
• Mental Health Counseling(S): GPA ~3.50; GRE 1000; Interview.
• School Counseling(M): GPA ~3.00; GRE ~1000; Interview.
• School Counseling(S): GPA ~3.00; GRE 1000; Interview.
• Marriage and Family Counseling(S): GPA ~3.50; GRE 1000.
• Rehabilitation Counseling(M): GPA ~3.00; GRE ~1000; Interview.

Enrollment
• Mental Health Counseling(M & S): 50 Admitted yearly; 20 Graduated yearly; 20 Female; 10 Male.
• School Counseling(M & S): 50 Admitted yearly; 20 Graduated yearly; 10 Male.
• Marriage and Family Counseling(S): 3 Admitted yearly.
• Rehabilitation Counseling(M): 10 Admitted yearly; 5 Graduated yearly; 7 Female; 3 Male.

Diversity
• African-American; Asian-American; Caucasian; Hispanic; Multiracial; Other.

Graduation
Requirements
• Mental Health Counseling(M): 48 Class hours; 400 Practicum hours; 600 Internship hours.
• Mental Health Counseling(S): 33 Class hours; 33+ Practicum hours.
• School Counseling(M): 60 Class hours; 150 Practicum hours; 600 Internship hours; Portfolio.
• School Counseling(S): 33 Class hours; 33+ Practicum hours; Portfolio.
• Marriage and Family Counseling(S): 33 Class hours; 33+ Practicum hours.
• Rehabilitation Counseling(M): 60 Class hours; 150 Practicum hours; 600 Internship hours.

Postgraduation activity: Advanced education and employment setting percentages.
• Mental Health Counseling(M & S): 5 Advanced education; 30 Managed care; 05 Private practice; 60 Agency practice.
• School Counseling(M & S): 5 Advanced education; 30 Elementary school; 30 Middle school; 40 Secondary school.
• Marriage and Family Counseling(S).
• Rehabilitation Counseling(M): 20 Private practice; 70 Agency practice.

Planned Program Modifications
Courses

Drop	Add
• Career/Life Planning	• NP.
• Marriage and Family Counseling	
• Play Therapy	
• Psychopharmocology.	

Other	Decrease	Increase
	• NP.	• Course Offerings
		• Diversity Recruiting of Faculty
		• Diversity Recruiting of Students
		• Financial Aid
		• National Accreditation
		• Number of Distance Education Courses
		• Number of Off-Campus Courses
		• Number of On-Line Courses.

Related Programs Clinical Social Workers
Psychology

Faculty

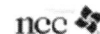 Percent of faculty reported with NCC certification: 67%. ncc

Percent in professional counseling practice: 100%.

Research interests 1. Effectiveness of school counseling programs in promoting student academic and social competencies; 2. Treatment effectiveness in child, adolescent and family counseling; 3. Career and occupational transitions for youth, adults and disabled individuals.

Diversity • Caucasian; Hispanic.

Name, Degree, Rank, State/National Credentials, % time devoted to program, email
• Brigman, Greg; PhD; Assoc.; NCC; >81%; *gbrigman@fau.edu*
• Kontosh, Larry; PhD; Assist.; LPC, CRC; >81%;
• Campbell, Chari; PhD; Assoc.; NCC; >81%; *ccampbel@fau.edu*
• Webb, Linda; PhD; Assist.; NCC; >81%; *lwebb@fau.edu*
• Nicoll, William G; PhD; Full Prof.; LPC, NCC; >81%; *nicoll@fau.edu*
• Miranda, Alex O; PhD; Assoc.; LMHC; >81%; *amiranda@fau.edu*

Has CHI SIGMA IOTA (International Counseling Society) chapter.

FL: Florida State University

307 Stone Building
Tallahassee, FL 32306-4453
United States
Dean   Richard Kunkel
Administrator   Gary W. Peterson, Program Coordinator
           Department   Educational Psychology and Learning Systems
                    (850) 644-4592, fax (850) 644-8776, gpeterso@admin.fsu.edu

Key   See key for Data on Each Department (this section) on page 79.

Program

Accreditation   Regional Accreditation, **CACREP:** Career Counseling, **CACREP:** Mental Health Counseling,
          CACREP: School Counseling

Uniqueness   We have CACREP-approved programs in mental health counseling, school counseling and
          career counseling

Degrees   • Mental Health Counseling: S.
          • School Counseling: S.
          • Career Counseling: S.

Contact   • Mental Health Counseling: S = Steve Rollin.
          • School Counseling: S = Don Kelly.
          • Career Counseling: S = Robert Reardon.

Admission and Graduation Data

Admission
Requirements   • Mental Health Counseling(S): GPA 3.00; GRE 1000.
          • School Counseling(S): GPA 3.00; GRE 1000.
          • Career Counseling(S): GPA 3.00; GRE 1000.

Enrollment   • Mental Health Counseling(S): 16 Admitted yearly; 14 Graduated yearly.
          • School Counseling(S): 9 Admitted yearly; 8 Graduated yearly.
          • Career Counseling(S): 5 Admitted yearly; 4 Graduated yearly.

Diversity   • African-American; Asian-American; Caucasian; Hispanic.

Graduation
Requirements   • Mental Health Counseling(S): 72 Class hours; 100 Practicum hours; 900 Internship hours;
          Comprehensive exam.
          • School Counseling(S): 72 Class hours; 100 Practicum hours; 600 Internship hours;
          Comprehensive exam.
          • Career Counseling(S): 72 Class hours; 100 Practicum hours; 600 Internship hours;
          Comprehensive exam.

Postgraduation activity: Advanced education and employment setting percentages.
          • Mental Health Counseling(S): 20 Advanced education; 10 Managed care; 10 Private
          practice; 50 Agency practice; 10 Other.
          • School Counseling(S): 10 Advanced education; 10 Elementary school; 40 Middle school;
          40 Secondary school.
          • Career Counseling(S): 25 Advanced education; 10 Agency practice; 10 Middle school; 10
          Secondary school; 45 Student affairs; 10 Other.

Planned Program Modifications

Courses   Drop   Add
                   • NP.   • NP.

Other   Decrease   Increase
                   • NP.   • Clinical Supervision
                                      • Diversity Recruiting of Faculty
                                      • Faculty FTE.

Related Programs Clinical Social Workers
          Marriage and Family Therapists
          Psychology
          Arts Therapists
          Psychiatric Nurses
          Human Resource Personnel
          Communications

Faculty

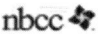 Percent of faculty reported with NCC certification: 29%.

Percent in professional counseling practice: 13%.

Research interests Career development and decision-making; interventions for at-risk youth ; use of
                            technology in counseling and career development

Diversity   • Caucasian.

Name, Degree, Rank, State/National Credentials, % time devoted to program, email
• Kelly, Donald F; PhD; Assoc.; 61-80%; *kelly@coe.fsu.edu*
• Peterson, Gary W; PhD; Full Prof.; 41-60%; *gpeterson@admin.fsu.edu*
• Prevatt, Frances; PhD; Assoc.; <21%; *prevatt@coe.fsu.edu*
• Reardon, Robert C; PhD; Full Prof.; NCC; 41-60%; *reardon@admin.fsu.edu*
• Rollin, Steven; EdD; Full Prof.; <21%; *rollin@coe.fsu.edu*
• Sampson, James P; PhD; Full Prof.; NCC; >81%; *jpsampso@garret.acns.fsu.edu*
• Proctor, Briley; PhD; Assist.; <21%; *proctor@coe.fsu.edu*

FL: Rollins College

	1000 Holt Ave. - 2726
	Winter Park, FL 32789-4499
	USA
Dean	Patricia Lancaster, Hamilton Holt School
Administrator	Kathryn L. Norsworthy, Associate Professor and Chair
	Department Graduate Studies in Counseling
	(407) 691-1708, fax (407) 646-1546, wdigerlando@rollins.edu,
	www.ric.edu/cep

Key   See key for Data on Each Department (this section) on page 79.

Program

Accreditation   Regional Accreditation, **CACREP:** Mental Health Counseling, **CACREP:** School Counseling

Uniqueness   Focus on social justice and multiculturalism in counseling. Offers a Master Therapist series as the capstone experience for students in final year. Requires personal counseling experience for all students. Family and relationship counseling and group counseling sequences required.

Degrees
- Mental Health Counseling: M.
- School Counseling: M.

Contact
- Mental Health Counseling: M = Kathryn L. Norsworthy, Ph.D.
- School Counseling: M = Kathryn L. Norsworthy, Ph.D.

Admission and Graduation Data

Admission

Requirements
- Mental Health Counseling(M): GPA 3.00; GRE 1000; MAT 50; 2 Years work experience.
- School Counseling(M): GPA 3.00; GRE 1000; MAT 50; 2 Years work experience.

Enrollment
- Mental Health Counseling(M): 30 Admitted yearly; 20 Graduated yearly; 85 Female; 5 Male.
- School Counseling(M): 5 Admitted yearly; 5 Graduated yearly; 4 Female; 1 Male.

Diversity
- African-American; Asian-American; Caucasian; Hispanic; Native American; Pacific Islander; Multiracial; Other.

Graduation

Requirements
- Mental Health Counseling(M): 60 Class hours; 250 Practicum hours; 750 Internship hours.
- School Counseling(M): 48 Class hours; 100 Practicum hours; 600 Internship hours.

Postgraduation activity: Advanced education and employment setting percentages.
- Mental Health Counseling(M): 10 Advanced education; 5 Managed care; 70 Agency practice; 15 Other.
- School Counseling(M): 5 Advanced education; 45 Elementary school; 10 Middle school; 30 Secondary school; 10 Other.

Planned Program Modifications

Courses	Drop	Add
	• NP.	• NP.

Other	Decrease	Increase
	• NP.	• Diversity Recruiting of Faculty
		• Diversity Recruiting of Students.

Related Programs Organizational Beaviorists

Faculty

nbcc ❧   Percent of faculty reported with NCC certification: **100**%.   ncc ❧

Percent in professional counseling practice: 50%.

Research interests Provost: MBTI, Jungian-based dreamwork, and play and leisure over the lifespan; Homrich: Family resiliency, divorcing families, human sexuality; Shafe: Eating disorders, human development, and women's issues; Norsworthy: International and social justice applications in counseling and psychology, feminist theory and practice, clinical hypnosis, and Buddhist applications in counseling and counselor education

Diversity   • Asian-American; Caucasian; Hispanic.

Name, Degree, Rank, State/National Credentials, % time devoted to program, email
- Shafe, Marie C; EdD; Full Prof.; LPC, NCC; >81%; *mcshafe@aol.com*
- Provost, Judith A; EdD; Full Prof.; LPC, NCC; >81%; *jprovost@rollins.edu*
- Homrich, Alicia M; PhD; Assist.; NCC, Licensed Psychologist; >81%; *ahomrich@rollins.edu*
- Norsworthy, Kathryn L; PhD; Assoc.; NCC, Licensed Psychologist; >81%; *Knorswor@rollins.edu*

Has CHI SIGMA IOTA (International Counseling Society) chapter.

FL: University of Central Florida

PO Box 161250
Orlando, FL 32816-1250
USA
Dean   Dr. Sandra L. Robinson, Dean College of Education
Administrator   E.H. Mike Robinson, III Ph.D. NCC, Coordinator, Programs in Counselor Education
                    Department   Child, Family and Community Sciences
                    (407) 823-3063, fax (407) 823-0044, counsel@mail.ucf.edu,
                    http://edcollege.ucf.edu/mod_depts/

Key   See key for Data on Each Department (this section) on page 79.

Program
Accreditation   Regional Accreditation, **CACREP:** Counselor Education and Supervision, **CACREP:** Mental
                Health Counseling, **CACREP:** School Counseling

CACREP

Uniqueness   Diversity of the students and faculty, certificate programs in Play Therapy, Marriage and
            Family Therapy and pending programs in Career and College Counseling. Variety of Clinical
            experiences including extensive practicum in the College of Education Community Counseling
            Clinic. Collaborative work and research opportunities in the Tony Jennings Exceptional
            Education Institute and the UCF Academy for Teaching, Learning and Leadership.

Degrees   • Mental Health Counseling: M.
            • School Counseling: M, S.
            • Counselor Education: PhD.

Contact   • Mental Health Counseling: M = Mark Young.
            • School Counseling: M, S = B. Grant Hayes.
            • Counselor Education: D = E.H. Mike Robinson, III.

Admission and Graduation Data
Admission
Requirements • Mental Health Counseling(M): GRE 1000; GRE V 500; GRE Q 500; GRE A NA; Interview.
            • School Counseling(M): GRE 1000; GRE V 500; GRE Q 500; GRE A NA; Interview.
            • School Counseling(S): GRE 1000; GRE V 500; GRE Q 500; GRE A NA; Interview.
            • Counselor Education(D): Masters and GPA 3.00; GRE 1000; GRE V 500; GRE Q 500;
              GRE A NA.

Enrollment   • Mental Health Counseling(M): 25/30 Admitted yearly; 22 Graduated yearly; 54 Female;
              8 Male.
            • School Counseling(M & S): 25/30 Admitted yearly; 23 Graduated yearly; 52 Female;
              7 Male.
            • Counselor Education(D): 6 Admitted yearly; 6 Graduated yearly; 12 Female; 7 Male.

Diversity   • African-American; Asian-American; Caucasian; Hispanic; Native American.

Graduation
Requirements • Mental Health Counseling(M): 63 Class hours; 200 Practicum hours; 1000 Internship
              hours; CPCE; Portfolio.
            • School Counseling(M): 51/60 Class hours; 150 Practicum hours; 600 Internship hours;
              CPCE; Portfolio.
            • School Counseling(S): 48 Class hours; 150 Practicum hours; 600 Internship hours; CPCE;
              Portfolio.
            • Counselor Education(D): 84 Class hours; 300 Practicum hours; 900 Internship hours;
              Comprehensive exam; Oral exam; Dissertation.

Postgraduation activity: Advanced education and employment setting percentages.
            • Mental Health Counseling(M): 15 Advanced education; 10 Managed care; 05 Private
              practice; 65 Agency practice; 10 Other.
            • School Counseling(M & S): 10 Advanced education; 15 Elementary school; 25 Middle
              school; 40 Secondary school; 10 Other.
            • Counselor Education(D): 16.7 Agency practice; 16.7 Elementary school; 66.6 Student
              affairs.

Planned Program Modifications

Courses

Drop	Add
• Adventure Counseling	• NP.
• Career/Life Planning	
• Consultation	
• Crisis/Violence Counseling	
• Marriage and Family Counseling	
• Play Therapy	
• Wellness.	

Other

Decrease	Increase
• NP.	• Course Offerings
	• Diversity Recruiting of Students
	• Graduation Requirements
	• Number of Degree Majors.

Related Programs Clinical Social Workers
Psychology

Faculty

 nbcc ❧   Percent of faculty reported with NCC certification: 27%.   ncc ❧

Percent in professional counseling practice: NP.

Research interests

Diversity   • African-American; Caucasian; Hispanic; Native American.

Name, Degree, Rank, State/National Credentials, % time devoted to program, email
• Balado, Carl; EdD; Assoc.; 41-60%; *balado@mail.ucf.edu*
• Bollet, Robert; EdD; Assoc.; LMHC; 22-40%; *bollet@mail.ucf.edu*
• Casado, Montse; PhD; Assist.; LMFT, RPT; >81%; *mcasado@mail.ucf.edu*
• Daire, Andrew P; PhD; Assist.; LMHC; >81%; *adaire@mail.ucf.edu*
• Hayes, Grant; PhD; Assist.; LPC; >81%; *ghayes@mail.ucf.edu*
• Jones, Dayle K; PhD; Assist.; NCC, LMHC; >81%; *kjones@mail.ucf.edu*
• Jones, Leslie; PhD; Assist.; RPT; >81%; *ljones@mail.ucf.edu*
• Robinson,III, E H Mike; PhD; Full Prof.; NCC; >81%; *erobinso@mail.ucf.edu*
• Rasmus, Scott D; MA; Instructor; LMFT; >81%; *srasmus@mail.ucf.edu*
• Young, Mark; PhD; Full Prof.; NCC, LMHC, LMFT; >81%; *myoung@mail.ucf.edu*
• Taub, Gordon; PhD; Assist.; 22-40%; *gtaub@mail.ucf.edu*

Has CHI SIGMA IOTA (International Counseling Society) chapter.

FL: University of Florida

1215 Norman Hall, P. O. Box 117046
Gainesville, FL 32611-7046
USA

Dean   Dean K. Emihovich
Administrator   M. Harry Daniels, Chairperson & Professor
             Department   Counselor Education Department
             (352) 392-0731 Ext. 200, fax (352) 846-2697, harryd@coe.ufl.edu,
             www.coe.ufl.edu/counselor/ced/index.html

Key   See key for Data on Each Department (this section) on page 79.

Program
Accreditation   Regional Accreditation, **CACREP:** Marriage and Family Counseling, **CACREP:** Mental Health
             Counseling, **CACREP:** School Counseling, **CACREP:** Counselor Education and Supervision

CACREP

Uniqueness   Refer to Dept. Website www.coe.ufl.edu/counselor/ced/index.html

Degrees   • Mental Health Counseling: M, S, EdD, PhD.
            • School Counseling: M, S, EdD, PhD.
            • Marriage and Family Counseling: M, S, EdD, PhD.

Contact   • Mental Health Counseling: M, S, D = M. Harry Daniels.
            • School Counseling: M, S, D = M. Harry Daniels.
            • Marriage and Family Counseling: M, S, D = M. Harry Daniels.

Admission and Graduation Data
Admission
Requirements   • Mental Health Counseling(M): GPA 3.00; GRE 1000; GRE V 500; GRE Q 500; Interview.
            • Mental Health Counseling(S): GPA 3.00; GRE 1000; GRE V 500; GRE Q 500; Interview.
            • Mental Health Counseling(D): Masters and GPA 3.20; GRE 1100; GRE V 550; GRE Q 550.
            • School Counseling(M): GPA 3.00; GRE 1000; GRE V 500; GRE Q 500; Interview.
            • School Counseling(S): GPA 3.00; GRE 1000; GRE V 500; GRE Q 500; Interview.
            • School Counseling(D): Masters and GPA 3.20; GRE 1100; GRE V 550; GRE Q 550.
            • Marriage and Family Counseling(M): GPA 3.00; GRE 1000; GRE V 500; GRE Q 500;
              Interview.
            • Marriage and Family Counseling(S): GPA 3.00; GRE 1000; GRE V 500; GRE Q 500;
              Interview.
            • Marriage and Family Counseling(D): Masters and GPA 3.20; GRE 1100; GRE V 550;
              GRE Q 550.

Enrollment   • Mental Health Counseling(M & S): 18 Admitted yearly; 12 Graduated yearly.
            • Mental Health Counseling(D): 7 Admitted yearly; 5 Graduated yearly.
            • School Counseling(M & S): 18 Admitted yearly; 16 Graduated yearly.
            • School Counseling(D): 3 Admitted yearly; 2 Graduated yearly.
            • Marriage and Family Counseling(M & S): 16 Admitted yearly; 11 Graduated yearly.
            • Marriage and Family Counseling(D): 3 Admitted yearly; 5 Graduated yearly.

Diversity   • NP.

Graduation
Requirements   • Mental Health Counseling(M): 3 Class hours; 400 Practicum hours; 600 Internship hours;
              Oral exam.
            • Mental Health Counseling(S): 72 Class hours; 400 Practicum hours; 600 Internship hours;
              Oral exam.
            • Mental Health Counseling(D): 120 Class hours; 1200 Internship hours; Comprehensive
              exam; Oral exam; Dissertation.
            • School Counseling(M): 3 Class hours; 300 Practicum hours; 600 Internship hours; Oral
              exam.
            • School Counseling(S): 72 Class hours; 300 Practicum hours; 600 Internship hours; Oral
              exam.
            • School Counseling(D): 120 Class hours; 1200 Internship hours; Oral exam; Dissertation.
            • Marriage and Family Counseling(M): 3 Class hours; 400 Practicum hours; 600 Internship
              hours; Oral exam.
            • Marriage and Family Counseling(S): 72 Class hours; 400 Practicum hours; 600 Internship
              hours; Oral exam.
            • Marriage and Family Counseling(D): 120 Class hours; 1200 Internship hours;
              Comprehensive exam; Oral exam; Dissertation.

Postgraduation activity: Advanced education and employment setting percentages.
- Mental Health Counseling(M & S): 25 Advanced education; 10 Managed care; 15 Private practice; 50 Agency practice.
- Mental Health Counseling(D):
- School Counseling(M & S): 10 Advanced education; 30 Elementary school; 30 Middle school; 30 Secondary school.
- School Counseling(D):
- Marriage and Family Counseling(M & S): 25 Advanced education; 10 Managed care; 15 Private practice; 50 Agency practice.
- Marriage and Family Counseling(D):

Planned Program Modifications

Courses   Drop   Add
- NP.   • NP.

Other   Decrease   Increase
- Faculty FTE   • NP.
- Number of Degree Majors.

Related Programs Psychology
Psychiatric Nurses
Psychiatrists

Faculty

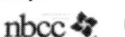 Percent of faculty reported with NCC certification: 50%.

Percent in professional counseling practice: 100%.

Research interests Refer to Dept. Website: www.coe.ufl.edu/counselor/ced/index.html

Diversity   • African-American; Caucasian; Hispanic; Multiracial.

Name, Degree, Rank, State/National Credentials, % time devoted to program, email
- Daniels, M. Harry; PhD; Full Prof.; NCC; >81%; *harryd@coe.ufl.edu*
- Amatea, Ellen S; PhD; Full Prof.; >81%; *eamatea@coe.ufl.edu*
- Archer, James; PhD; Full Prof.; >81%; *jarcher@coe.ufl.edu*
- Clark, Mary A; PhD; Assist.; NCC; >81%; *maclark@coe.ufl.edu*
- Doan, Silvia E; PhD; Assoc.; >81%; *silvia@coe.ufl.edu*
- Loesch, Larry C; PhD; Full Prof.; NCC; >81%; *lloesch@coe.ufl.edu*
- Myrick, Robert; PhD; Full Prof.; >81%; *rmyrick@coe.ufl.edu*
- Parker, Woodrow; PhD; Full Prof.; >81%; *mparker@coe.ufl.edu*
- Pitts, James; PhD; Assoc.; >81%; *jpitts@coe.ufl.edu*
- Sherrard, Peter A; EdD; Assoc.; NCC, LMFT, LMHC; >81%; *psherrard@coe.ufl.edu*
- Smith, Sondra; PhD; Assist.; NCC; >81%; *ssmith@coe.ufl.edu*
- Wittmer, Joe; PhD; Full Prof.; NCC; >81%; *jwittmer@coe.ufl.edu*

Has CHI SIGMA IOTA (International Counseling Society) chapter.

FL: University of North Florida

4567 St. Johns Bluff Rd. South
Jacksonville, FL 32224-2676
United States
Dean   John Venn
Administrator   Lynne Carroll & Carolyn Stone, Associate Professors/ Co-program leaders
                    Department   Department of Counselor Education
                    (904) 620-2838, fax (904) 620-2982, http://www.unf.edu/coehs/

Key   See key for Data on Each Department (this section) on page 79.

Program

Accreditation   Regional Accreditation, **CACREP:** Mental Health Counseling, **CACREP:** School Counseling

Uniqueness   Comprehensive 60 hr. mental health counseling track and innovative school counseling track which follows a cohort model. 100% placement of graduates of both tracks.

Degrees   • Mental Health Counseling: M.
          • School Counseling: M.

Contact   • Mental Health Counseling: M = Lynne Carroll.
          • School Counseling: M = Carolyn Stone.

Admission and Graduation Data

Admission
Requirements   • Mental Health Counseling(M): GPA 3.00; GRE 1000; 1 Year work experience; Interview.
               • School Counseling(M): GPA 3.00; GRE 1000; 1 Year work experience; Interview.

Enrollment   • Mental Health Counseling(M): 25 Admitted yearly; 25 Graduated yearly.
             • School Counseling(M): 30 Admitted yearly; 30 Graduated yearly.

Diversity   • African-American; Caucasian; Hispanic.

Graduation
Requirements   • Mental Health Counseling(M): 60 Class hours; 100 Practicum hours; 900 Internship hours.
               • School Counseling(M): 51 Class hours; 100 Practicum hours; 600 Internship hours.

Postgraduation activity: Advanced education and employment setting percentages.
               • Mental Health Counseling(M): 5 Advanced education; 5 Managed care; 90 Agency practice.
               • School Counseling(M): 50 Elementary school; 25 Middle school; 25 Secondary school.

Planned Program Modifications

Courses   Drop   Add
             • NP.   • NP.

Other   Decrease   Increase
             • NP.   • NP.

Related Programs

Faculty

   Percent of faculty reported with NCC certification: 50%.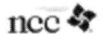

Percent in professional counseling practice: NP.

Research interests

Diversity   • Caucasian.

Name, Degree, Rank, State/National Credentials, % time devoted to program, email
• Carroll, Lynne; PhD; Assoc.; >81%; *lcarroll@unf.edu*
• Schumacher, Rebecca; EdD; Assist.; >81%; *rschumach@unf.edu*
• Pepper, Barbara; PhD; Adjunct; LPC, NCC; 41-60%; *bpepper@unf.edu*
• Hansford, Sandra; EdD; Assoc.; NCC; 41-60%; *zipper@mediaone.net*
• Lombana, Judy; EdD; Full Prof.; NCC; >81%; *jlombana@uaf.edu*
• Stone, Carolyn; EdD; Assoc.; >81%; *Cstone@uaf.edu*

GA: Columbus State University

	4225 University Avenue
	Columbus, GA 36874-5645
	United States
Dean	Thomas Harrison, Dean, College of Education
Administrator	H.T. Ford, Jr., Department Chair
	Department Counseling, Educational Leadership and Professional Studies
	(706) 568-2222, fax (706) 568-5088, http://celps.colstate.edu

Key   See key for Data on Each Department (this section) on page 79.

Program

Accreditation   Regional Accreditation, **CACREP:** Community Counseling, **CACREP:** School Counseling

Uniqueness   NP.

Degrees
- Community Counseling: M.
- School Counseling: M, S.

Contact
- Community Counseling: M = NP.
- School Counseling: M, S = NP.

Admission and Graduation Data

Admission

Requirements
- Community Counseling(M): GPA 2.70; GRE 800; MAT 44; Interview.
- School Counseling(M): GPA 2.70; GRE 800; MAT 44; 2 Years work experience; Interview.
- School Counseling(S): GPA 2.70; GRE 800; MAT 44; 2 Years work experience; Interview.

Enrollment
- Community Counseling(M): 60 Admitted yearly; 30 Graduated yearly; 20 Female; 10 Male.
- School Counseling(M & S): 40 Admitted yearly; 15 Graduated yearly; 10 Female; 5 Male.

Diversity
- African-American; Asian-American; Caucasian; Multiracial.

Graduation

Requirements
- Community Counseling(M): 48 Class hours; 100 Practicum hours; 600 Internship hours; Comprehensive exam; Portfolio.
- School Counseling(M): 48 Class hours; 100 Practicum hours; 600 Internship hours; Comprehensive exam; Portfolio.
- School Counseling(S): 30 Class hours; VAR Internship hours.

Postgraduation activity: Advanced education and employment setting percentages.
- Community Counseling(M): 15 Advanced education; 20 Managed care; 5 Private practice; 60 Agency practice.
- School Counseling(M & S): 40 Elementary school; 20 Middle school; 40 Secondary school.

Planned Program Modifications

Courses	Drop		Add
	• NP.	• NP.	

Other	Decrease		Increase
	• NP.	• NP.	

Related Programs

Faculty

nbcc ✦   Percent of faculty reported with NCC certification: 88%.   ncc ✦

Percent in professional counseling practice: NP.

Research interests

Diversity
- Caucasian.

Name, Degree, Rank, State/National Credentials, % time devoted to program, email
- Baltimore, Michael; PhD; LPC, NCC, LMFT; >81%; *baltimore_michael@colstate.edu*
- Gillam, Lenior; PhD; LPC, NCC; >81%; *gillam_lenoir@colstate.edu*
- Godwin, Opal; Other; LCSW; <21%;

- Hornbuckle, David; PhD; LPC, NCC; >81%; *hornbuckle_david@colstate.edu*
- Muse, Stephen; PhD; NCC; <21%;
- Hardin, Delilah; Other; LPC, NCC;
- Fitch, Trey; LPC, NCC; >81%; *fitch_trey@colstate.edu*
- Hickson, Joyce; EdD; LPC, NCC; *hickson_joyce@colstate.edu*

Has CHI SIGMA IOTA (International Counseling Society) chapter.

GA: Georgia State University

	30 Pryor Street
	Atlanta, GA 30303-3083
	United States
Dean	Ronald Colarusso, Ph.D. College of Education
Administrator	JoAnna White, Chair
	Department Counseling and Psychological Services
	(404) 651-2550, fax (404) 651-1160, http://education.gsu.edu/cps/index.htm

Key   See key for Data on Each Department (this section) on page 79.

Program
Accreditation   Regional Accreditation, **CACREP:** Community Counseling, **CACREP:** School Counseling, CORE: Rehabilitation Counseling, **CACREP:** Counselor Education and Supervision

CACREP

Uniqueness   Course listing and website information use the term Professional Counseling to refer to Community Counseling.

Degrees
- Community Counseling: M, S.
- School Counseling: M, S.
- Counselor Education: PhD.

Contact
- Community Counseling: M, S = Gary L. Arthur, Ed.D..
- School Counseling: M, S = Fran Mullis, Ph.D..
- Counselor Education: D = Roy M. Kern, Ed.D..

Admission and Graduation Data
Admission
Requirements
- Community Counseling(M): GPA 2.50; GRE 800; GRE V NA; GRE Q NA; GRE A NA; MAT NA; 6 Years work experience.
- Community Counseling(S): GPA 2.50; GRE 900; GRE V NA; GRE Q NA; GRE A NA; MAT NA; 6 Years work experience.
- School Counseling(M): GPA 2.50; GRE 800; GRE V NA; GRE Q NA; GRE A NA; MAT NA; 1 Year work experience.
- School Counseling(S): GPA 2.50; GRE 900; GRE V NA; GRE Q NA; GRE A NA; MAT NA; 1 Year work experience.
- Counselor Education(D): Masters and GPA 3.25; GRE 1000; GRE V 500; GRE Q 500; GRE A 500; MAT NA; 1 Year work experience.

Enrollment
- Community Counseling(M & S): 150 Admitted yearly; 115 Graduated yearly; 245 Female; 52 Male.
- School Counseling(M & S): 28 Admitted yearly; 23 Graduated yearly; 63 Female; 2 Male.
- Counselor Education(D): 4-6 Admitted yearly; 2-4 Graduated yearly; 12 Female; 4 Male.

Diversity
- African-American; Asian-American; Caucasian; Hispanic; Native American; Pacific Islander; Multiracial.

Graduation
Requirements
- Community Counseling(M): 48 Class hours; 100 Practicum hours; 600 Internship hours; Comprehensive exam.
- Community Counseling(S): 30 Class hours; 300 Practicum hours; NA Internship hours; Portfolio.
- School Counseling(M): 48 Class hours; 100 Practicum hours; 600 Internship hours; Comprehensive exam.
- School Counseling(S): 30 Class hours; 300 Practicum hours; NA Internship hours; Portfolio.
- Counselor Education(D): 97 Class hours; 360 Practicum hours; 600 Internship hours; Comprehensive exam; Dissertation; Portfolio.

Postgraduation activity: Advanced education and employment setting percentages.
- Community Counseling(M & S): 16 Advanced education; 3 Managed care; 1 Private practice; 76 Agency practice; 4 Other.
- School Counseling(M & S): 5 Advanced education; 60 Elementary school; 15 Middle school; 20 Secondary school.
- Counselor Education(D): 10 Managed care; 10 Private practice; 20 Agency practice; 20 Elementary school; 10 Middle school; 10 Secondary school; 20 Student affairs.

Planned Program Modifications

Courses	Drop	Add
	• NP.	• Addictions
		• Psychodiagnosis.

Other	Decrease	Increase
	• NP.	• NP.

Related Programs Psychology
Psychiatric Nurses
International Studies

Faculty

nbcc ❖ Percent of faculty reported with NCC certification: 35%. ncc ❖

Percent in professional counseling practice: 10%.

Research interests

Diversity • African-American; Asian-American; Caucasian; Multiracial.

Name, Degree, Rank, State/National Credentials, % time devoted to program, email
- Ancis, Julie R; PhD; Assoc.; >81%; *jancis@gsu.edu*
- Arthur, Gary L; EdD; Full Prof.; LPC, NCC; >81%; *garthur@gsu.edu*
- Ashby, Jeffrey S; PhD; Assoc.; LP; 41-60%; *jashby2@gsu.edu*
- Brack, Gregory; PhD; Assoc.; LP; 61-80%; *gbrack@gsu.edu*
- Chang, Catherine; PhD; Assist.; LPC, NCC; >81%; *cchang@gsu.edu*
- Chung, Barry; PhD; Assoc.; >81%; *bchung@gsu.edu*
- Draper, Kay; PhD; Assist.; LPC, NCC; >81%; *kdraper@gsu.edu*
- Edwards, Dana L; PhD; Assist.; LPC; >81%; *dedwards3@gsu.edu*
- Hill, Joseph; PhD; Assist.; LPC, CRC, LAP; 61-80%; *jhill@gsu.edu*
- Katrin, Susan; PhD; Assoc.; LPC, NCC, LP, CGP, CCMHC; >81%; *skatrin@gsu.edu*
- Kern, Roy M; EdD; Full Prof.; LPC, LMFT, AAMFT; >81%; *rkern@gsu.edu*
- Matheny, Kenneth B; PhD; Full Prof.; LAP; >81%; *kmatheny@gsu.edu*
- Mullis, Francis Y; PhD; Assoc.; LPC, NCC, NCSC; >81%; *fmullis@gsu.edu*
- Perkins-Dock, Robin; PhD; Assist.; LPC; >81%; *rgordon2@gsu.edu*
- Ripley, Karen; PhD; Assist.; LPC, NCC, REB Therapist; >81%; *kripley@gsu.edu*
- Sampson, Stephen; PhD; Assist.; LP; >81%; *ssampson@gsu.edu*
- Weed, Roger O; PhD; Full Prof.; CRC, CDMS, CCM, CLCP; <21%; *rweed@gsu.edu*
- White, JoAnna; EdD; Full Prof.; LPC, CPTS; >81%; *jwhite@gsu.edu*
- Dew, Brian; PhD; Assist.; LPC, NCC, SAC; >81%;
- Cadenhead, Catherine P; PhD; Assist.; LP, CSP; 22-40%; *cfortner@gsu.edu*

Has CHI SIGMA IOTA (International Counseling Society) chapter.

GA: State University of West Georgia

	Education Center Annex #237
	Carrolton, GA 30118-4160
	United States
Dean	Kent Layton, Ph.D.; College of Education
Administrator	Brent M. Snow, Ph.D., Professor & Chair
	Department Department of Counseling & Educational Psychology
	(770) 836-6554, fax (770) 836-4645, bsnow@westga.edu, coe.westga.edu/cep

Key   See key for Data on Each Department (this section) on page 79.

Program

Accreditation   Regional Accreditation, **CACREP:** Community Counseling, **CACREP:** School Counseling

Uniqueness   Department faculty are leaders in the national initiative to transform school counseling. Very large and active chapter of Chi Sigma Iota (honorary society in counseling).

Degrees
- Community Counseling: M, S.
- School Counseling: M, S.

Contact
- Community Counseling: M, S = Dr. Snow.
- School Counseling: M, S = Dr. Snow.

Admission and Graduation Data

Admission

Requirements
- Community Counseling(M): GPA 2.70; GRE 900; GRE V 450; GRE Q 450; GRE A 450; Interview.
- Community Counseling(S): GPA 2.70; GRE 900; GRE V 450; GRE Q 450; GRE A 450; Interview.
- School Counseling(M): GPA 2.70; GRE 900; GRE V 450; GRE Q 450; GRE A 450; Interview.
- School Counseling(S): GPA 2.70; GRE 900; GRE V 450; GRE Q 450; GRE A 450; Interview.

Enrollment
- Community Counseling(M & S): 15 Admitted yearly; 15 Graduated yearly; 10 Female; 5 Male.
- School Counseling(M & S): 70 Admitted yearly; 45 Graduated yearly; 40 Female; 5 Male.

Diversity
- African-American; Asian-American; Caucasian; Multiracial.

Graduation

Requirements
- Community Counseling(M): 48 Class hours; 150 Practicum hours; 600 Internship hours; Comprehensive exam; CPCE.
- Community Counseling(S): 27 Class hours; VAR Internship hours; Oral exam.
- School Counseling(M): 48 Class hours; 100 Practicum hours; 600 Internship hours; Comprehensive exam; CPCE.
- School Counseling(S): 27 Class hours; VAR Internship hours; Oral exam.

Postgraduation activity: Advanced education and employment setting percentages.
- Community Counseling(M & S): 20 Advanced education; 5 Private practice; 75 Agency practice.
- School Counseling(M & S): 10 Advanced education; 30 Elementary school; 30 Middle school; 30 Secondary school.

Planned Program Modifications

Courses	Drop	Add
	• NP.	• Addictions
		• Advocacy
		• Grief Counseling
		• Eating Disorders.

Other	Decrease	Increase
	• NP.	• Number of On-Line Courses.

Related Programs Psychology

Faculty

 Percent of faculty reported with NCC certification: 33%.

Percent in professional counseling practice: NP.

Research interests   Research interests of faculty are broad, culminating in many publications and presentations. Faculty are actively involved with significant agendas, leadership positions, service, innovative teaching, and consultation.

Diversity   • African-American; Asian-American; Caucasian.

Name, Degree, Rank, State/National Credentials, % time devoted to program, email
- Boes, Susan R; PhD; Assoc.; LPC, NCC; >81%; *sboes@westga.edu*
- Charlesworth, John R; PhD; Assist.; Psychologist; >81%; *jcharles@westga.edu*
- Jackson, Constance M; EdD; Assist.; LPC, NCC; >81%; *mjacks@westga.edu*
- Painter, Linda C; PhD; Assoc.; LPC; >81%; *lpainter@westga.edu*
- Phillips, Paul L; EdD; Assoc.; 61-80%; *pphillip@westga.edu*
- Rolle, George E; PhD; Full Prof.; LPC; >81%; *grolle@westga.edu*
- Snow, Brent M; PhD; Full Prof.; LPC, NCC; >81%; *bsnow@westga.edu*
- Stanard, Rebecca A; PhD; Assoc.; LPC; >81%; *rstanard@westga.edu*
- Wulff, Mary B; PhD; Assoc.; 41-60%; *mwulff@westga.edu*
- Cao, Li; PhD; Assist.; 41-60%; *lcao@westga.edu*
- Nietfeld, John L; PhD; Assist.; 41-60%; *jnietfel@westga.edu*
- Smith, Cheri; PhD; Assist.; LPC, NCC; >81%; *cheris@westga.edu*

Has CHI SIGMA IOTA (International Counseling Society) chapter.

IA: Iowa State University

	N221 Lagomarcino Hall
	Ames, IA 50011-3195
	USA
Dean	Dean Walter Gmelch
Administrator	John M. Littrell, Program Coordinator
	Department Educational Leadership & Policy Studies
	(515) 294-5746, fax (515) 294-4941, jlittrel@iastate.edu,
	http://www.educ.iastate.edu/elps/coed/hmpg.htm

Key   See key for Data on Each Department (this section) on page 79.

Program

Accreditation   Regional Accreditation

Uniqueness   Our newly revised and innovative curriculum focuses on three major modules: (1) counseling individuals, (2) facilitating groups, and (3) enhancing schools and communities. Traditional counseling courses are infused into the three modules. The mission of school counseling at Iowa State University is to: (a) nurture the talents and strengths of counselors as educational leaders in their schools, (b) champion school counselors working in collaborative, learner-centered teams as they advocate for all students, and (c) encourage innovative and solution-focused approaches in meeting life's challenges.

Degrees   • School Counseling: M.

Contact   • School Counseling: M = John M. Littrell.

Admission and Graduation Data

Admission

Requirements   • School Counseling(M): GPA 3.20; 2 Years work experience; Interview.

Enrollment   • School Counseling(M): 12-15 Admitted yearly; 12-15 Graduated yearly; 20 Female; 10 Male.

Diversity   • African-American; Caucasian; Hispanic; Multiracial.

Graduation

Requirements   • School Counseling(M): 36-42 Class hours; 100 Practicum hours; 400 Internship hours; Oral exam; Portfolio.

Postgraduation activity: Advanced education and employment setting percentages.
   • School Counseling(M): 30 Elementary school; 20 Middle school; 50 Secondary school.

Planned Program Modifications

Courses	Drop	Add
	• NP.	• NP.

Other	Decrease	Increase
	• NP.	• Diversity Recruiting of Faculty
		• Diversity Recruiting of Students
		• Faculty FTE.

Related Programs Marriage and Family Therapists
                 Psychology

Faculty

nbcc   Percent of faculty reported with NCC certification: 75%.   **ncc**

Percent in professional counseling practice: 0%.

Research interests brief counseling, meaningful intergenerational connections, school counseling issues, body image, social and cultural issues

Diversity   • Caucasian.

Name, Degree, Rank, State/National Credentials, % time devoted to program, email
• Littrell, John M; EdD; Full Prof.; NCC; >81%; *jlittrel@iastate.edu*
• Bartlett, Jan R; PhD; Assist.; >81%; *jbartlet@iastate.edu*
• Kuhl, Jan; MS; Instructor; NCC; <21%; *kuhljan@yahoo.com*
• Bisignano, Penny; MS; Instructor; NCC; <21%; *pbisignano@aea11.k12.ia.us*

Has CHI SIGMA IOTA (International Counseling Society) chapter.

IA: The University of Iowa

338 Lindquist Center N.
Iowa City, IA 52242-1529
United States

Dean   Dean Sandra Bowman Damico, College of Education
Administrator Dennis R. Maki, Chairperson
          Department   Division of Co. Rehab & Stu Dev
                           (319) 335-5275, fax (319) 335-5921, dennis-maki@uiowa.edu,
                           http://coe164.education.uiowa.edu:8180/crsd/

Key   See key for Data on Each Department (this section) on page 79.

Program

Accreditation   Regional Accreditation, **CACREP:** Community Counseling, **CACREP:** Counselor Education
                   and Supervision, **CACREP:** School Counseling, **CACREP:** Student Affairs - Professional
                   Practice, CORE: Rehabilitation Counseling

CACREP

Uniqueness   NP.

Degrees   • Community Counseling: M.
                • School Counseling: M.
                • Rehabilitation Counseling: M, PhD.
                • Student Affairs: M, PhD.
                • Counselor Education: PhD.

Contact   • Community Counseling: M = Vilia M. Tarvydas.
                • School Counseling: M = David A. Jepsen.
                • Rehabilitation Counseling: M, D = Vilia Tarvydas.
                • Student Affairs: M, D = Elizabeth Whitt.
                • Counselor Education: D = David A.Jepsen.

Admission and Graduation Data

Admission

Requirements   • Community Counseling(M): GPA 3.00; GRE 1000; 1 Year work experience; Interview.
                • School Counseling(M): GPA 3.00; GRE 1000; Interview.
                • Rehabilitation Counseling(M): GPA 3.00; GRE 1000; GRE Q 0; 1 Year work experience;
                  Interview.
                • Rehabilitation Counseling(D): Masters and GPA 3.00; GRE 1100; 1 Year work experience.
                • Student Affairs(M): GPA 3.00; GRE 1000; 1 Year work experience; Interview.
                • Student Affairs(D): Masters and GPA 3.00; GRE 1100.
                • Counselor Education(D): Masters and GPA 3.00; GRE 1100.

Enrollment   • Community Counseling(M): 15 Admitted yearly; 15 Graduated yearly.
                • School Counseling(M): 20 Admitted yearly; 20 Graduated yearly; 25 Female; 5 Male.
                • Rehabilitation Counseling(M): 15 Admitted yearly; 15 Graduated yearly; 28 Female;
                  2 Male.
                • Rehabilitation Counseling(D): 3 Admitted yearly; 3 Graduated yearly; 6 Female; 3 Male.
                • Student Affairs(M): 15 Admitted yearly; 15 Graduated yearly; 12 Female; 3 Male.
                • Student Affairs(D): 4 Admitted yearly; 7 Female; 1 Male.
                • Counselor Education(D): 3 Admitted yearly; 3 Graduated yearly; 8 Female; 7 Male.

Diversity   • African-American; Caucasian; Hispanic; Multiracial.

Graduation

Requirements   • Community Counseling(M): 60 Class hours; 300 Practicum hours; 600 Internship hours;
                  Comprehensive exam.
                • School Counseling(M): 48-61 Class hours; 100 Practicum hours; 600 Internship hours;
                  Comprehensive exam; Portfolio.
                • Rehabilitation Counseling(M): 60 Class hours; 350 Practicum hours; 600 Internship hours;
                  Comprehensive exam.
                • Rehabilitation Counseling(D): 96 Class hours; 180 Practicum hours.
                • Student Affairs(M): 48 Class hours; 100 Practicum hours; 600 Internship hours.
                • Student Affairs(D): 96 Class hours; 180 Practicum hours; 600 Internship hours.
                • Counselor Education(D): 96 Class hours; 180 Practicum hours; 600 Internship hours;
                  Comprehensive exam; Oral exam; Dissertation.

Postgraduation activity: Advanced education and employment setting percentages.
                • Community Counseling(M): 10 Advanced education; 10 Managed care; 10 Private practice;
                  70 Agency practice.
                • School Counseling(M): 5 Advanced education; 60 Elementary school; 5 Middle school; 30
                  Secondary school.

- Rehabilitation Counseling(M): 10 Advanced education; 10 Managed care; 40 Private practice; 40 Agency practice.
- Rehabilitation Counseling(D): 10 Managed care; 10 Private practice; 20 Agency practice; 60 Student affairs.
- Student Affairs(M): 25 Advanced education; 75 Other.
- Student Affairs(D): 10 Private practice; 55 Student affairs; 35 Other.
- Counselor Education(D): 20 Private practice; 15 Agency practice; 65 Student affairs.

Planned Program Modifications

Courses	Drop	Add
	• NP.	• NP.

Other	Decrease Increase	
	• NP.	• Diversity Recruiting of Faculty
		• Diversity Recruiting of Students
		• Faculty FTE.

Related Programs Clinical Social Workers
Psychology
Psychiatric Nurses
Psychiatrists
Organizational
Behaviorists
Communications
International Studies

Faculty

 Percent of faculty reported with NCC certification: 14%.

Percent in professional counseling practice: 25%.

Research interests NP.

Diversity • African-American; Caucasian; Hispanic; Native American.

Name, Degree, Rank, State/National Credentials, % time devoted to program, email
- Claar, Joan; PhD; Adjunct; <21%;
- Cocco, Karen; PhD; Assist.; >81%; *karen-cocco@uiowa.edu*
- Colangelo, Nicholas; PhD; Full Prof.; <21%; *nick-colangelo@uiowa.edu*
- Watt, Sherry; PhD; Assist.; <21%; *sherry-watt@uiowa.edu*
- Eichinger, Leanne; MA; Lecturer; <21%; *leanne.eichinger@doc.state.ia.us*
- Grady, David; PhD; Adjunct; <21%; *david-grady@uiowa.edu*
- Grajeles, Elisa; PhD; Adjunct; <21%; *elisa-grajales@uiowa.edu*
- Harper, Dennis; PhD; Full Prof.; ABPP; <21%; *dennis-harper@uiowa.edu*
- Whitt, Elizabeth; PhD; Full Prof.; 41-60%; *elizabeth-whitt@uiowa.edu*
- Jepsen, David A; PhD; Full Prof.; >81%; *david-jepsen-@uiowa.edu*
- Liddell, Debora; EdD; Assoc.; >81%; *debora-liddell@uiowa.edu*
- Maki, Dennis R; PhD; Full Prof.; NCC, CRC,ACS,LMHC; >81%; *dennis-maki@uiowa.edu*
- Margolin, Leslie; PhD; Full Prof.; 41-60%; *leslie-margolin@uiowa.edu*
- Milsom, Amy; EdD; Assist.; NCC; >81%; *amy-milsom@uiowa.edu*
- O'Rourke, Barbara; PhD; Adjunct; <21%; *borouyke@blue.weeg.uiowa.edu*
- Pascarella, Ernie; PhD; Full Prof.; <21%; *ernest-pascarella@uiowa.edu*
- Portman, Tarrell; PhD; Assist.; NCC, LMHC; <21%; *tarrell-portman@uiowa.edu*
- Rosenthal, David; PhD; Assist.; <21%; *david-rosenthal@uiowa.edu*
- Tarvydas, Vilia; PhD; Full Prof.; CRC,LMHC; <21%; *vilia-tarvydas@uiowa.edu*
- Serrato, Carlos; MA; Adjunct; <21%; *carlos-serrato@uiowa.edu*
- Sims, Johnnie; PhD; Adjunct; <21%; *johnnie-sims@uiowa.edu*

Has CHI SIGMA IOTA (International Counseling Society) chapter.

IA: University of North Iowa

514 Schindler Ed Center, UNI
Cedar Falls, IA 50614-0604
United States

Dean   Dean William Callahan, Schindler Ed Center
Administrator   Ann Vernon, PhD, LMHC, NCC, Professor and Coordinator of Counseling
                    Department   Educational Leadership, Counseling and Postsecondary Education
                                      (319) 273-2605, fax (319) 273-5175, Ann.Vernon@uni.edu

Key   See key for Data on Each Department (this section) on page 79.

Program
Accreditation   Regional Accreditation, **CACREP:** Mental Health Counseling, **CACREP:** School Counseling

Uniqueness   • NP.

Degrees   • Mental Health Counseling: M.
                  • School Counseling: M.

Contact   • Mental Health Counseling: M = Dr. Ann Vernon.
                  • School Counseling: M = Dr. Ann Vernon.

Admission and Graduation Data
Admission
Requirements   • Mental Health Counseling(M): GPA 3.00; GRE NR.
                  • School Counseling(M): GPA 3.00; GRE NR.

Enrollment   • Mental Health Counseling(M): 30-40 Admitted yearly; 10-15 Graduated yearly; 40 Female;
                    30 Male.
                  • School Counseling(M): 30-40 Admitted yearly; 10-15 Graduated yearly; 60 Female;
                    15 Male.

Diversity   • African-American; Asian-American; Caucasian.

Graduation
Requirements   • Mental Health Counseling(M): 62 Class hours; 100 Practicum hours; 900 Internship hours;
                    Comprehensive exam; Thesis.
                  • School Counseling(M): 56 or 62 for nonteaching majors Class hours; 150 Practicum hours;
                    600 Internship hours; Comprehensive exam; Thesis.

Postgraduation activity: Advanced education and employment setting percentages.
                  • Mental Health Counseling(M): 2 Advanced education; 3 Managed care; 5 Private practice;
                    80 Agency practice; 10 Other.
                  • School Counseling(M): 40 Elementary school; 30 Middle school; 30 Secondary school.

Planned Program Modifications
Courses   Drop   Add
                  • NP.   • NP.

Other   Decrease   Increase
                  • NP.   • NP.

Related Programs

Faculty

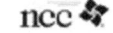   Percent of faculty reported with NCC certification: 60%.   ncc

Percent in professional counseling practice: 60%.

Research interests REBT, counseling children & adolescents, multicultural counseling, counseling theory,
            group work

Diversity   • Asian-American; Caucasian; Hispanic.

Name, Degree, Rank, State/National Credentials, % time devoted to program, email
• Clemente, Roberto; PhD; Assist.; >81%; *Roberto.Clemente@uni.edu*
• Murgatroyd, Wanpen; PhD; Assist.; >81%; *Wanpen.Murgatroyd@uni.edu*
• Halbur, Duane A; PhD; Assist.; NCC, LMHC; >81%; *Duane.Halbur@uni.edu*
• Vess, Kimberly A; PhD; Assist.; NCC, LMHC; >81%; *Kimberly.Vess@uni.edu*
• Vernon, Ann S; PhD; Full Prof.; NCC, LMHC; >81%; *Ann.Vernon@uni.edu*

ID: Boise State University

	1910 University Avenue, Education 612
	Boise, ID 83725
	USA
Dean	Dean Joyce Garrett, College of Education
Administrator	Dr. Ken Coll, Chair
	Department Counselor Education
	(208) 426-1219, kcoll@boisestate.edu, http://education.boisestate.edu/counseling

Key   See key for Data on Each Department (this section) on page 79.

Program
Accreditation   Regional Accreditation, **CACREP:** School Counseling

Uniqueness   60-credit degree focusing on School Counseling with optional Addiction Studies track, leading to state certification and/or licensure and addictions credentials. Courses offered primarily nights and weekends to accommodate employed persons. Companion Institution to The Education Trust counseling reform initiative.

Degrees   • School Counseling: M.

Contact   • School Counseling: M = Dr. Bobbie Birdsall.

Admission and Graduation Data
Admission
Requirements   • School Counseling(M): Interview.

Enrollment   • School Counseling(M): 15-18 Admitted yearly; 15-16 Graduated yearly; 32 Female; 19 Male.

Diversity   • African-American; Asian-American; Caucasian; Hispanic; Native American.

Graduation
Requirements   • School Counseling(M): 60 Class hours; 100 Practicum hours; 700 Internship hours; Comprehensive exam; Portfolio.

Postgraduation activity: Advanced education and employment setting percentages.
      • School Counseling(M): 10 Private practice; 15 Agency practice; 20 Elementary school; 30 Middle school; 15 Secondary school; 10 Other.

Planned Program Modifications

Courses	Drop	Add
	• NP.	• Computer and Related Technology.

Other	Decrease	Increase
	• NP.	• Number of Distance Education Courses
		• Number of Off-Campus Courses
		• Number of On-Line Courses.

Related Programs Clinical Social Workers
                         Communications
                         Other

Faculty

nbcc ✦   Percent of faculty reported with NCC certification: 75%.   ncc ✦

Percent in professional counseling practice: 100%.

Research interests Birdsall (NCC, NCSC, LPCP) research areas are family counseling in school settings, spirituality in counseling and school counseling reform. She is an appointed member of the Idaho Licensure Board. Coll (NCC, LPCP) research areas are addictions prevention, effective assessment and interventions for adolescents, and outcome based evaluation. He is a successful grant writer in Addictions Studies. Miller (NCC, NCSC, LPC, LCPC) research areas are equity and ethical practice in a multicultural society and the role of counselors in education reform. She is an appointed member of the Idaho Counseling Advisory Committee. Nelson (LPC) research areas are story telling and mythology as tools in counseling. She is current president of the Idaho Psychological Association.

Diversity   •   Caucasian.

Name, Degree, Rank, State/National Credentials, % time devoted to program, email
*   Birdsall, Bobbie; PhD; Assoc.; LPC, NCC; >81%; *bbirdsa@boisestate.edu*
*   Coll, Ken M; PhD; Full Prof.; LPC, NCC; 41-60%; *kcoll@boisestate.edu*
*   Miller, Maggie; PhD; Full Prof.; LPC, NCC; >81%; *mmiller@boisestate.edu*
*   Nelson, AnneMarie; PhD; Assoc.; LPC; >81%; *anelson@boisestate.edu*

Has CHI SIGMA IOTA (International Counseling Society) chapter.

ID: Idaho State University

	ISU Box 8120 Pocatello, ID 83209 8120 USA
Dean	L.C. Hatzenbueller Dean, Kasiska College of Health Professions
Administrator	Stephen S. Feit, Chair
	Department Dept. of Counseling
	(208) 282-3156, fax (208) 282-2583, lemmcher@isu.edu, www.isu.edu/hpcounsl

Key   See key for Data on Each Department (this section) on page 79.

Program

Accreditation   Regional Accreditation, **CACREP:** Counselor Education and Supervision, **CACREP:** Marriage and Family Counseling, **CACREP:** Mental Health Counseling, **CACREP:** School Counseling, **CACREP:** Student Affairs - Counseling

Uniqueness   All programs CACREP approved (School Counseling, Mental Health Counseling, Marriage and Family, Student Affairs and College Counseling, Doctoral program).

Degrees
- Mental Health Counseling: M.
- School Counseling: M.
- Marriage and Family Counseling: M.
- Student Affairs: M.
- Counselor Education: PhD.

Contact
- Mental Health Counseling: M = Dr Nicole Hill.
- School Counseling: M = Dr Virginia Allen.
- Marriage and Family Counseling: M = Dr David Kleist.
- Student Affairs: M = Dr Don Paulson.
- Counselor Education: D = Dr Stephen Feit.

Admission and Graduation Data

Admission

Requirements
- Mental Health Counseling(M): GPA 3.00; MAT 42; Interview.
- School Counseling(M): GPA 3.00; MAT 42; Interview.
- Marriage and Family Counseling(M): GPA 3.00; MAT 42; Interview.
- Student Affairs(M): GPA 3.00; MAT 42; Interview.
- Counselor Education(D): MAT 42.

Enrollment
- Mental Health Counseling(M): 10 Admitted yearly; 10 Graduated yearly; 14 Female; 6 Male.
- School Counseling(M): 10 Admitted yearly; 10 Graduated yearly; 14 Female; 6 Male.
- Marriage and Family Counseling(M): 10 Admitted yearly; 10 Graduated yearly; 14 Female; 6 Male.
- Student Affairs(M): 3 Admitted yearly; 3 Graduated yearly; 1 Female; 2 Male.
- Counselor Education(D): 4 Admitted yearly; 4 Graduated yearly; 7 Female; 3 Male.

Diversity
- African-American; Asian-American; Caucasian; Hispanic; Native American; Other.

Graduation

Requirements
- Mental Health Counseling(M): 60 Class hours; 150 Practicum hours; 850 Internship hours; Comprehensive exam; Oral exam.
- School Counseling(M): 48 Class hours; 150 Practicum hours; 600 Internship hours; Comprehensive exam; Oral exam.
- Marriage and Family Counseling(M): 64 Class hours; 150 Practicum hours; 850 Internship hours; Oral exam.
- Student Affairs(M): 48 Class hours; 150 Practicum hours; 600 Internship hours; Oral exam.
- Counselor Education(D): 96 Class hours; 150 Practicum hours; 1000 Internship hours; Comprehensive exam; Dissertation.

Postgraduation activity: Advanced education and employment setting percentages.
- Mental Health Counseling(M): 10 Advanced education; 90 Agency practice.
- School Counseling(M): 10 Advanced education; 40 Elementary school; 40 Middle school; 20 Secondary school.
- Marriage and Family Counseling(M): 10 Advanced education; 90 Agency practice.
- Student Affairs(M): 100 Other.
- Counselor Education(D): 90 Advanced education; 10 Private practice.

Planned Program Modifications

Courses   Drop   Add
                                    •   NP.   •   Addictions
                                                                 •   Play Therapy.

Other   Decrease   Increase
                                    •   NP.   •   Course Offerings.

Related Programs Psychology

Faculty

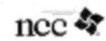 nbcc   Percent of faculty reported with NCC certification: 63%.   ncc

Percent in professional counseling practice: 20%.

Research interests •   NP.

Diversity   •   NP.

Name, Degree, Rank, State/National Credentials, % time devoted to program, email
•   Allen, Virginia; EdD; Full Prof.; LPC, NCC; >81%; *Allevirg@isu.edu*
•   Feit, Stephen; EdD; Full Prof.; LPC, NCC; >81%; *Feitstep@isu.edu*
•   Hill, Nicole; PhD; Assist.; LPC; >81%; *Hillnico@isu.edu*
•   Crews, Judith; PhD; Assist.; LPC, NCC; >81%; *Crewj@isu.edu*
•   Kleist, David; PhD; Assoc.; LPC, NCC; >81%; *Kleidavi@isu.edu*
•   Paulson, Don; PhD; Assist.; LPC; <21%; *Pauldona@isu.edu*
•   Singarajah, Thana; EdD; Assist.; LPC; 41-60%; *Singthan@isu.edu*
•   Stinchfield, Tracy; EdD; Assist.; LPC, NCC; >81%; *Stintrac@isu.edu*

Has CHI SIGMA IOTA (International Counseling Society) chapter.

ID: Northwest Nazarene University

	623 Holly St.
	Nampa, ID 83686
	USA
Dean	Dennis Cartwright, Dean of School of Applied Studies
Administrator	Brenda Freeman, Program Head, Counseling
	Department Education
	(208) 467-8345, fax (208) 467-8339, bdkrohn@nnu.edu, www.nnu.edu

Key   See key for Data on Each Department (this section) on page 79.

Program
Accreditation   Regional Accreditation, **CACREP:** School Counseling

Uniqueness   NNU is a liberal arts institution with a commitment to a service orientation toward students and academic excellence.

Degrees   • School Counseling: M.

Contact   • School Counseling: M = Brenda Freeman.

Admission and Graduation Data
Admission
Requirements   • School Counseling(M): GPA 3.00; Interview.

Enrollment   • School Counseling(M): 13 Admitted yearly; 10 Graduated yearly; 10 Male.

Diversity   • Asian-American; Caucasian; Hispanic.

Graduation
Requirements   • School Counseling(M): 53 Class hours; 200 Practicum hours; 600 Internship hours; Comprehensive exam; Portfolio.

Postgraduation activity: Advanced education and employment setting percentages.
• School Counseling(M): 40 Elementary school; 35 Middle school; 18 Secondary school; 7 Other.

Planned Program Modifications
Courses	Drop	Add
	• NP.	• Adventure Counseling
		• Career/Life Planning
		• Human Sexuality
		• Marriage and Family Counseling
		• Play Therapy.

Other	Decrease	Increase
	• NP.	• Course Offerings
		• Faculty FTE
		• Number of Degree Majors.

Related Programs Clinical Social Workers

Faculty

nbcc ✲   Percent of faculty reported with NCC certification: 57%.   ncc ✲

Percent in professional counseling practice: NP.

Research interests Research and service related to mental health projects for Native American youth and families; play therapy; Adlerian approaches to working with children; strategies of clinical supervision.

Diversity   • Caucasian; Hispanic.

Name, Degree, Rank, State/National Credentials, % time devoted to program, email
• Townsend, Darlene C; EdD; Full Prof.; LPC, NCC, IMFC; >81%; *dctownsend@nnu.edu*
• Craig, Dick R; EdD; Full Prof.; LPC, NCC, IMFC; >81%; *rdcraig@nnu.edu*
• Hills, Ken D; PhD; Full Prof.; 22-40%; *kdhills@nnu.edu*
• Freeman, Brenda J; PhD; Full Prof.; LPC, NCC; >81%; *bjfreeman@nnu.edu*
• Riley, Riley D; MSW; Instructor; lsw; <21%; *rosiedr@aol.com*
• Filer, Steve; MEd; Instructor; LPC, NCC, CADC; <21%; *filers@meridianschools.org*
• Thuerer, John; PhD; Instructor; LPC; <21%; *jthuerer@albertsons.edu*

Has CHI SIGMA IOTA (International Counseling Society) chapter.

ID: University of Idaho

P.O. BOX 303
Moscow, ID 83844-3083
US

Dean Dr. Jeanne Christiansen, College of Education
Administrator Dr. Jim Gregson, Division Director
Department   Adult, Counselor and Technology Education
(208) 885-2768, fax (208) 885-6869, jfischer@uidaho.edu

Key   See key for Data on Each Department (this section) on page 79.

Program
Accreditation   Regional Accreditation

Uniqueness   The University of Idaho Counseling and School Psychology Program provide two very unique degrees. The School Counseling/School Psychology degree which allows students to pursue both areas in a school setting. The Rehabilitation/Community Counseling degree which prepares students to be Certified Rehabilitation Counselors and Licensed Professional Counselors in Idaho.

Degrees
- Community Counseling: M, S.
- School Counseling: M, S.
- Other: M, S.
- Rehabilitation Counseling: M, S.
- Counselor Education: PhD.

Contact
- Community Counseling: M, S = NP.
- School Counseling: M = Dr. Tom Fairchild.; S = NP.
- Other: M = Dr. Tom Fairchild.; S = NP.
- Rehabilitation Counseling: M = Dr. Jerry Fischer.; S = NP.
- Counselor Education: D = Dr. Tom Trotter.

Admission and Graduation Data
Admission
Requirements
- Community Counseling(M): GPA 3.00; Interview.
- Community Counseling(S): GPA 3.00; Interview.
- School Counseling(M): GPA 3.00; Interview.
- School Counseling(S): GPA 3.00; Interview.
- Other(M): GPA 3.00; Interview.
- Other(S): GPA 3.00; Interview.
- Rehabilitation Counseling(M): GPA 3.00; Interview.
- Rehabilitation Counseling(S): GPA 3.00; Interview.
- Counselor Education(D): Masters and GPA 3.50; GRE 1100; GRE V 550; GRE Q 550.

Enrollment
- Community Counseling(M & S): 6 Admitted yearly.
- School Counseling(M & S): 6 Admitted yearly.
- Other(M & S): 12 Admitted yearly.
- Rehabilitation Counseling(M & S): 6 Admitted yearly.
- Counselor Education(D): NP.

Diversity
- African-American; Asian-American; Caucasian; Hispanic; Native American.

Graduation
Requirements
- Community Counseling(M): 60 Class hours; 100 Practicum hours; 900 Internship hours; Oral exam; Portfolio.
- Community Counseling(S): 72 Class hours; Comprehensive exam.
- School Counseling(M): 60 Class hours; 100 Practicum hours; 900 Internship hours; Oral exam; Portfolio.
- School Counseling(S): 72 Class hours; Comprehensive exam.
- Other(M): 60 Class hours; 100 Practicum hours; 900 Internship hours; Oral exam; Portfolio.
- Other(S): 72 Class hours; Comprehensive exam.
- Rehabilitation Counseling(M): 60 Class hours; 100 Practicum hours; 900 Internship hours; Oral exam; Portfolio.
- Rehabilitation Counseling(S): 72 Class hours; Comprehensive exam.
- Counselor Education(D): 124 Class hours; 100 Practicum hours; 500 Internship hours; CPCE; Dissertation.

Postgraduation activity: Advanced education and employment setting percentages.
- Community Counseling(M & S): 100 Advanced education; 100 Agency practice.
- School Counseling(M & S): 100 Advanced education; 30 Elementary school; 30 Middle school; 30 Secondary school.
- Other(M & S): 100 Advanced education; 30 Middle school; 30 Secondary school; 30 Student affairs.
- Rehabilitation Counseling(M & S): 100 Advanced education; 100 Agency practice.
- Counselor Education(D): 100 Private practice.

Planned Program Modifications

Courses | Drop | Add
- NP. | - NP.

Other | Decrease | Increase
- NP. | - NP.

Related Programs

Faculty

 Percent of faculty reported with NCC certification: 0%. ncc

Percent in professional counseling practice: 20%.

Research interests Multicultural counseling, Ethics, Parents of Children with Disabilities, School Psychologist Accountability hypnotherapy, youth at risk

Diversity • Caucasian; Hispanic.

Name, Degree, Rank, State/National Credentials, % time devoted to program, email
- Trotter, Thomas; PhD; Full Prof.; 41-60%; *trotter@uidaho.edu*
- Fairchild, Thomas; PhD; Full Prof.; >81%; *thomasf@uidaho.edu*
- Biller, Ernest; PhD; Assoc.; >81%; *ernieb@uidaho.edu*
- Fischer, Jerry; PhD; Full Prof.; LPC, CRC; >81%; *jfischer@uidaho.edu*
- Ortiz, Deanna; MS; Instructor; LPC; *dortiz@uidaho.edu*

IL: College of Arts and Sciences (CAS)-National Louis University

	200 S. Naperville Road
	Wheaton, IL 60187-5422
	USA
Dean	Dr. Martha Cazazza (CAS) 122 S. Michigan Ave. Chicago, IL 60603
Administrator	Susan Thorne-Devin, Department Chair
	Department Human Services
	(630) 668-3838, fax (630) 668-5883

Key See key for Data on Each Department (this section) on page 79.

Program

Accreditation   Regional Accreditation

Uniqueness   Program is located on 5 campuses throughout Chicago Area to meet the needs of adult, non-traditional students who are working and returning to school; program ephasizes adult learning model of education; cohort delivery model holds classes one night a week; classroom model of teaching is diadectic and experiential building on students professional work experiences and personal life experiences; mulitdisciplinary faculty; philosophy of program; strong multicultural and family system approach; certificates in Career Counseling(21-24SH); Community Wellness and Prevention (18SH); Counseling Studies for Psychology Students (18-24 SH)

Degrees
- Community Counseling: M.
- Gerontological Counseling: M.
- Other: M.

Contact
- Community Counseling: M = Susan Thorne-Devin.
- Gerontological Counseling: M = Jim Ellor.
- Other: M = Pat McGrath/Community Wellness and Janice Guerriero/Career Counseling.

Admission and Graduation Data

Admission

Requirements
- Community Counseling(M): GPA 3.00; Interview.
- Gerontological Counseling(M): GPA 3.00; Interview.
- Other(M): GPA 3.00; Interview.

Enrollment
- Community Counseling(M): 120 Admitted yearly; 60 Graduated yearly; 100 Female; 20 Male.
- Gerontological Counseling(M): 10 Admitted yearly; 5 Graduated yearly; 10 Female.
- Other(M): 10 Admitted yearly; 5 Graduated yearly; 10 Female.

Diversity
- African-American; Asian-American; Caucasian; Hispanic; Multiracial.

Graduation

Requirements
- Community Counseling(M): 48 Class hours; 600 Internship hours; CPCE; Portfolio.
- Gerontological Counseling(M): 48 Class hours; 600 Internship hours; CPCE; Portfolio.
- Other(M): 48 Class hours; 600 Internship hours; CPCE; Portfolio.

Postgraduation activity: Advanced education and employment setting percentages.
- Community Counseling(M): 10 Advanced education; 10 Managed care; 5 Private practice; 65 Agency practice; 10 Elementary school.
- Gerontological Counseling(M): 5 Advanced education; 15 Managed care; 5 Private practice; 75 Agency practice; 5 Elementary school.
- Other(M): 5 Advanced education; 10 Managed care; 80 Agency practice; 5 Elementary school.

Planned Program Modifications

Courses	Drop	Add
	• NP.	• Abuse of Individual
		• Consultation
		• Diversity
		• Gender Studies
		• Grief Counseling
		• Life Coaching
		• Play Therapy
		• School Counseling
		• Special Needs Populations
		• Supervision
		• Teaming.

Other	Decrease	Increase
	• NP.	• Course Offerings
		• Diversity Recruiting of Faculty
		• Faculty FTE
		• Graduation Requirements
		• National Accreditation
		• Number of Off-Campus Courses.

Related Programs Other

Faculty

nbcc Percent of faculty reported with NCC certification: 31%. **ncc**

Percent in professional counseling practice: 50%.

Research interests Gender-sensitive counseling; LGBT Issues -current project: Interviewing lesbian widows about their experiences; Clinical Supervision -developing workshops for supervisors; Domestic Abuse; Post-traumatic Stress, and the impact of September 11th International Children's Study - fears of children and how children manage their fears; On-line teaching; Career Counseling; Executive Coaching; Adapting Career Assessments for Diverse Client Needs; Gerontology - Assessment of Needs of the Aging; Grief Counseling; Community Wellness; Assessment - Reviewing of Course Evaluations; EMDR School Counseling; Human Services Administration

Diversity   • Caucasian.

Name, Degree, Rank, State/National Credentials, % time devoted to program, email
• Bracki, Marie; PsyD; Assoc.; NCC, LCPC;NCSP; ACS; 41-60%; *mbracki@nl.ewdu*
• Bracki, Robert; MS; Assist.; <21%; *rbraqcki@nl.edu*
• Clemmer, Chris; DMin; Assoc.; <21%; *cclemmer@nl.edu*
• Ellor, James; PhD; Full Prof.; LCSW;DCSW; >81%; *jellor@nl.edu*
• Frankel, Penina; PhD; Assoc.; NCC, LCPC; *pfrankel@nl.edu*
• Guerriero, Janice; PhD; Assoc.; NCC, LCPC;NCCC;CSW;CADC;ACS; >81%; *jguerriero@nl.edu*
• Kerstein, Susan; MSW; Assoc.; LSW; 22-40%; *skerstein@nl,edu*
• Lanni-Ruggeri, Judith; MSW; Assist.; LSW; 41-60%; *jlruggeri@nl.edu*
• McGrath, Patrick; EdD; Full Prof.; NCC, AAMFT; >81%; *PMcGrath@nl.edu*
• Nesbitt, Sue; PhD; Assoc.; LCSW;LCPC; >81%; *snesbitt@nl.edu*
• Tarnoff, Eileen; MA; Assist.; LCSW;ACSW; BCD; >81%; *etarnoff@nl.edu*
• Thorne-Devin, Susan; MSW; Assist.; LCSW; >81%; *stdevin@nl.edu*
• Whipple, Vicky; EdD; Assoc.; LCPC;ACS; >81%; *vwhipple@nl.edu*

IL: Concordia University

7400 Augusta
River Forest, IL 60305
USA
Dean   Dr. Marvin Bartell, Dean College of Arts and Science
Administrator   Dr. Michael Smith, Department Chair
Department   Psychology (708) 209-3448, fax (708) 209-3176, www.curf.edu

Key   See key for Data on Each Department (this section) on page 79.

Program
Accreditation   Regional Accreditation, **CACREP:** Community Counseling, **CACREP:** School Counseling

Uniqueness

Degrees   • Community Counseling: M.
          • School Counseling: M.

Contact   • Community Counseling: M = Dr. Michael Smith.
          • School Counseling: M = Dr. Dale J. Septeowski.

Admission and Graduation Data
Admission
Requirements   • Community Counseling(M): GPA 3.00.
               • School Counseling(M): GPA 3.00.

Enrollment   • Community Counseling(M): 15 Admitted yearly; 7 Graduated yearly.
             • School Counseling(M): 7 Admitted yearly; 3 Graduated yearly.

Diversity   • African-American; Asian-American; Caucasian; Hispanic; Native American.

Graduation
Requirements   • Community Counseling(M): 48 Class hours; 100 Practicum hours; 600 Internship hours; Comprehensive exam; Oral exam.
               • School Counseling(M): 48 Class hours; 100 Practicum hours; 600 Internship hours; Oral exam; Portfolio.

Postgraduation activity: Advanced education and employment setting percentages.
               • Community Counseling(M): 10 Advanced education; 90 Agency practice.
               • School Counseling(M): 10 Elementary school; 10 Middle school; 80 Secondary school.

Planned Program Modifications
Courses   Drop   Add
                   • NP.   • NP.

Other   Decrease   Increase
                   • Faculty FTE.
                   • Number of Off-Campus Courses.

Related Programs

Faculty

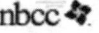   Percent of faculty reported with NCC certification: 20%.

Percent in professional counseling practice: 75%.

Research interests NP.

Diversity   • Asian-American; Caucasian.

Name, Degree, Rank, State/National Credentials, % time devoted to program, email
• Septeowski, Dale J; EdD; Full Prof.; LPC, NCC; >81%; *crfsepteodj@curf.edu*
• Smith, Michael; PhD; Assoc.; LCPC; 61-80%;
• Rahn, Julia; PhD; Assist.; 41-60%;
• Patrick, Shawn; EdD; Assist.; 22-40%;
• Bekenbach, John; EdD; Assist.; 22-40%;

IL: Eastern Illinois University

	600 Lincoln Ave.
	Charleston, IL 61920-3099
	United States
Dean	Charles Rohn, College of Education and Professional Studies
Administrator	Richard L. Roberts, Ph.D., Chair
	Department Department of Counseling and Student Development
	(217) 581-2400, fax (217) 581-7800, cfrlr@eiu.edu, www.eiu.edu/~eiucsd

Key   See key for Data on Each Department (this section) on page 79.

Program

Accreditation   Regional Accreditation, **CACREP:** Community Counseling, **CACREP:** School Counseling

Uniqueness   The Department of Counseling and Student Development has a collegial faculty dedicated to training counselors for the 21st century.

Degrees
- Community Counseling: M.
- School Counseling: M.

Contact
- Community Counseling: M = Dr. Roberts.
- School Counseling: M = Dr. Roberts.

Admission and Graduation Data

Admission

Requirements
- Community Counseling(M): GPA 2.75; Interview.
- School Counseling(M): GPA 2.75; Interview.

Enrollment
- Community Counseling(M): 20 Admitted yearly; 20 Graduated yearly.
- School Counseling(M): 20 Admitted yearly; 20 Graduated yearly.

Diversity
- African-American; Asian-American; Caucasian; Hispanic; Multiracial.

Graduation

Requirements
- Community Counseling(M): 48 Class hours; 100 Practicum hours; 600 Internship hours; Comprehensive exam.
- School Counseling(M): 48 Class hours; 100 Practicum hours; 600 Internship hours; Comprehensive exam.

Postgraduation activity: Advanced education and employment setting percentages.
- Community Counseling(M): 5 Advanced education; 90 Agency practice; 5 Other.
- School Counseling(M): 10 Elementary school; 15 Middle school; 70 Secondary school.

Planned Program Modifications

Courses	Drop		Add
	• NP.		• NP.

Other	Decrease		Increase
	• NP.		• Diversity Recruiting of Students
			• Number of On-Line Courses.

Related Programs Psychology

Faculty

 Percent of faculty reported with NCC certification: 20%.   ncc

Percent in professional counseling practice: 10%.

Research interests Multiculturalism and technology.

Diversity
- African-American; Caucasian.

Name, Degree, Rank, State/National Credentials, % time devoted to program, email
- Conn, Steve; PhD; Assist.; >81%; *cfscr@eiu.edu*
- Eberly, Charles G; PhD; Full Prof.; 22-40%; *cfcge@eiu.edu*
- Fraker, French L; PhD; Full Prof.; NCC; >81%; *cfflf@eiu.edu*
- Kaser, Lynda L; EdD; Full Prof.; NCC; >81%; *cflk2@eiu.edu*
- Leitschuh, Gloria A; PhD; Full Prof.; >81%; *cfgl@eiu.edu*

- Lyles, Judith W; EdD; Full Prof.; >81%; *cfjll@eiu.edu*
- Farber, Nancy; PhD; Assist.; >81%; *cfkem@eiu.edu*
- Powell, Barbara M; PhD; Assoc.; 61-80%; *cfbmp@eiu.edu*
- Roberts, Richard L; PhD; Full Prof.; *cfrlr@eiu.edu*
- Wallace, James A; PhD; Assist.; <21%; *cfkfw@eiu.edu*

Has CHI SIGMA IOTA (International Counseling Society) chapter.

IL: Illinois Institute of Technology

3101 S. Dearborn St.
Chicago, IL 60616
USA

Dean Dr. Ellen M. Mitchell/Psychology
Administrator Dr. Chow S. Lam, Professor/Program Director
Department   Institute of Psychology
(312) 567-3515, fax (312) 567-3493, Lam@iit.edu,
http://www.iit.edu/colleges/psych/

Key See key for Data on Each Department (this section) on page 79.

Program

Accreditation Regional Accreditation, CORE: Rehabilitation Counseling

Uniqueness A CORE accredited 60-hour program training students as rehabilitation counselors to work with persons with disabilities. Graduates are eligible to become CRC and LPC in Illinois. Scholarships are available for qualified students, especially for students with disabilities and minorities.

Degrees • Rehabilitation Counseling: M, PhD.

Contact • Rehabilitation Counseling: M, D = Dr. Chow S. Lam.

Admission and Graduation Data
Admission
Requirements • Rehabilitation Counseling(M): GPA 3.00; Interview.
 • Rehabilitation Counseling(D): Masters and GPA 3.50; GRE 1000.

Enrollment • Rehabilitation Counseling(M): 15 Admitted yearly; 12 Graduated yearly; 12 Female; 3 Male.
 • Rehabilitation Counseling(D): 3 Admitted yearly; 2 Graduated yearly; 2 Female; 1 Male.

Diversity • African-American; Asian-American; Caucasian; Hispanic.

Graduation
Requirements • Rehabilitation Counseling(M): 60 Class hours; 200 Practicum hours; 600 Internship hours; Thesis.
 • Rehabilitation Counseling(D): 110 Class hours; 900 Practicum hours; 2000 Internship hours; Oral exam; Dissertation.

Postgraduation activity: Advanced education and employment setting percentages.
 • Rehabilitation Counseling(M): 100 Agency practice.
 • Rehabilitation Counseling(D):

Planned Program Modifications

Courses	Drop	Add
	• NP.	• NP.

Other	Decrease	Increase
	• NP.	• NP.

Related Programs Psychology

Faculty

nbcc Percent of faculty reported with NCC certification: 0%.   **ncc**

Percent in professional counseling practice: NP.

Research interests Vocational rehabilitation, rehabilitation for persons with TBI, chronic mental illness, assistive technology, cross-cultural rehabilitation counseling, psychosocial adjustment of disability and chronic illness, stages of change and treatment matching, QOL of persons with disabilities.

Diversity • Asian-American; Caucasian.

Name, Degree, Rank, State/National Credentials, % time devoted to program, email
• Bard, Christine; PhD; Assist.; >81%; *bard@iit.edu*
• Geist, Glen O; PhD; Full Prof.; CRC; >81%; *geist@iit.edu*
• Hilburger, John; PhD; Assist.; LPC, CRC; >81%; *hilburger@iit.edu*
• Lam, Chow S; PhD; Full Prof.; LPC, CRC; >81%; *Lam@iit.edu*
• Merbitz, Charles; PhD; Assoc.; CRC; >81%; *cmerbitz@iit.edu*

IL: Lewis University

	One University Parkway
	Romeoville, IL 60446
	USA
Dean	Acting Dean Angela Durante
Administrator	Edmund M. Kearney, Ph.D., Graduate Program Director
	Department Psychology
	(815) 836-5594, www.lewisu.edu

Key   See key for Data on Each Department (this section) on page 79.

Program
Accreditation   Regional Accreditation

Uniqueness   Our counseling program provides a skill based training program for individuals who want to work with children, adolescents, or adults in mental health and educational setting.

Degrees
- Community Counseling: M.
- Mental Health Counseling: M.
- School Counseling: M.

Contact
- Community Counseling: M = Edmund Kearney.
- Mental Health Counseling: M = Ann Barich.
- School Counseling: M = Richard Guerra.

Admission and Graduation Data
Admission
Requirements
- Community Counseling(M): GPA 3.00.
- Mental Health Counseling(M): GPA 3.00.
- School Counseling(M): GPA 3.00.

Enrollment
- Community Counseling(M): 15 Admitted yearly; 7 Graduated yearly; 90% Female; 10% Male.
- Mental Health Counseling(M): 15 Admitted yearly; 7 Graduated yearly; 90% Female; 10% Male.
- School Counseling(M): 40 Admitted yearly; 20 Graduated yearly; 75% Female; 25% Male.

Diversity
- African-American; Asian-American; Caucasian; Hispanic; Multiracial.

Graduation
Requirements
- Community Counseling(M): 48 Class hours; 100 Practicum hours; 600 Internship hours; Comprehensive exam; Portfolio.
- Mental Health Counseling(M): 48 Class hours; 100 Practicum hours; 600 Internship hours; Comprehensive exam; Portfolio.
- School Counseling(M): 40 Class hours; 100 Practicum hours; 300 Internship hours; Comprehensive exam.

Postgraduation activity: Advanced education and employment setting percentages.
- Community Counseling(M): 5 Advanced education; 10 Private practice; 50 Agency practice; 5 Student affairs; 30 Other.
- Mental Health Counseling(M): 5 Advanced education; 10 Private practice; 50 Agency practice; 5 Student affairs; 30 Other.
- School Counseling(M): 5 Elementary school; 5 Middle school; 90 Secondary school.

Planned Program Modifications
Courses	Drop	Add
	• NP.	• Consultation
		• Internet Use
		• Play Therapy
		• Supervision.

| Other | Decrease | Increase |
| | • NP. | • Faculty FTE. |

Related Programs

Faculty

nbcc ❖   Percent of faculty reported with NCC certification: 0%.   ncc ❖

Percent in professional counseling practice: 50%.

Research interests ADHD; Professional Identity; Teaching; Work-Family Conflict; Multicultural Issues in Training and education

Diversity   • African-American; Asian-American; Caucasian.

Name, Degree, Rank, State/National Credentials, % time devoted to program, email
- Kearney, Edmund; PhD; Full Prof.; Clinical Psychologist-Illinois; 61-80%; *kearneed@lewisu.edu*
- Barich, Ann; PhD; Assoc.; Psychologist-Wisconsin; 41-60%; *barichan@lewisu.edu*
- Helm, Katherine; PhD; Assist.; 41-60%; *helmka@lewisu.edu*
- Guerra, Richard; PhD; Assoc.; Clinical Psychologist-Illinois and CSC; 61-80%; *guerrari@lewisu.edu*
- Vandendorpe, Mary; PhD; Full Prof.; 22-40%;
- Sheffer, Susan; PhD; Assist.; <21%;

IL: Southern Illinois University Carbondale

EPSE, SIUC
Carbondale, IL 62901-4618
USA

Dean   Keith Hillkirk, Wham 115
Administrator   Karen K. Prichard, Coordinator
                    Department   Educational Psychology & Special Education
                                  (618) 536-7763, fax (618) 453-7110, lwhite@siu.edu,
                                  http://www.siu.edu/departments/coe/epse/

Key   See key for Data on Each Department (this section) on page 79.

Program

Accreditation   Regional Accreditation, **CACREP:** Community Counseling, **CACREP:** Counselor Education
                and Supervision, **CACREP:** Marriage and Family Counseling, **CACREP:** School Counseling

CACREP

Uniqueness   A Masters with a 3.5 GPA or a GRE (V+Q) of 1000 is required for admission to the counselor
                education doctoral program.

Degrees   • Community Counseling: M.
                • School Counseling: M.
                • Marriage and Family Counseling: M.
                • Counselor Education: PhD.

Contact   • Community Counseling: M = Dr. Kim Asner-Self.
                • School Counseling: M = Dr. David Duys.
                • Marriage and Family Counseling: M = Dr. Jane Cox.
                • Counselor Education: D = Dr. Karen Prichard.

Admission and Graduation Data

Admission

Requirements   • Community Counseling(M): GPA 2.70.
                • School Counseling(M): GPA 2.70.
                • Marriage and Family Counseling(M): GPA 2.70.
                • Counselor Education(D): NP.

Enrollment   • Community Counseling(M): 15 Admitted yearly; 13 Graduated yearly; 12 Female; 3 Male.
                • School Counseling(M): 20 Admitted yearly; 18 Graduated yearly; 19 Female; 1 Male.
                • Marriage and Family Counseling(M): 12 Admitted yearly; 6 Graduated yearly; 10 Female;
                  2 Male.
                • Counselor Education(D): 10 Admitted yearly; 8 Graduated yearly; 15 Female; 3 Male.

Diversity   • African-American; Asian-American; Caucasian; Hispanic; Native American; Other.

Graduation

Requirements   • Community Counseling(M): 48 Class hours; 100 Practicum hours; 600 Internship hours;
                  Comprehensive exam.
                • School Counseling(M): 48 Class hours; 100 Practicum hours; 600 Internship hours;
                  Comprehensive exam.
                • Marriage and Family Counseling(M): 60 Class hours; 150 Practicum hours; 600 Internship
                  hours.
                • Counselor Education(D): 80 Class hours; 180 Practicum hours; 600 Internship hours;
                  Comprehensive exam; Dissertation.

Postgraduation activity: Advanced education and employment setting percentages.
                • Community Counseling(M): 20 Advanced education; 10 Private practice; 50 Agency
                  practice; 10 Other.
                • School Counseling(M): 10 Advanced education; 5 Other.
                • Marriage and Family Counseling(M): 20 Advanced education; 10 Private practice; 70
                  Agency practice.
                • Counselor Education(D): 75 Advanced education; 5 Private practice; 10 Agency practice;
                  10 Other.

Planned Program Modifications

Courses   Drop   Add
                           • NP.   • NP.

Other   Decrease   Increase
                           • NP.   • Number of Off-Campus Courses.

Related Programs Clinical Social Workers
Psychology
Other

Faculty

nbcc ❧ Percent of faculty reported with NCC certification: 83%. ncc ❧

Percent in professional counseling practice: 0%.

Research interests Multicultural counseling, supervision, group work, constructive developmental approaches to school counseling.

Diversity • Caucasian.

Name, Degree, Rank, State/National Credentials, % time devoted to program, email
- Asner-Self, Kimberly K; EdD; Assist.; LPC, NCC; >81%; *kasner@siu.edu*
- Cox, Jane A; PhD; Assist.; NCC; >81%; *janecox@siu.edu*
- Duys, David K; PhD; Assist.; LPC; >81%; *duys@siu.edu*
- Brown, Beverly M; PhD; Full Prof.; NCC; >81%; *bevbrown@siu.edu*
- Prichard, Karen K; PhD; Assoc.; NCC; >81%; *prichard@siu.edu*
- White, Lyle J; PhD; Full Prof.; LPC, NCC, licensed marriage & family therapist; 41-60%; *lwhite@siu.edu*

Has CHI SIGMA IOTA (International Counseling Society) chapter.

IL: Western Illinois University

3561 60th Street
Moline, IL 61265-5881
United States
Dean   Bonnie Smith, College of Education & Human Services
Administrator   Melanie E. Rawlins, Chair and Professor
Department   Counselor Education
(309) 762-1876, fax (309) 762-6989, m-Rawlins1@wiu.edu,
www.wiu.edu/counselored

Key   See key for Data on Each Department (this section) on page 79.

Program
Accreditation   Regional Accreditation, **CACREP:** Community Counseling, **CACREP:** School Counseling

Uniqueness   Program also contains a certificate program in Marriage and Family Counseling

Degrees   • Community Counseling: M.
                • School Counseling: M.

Contact   • Community Counseling: M = Melanie Rawlins.
                • School Counseling: M = Melanie Rawlins.

Admission and Graduation Data
Admission
Requirements   • Community Counseling(M): GPA 2.50; Interview.
                • School Counseling(M): GPA 2.50; Interview.

Enrollment   • Community Counseling(M): NP.
                • School Counseling(M): NP.

Diversity   • African-American; Asian-American; Caucasian; Hispanic; Pacific Islander; Multiracial.

Graduation
Requirements   • Community Counseling(M): 48 Class hours; 100 Practicum hours; 600 Internship hours.
                • School Counseling(M): 48 Class hours; 100 Practicum hours; 600 Internship hours.

Postgraduation activity: Advanced education and employment setting percentages.
                • Community Counseling(M): 30 Managed care; 70 Agency practice.
                • School Counseling(M): 15 Elementary school; 20 Middle school; 65 Secondary school.

Planned Program Modifications
Courses   Drop   Add
                • NP.   • NP.

Other   Decrease   Increase
                • NP.   • Number of Distance Education Courses
                                           • Number of On-Line Courses.

Related Programs

Faculty

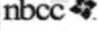   Percent of faculty reported with NCC certification: 0%.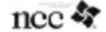

Percent in professional counseling practice: 25%.

Research interests multi-racial, career & lifestyle, baby boomers, developmental counseling.

Diversity   • Caucasian; Multiracial.

Name, Degree, Rank, State/National Credentials, % time devoted to program, email
• Hamann, Edward E; EdD; Full Prof.; >81%;
• McFarland, William P; EdD; Full Prof.; >81%;
• Henriksen, Richard C; PhD; Full Prof.; >81%;
• O'Ryan, Leslie W; EdD; Assist.; >81%;
• Rawlins, Melanie; PhD; Full Prof.; >81%

Has CHI SIGMA IOTA (International Counseling Society) chapter.

IN: Ball State University

	Teachers College 622
	Muncie, IN 47306-0585
	United States
Dean	Roy A. Weaver, Teachers College
Administrator	Sharon L. Bowman, Ph.D., Chairperson
	Department Department of Counseling Psychology and Guidance Services
	(765) 285-8040, fax (765) 285-2067, sbowman@bsu.edu,
	www.bsu.edu/counselingpsych

Key See key for Data on Each Department (this section) on page 79.

Program

Accreditation Regional Accreditation, **CACREP:** Community Counseling, **CACREP:** School Counseling;
CORE: Rehabilitation Counseling

CACREP

Uniqueness Large faculty with diverse interests; balance of research and experiential components.

Degrees
- Community Counseling: M.
- Mental Health Counseling: M.
- School Counseling: M.
- Other: PhD.
- Rehabilitation Counseling: M.

Contact
- Community Counseling: M = Phyllis Gordon.
- Mental Health Counseling: M = Phyllis Gordon.
- School Counseling: M = Charlene Alexander.
- Other: D = Lawrence Gerstein.
- Rehabilitation Counseling: M = Phyllis Gordon.

Admission and Graduation Data

Admission

Requirements
- Community Counseling(M): GPA 2.75.
- Mental Health Counseling(M): GPA 2.75.
- School Counseling(M): GPA 2.75.
- Other(D): GPA 3.20; GRE 1000.
- Rehabilitation Counseling(M): GPA 2.75.

Enrollment
- Community Counseling(M): 10 Admitted yearly; 10 Graduated yearly.
- Mental Health Counseling(M): 20 Admitted yearly; 15 Graduated yearly.
- School Counseling(M): 12 Admitted yearly; 10 Graduated yearly.
- Other(D): 10 Admitted yearly; 7 Graduated yearly; 31 Female; 11 Male.
- Rehabilitation Counseling(M): 12 Admitted yearly; 11 Graduated yearly.

Diversity
- African-American; Asian-American; Caucasian; Hispanic; Multiracial; Other.

Graduation

Requirements
- Community Counseling(M): 48 Class hours; 200 Practicum hours; 600 Internship hours;
  Comprehensive exam.
- Mental Health Counseling(M): 60 Class hours; 200 Practicum hours; 900 Internship hours;
  Comprehensive exam.
- School Counseling(M): 48 Class hours; 200 Practicum hours; 600 Internship hours;
  Comprehensive exam; Portfolio.
- Other(D): 97 Class hours; 400 Practicum hours; 1500 Internship hours; Comprehensive
  exam; Oral exam; Dissertation; Portfolio.
- Rehabilitation Counseling(M): 48 Class hours; 100 Practicum hours; 600 Internship hours;
  Comprehensive exam.

Postgraduation activity: Advanced education and employment setting percentages.
- Community Counseling(M): 25 Advanced education; 10 Managed care; 15 Private practice;
  50 Agency practice.
- Mental Health Counseling(M): NP.
- School Counseling(M): 5 Advanced education; 30 Elementary school; 20 Middle school; 40
  Secondary school; 5 Other.
- Other(D): 20 Managed care; 25 Private practice; 25 Agency practice; 20 Student affairs; 10
  Other.
- Rehabilitation Counseling(M): 10 Advanced education; 5 Managed care; 20 Private
  practice; 60 Agency practice; 5 Other.

Planned Program Modifications
Courses

Drop	Add
• NP.	• NP.

Other

Decrease	Increase
• Number of Off-Campus Courses.	• National Accreditation.

Related Programs Psychology
　　　　　　　　Other

Faculty

 Percent of faculty reported with NCC certification: 0%.

Percent in professional counseling practice: 33%.

Research interests Multicultural Issues; Psycho-Social Oncology

Diversity　　　• African-American; Caucasian; Multiracial.

Name, Degree, Rank, State/National Credentials, % time devoted to program, email
- Alexander, Charlene; PhD; Assoc.; School Counselor; 61-80%; *calexander@bsu.edu*
- Bowman, Sharon; PhD; Full Prof.; LMHC, HSPP; 41-60%; *sbowman@bsu.edu*
- Dixon, David; PhD; Full Prof.; <21%; *ddixon@bsu.edu*
- Gerstein, Lawrence; PhD; Full Prof.; Psychologist; 61-80%; *rangzen@aol.com*
- Gordon, Phyllis; PhD; Full Prof.; CRC; 61-80%; *pgordon@bsu.edu*
- Kruczek, Theresa; PhD; Assist.; HSPP; 61-80%; *tkruczek@bsu.edu*
- Nicholas, Donald; PhD; Full Prof.; HSPP; 61-80%; *dnichola@bsu.edu*
- Perrone, Kristin; PhD; Assoc.; LMHC; HSPP; 61-80%; *kshea@bsu.edu*
- Spengler, Paul; PhD; Assoc.; LMHC; 61-80%; *pspengle@bsu.edu*
- White, Michael; PhD; Full Prof.; Psychologist; *mwhite2@bsu.edu*
- Aegisdottir, Stefania; PhD; Assist.; 61-80%; *stefaegis@bsu.edu*
- Tschopp, Molly; PhD; Assist.; CRC; 61-80%; *mktschopp@bsu.edu*

IN: Butler University

Dean	4600 Sunset Avenue Indianapolis, IN 46208-3485 United States Dr. Robert Rider- Jordan Hall 171
Administrator	Ronald W. Goodman, Program Director
	Department Department of Cont Education
	(317) 940-9501, fax (317) 940-6481, rgoodman@Butler.edu

Key   See key for Data on Each Department (this section) on page 79.

Program

Accreditation   Regional Accreditation, **CACREP:** School Counseling

Uniqueness   Unit Assessment systems; cohort model; partnership with Brooke and Place for grieving young people.

Degrees   • School Counseling: M.

Contact   • School Counseling: M = Dr.Ron Goodman.

Admission and Graduation Data
Admission

Requirements   • School Counseling(M): GPA 3.00; GRE 875; MAT 40; Interview.

Enrollment   • School Counseling(M): 24 Admitted yearly; 20 Graduated yearly; 55 Female; 15 Male.

Diversity   • African-American; Caucasian.

Graduation

Requirements   • School Counseling(M): 48 Class hours; 100 Practicum hours; 600 Internship hours; CPCE; Portfolio.

Postgraduation activity: Advanced education and employment setting percentages.
   • School Counseling(M): 10 Agency practice; 30 Elementary school; 20 Middle school; 40 Secondary school.

Planned Program Modifications

Courses	Drop	Add
	• NP.	• Grief Counseling.

Other	Decrease	Increase
	• NP.	• NP.

Related Programs

Faculty

nbcc ❧.   Percent of faculty reported with NCC certification: 60%.   **ncc** ❧

Percent in professional counseling practice: 20%.

Research interests Technology applications; credentialing issues; grief counseling.

Diversity   • Caucasian.

Name, Degree, Rank, State/National Credentials, % time devoted to program, email
• Bloom, John W; PhD; Full Prof.; NCC, ACS LMHC; >81%; *jbloom@butler.edu*
• Goodman, Ronald W; EdD; Full Prof.; NCC, ACS LMHC LMFT; >81%; *rgoodman@butler.edu*
• Keller, Thomas J; EdD; Assoc.; NCC, ACS LMHC; >81%; *tkeller@butler.edu*
• Lauri, Waldner; EdS; Adjunct; School Counselor School Psychologist; <21%;
• Wright, Pam; MS; Adjunct; LMFT; <21%

Has CHI SIGMA IOTA (International Counseling Society) chapter.

IN: Indiana State University

	School of Education
	Terre Haute, IN 47809
	USA
Dean	Jack Maynard
Administrator	Michele C. Boyer, Chair
	Department Counseling
	(812) 237-2870, fax (812) 237-2870, Counseling@indstate.edu,
	http://counseling.indstate.edu/

Key   See key for Data on Each Department (this section) on page 79.

Program

Accreditation   Regional Accreditation

Uniqueness   The Department of Counseling has 8 full time faculty and uses University and community experts as adjunct faculty. There are approximately 155 graduate students within the department's four Master's and one Doctoral program. The faculty and students provide direct services and consultation to many individuals and organizations and coordinate several on-going projects.

Degrees
- Mental Health Counseling: M.
- School Counseling: M.
- Marriage and Family Counseling: M.
- Student Affairs: M.

Contact
- Mental Health Counseling: M = NP.
- School Counseling: M = NP.
- Marriage and Family Counseling: M = NP.
- Student Affairs: M = NP.

Admission and Graduation Data

Admission

Requirements
- Mental Health Counseling(M): GPA 3.25; GRE 1455; GRE V 440; GRE Q 515; GRE A 500; Interview.
- School Counseling(M): GPA 2.50; Interview.
- Marriage and Family Counseling(M): GPA 2.75; GRE 1455; GRE V 440; GRE Q 515; GRE A 500; Interview.
- Student Affairs(M): GPA 2.50; GRE 1455; GRE V 440; GRE Q 515; GRE A 500; Interview.

Enrollment
- Mental Health Counseling(M): 20 Admitted yearly; 20 Graduated yearly; 35 Female; 4 Male.
- School Counseling(M): 20 Admitted yearly; 17 Graduated yearly; 32 Female; 8 Male.
- Marriage and Family Counseling(M): 8 Admitted yearly; 7 Graduated yearly; 8 Female; 2 Male.
- Student Affairs(M): 20 Admitted yearly; 15 Graduated yearly; 20 Female; 15 Male.

Diversity
- African-American; Asian-American; Caucasian; Hispanic; Native American; Pacific Islander; Multiracial.

Graduation

Requirements
- Mental Health Counseling(M): 60 Class hours; 100 Practicum hours; 900 Internship hours; Comprehensive exam; CPCE; Oral exam.
- School Counseling(M): 52 Class hours; 100 Practicum hours; 600 Internship hours; Oral exam; Portfolio.
- Marriage and Family Counseling(M): 60 Class hours; 100 Practicum hours; 400 Internship hours.
- Student Affairs(M): 48 Class hours; 100 Practicum hours; 600 Internship hours.

Postgraduation activity: Advanced education and employment setting percentages.
- Mental Health Counseling(M): 30 Advanced education; 10 Managed care; 10 Private practice; 50 Agency practice.
- School Counseling(M): 5 Agency practice; 30 Elementary school; 30 Middle school; 30 Secondary school.
- Marriage and Family Counseling(M): 10 Advanced education; 10 Managed care; 10 Private practice; 70 Agency practice.
- Student Affairs(M): 100 Other.

Planned Program Modifications

Courses	Drop	Add
	• NP.	• NP.

Other	Decrease	Increase
	• NP.	• NP.

Related Programs

Faculty

Percent of faculty reported with NCC certification: 25%.

Percent in professional counseling practice: 100%.

Research interests See web site for information on individual faculty

Diversity   • African-American; Caucasian; Hispanic.

Name, Degree, Rank, State/National Credentials, % time devoted to program, email
- Barratt, William; PhD; Assoc.; 61-80%; *egbarra@isugw.indstate.edu*
- Boyer, Michele C; PhD; Full Prof.; <21%; *egboyer@isugw.indstate.edu*
- Campbell, James L; PhD; Assoc.; NCC; 61-80%; *egcampb@isugw.indstate.edu*
- Chaney, Reece; PhD; Full Prof.; 61-80%; *egchane@isugw.indstate.edu*
- Hines, Peggy L; EdD; Assoc.; 41-60%; *eghines@isugw.indstate.edu*
- Passmore, J. L; PhD; Full Prof.; 41-60%; *egpassm@isugw.indstate.edu*
- Shuff, I M; PhD; Assoc.; NCC; 22-40%; *egshuff@isugw.indstate.edu*

IN: Indiana University

201 N. Rose
Bloomington, IN 47405-1006
US

Dean   Dr. Gerardo Gonzalez IU School of Education
Administrator Susan Whiston, Program Coordinator
                  Department   Counseling and Eduational Psychology
                                (812) 856-8323, fax (812) 856-8333, cep@indiana.edu,
                                http://education.indiana.edu/~counsel/

Key   See key for Data on Each Department (this section) on page 79.

Program
Accreditation   Regional Accreditation, **CACREP:** Community Counseling, **CACREP:** Mental Health
                Counseling, **CACREP:** School Counseling

Uniqueness   The counseling program has a long history of being a top-rated program, using state-of-art
                technology, and many highly recognized faculty who are implementing a scientist-practitioner
                model with an emphasis on change across therapeutic settings.

Degrees   • Community Counseling: M.
                • Mental Health Counseling: S, PhD.
                • School Counseling: M.

Contact   • Community Counseling: M = Dr. Sue Whiston.
                • Mental Health Counseling: S = Dr. Sue Whiston.; D = Dr. Chalmer Thompson.
                • School Counseling: M = Dr. Sue Whiston.

Admission and Graduation Data
Admission
Requirements   • Community Counseling(M): GPA 2.75; GRE 1300.
                • Mental Health Counseling(S): GPA 2.75; GRE 1300.
                • Mental Health Counseling(D): GPA 3.00; GRE V 600; GRE Q 600; GRE A 600.
                • School Counseling(M): GPA 2.75; GRE 1300.

Enrollment   • Community Counseling(M): 25 Admitted yearly; 22 Graduated yearly.
                • Mental Health Counseling(S): 10 Admitted yearly; 10 Graduated yearly.
                • Mental Health Counseling(D): 5-8 Admitted yearly; 5-8 Graduated yearly; 22 Female;
                  20 Male.
                • School Counseling(M): 25 Admitted yearly; 22 Graduated yearly.

Diversity   • African-American; Asian-American; Caucasian; Hispanic; Pacific Islander; Multiracial;
                  Other.

Graduation
Requirements   • Community Counseling(M): 48 Class hours; 100 Practicum hours; 600 Internship hours.
                • Mental Health Counseling(S): 65 Class hours; 100 Practicum hours; 900 Internship hours;
                  Comprehensive exam.
                • Mental Health Counseling(D): 96 Class hours; 150-500 Practicum hours; 2000 Internship
                  hours; Comprehensive exam; Oral exam; Dissertation.
                • School Counseling(M): 48 Class hours; 100 Practicum hours; 600 Internship hours.

Postgraduation activity: Advanced education and employment setting percentages.
                • Community Counseling(M): 30 Advanced education; 60 Agency practice; 10 Other.
                • Mental Health Counseling(S): 5 Advanced education; 15 Managed care; 10 Private
                  practice; 60 Agency practice; 5 Other.
                • Mental Health Counseling(D): 40 Agency practice; 40 Student affairs; 20 Other.
                • School Counseling(M): 10 Advanced education; 20 Elementary school; 35 Middle school;
                  35 Secondary school.

Planned Program Modifications
Courses	Drop	Add
	• NP.	• Psychopharmocology.

Other	Decrease	Increase
	• NP.	• Course Offerings
		• Diversity Recruiting of Students
		• Number of Distance Education Courses
		• Number of On-Line Courses.

Related Programs Clinical Social Workers
Psychology

Faculty

nbcc ❧   Percent of faculty reported with NCC certification: 9%.   ncc ❧

Percent in professional counseling practice: NP.

Research interests All faculty have active research agendas including career counseling, family therapy, multicultural counseling, prevention interventions, school counseling, and social justice issues.

Diversity   • African-American; Caucasian; Hispanic.

Name, Degree, Rank, State/National Credentials, % time devoted to program, email
* Daniels, Jeff; PhD; Assist.; >81%; *jedaniels@indiana.edu*
* Delgado-Romero, Edward; PhD; Assist.; >81%; *edelgado@indiana.edu*
* Gonzalez, Gerardo; PhD; Full Prof.; <21%;
* Morran, Keith; PhD; Full Prof.; >81%; *KMORRAN@IUPUI>EDU*
* Ridley, Charles; PhD; Full Prof.; 61-80%; *cridley@indiana.edu*
* Robison, Floyd; PhD; Assoc.; >81%; *FLIP@IUPUI.EDU*
* Sexton, Tom; PhD; Full Prof.; >81%; *thsexton@indiana.edu*
* Stockton, Rex; PhD; Full Prof.; LPC, NCC; >81%; *stocktor@indiana.edu*
* Thompson, Chalmer; PhD; Assoc.; >81%; *chathomp@indiana.edu*
* Tracy, Michael; PhD; Assoc.; >81%; *tracy@indiana.edu*
* Whiston, Sue; PhD; Full Prof.; >81%; *swhiston@indiana.edu*

IN: Indiana Wesleyan University

4201 S. Washington Street
Marion, IN 46953
USA
Dean James O. Fuller, Ph.D., Indiana Wesleyan University
Administrator Jerry E. Davis, Ph.D., Director of Graduate Counseling Program
Department   Graduate Counseling Program
(765) 677-2995, fax (765) 677-2504, grcns.office@indwes.edu,
http://graduatecounseling.indwes.edu/

Key   See key for Data on Each Department (this section) on page 79.

Program

Accreditation   Regional Accreditation, **CACREP:** Community Counseling, **CACREP:** Marriage and Family
Counseling

Uniqueness   intregration of Christian faith and values with integrity into the counseling profession. Faculty
who are doctorally trained, licensed and practicing in the field.

Degrees
- Community Counseling: M.
- Marriage and Family Counseling: M.

Contact
- Community Counseling: M = NP.
- Marriage and Family Counseling: M = NP.

Admission and Graduation Data

Admission
Requirements
- Community Counseling(M): GPA 3.00; GRE 1000.
- Marriage and Family Counseling(M): GPA 3.00; GRE 1000.

Enrollment
- Community Counseling(M): NP.
- Marriage and Family Counseling(M): NP.

Diversity
- African-American; Caucasian; Native American; Multiracial.

Graduation
Requirements
- Community Counseling(M): 48-60 Class hours; 100 Practicum hours; 600-900 Internship
hours; Portfolio.
- Marriage and Family Counseling(M): 60 Class hours; 100 Practicum hours; 900 Internship
hours; Portfolio.

Postgraduation activity: Advanced education and employment setting percentages.
- Community Counseling(M): NP.
- Marriage and Family Counseling(M): NP.

Planned Program Modifications

Courses	Drop	Add
• NP.		• NP.

Other	Decrease	Increase
• NP.		• NP.

Related Programs

Faculty

Percent of faculty reported with NCC certification: 17%.

Percent in professional counseling practice: 100%.

Research interests cultural re-entry, blamer softening, effects of spirituality on counseling, multicultural issues

Diversity
- Caucasian.

Name, Degree, Rank, State/National Credentials, % time devoted to program, email
- Davis, Jerry E; PhD; Full Prof.; LMFT, LCSW, LMFT; >81%; *jerry.davis@indwes.edu*
- Fuller, James O; PhD; Assoc.; NCC, NSCS; 41-60%; *jim.fuller@indwes.edu*
- Bradley, Brent A; PhD; Assist.; >81%; *brent.bradley@indwes.edu*
- Riggs, Barbara; PhD; Instructor; 41-60%; *barbara.riggs@indwes.edu*
- Bolding, Nancy; PsyD; Adjunct; <21%; *nkbolding@insightbb.com*
- Gaff-Clark, Carla; PhD; Adjunct; <21%; *cgaff@inetdirect.net*

Has CHI SIGMA IOTA (International Counseling Society) chapter.

IN: Indiana-Purdue University at Fort Wayne

	2101 E. Coliseum Blvd.
	Fort Wayne, IN 46805-1499
	USA
Dean	Dr. Weiner, School of Education
Administrator	William E. Utesch, Chair Professional Studies & Director of Counselor Education Program
	Department Counselor Education Program
	(260) 481-6003, fax (260) 481-5408, utesch@ipfw.edu, Education@ipfw.edu

Key   See key for Data on Each Department (this section) on page 79.

Program

Accreditation   Regional Accreditation

Uniqueness   The department consists of two master's degrees that have as their foundation systemic training.

Degrees
- School Counseling: M.
- Marriage and Family Counseling: M.

Contact
- School Counseling: M = William E. Utesch.
- Marriage and Family Counseling: M = Jim Burg.

Admission and Graduation Data

Admission

Requirements
- School Counseling(M): GPA 3.20; Interview.
- Marriage and Family Counseling(M): GPA 3.20; Interview.

Enrollment
- School Counseling(M): 14 Admitted yearly; 12 Graduated yearly; 34 Female; 18 Male.
- Marriage and Family Counseling(M): 14 Admitted yearly; 12 Graduated yearly; 32 Female; 22 Male.

Diversity
- African-American; Caucasian; Hispanic.

Graduation

Requirements
- School Counseling(M): 51 Class hours; 100 Practicum hours; nine month Internship hours; Comprehensive exam; Portfolio.
- Marriage and Family Counseling(M): 57 Class hours; 132 Practicum hours; 400 Internship hours; Portfolio.

Postgraduation activity: Advanced education and employment setting percentages.
- School Counseling(M): 35 Elementary school; 40 Middle school; 25 Secondary school.
- Marriage and Family Counseling(M): 2 Advanced education; 13 Managed care; 5 Private practice; 80 Agency practice.

Planned Program Modifications

Courses	Drop	Add
	• NP.	• Addictions
		• Gerontological Counseling
		• Play Therapy.

Other	Decrease	Increase
	• NP.	• Course Offerings
		• Diversity Recruiting of Faculty
		• Diversity Recruiting of Students
		• National Accreditation
		• Number of Distance Education Courses
		• Number of Off-Campus Courses.

Related Programs

Faculty

nbcc ❧   Percent of faculty reported with NCC certification: 57%.   **ncc** ❧

Percent in professional counseling practice: 60%.

Research interests   Research interests range from systems applications for multiple human system functioning to Marital Enrichment.

Diversity
- African-American; Caucasian.

Name, Degree, Rank, State/National Credentials, % time devoted to program, email
- Keri, Gabe; PhD; Assist.; NCC; >81%; *keri@ipfw.edu*
- Utesch, William; PhD; Assoc.; LPC, NCC, LMFT; >81%; *utesch@ipfw.edu*
- Burg, Jim; PhD; Assist.; LMFT; >81%;
- Gordon, Tom; MA; Adjunct; 22-40%;
- Weaver, Ken; MA; Adjunct; LPC, LMFT,LCSW; 22-40%;
- Goller, Martha; MS; Adjunct; LPC, NCC; <21%;
- Smith, Linda; MS; Adjunct; LPC, NCC, LMFT; <21%;

Has CHI SIGMA IOTA (International Counseling Society) chapter.

IN: Purdue University

Beering Hall of Liberal Arts & Education; 100 N University St.
West Lafayette, IN 47907-2067
Tippicanoe
Dean George Hynd; School of Education
Administrator Kevin Kelly, Department Head
Department   Educational Studies
               (765) 494-9170, fax (765) 496-1228,
               http://www.edst.purdue.edu/overview/welcome.html

Key   See key for Data on Each Department (this section) on page 79.

Program
Accreditation   Regional Accreditation, **CACREP:** Mental Health Counseling, **CACREP:** School Counseling

Uniqueness   Programs are small, which facilitates close working relationships with faculty.
               http://www.edst.purdue.edu/cd/development/cdmain.html.

Degrees
- Mental Health Counseling: M.
- School Counseling: M.
- Student Affairs: M.

Contact
- Mental Health Counseling: M = M. Carole Pistole.
- School Counseling: M = Jean Peterson.
- Student Affairs: M = Deborah J. Taub.

Admission and Graduation Data
Admission
Requirements
- Mental Health Counseling(M): GPA 3.00; GRE 1000; GRE V 500; GRE Q 500; GRE W 3.5.
- School Counseling(M): GPA 3.00; GRE 1000; GRE V 500; GRE Q 500; GRE W 3.5.
- Student Affairs(M): GPA 3.00; GRE 1000; GRE V 500; GRE Q 500; GRE W 3.5.

Enrollment
- Mental Health Counseling(M): 10 Admitted yearly; 7-8 Graduated yearly; 10 Female; 5 Male.
- School Counseling(M): 10 Admitted yearly; 8-10 Graduated yearly; 19 Female; 1 Male.
- Student Affairs(M): 10 Admitted yearly; 8 Graduated yearly; 11 Female; 5 Male.

Diversity
- African-American; Asian-American; Caucasian; Hispanic; Other.

Graduation
Requirements
- Mental Health Counseling(M): 60 Class hours; 100 Practicum hours; 900 Internship hours.
- School Counseling(M): 48 Class hours; 100 Practicum hours; 600 Internship hours.
- Student Affairs(M): 42 Class hours; 100 Practicum hours; 200 Internship hours.

Postgraduation activity: Advanced education and employment setting percentages.
- Mental Health Counseling(M): NP.
- School Counseling(M): NP.
- Student Affairs(M): 100 Other.

Planned Program Modifications
Courses   Drop   Add
               • NP.   • NP.

Other   Decrease   Increase
               • NP.   • Diversity Recruiting of Faculty
                                              • Diversity Recruiting of Students.

Related Programs Marriage and Family Therapists
                        Psychology

Faculty

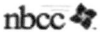   Percent of faculty reported with NCC certification: 14%.   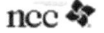

Percent in professional counseling practice: 14%.

Research interests Haring: Career development — nontraditional, barriers, mentoring; Kelly: Career assessment and development; Kwan: Multicultural assessment, racial & ethnic identity development; Peterson: Social/emotional concerns of high ability youth and underachievement, training & professional development of school counselors Pistole: Attachment theory in adult & counseling relationships Servaty-Seib: Developmental aspects of grief; death-related attitudes & beliefs; loss as a general intervention model Taub: Student development theory; college student affairs; women's issues; multicutural issues

Diversity   • Caucasian; Other.

Name, Degree, Rank, State/National Credentials, % time devoted to program, email
• Kelly, Kevin; PhD; Full Prof.; IN psych licensure; 22-40%; *kkelly@purdue.edu*
• PIstole, M. Carole; PhD; Assoc.; NJ psych liscensure; 22-40%; *pistole@purdue.edu*
• Kwan, Karl; PhD; Assoc.; *kkwan@purdue.edu*
• Peterson, Jean; PhD; Assoc.; NCC, LMHC; >81%; *jeanp@purdue.edu*
• Taub, Deborah; PhD; Assoc.; >81%; *dtaub@purdue.edu*
• Servaty-Seib, Heather; PhD; Assist.; IN psych liscensure; 41-60%; *servaty@purdue.edu*
• Haring, Marilyn; PhD; Full Prof.; 22-40%; *haringm@purdue.edu*

KS: Emporia State University

	Campus Box 4036, 1200 Commercial St.
	Emporia, KS 66801-5087
	USA
Dean	Dr. Tes Mehring
Administrator	David M. Kaplan, PhD, Chair
	Department Counselor Education and Rehabilitation Programs
	(620) 341-5220, fax (620) 341-6200, kaplanda@emporia.edu,
	www.emporia.edu/counre

Key   See key for Data on Each Department (this section) on page 79.

Program

Accreditation   **CACREP:** Mental Health Counseling, **CACREP:** School Counseling, **CACREP:** Student Affairs - Counseling, **CACREP:** Student Affairs - Professional Practice, **CORE:** Rehabilitation Counseling

Uniqueness   ESU is the only school in the region to have four nationally accredited CACREP or CORE masters programs. Forty-four percent of licensed counselors in Kansas whose licensure is based on a counseling degree from a Kansas institution are graduates of our department. Also, more school counselors in Kansas graduate from ESU than from any other institution.The department has a unique dual degree program in Mental Health Counseling and Art Therapy.

Degrees
- Mental Health Counseling: M.
- School Counseling: M.
- Other: M.
- Rehabilitation Counseling: M.

Contact
- Mental Health Counseling: M = Dr. Wendy Enochs.
- School Counseling: M = Dr. Dennis Pelsma.
- Other: M = Dr. Wendy Enochs.
- Rehabilitation Counseling: M = Dr. Marvin Kuehn.

Admission and Graduation Data

Admission

Requirements
- Mental Health Counseling(M): GPA 3.00; GRE 850; MAT 40; Interview.
- School Counseling(M): GPA 3.00; GRE 850; MAT 40; Interview.
- Other(M): GPA 3.00; GRE 850; MAT 40; Interview.
- Rehabilitation Counseling(M): GPA 3.00; GRE 850; MAT 40; Interview.

Enrollment
- Mental Health Counseling(M): 7-12 Admitted yearly; 7-12 Graduated yearly; 4-8 Female; 3-4 Male.
- School Counseling(M): 10-20 Admitted yearly; 10-20 Graduated yearly; 3-6 Male.
- Other(M): 7-12 Admitted yearly; 7-12 Graduated yearly; 4-6 Female; 3-6 Male.
- Rehabilitation Counseling(M): 7-12 Admitted yearly; 7-12 Graduated yearly; 4-6 Female; 3-6 Male.

Diversity
- African-American; Asian-American; Caucasian; Hispanic; Native American; Multiracial; Other.

Graduation

Requirements
- Mental Health Counseling(M): 60 Class hours; 100 Practicum hours; 900 Internship hours; Comprehensive exam.
- School Counseling(M): 48 Class hours; 100 Practicum hours; Comprehensive exam.
- Other(M): 48 Class hours; 100 Practicum hours; 600 Internship hours; Comprehensive exam.
- Rehabilitation Counseling(M): 60 Class hours; 100 Practicum hours; 600 Internship hours; Comprehensive exam.

Postgraduation activity: Advanced education and employment setting percentages.
- Mental Health Counseling(M): 10 Advanced education; 90 Agency practice.
- School Counseling(M): 25 Elementary school; 15 Middle school; 60 Secondary school.
- Other(M): 10 Advanced education; 90 Student affairs.
- Rehabilitation Counseling(M): 10 Advanced education; 10 Agency practice; 80 Other.

Planned Program Modifications

Courses	Drop	Add
	• NP.	• NP.

Other	Decrease	Increase
	• NP.	• Number of On-Line Courses.

Related Programs Psychology
Arts Therapists
Communications

Faculty

nbcc ♣.   Percent of faculty reported with NCC certification: 27%.   ncc ♣

Percent in professional counseling practice: 10%.

Research interests The faculty include the 2002-03 president of The American Counseling Association and past presidents of such organizations as the Council On Rehabilitation Education, Kansas Counseling Association, Kansas Career Development Association, and Kansas Rehabilitation Association.

Diversity   • Caucasian; Hispanic; Other.

Name, Degree, Rank, State/National Credentials, % time devoted to program, email
- Costello, James J; PhD; Assist.; CRC; 61-80%; *costellj@emporia.edu*
- Currier, Kenneth F; PhD; Assist.; CRC; 61-80%; *currierk@emporia.edu*
- Enochs, Wendy K; PhD; Assist.; LPC; >81%; *enochswe@emporia.edu*
- Etzbach, Colleen A; RhD; Assist.; CRC; 61-80%; *etzbachc@emporia.edu*
- Kaplan, David M; PhD; Full Prof.; NCC, NCCC, Licensed Psychologist (NY), CFT, MCC; >81%; *kaplanda@emporia.edu*
- Kuehn, Marvin D; EdD; Full Prof.; CRC; >81%; *kuehnmar@emporia.edu*
- Neufeld, Patricia J; PhD; Assoc.; LPC, NCC, CSC (KS); >81%; *neufeldp@emporia.edu*
- Pelsma, Dennis M; PhD; Assoc.; LPC, Certified Psychologist (KS & MO), CSC (KS); >81%; *pelsmade@emporia.edu*
- Sasser, Judith S; PhD; Assist.; CSC (KS); >81%; *sasserju@emporia.edu*
- Strohm, David A; ABD; Assist.; CSC (KS); >81%; *strohmda@emporia.edu*
- Wurtz, Philip J; PhD; Full Prof.; LPC, NCC, CCMHC, CADAC (KS); >81%; *wurtzphi@emporia.edu*

Has CHI SIGMA IOTA (International Counseling Society) chapter.

KS: Kansas State University

	1100 Mid-Campus Dr., Rm. 36
	Manhattan, KS 66506-5312
	United States
Dean	Michael C. Holen
Administrator	Fred Bradley, Program Director
	Department Department of Counseling & Educ. Psy
	(785) 532-5541, fax (785) 532-7304, fbradley@ksu.edu, http://coe.ksu.edu

Key   See key for Data on Each Department (this section) on page 79.

Program

Accreditation   Regional Accreditation, **CACREP:** Counselor Education and Supervision, **CACREP:** Community Counseling

CACREP

Uniqueness   At the M.S. level students receive extensive experience in the schools. At the Ph. D. level students have considerable latitude in designing elements of their curriculum.

Degrees
- School Counseling: M, EdD.
- Student Affairs: M, PhD.
- Counselor Education: PhD.

Contact
- School Counseling: M = Dr. Judith Hughey.; D = Dr. Ken Hughey.
- Student Affairs: M = Dr. Adrienne Leslie-Toogood-.; D = Dr. Doris Wright-Carroll.
- Counselor Education: D = Dr. Fred Bradley.

Admission and Graduation Data

Admission

Requirements
- School Counseling(M): GPA 3.00; GRE 970; GRE V 485; GRE Q 485; GRE A 0; MAT 50; 1 Year work experience.
- School Counseling(D): Masters and GPA 3.00; GRE 1000; GRE V 500; GRE Q 500; GRE A 0; 2 Years work experience.
- Student Affairs(M): GPA 3.00; GRE 1000; GRE V 500; GRE Q 500; GRE A 0; MAT 50.
- Student Affairs(D): Masters and GPA 3.00; GRE 1000; GRE V 500; GRE Q 500; GRE A 0.
- Counselor Education(D): Masters and GPA 3.00; GRE 1000; GRE V 500; GRE Q 500; GRE A 0; 2 Years work experience.

Enrollment
- School Counseling(M): 25 Admitted yearly; 15 Graduated yearly; 40 Female; 8 Male.
- School Counseling(D): 2 Admitted yearly; 2 Female; 1 Male.
- Student Affairs(M): 20 Admitted yearly; 10 Graduated yearly; 20 Female; 20 Male.
- Student Affairs(D): 3 Admitted yearly; 1 Graduated yearly; 3 Female; 1 Male.
- Counselor Education(D): 5 Admitted yearly; 2 Graduated yearly; 14 Female; 5 Male.

Diversity
- African-American; Caucasian; Hispanic.

Graduation

Requirements
- School Counseling(M): 48 Class hours; 100 Practicum hours; 600 Internship hours; Comprehensive exam.
- School Counseling(D): 94 Class hours; 300 Internship hours; Dissertation.
- Student Affairs(M): 39 Class hours; 50 Practicum hours; 160 Internship hours.
- Student Affairs(D): 120 Class hours; 50 Practicum hours; 160 Internship hours; Comprehensive exam; Dissertation.
- Counselor Education(D): 120 Class hours; 100 Practicum hours; 600 Internship hours; Comprehensive exam; Dissertation.

Postgraduation activity: Advanced education and employment setting percentages.
- School Counseling(M): 35 Elementary school; 20 Middle school; 45 Secondary school.
- School Counseling(D): 40 Middle school; 40 Student affairs; 20 Other.
- Student Affairs(M): 10 Advanced education; 90 Other.
- Student Affairs(D): 100 Student affairs.
- Counselor Education(D): 10 Agency practice; 5 Middle school; 5 Student affairs; 90 Other.

Planned Program Modifications

Courses	Drop	Add
	• NP.	• Psychodiagnosis.

Other	Decrease	Increase
	• NP.	• Diversity Recruiting of Students
		• Number of Distance Education Courses
		• Number of On-Line Courses.

Related Programs Marriage and Family Therapists

Faculty

nbcc ✦.   Percent of faculty reported with NCC certification: 31%.   ncc ✦

Percent in professional counseling practice: NP.

Research interests Alcohol and Drug Abuse Prevention, Career Developent in Schools, and Counseling
                  Support for Culturally and Linguistically Diverse Students.

Diversity   • African-American; Caucasian.

Name, Degree, Rank, State/National Credentials, % time devoted to program, email
*   Benton, Stephen L; PhD; Full Prof.; 22-40%; *leroy@ksu.edu*
*   Bradley, Fred O; PhD; Full Prof.; NCC, LCPC; >81%; *fbradley@ksu.edu*
*   Benton, Sheryl A; PhD; Assist.; Licensed Psychologist; <21%; *benton@ksu.edu*
*   Hanna, Gerald S; EdD; Full Prof.; >81%; *ghanna@ksu.edu*
*   Hoyt, Kenneth B; PhD; Full Prof.; <21%; *khoyt@ksu.edu*
*   Hughey, Judith K; EdD; Assoc.; NCC, LCPC; >81%; *jhughey@ksu.edu*
*   Hughey, Kenneth F; PhD; Full Prof.; NCC, Licensed Clinical Professional Counselor; >81%;
    khughey@ksu.edu
*   Lynch, Michael L; EdD; Assoc.; <21%; *mlynch@ksu.edu*
*   Leslie-Toogood, Adrienne; PhD; Assist.; Licensed Psychologist; >81%; *atoogood@ksu.edu*
*   Newton, Fred B; PhD; Full Prof.; Licensed Psychologist; 22-40%; *newtonf@ksu.edu*
*   Jones, Carla E; PhD; Assist.; <21%; *cjones@ksu.edu*
*   Wright-Carrroll, Doris; PhD; Assoc.; NCC, Licensed Psychologist; >81%; *djwright@ksu.edu*
*   Nutt, Charles L; PhD; Adjunct; <21%; *cnutt@ksu.edu*

KS: Pittsburg State University

	1701 S. Broadway
	Pittsburg, KS 66762-7557
	United States
Dean	Steve Scott, College of Education
Administrator	Dr. David P. Hurford, Chair
	Department Department of Psy & Counseling
	(316) 235-4522, fax (316) 235-4520, psych@pittstate.edu,
	www.pittstate.edu/psych

Key   See key for Data on Each Department (this section) on page 79.

Program

Accreditation   Regional Accreditation, **CACREP:** Community Counseling

Uniqueness   The department offers an eclectic approach that is highly applied.

Degrees
* Community Counseling: M, S.
* School Counseling: M, S.
* Marriage and Family Counseling: M, S.

Contact
* Community Counseling: M, S = Donald Ward.
* School Counseling: M, S = Becky Brannock.
* Marriage and Family Counseling: M, S = Robert Sheverbush.

Admission and Graduation Data

Admission

Requirements
* Community Counseling(M): GPA 3.00; GRE 1200; GRE V 400; GRE Q 400; GRE A 400.
* Community Counseling(S): GPA 3.00; GRE 1200; GRE V 400; GRE Q 400; GRE A 400.
* School Counseling(M): GPA 3.00; GRE 1200; GRE V 400; GRE Q 400; GRE A 400.
* School Counseling(S): GPA 3.00; GRE 1200; GRE V 400; GRE Q 400; GRE A 400.
* Marriage and Family Counseling(M): GPA 3.00; GRE 1200; GRE V 400; GRE Q 400; GRE A 400.
* Marriage and Family Counseling(S): GPA 3.00; GRE 1200; GRE V 400; GRE Q 400; GRE A 400.

Enrollment
* Community Counseling(M & S): 20 Admitted yearly; 20 Graduated yearly.
* School Counseling(M & S): 20 Admitted yearly; 20 Graduated yearly.
* Marriage and Family Counseling(M & S): 10 Admitted yearly; 10 Graduated yearly.

Diversity
* African-American; Asian-American; Caucasian; Hispanic; Native American; Pacific Islander.

Graduation

Requirements
* Community Counseling(M): 59 Class hours; 150 Practicum hours; 450 Internship hours.
* Community Counseling(S): 30 Class hours.
* School Counseling(M): 48 Class hours; 150 Practicum hours; 300 Internship hours.
* School Counseling(S): 30 Class hours.
* Marriage and Family Counseling(M): 32 Class hours; 450 Practicum hours; 150 Internship hours.
* Marriage and Family Counseling(S): 30 Class hours.

Postgraduation activity: Advanced education and employment setting percentages.
* Community Counseling(M & S): 5 Advanced education; 95 Agency practice.
* School Counseling(M & S): 25 Elementary school; 15 Middle school; 60 Secondary school.
* Marriage and Family Counseling(M & S): 5 Advanced education; 25 Private practice; 70 Agency practice.

Planned Program Modifications

Courses	Drop	Add
	• NP.	• NP.

Other	Decrease	Increase
	• NP.	• NP.

Related Programs Psychology

Faculty

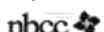   Percent of faculty reported with NCC certification: 60%.

Percent in professional counseling practice: 60%.

Research interests Social cognitiion, sexual aggression, psychology of law, gender issues, school guidance counseling in athletics, learning, psychopharmacology, cognitive-behavioral therapy, life-span development, moral development, moral reasoning, psychology of religion, human development, research design & methodology, reading disabiliites, phonemic processing in chidren, psychopathology, personality assessment, rural mental health services, infant health & development, school psychological services, behavior disorders, consultation, assessment, personality, sexual harassment, family systems counseling, multicultural counseling, marriage counseling, community counseling, group processes, group dynamics, group counseling, team building, theories and techniques of counseling and psychotherapy

Diversity   • Caucasian; Pacific Islander.

Name, Degree, Rank, State/National Credentials, % time devoted to program, email
- Brannock, Becky S; PhD; Assoc.; LPC; >81%; *rbrannoc@pittstate.edu*
- Sharp, Conni K; EdD; Assoc.; LPC, NCC; >81%; *csharp@pittstate.edu*
- Sheverbush, Robert L; EdD; Full Prof.; LPC, NCC; >81%; *rsheverb@pittstate.edu*
- Sparks, Rozanne R; EdD; Full Prof.; <21%; *rsparks@pittstate.edu*
- Ward, Donald E; EdD; Full Prof.; LPC, NCC; >81%; *dward@pittstate.edu*

Has CHI SIGMA IOTA (International Counseling Society) chapter.

KS: University of Kansas

621 Joseph R. Pearson Hall, 1122 West Campus Road
Lawrence, KS 66045
United States
Dean   Angela Lumpkin
Administrator   James W. Lichtenberg, Chairperson
Department   Psych & Research in Education
(785) 864-3931, fax (785) 864-3820, jlicht@ku.edu, www.soe.ku.edu

Key   See key for Data on Each Department (this section) on page 79.

Program
Accreditation   Regional Accreditation

Uniqueness   Program offers quality scientist-practitioner training.

Degrees
- School Counseling: M.
- Other: M.

Contact
- School Counseling: M = NP.
- Other: M = NP.

Admission and Graduation Data
Admission
Requirements
- School Counseling(M): NP.
- Other(M): NP.

Enrollment
- School Counseling(M): 15 Admitted yearly; 15 Graduated yearly.
- Other(M): 15 Admitted yearly; 15 Graduated yearly.

Diversity
- NP.

Graduation
Requirements
- School Counseling(M): 50 Practicum hours.
- Other(M): 50 Practicum hours.

Postgraduation activity: Advanced education and employment setting percentages.
- School Counseling(M): NP.
- Other(M): NP.

Planned Program Modifications
Courses	Drop	Add
• NP.		• NP.

Other	Decrease	Increase
• NP.		• NP.

Related Programs

Faculty

    Percent of faculty reported with NCC certification: 0%.

Percent in professional counseling practice: NP.

Research interests Vocational decision-making, test interpretation, positive psychology

Diversity
- Caucasian; Hispanic.

Name, Degree, Rank, State/National Credentials, % time devoted to program, email
- NP.

KY: Eastern Kentucky University

521 Lancaster Ave, 406 Bert Combs
Richmond, KY 40475-3102
United States
Dean   Mark Wasicsko 420 Bert Combs
Administrator   Dr. Patricia W. Stevens, Chair
                      Department   Counseling and Educational Leadership
                                      (859) 622-1124, fax (859) 622-1126, patricia.stevens@eku.edu,
                                      www.education.eku.edu/cel

Key   See key for Data on Each Department (this section) on page 79.

Program
Accreditation   Regional Accreditation, **CACREP:** School Counseling, **CACREP:** Mental Health Counseling

Uniqueness   A program faculty invested in mentoring students in their professional careers. Involvement in
                professional organizations is supported and opportunities for presentations at conferences
                are regularly provided for students.

Degrees   • Mental Health Counseling: M.
                • School Counseling: M.
                • Other: M.

Contact   • Mental Health Counseling: M = Patricia Stevens.
                • School Counseling: M = Patricia Stevens.
                • Other: M = Patricia Stevens.

Admission and Graduation Data
Admission
Requirements   • Mental Health Counseling(M): GPA 3.00; GRE V 400; GRE Q 400; GRE A 400; MAT 30.
                • School Counseling(M): GPA 3.00; GRE V 400; GRE Q 400; GRE A 400; MAT 30.
                • Student Affairs(M): GPA 2.50; GRE V 400; GRE Q 400; GRE A 400; MAT 30.

Enrollment   • Mental Health Counseling(M): 14 Admitted yearly.
                • School Counseling(M): 30 Admitted yearly.
                • Other (M): NP.

Diversity   • African-American; Asian-American; Caucasian.

Graduation
Requirements   • Mental Health Counseling(M): 60 Class hours; 100 Practicum hours; 900 Internship hours;
                  Comprehensive exam; CPCE.
                • School Counseling(M): 48 Class hours; 100 Practicum hours; 600 Internship hours;
                  Comprehensive exam; CPCE.
                • Other (M): 36 Class hours; Comprehensive exam.

Postgraduation activity: Advanced education and employment setting percentages.
                • Mental Health Counseling(M): 5 Advanced education; 5 Managed care; 5 Private practice;
                  80 Agency practice; 5 Other.
                • School Counseling(M): 2 Advanced education; 32.6 Elementary school; 32.6 Middle
                  school; 32.6 Secondary school.
                • Other (M): 8 Advanced education; 2 Agency practice; 90 Other.

Planned Program Modifications
Courses   Drop   Add
                        • NP.   • Crisis/Violence Counseling
                                                            • Gerontological Counseling
                                                            • Marriage and Family Counseling.

Other   Decrease   Increase
                        • Faculty FTE   • Diversity Recruiting of Faculty
                        • Number of Distance Education   • Diversity Recruiting of Students
                          Courses.   • National Accreditation
                                                            • Number of Off-Campus Courses
                                                            • Number of On-Line Courses.

Related Programs Clinical Social Workers
                     Psychology
                     Other

Faculty

 Percent of faculty reported with NCC certification: 33%.

Percent in professional counseling practice: NP.

Research interests Gender, ethical, and legal issues; crisis/violence counseling.

Diversity   • African-American; Caucasian.

Name, Degree, Rank, State/National Credentials, % time devoted to program, email
* Callahan, Connie J; PhD; Assoc.; LPC, LMFT; >81%; *connie.callahan@eku.edu*
* Erickson, Paul; PhD; Assist.; 61-80%; *paul.erickson@eku.edu*
* Gray, Neal D; PhD; Assist.; LPC, LMFT, CSC, CCDC III; >81%; *neal.gray@eku.edu*
* Naugle, Kim A; PhD; Assoc.; LPC, NCC, Licensed Psy; >81%; *kim.naugle@eku.edu*
* Stockburger, Muriel; EdD; Assist.; LPC; >81%; *muriel.stockburger@eku.edu*
* Stevens, Patricia W; PhD; Full Prof.; LPC, NCC, LMFT, LMFT Supv., LPC, NCC.; 61-80%; *patricia.stevens@eku.edu*
* Strong, Connie S; PhD; Full Prof.; LPC, NCC; 22-40%; *sue.strong@eku.edu*
* Sexton, Larry C; EdD; Full Prof.; LPC; 22-40%; *larry.sexton@eku.edu*
* Chapman, Ann; PhD; >81%; *ann.chapman@eku.edu*

Has CHI SIGMA IOTA (International Counseling Society) chapter.

KY: University of Kentucky

	224 Taylor Education Bldg. Lexington, KY 40506USA
Dean	Dean James Cilbuka
Administrator	Ralph M. Crystal, Professor and Coordinator
	Department Special Education and Rehabilitation Counseling
	(859) 257-3834, fax (859) 257-3835, crystal@uky.edu, www.uky.edu

Key   See key for Data on Each Department (this section) on page 79.

Program

Accreditation	Regional Accreditation, CORE: Rehabilitation Counseling
Uniqueness	The program values diversity, research, multi-disciplinary training, on a competency based model of rehabilitation education.
Degrees	• Rehabilitation Counseling: M.
Contact	• Rehabilitation Counseling: M = Ralph M. Crystal.

Admission and Graduation Data

Admission

Requirements	• Rehabilitation Counseling(M): GPA 2.75; GRE 1200; GRE V 400; GRE Q 400; GRE A 400; Interview.
Enrollment	• Rehabilitation Counseling(M): 20 Admitted yearly; 20 Graduated yearly; 15 Female; 5 Male.
Diversity	• African-American; Asian-American; Caucasian; Hispanic; Native American; Pacific Islander.

Graduation

Requirements	• Rehabilitation Counseling(M): 55-60 Class hours; 300 Practicum hours; 600 Internship hours; Comprehensive exam; Oral exam.

Postgraduation activity: Advanced education and employment setting percentages.
  • Rehabilitation Counseling(M): 10 Advanced education; 10 Private practice; 80 Agency practice.

Planned Program Modifications

Courses	Drop	Add
	• NP.	• Legal/Ethical Issues.

Other	Decrease	Increase
	• NP.	• Course Offerings • Diversity Recruiting of Students • Financial Aid • Number of Degree Majors • Number of Distance Education Courses • Number of Off-Campus Courses • Number of On-Line Courses.

Related Programs Clinical Social Workers
Marriage and Family Therapists
Psychology
Psychiatric Nurses
Psychiatrists
Organizational Behaviorists
Communications
International Studies

Faculty

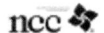 Percent of faculty reported with NCC certification: 40%.

Percent in professional counseling practice: 20%.

Research interests HIV/AIDS; Epilepsy and Quality of Life; Migrant and Seasonal Farmworkers; Cultural Diversity and Women's Issues

Diversity	• African-American; Caucasian.

Name, Degree, Rank, State/National Credentials, % time devoted to program, email
- Crystal, Ralph M; PhD; Full Prof.; LPC, NCC, CRC; >81%; *crystal@uky.edu*
- Feist-Price, Sonja M; RhD; Assoc.; LPC, CRC; >81%; *smfeis@uky.edu*
- Harley, Debra A; PhD; Assoc.; LPC, NCC, CRC; >81%; *dhar100@uky.edu*
- Bishop, Malachy; PhD; Assist.; CRC; >81%; *mbishop@uky.edu*
- Rogers, Jackie B; PhD; Assist.; LPC, CRC; <21%; *jbroge2@uky.edu*

Has CHI SIGMA IOTA (International Counseling Society) chapter.

KY: Western Kentucky University

1 Big Red Way, Col of Ed & Behav Sci
Bowling Green, KY 42101-5576
United States

Dean
Administrator   Donald R. Nims, Interim Department Head
                       Department   Department of Counseling and Student Affairs
                                       (270) 745-4953, fax (270) 745-5301, counseling.program@wku.edu

Key   See key for Data on Each Department (this section) on page 79.

Program
Accreditation   NP.

Uniqueness   Most of the graduate students in our counseling programs are employed and attend our
                 classes on a part-time basis.

Degrees   • Mental Health Counseling: M.
                 • Marriage and Family Counseling: M.
                 • Student Affairs: M.

Contact   • Mental Health Counseling: M = Fred Stickle.
                 • Marriage and Family Counseling: M = NP.
                 • Student Affairs: M = Aaron Hughey.

Admission and Graduation Data
Admission
Requirements   • Mental Health Counseling(M): GRE 1350.
                 • Marriage and Family Counseling(M): NP.
                 • Student Affairs(M): GPA 2.75.

Enrollment   • Mental Health Counseling(M): 30 Admitted yearly; 10 Graduated yearly.
                 • Marriage and Family Counseling(M): 15 Admitted yearly; 10 Graduated yearly.
                 • Student Affairs(M): 15 Admitted yearly; 13 Graduated yearly.

Diversity   • NP.

Graduation
Requirements   • Mental Health Counseling(M): 60 Class hours; 100 Practicum hours; 600 Internship hours.
                 • Marriage and Family Counseling(M): 60 Class hours; 100 Practicum hours; 600 Internship
                   hours.
                 • Student Affairs(M): 48 Class hours; 100 Practicum hours; 600 Internship hours.

Postgraduation activity: Advanced education and employment setting percentages.
                 • Mental Health Counseling(M): 5 Advanced education; 50 Managed care; 15 Private
                   practice; 25 Agency practice; 5 Other.
                 • Marriage and Family Counseling(M): NP.
                 • Student Affairs(M): 4 Advanced education; 96 Other.

Planned Program Modifications
Courses   Drop   Add
                 • NP.   • NP.

Other   Decrease   Increase
                 • NP.   • NP.

Related Programs

Faculty

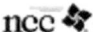   Percent of faculty reported with NCC certification: 50%.

Percent in professional counseling practice: NP.

Research interests NP.

Diversity   • NP.

Name, Degree, Rank, State/National Credentials, % time devoted to program, email
• Dinkmeyer, Jr., Don C; PhD; Full Prof.; NCC; >81%;
• Greenwalt, Bill C; EdD; Assist.; NCC; >81%;
• Hayden, Delbert J; PhD; Full Prof.; >81%;
• Hughey, Aaron W; EdD; Assoc.; >81%;

- James, Susan M; EdD; Assoc.; >81%;
- Mason, Cynthia P; EdD; Assoc.; >81%;
- Minatrea, Neresa B; PhD; Assoc.; NCC; >81%;
- Nims, Donald R; EdD; Assoc.; NCC; >81%;
- Schnacke, Stephen B; EdD; Full Prof.; NCC; >81%;
- Sheeley, Vernon Lee; PhD; Full Prof.; >81%;
- Stickle, Fred E; PhD; Full Prof.; NCC; >81%;
- Westbrooks, Karen L; PhD; Full Prof.; >81%;

LA: Louisiana State University

122 Peabody Hall
Baton Rouge, LA 70803-4721
USA

Dean   Dean Barbara Fuhrmann, College of Education, 221 Peabody Hall
Administrator Gary G. Gintner, Ph.D., Coordinator of Counselor Education and Assistant Professor
Department   Educational Leadership, Research and Counseling
(225) 578-2197, gintner@lsu.edu, http://asterix.ednet.lsu.edu/'elrcweb/

Key   See key for Data on Each Department (this section) on page 79.

Program

Accreditation   Regional Accreditation, **CACREP:** Community Counseling, **CACREP:** School Counseling

CACREP

Uniqueness   The program emphasizes close collaboration between students and faculty. There is a strong
emphasis on practical in-class and out-of-class clinical experiences in each course.

Degrees   • Community Counseling: M, S.
              • School Counseling: M, S.

Contact   • Community Counseling: M = Laura G. Hensley, Ph.D..; S = Gary G. Gintner, Ph.D..
              • School Counseling: M, S = David A. Spruill, Ph.D..

Admission and Graduation Data

Admission
Requirements • Community Counseling(M): GPA 3.00; GRE 1000; GRE V 500; GRE Q 500.
              • Community Counseling(S): GPA 3.00; GRE 1000; GRE V 500; GRE Q 500.
              • School Counseling(M): GPA 3.00; GRE 1000; GRE V 500; GRE Q 500.
              • School Counseling(S): GPA 3.00; GRE 1000; GRE V 500; GRE Q 500.

Enrollment   • Community Counseling(M & S): 10 Admitted yearly; 9 Graduated yearly; 22 Female; 1
                Male.
              • School Counseling(M & S): 5 Admitted yearly; 5 Graduated yearly; 10 Female.

Diversity   • African-American; Asian-American; Caucasian.

Graduation
Requirements • Community Counseling(M): 48 Class hours; 100 Practicum hours; 600 Internship hours;
                Comprehensive exam.
              • Community Counseling(S): 60 Class hours; 300 Internship hours; Comprehensive exam.
              • School Counseling(M): 48 Class hours; 100 Practicum hours; 600 Internship hours;
                Comprehensive exam.
              • School Counseling(S): 60 Class hours; 300 Internship hours; Comprehensive exam.

Postgraduation activity: Advanced education and employment setting percentages.
              • Community Counseling(M & S): 10 Advanced education; 70 Agency practice; 20 Other.
              • School Counseling(M & S): 40 Elementary school; 20 Middle school; 40 Secondary school.

Planned Program Modifications

Courses   Drop   Add
                  • NP.   • Addictions
                                                 • Career/Life Planning
                                                 • Teaming
                                                 • Theory Component.

Other   Decrease   Increase
                  • NP.   • Number of Off-Campus Courses.

Related Programs Clinical Social Workers
                     Psychology
                     Communications

Faculty

nbcc ❖.   Percent of faculty reported with NCC certification: **100**%.   ncc ❖

Percent in professional counseling practice: 100%.

Research interests Gary G. Gintner, Ph.D.: Designing effective treatment plans, practice guidelines for psychiatric disorders, and effectiveness of motivational interviewing for substance use problems.David A. Spruill, Ph.D.: Training issues in marriage and family counseling, professional development issues, and ethics.Laura G. Hensley, Ph.D.: Women's issues, sexual assault, college counseling, and group work.

Diversity • Caucasian.

Name, Degree, Rank, State/National Credentials, % time devoted to program, email
- Gintner, Gary G; PhD; Assoc.; LPC, NCC; >81%; *gintner@lsu.edu*
- Spruill, David A; PhD; Assoc.; LPC, NCC, LMFT; >81%; *dspruill@lsu.edu*
- Hensley, Laura G; PhD; Assist.; LPC, NCC; >81%; *lhensley@lsu.edu*

Has CHI SIGMA IOTA (International Counseling Society) chapter.

LA: Louisiana State University in Shreveport

	One University Place
	Shreveport, LA 71115-2399
	USA
Dean	Gale Bridger, College of Education and Human Development
Administrator	Meredith Nelson, PhD, MSCP Program Coordinator
	Department Psychology
	(318) 797-5044, fax (318) 798-4171, mnelson@pilot.lsus.edu, www.lsus.edu

Key   See key for Data on Each Department (this section) on page 79.

Program
Accreditation   Regional Accreditation

Uniqueness   NP.

Degrees
- Community Counseling: M.
- Other: S.

Contact
- Community Counseling: M = Meredith Nelson.
- Other: S = Merikay Ringer.

Admission and Graduation Data
Admission
Requirements
- Community Counseling(M): GPA 2.75; GRE 800; GRE V 400; GRE Q 400.
- Other(S):

Enrollment
- Community Counseling(M): 20 Admitted yearly; 15 Graduated yearly; 65% Female; 35% Male.
- Other(S).

Diversity
- African-American; Caucasian; Native American; Multiracial.

Graduation
Requirements
- Community Counseling(M): 48 Class hours; 100 Practicum hours; 600 Internship hours; Comprehensive exam; CPCE; Portfolio.
- Other(S): 70 Class hours; 300 Practicum hours; 1000 Internship hours; Comprehensive exam; Oral exam; Portfolio.

Postgraduation activity: Advanced education and employment setting percentages.
- Community Counseling(M): 15 Advanced education; 30 Managed care; 20 Private practice; 20 Agency practice; 5 Student affairs; 10 Other.
- Other(S).

Planned Program Modifications
Courses	Drop	Add
	• NP.	• Addictions
		• Crisis/Violence Counseling
		• Experiential Component
		• Forensic Counseling
		• Gerontological Counseling
		• Marriage and Family Counseling
		• Play Therapy
		• Psychopharmocology
		• School Counseling.

Other	Decrease	Increase
	• NP.	• Course Offerings
		• Diversity Recruiting of Faculty
		• Diversity Recruiting of Students
		• Faculty FTE
		• National Accreditation
		• Number of Degree Majors
		• Number of Distance Education Courses
		• Number of On-Line Courses.

Related Programs

Faculty

 Percent of faculty reported with NCC certification: 12%.

Percent in professional counseling practice: 30%.

Research interests

Diversity   •   African-American; Asian-American; Caucasian.

Name, Degree, Rank, State/National Credentials, % time devoted to program, email
- Nelson, Meredith G; PhD; Assist.; LPC, NCC, LMFT; >81%; *mnelson@pilot.lsus.edu*
- Yong, Dai; PhD; Assoc.; 61-80%; *ydai@pilot.lsus.ed*
- Hollenshead, Jean; PhD; Assoc.; 61-80%; *jhollens@pilot.lsus.edu*
- Stanley, Patricia D.; PhD; Full Prof.; 22-40%; *pstanley@pilot.lsus.edu*
- Nolan, Rebecca; PhD; Full Prof.; <21%; *rnolan@pilot.lsus.edu*
- Evans, James; MA; Instructor; *jevans@pilot.lsus.edu*
- Ringe, Merikayr; PhD; Assoc.; 22-40%; *mringer@pilot.lsus.edu*
- Adomaitus, Ray; PhD; Assist.; >81%

LA: Loyola University

6363 St. Charles Avenue
New Orleans, LA 70118
United States

Dean
Administrator   Justin E. Levitov, Director
                      Department   Department of Education & Counseling
                                      (504) 864-7840, fax (504) 864-7844, Educate@Loyno.Edu

Key   See key for Data on Each Department (this section) on page 79.

Program
Accreditation   NP.

Uniqueness   Loyola's M.S. Program in counseling includes both a strong theoretical emphases and live
                practice situations where client actors are used to train students. A low student teacher ratio
                ensures individual attention.

Degrees   • Community Counseling: M.

Contact   • Community Counseling: M = NP.

Admission and Graduation Data
Admission
Requirements   • Community Counseling(M): GPA 3.00; GRE 1600; GRE V 550; GRE Q 550; GRE A 500;
                  MAT 45; Interview.

Enrollment   • Community Counseling(M): 20 Admitted yearly; 10 Graduated yearly; 85% Female;
                  15% Male.

Diversity   • African-American; Asian-American; Caucasian; Hispanic; Multiracial.

Graduation
Requirements   • Community Counseling(M): 48 Class hours; 140 Practicum hours; 600 Internship hours;
                  Comprehensive exam.

Postgraduation activity: Advanced education and employment setting percentages.
                • Community Counseling(M): 20 Advanced education; 40 Agency practice; 10 Middle school;
                  10 Secondary school; 10 Student affairs; 10 Other.

Planned Program Modifications
Courses   Drop   Add
                  • NP.   • NP.

Other   Decrease   Increase
                  • NP.   • National Accreditation.

Related Programs

Faculty

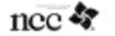 Percent of faculty reported with NCC certification: **100%**.

Percent in professional counseling practice: 100%.

Research interests NP.

Diversity   • Caucasian.

Name, Degree, Rank, State/National Credentials, % time devoted to program, email
• Fall, Kevin A; PhD; Assoc.; LPC, NCC; >81%; *kfall@loyno.edu*
• Levitov, Justin E; PhD; Full Prof.; LPC, NCC; >81%; *levitov@loyno.edu*
• Lyons, Christy E; PhD; Assist.; LPC, NCC; >81%; *clyons@loyno.edu*

Has CHI SIGMA IOTA (International Counseling Society) chapter.

LA: McNeese State University

	P.O. Box 91895
	Lake Charles, LA 70609-2895
	US
Dean	Dean Joe Savoie, Burton College of Education
Administrator	Jess Feist, EdD, Professor
	Department Psychology
	(337) 475-5457, fax (337) 475-5467, mdisney@acc.mcneese.edu,
	www.mcneese.edu

Key   See key for Data on Each Department (this section) on page 79.

Program

Accreditation   Regional Accreditation; Applied for CACREP: Mental Health Counseling, CACREP: School Counseling

Uniqueness   Faculty who teach the majority of counseling courses are clinicians/academicians. Each of these individuals has worked in the mental health field for more than 20 years in a variety of capacities. This brings a wealth of experience to the student population. Very early on in the program, students take their first experiential course where counseling is required under close supervision. Internship sites are varied in the area and most are paid placements. The Department operates the Kay Dore Counseling Clinic, a counseling service for low income families, where state of the art audio and video equipment is utilized by those in the experiential courses.

Degrees
- Mental Health Counseling: M.
- School Counseling: M.

Contact
- Mental Health Counseling: M = M. Janelle Disney.
- School Counseling: M = M. Janelle Disney.

Admission and Graduation Data

Admission

Requirements
- Mental Health Counseling(M): GPA ~3.00; GRE ~950; Interview.
- School Counseling(M): GPA ~2.70; GRE ~895; Interview.

Enrollment
- Mental Health Counseling(M): 5 Admitted yearly; 4 Graduated yearly; 4 Female; 1 Male.
- School Counseling(M): 4 Admitted yearly; 4 Graduated yearly.

Diversity
- African-American; Asian-American; Caucasian; Hispanic.

Graduation

Requirements
- Mental Health Counseling(M): 60 Class hours; 100 Practicum hours; 900 Internship hours; Comprehensive exam.
- School Counseling(M): 48 Class hours; 100 Practicum hours; 600 Internship hours; Comprehensive exam.

Postgraduation activity: Advanced education and employment setting percentages.
- Mental Health Counseling(M): 1 Advanced education; 5 Managed care; 94 Agency practice.
- School Counseling(M): 50 Elementary school; 50 Secondary school.

Planned Program Modifications

Courses	Drop	Add
	• NP.	• NP.

Other	Decrease	Increase
	• NP.	• Clinical Supervision
		• Diversity Recruiting of Faculty
		• Diversity Recruiting of Students
		• Financial Aid
		• National Accreditation.

Related Programs

Faculty

nbcc   Percent of faculty reported with NCC certification: 22%.   ncc

Percent in professional counseling practice: 33%.

Research interests Addictive disorders focusing mainly on alcohol and compulsive gambling; Neurological and
                    psychological effects of pollutants; Effects on families where one has been diagnosed with
                    cancer.

Diversity   • Caucasian.

Name, Degree, Rank, State/National Credentials, % time devoted to program, email
• Bartling, Carl; PhD; Full Prof.; 22-40%;
• Brannon, Linda; PhD; Full Prof.; Licensed psychologist; 22-40%; *lbrannon@laol.net*
• Dilks, Lawrence; PhD; Assoc.; LPC, NCC, Licensed psychologist; 61-80%;
• Disney, Janelle; PhD; Full Prof.; LPC, NCC, LMFT; >81%; *mdisney@mail.mcneese.edu*
• Odum-Gunn, Diana; PhD; Assist.; 22-40%;
• Melville, Cameron; PhD; Full Prof.; 22-40%; *melville@mail.mcneese.edu*
• Matzenbacher, Dena; PhD; Assist.; *dena@mail.mcneese.edu*
• Whiteman, Jerry; PhD; Assoc.; LPC, Licensed psychologist; >81%;
• Feist, Jess; EdD; Full Prof.; 61-80%;

LA: Northwestern State University

Student Personel Services Program
Natchitoches, LA 71497
USA

Dean   John Tollett, College of Education
Administrator   Robert L. Bowman, Ph. D; Chair, Stu Aff Prog
     Department   College of Education
     (318) 357-6289, fax (318) 357-6275, Bowmanr@nsula.edu,
     www.education.nsula.edu/sps/

Key   See key for Data on Each Department (this section) on page 79.

Program

Accreditation   Regional Accreditation, **CACREP:** Student Affairs - Counseling, **CACREP:** Student Affairs - Professional Practice

Uniqueness   Our program offers experiences unique to the college environment, numerous internship sites both on and off-campus and a collegial faculty while meeting requirements for the LPC credential.

Degrees
- College Counseling: M.
- Student Affairs: M.

Contact
- College Counseling: M = Robert Bowman.
- Student Affairs: M = Robert Bowman.

Admission and Graduation Data

Admission

Requirements
- College Counseling(M): GPA 2.50; GRE 800; GRE V 400; GRE Q 400; GRE A 0; Interview.
- Student Affairs(M): GPA 2.50; GRE 800; GRE V 400; GRE Q 400; GRE A 0; Interview.

Enrollment
- College Counseling(M): 20 Admitted yearly; 15 Graduated yearly.
- Student Affairs(M): 20 Admitted yearly; 15 Graduated yearly.

Diversity
- African-American; Asian-American; Caucasian; Native American; Multiracial.

Graduation

Requirements
- College Counseling(M): 48 Class hours; 100 Practicum hours; 600 Internship hours; Comprehensive exam.
- Student Affairs(M): 48 Class hours; 100 Practicum hours; 600 Internship hours.

Postgraduation activity: Advanced education and employment setting percentages.
- College Counseling(M): 15 Advanced education; 10 Private practice; 10 Agency practice; 65 Other.
- Student Affairs(M): 15 Advanced education; 10 Agency practice; 75 Other.

Planned Program Modifications

Courses   <u>Drop</u>   <u>Add</u>
     • NP.   • NP.

Other   <u>Decrease</u>   <u>Increase</u>
     • NP.   • Number of Distance Education Courses
                 • Number of Off-Campus Courses
                 • Number of On-Line Courses.

Related Programs

Faculty

 Percent of faculty reported with NCC certification: 57%.

Percent in professional counseling practice: NP.

Research interests NP.

Diversity
- Asian-American; Caucasian; Multiracial.

Name, Degree, Rank, State/National Credentials, % time devoted to program, email
- Bowman, Robert L; PhD; Full Prof.; NCC; >81%; *bowmanr@nsula.edu*
- Smith, Janice E; PhD; Assist.; NCC; >81%; *bowmany@nsula.edu*
- Curtis, Reagan M; PhD; Assist.; NCC; 22-40%; *hall@nsula.edu*
- Kher, Neelam; PhD; Full Prof.; 22-40%; *kher@nsula.edu*
- Pearson, Frances C; PhD; Assoc.; NCC; >81%; *pearson@nsula.edu*
- Teel, Faith; MA; Assist.; 22-40%;
- Christensen, Paula; PhD; Assoc.; 22-40%;

LA: Our Lady of Holy Cross

4123 Woodland Drive
New Orleans, LA 70131
United States

Dean
Administrator   Judith G. Miranti, Dean
                       Department   Division of Humanities, Educ & Counseling
                                     (504) 398-2214, fax (504) 391-2421, Jmiranti@olhec.edu

Key   See key for Data on Each Department (this section) on page 79.

Program
Accreditation   **CACREP:** Marriage and Family Counseling

Uniqueness   NP.

Degrees   • School Counseling: M.
                • Marriage and Family Counseling: M.
                • Community Counseling: M.

Contact   • School Counseling: M = Dr. Judith Miranti.
                • Marriage and Family Counseling: M = Dr. Judith Miranti.
                • Community Counseling: M = Dr. Judith Miranti.

Admission and Graduation Data
Admission
Requirements   • School Counseling(M): NP.
                • Marriage and Family Counseling(M): NP.
                • Community Counseling(M): NP.

Enrollment   • School Counseling(M): 10 Admitted yearly; 10 Graduated yearly.
                • Marriage and Family Counseling(M): 25 Admitted yearly; 25 Graduated yearly.
                • Community Counseling(M): 10 Admitted yearly; 5 Graduated yearly.

Diversity   • NP.

Graduation
Requirements   • School Counseling(M): 54 Class hours; 100 Practicum hours; 600 Internship hours.
                • Marriage and Family Counseling(M): 60 Class hours; 100 Practicum hours; 600 Internship
                  hours.
                • Community Counseling(M): 51 Class hours; 100 Practicum hours; 600 Internship hours.

Postgraduation activity: Advanced education and employment setting percentages.
                • School Counseling(M): NP.
                • Marriage and Family Counseling(M): NP.
                • Community Counseling(M): NP.

Planned Program Modifications
Courses   <u>Drop</u>   <u>Add</u>
                • NP.   • NP.

Other   <u>Decrease</u>   <u>Increase</u>
                • NP.   • NP.

Related Programs

Faculty

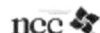   Percent of faculty reported with NCC certification: 0%.   ncc

Percent in professional counseling practice: NP.

Research interests NP.

Diversity   • NP.

Name, Degree, Rank, State/National Credentials, % time devoted to program, email
• NP.

Has CHI SIGMA IOTA (International Counseling Society) chapter.

LA: Southeastern Louisiana University

SLU 863
Hammond, LA 70402-0863
United States
Dean   Dr. Martha H. Thornhill, Interim Dean
Administrator   Brian Canfield, Department Head
                    Department   Department of Human Development
                                   (985) 549-2309, fax (985) 549-3758, bcanfield@selu.edu,
                                   http://www.selu.edu/Academics/Education/dhd/index.htm

Key   See key for Data on Each Department (this section) on page 79.

Program
Accreditation   Regional Accreditation, **CACREP:** Community Counseling, **CACREP:** School Counseling,
                    CACREP: Student Affairs - Counseling

Uniqueness   The faculty is committed to the highest standards of excellence. Future counselors receive an
                    abundance of individualized instruction from faculty who have a reputation of being accessible
                    and approachable.

Degrees   • Community Counseling: M.
                    • School Counseling: M.
                    • College Counseling: M.
                    • Marriage and Family Counseling: M.

Contact   • Community Counseling: M = Hunter Alessi.
                    • School Counseling: M = Mary Ballard.
                    • College Counseling: M = June Williams.
                    • Marriage and Family Counseling: M = Peter Emerson.

Admission and Graduation Data
Admission
Requirements   • Community Counseling(M): Letters; Interview.
                    • School Counseling(M): Letters; Interview.
                    • College Counseling(M): Letters; Interview.
                    • Marriage and Family Counseling(M): Interview.

Enrollment   • Community Counseling(M): NP.
                    • School Counseling(M): NP.
                    • College Counseling(M): NP.
                    • Marriage and Family Counseling(M): NP.

Diversity   • African-American; Asian-American; Caucasian; Hispanic.

Graduation
Requirements   • Community Counseling(M): 48 Class hours; 100 Practicum hours; 600 Internship hours;
                      Comprehensive exam; CPCE.
                    • School Counseling(M): 48 Class hours; 100 Practicum hours; 600 Internship hours;
                      Comprehensive exam; CPCE.
                    • College Counseling(M): 48 Class hours; 100 Practicum hours; 600 Internship hours;
                      Comprehensive exam; CPCE.
                    • Marriage and Family Counseling(M): 63 Class hours; 100 Practicum hours; 600 Internship
                      hours; Comprehensive exam; CPCE.

Postgraduation activity: Advanced education and employment setting percentages.
                    • Community Counseling(M): NP.
                    • School Counseling(M): NP.
                    • College Counseling(M): NP.
                    • Marriage and Family Counseling(M): NP.

Planned Program Modifications
Courses   Drop   Add
                    • NP.   • Grief Counseling.

Other   Decrease   Increase
                    • NP.   • Course Offerings
                                                     • Diversity Recruiting of Faculty
                                                     • Diversity Recruiting of Students
                                                     • Number of Distance Education Courses
                                                     • Number of Off-Campus Courses
                                                     • Number of On-Line Courses.

Related Programs Clinical Social Workers
Psychology

Faculty

nbcc ❖   Percent of faculty reported with NCC certification: 20%.   ncc ❖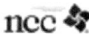

Percent in professional counseling practice: 100%.

Research interests NP.

Diversity   • Caucasian.

Name, Degree, Rank, State/National Credentials, % time devoted to program, email
• Alessi, Hunter D; PhD; Full Prof.; LPC, LMFT; >81%; *halessi@selu.edu*
• Ballard, Mary; PhD; Assoc.; LPC, LMFT; >81%; *mballard2@selu.edu*
• Canfield, Brian S; EdD; Full Prof.; LPC, LMFT, AAMFT Clinical Member; 61-80%; *bcanfield@selu.edu*
• Emerson, Peter M; EdD; Assoc.; LPC, NCC, LMFT, AAMFT Clinical Member; >81%; *pemerson@selu.edu*
• Williams, June M; PhD; Assist.; LPC, LMFT; >81%; *jwilliams@selu.edu*

Has CHI SIGMA IOTA (International Counseling Society) chapter.

LA: University of New Orleans

348 Education Building
New Orleans, LA 70148
USA

Dean Dr. James Meza, College of Education and Human Development
Administrator Dr. Diana Hulse-Killacky, Counseling Graduate Program Coordinator
Department   Educational Leadership, Counseling, and Foundations
(504) 280-6661, fax (504) 280-6453, dhulseki@uno.edu,
http://ed.uno.edu/~EDFR/Counseling/Programs.htm

Key   See key for Data on Each Department (this section) on page 79.

Program
Accreditation   Regional Accreditation, **CACREP:** Community Counseling, **CACREP:** Counselor Education
and Supervision, **CACREP:** Student Affairs - Counseling, **CACREP:** School Counseling

Uniqueness   The master's and doctoral degree programs in counseling at the University of New Orleans
emphasize the development of a strong professional identity in students. Faculty serve as role
models who are skilled counselors, active leaders in the profession, excellent teachers, and
recognized scholars. The program is rich in diversity with strong representation of African-
American, Hispanic, disabled, gay, lesbian, and bisexual students. The cultural richness of
New Orleans is reflected in the program's field placements, student backgrounds, and social
activities. Master's specializations are available in community, college, and school counseling.
The doctoral program emphasizes clinical supervision, teaching, professional leadership, and
research. Legal and ethical issues, multicultural counseling, group work, play therapy, and
counseling children are emphasized in courses. Assistantships that include in-state and out-
of-state tuition waivers are available for full-time graduate students. National speakers from
the counseling profession present to graduate students several times each year. The retention
and graduate rate of admitted master's and doctoral students is exceptionally high.

Degrees
- Community Counseling: M.
- School Counseling: M.
- College Counseling: M.
- Counselor Education: PhD.

Contact
- Community Counseling: M = Dr. Diana Hulse-Killacky.
- School Counseling: M = Dr. Diana Hulse-Killacky.
- College Counseling: M = Dr. Diana Hulse-Killacky.
- Counselor Education: D = Dr. Diana Hulse-Killacky.

Admission and Graduation Data
Admission
Requirements
- Community Counseling(M): GPA 2.50; GRE R.
- School Counseling(M): GPA 2.50; GRE R.
- College Counseling(M): GPA 2.50; GRE R.
- Counselor Education(D): Masters and GPA 3.00; GRE R.

Enrollment
- Community Counseling(M): 30 Admitted yearly; 30 Graduated yearly; 70 Female; 20 Male.
- School Counseling(M): 20 Admitted yearly; 20 Graduated yearly; 15 Male.
- College Counseling(M): 10 Admitted yearly; 10 Graduated yearly; 20 Female; 10 Male.
- Counselor Education(D): 15 Admitted yearly; 15 Graduated yearly; 30 Female; 18 Male.

Diversity
- African-American; Asian-American; Caucasian; Hispanic; Native American; Multiracial.

Graduation
Requirements
- Community Counseling(M): 60 Class hours; 100 Practicum hours; 600 Internship hours;
Comprehensive exam; CPCE.
- School Counseling(M): 60 Class hours; 100 Practicum hours; 600 Internship hours;
Comprehensive exam; CPCE.
- College Counseling(M): 60 Class hours; 100 Practicum hours; 600 Internship hours;
Comprehensive exam; CPCE.
- Counselor Education(D): 112 Class hours; 200 Practicum hours; 1200 Internship hours;
Comprehensive exam; CPCE; Oral exam; Dissertation.

Postgraduation activity: Advanced education and employment setting percentages.
- Community Counseling(M): 5 Managed care; 90 Agency practice.
- School Counseling(M): 5 Advanced education; 10 Elementary school; 40 Middle school; 50
Secondary school.
- College Counseling(M): 5 Advanced education; 95 Student affairs.
- Counselor Education(D): 5 Managed care; 20 Private practice; 50 Agency practice; 5
Secondary school; 20 Student affairs.

Planned Program Modifications

Courses	Drop	Add
	• NP.	• Advocacy
		• Crisis/Violence Counseling
		• Diversity
		• Legal/Ethical Issues
		• Play Therapy
		• School Counseling
		• Social Justice
		• Supervision.

Other	Decrease	Increase
	• NP.	• Admission Requirements
		• Course Offerings
		• Diversity Recruiting of Students
		• Financial Aid
		• Number of Distance Education Courses
		• Number of Off-Campus Courses.

Related Programs

Faculty

nbcc ❧.   Percent of faculty reported with NCC certification: 94%.   ncc ❧

Percent in professional counseling practice: 90%.

Research interests   Research interests of faculty include racial identity development, multicultural counseling, school counseling, employee assistance counseling, legal issues in counseling, ethical issues in counseling, counseling supervision, group work, play therapy, and counseling children and adolescents. Projects in the department include reporting suspected child abuse, counseling children victims of sexual abuse, counseling in a pastoral counseling center, supervision in a community mental health center, and assisting children who have failed academic tests for school promotion.

Diversity   • African-American; Caucasian.

Name, Degree, Rank, State/National Credentials, % time devoted to program, email
- Remley, Jr., Theodore P; PhD; Full Prof.; LPC, NCC; >81%; *tremley@uno.edu*
- Hulse-Killacky, Diana; EdD; Full Prof.; LPC, NCC; >81%; *dhulseki@uno.edu*
- Herlihy, Barbara; PhD; Full Prof.; LPC, NCC; >81%; *bherlihy@uno.edu*
- McCollum, Vivian; PhD; Assoc.; LPC, NCC; >81%; *vmccollu@uno.edu*
- Watson, Zarus; PhD; Assoc.; >81%; *zwatson@uno.edu*
- Christensen, Teresa; PhD; Assist.; LPC, NCC; >81%; *tchriste@uno.edu*
- Hightower, James; EdD; Lecturer; LPC, NCC; <21%; *jhightower@tmfi.org*
- Jarosinski, Jeffrey; PhD; Lecturer; LPC, NCC; <21%; *jeffrey.g.jarosinski@aexp.com*
- Lopez, Tiffany; PhD; Lecturer; LPC, NCC; <21%; *stsv-tml@nicholls.edu*
- Nguyen, Si; PhD; Lecturer; LPC, NCC; <21%; *singuyen98@yahoo.com*
- Oprea, Luane; PhD; Lecturer; LPC, NCC; <21%; *rnoprea@aol.com*
- Perry, Lucille; PhD; Lecturer; LPC, NCC; <21%; *lucilleperry@mindspring.com*
- Rosenbaum, William; PhD; Lecturer; LPC, NCC; <21%; *rosefau@bellsouth.net*
- Stokes, Larry; PhD; Lecturer; LPC, NCC; <21%; *lstokesphd@aol.com*
- Thorpe, Marilyn; PhD; Lecturer; LPC, NCC; <21%; *acivint@bellsouth.net*
- Roussel, Daniel; PhD; Lecturer; LPC, NCC; <21%; *rescuerover@aol.com*

Has CHI SIGMA IOTA (International Counseling Society) chapter.

MA: Bridgewater State College

233 Tillinghast Hall
Bridgewater, MA 02325
USA
Dean   Dr. Ed Minnock
Administrator   Dr. Victoria L. Bacon, Coordinator, Counseling Programs
                    Department   Counseling - SEPP
                    (508) 531-2836, fax (508) 531-6167, vbacon@bridgew.edu

Key   See key for Data on Each Department (this section) on page 79.

Program
   Accreditation   Regional Accreditation

   Uniqueness   Offers multiple counseling programs; faculty use contructivist framework, and mission
                    embraces professionalism, diversity and technology

   Degrees   • Mental Health Counseling: M, S.
                    • School Counseling: M.
                    • Student Affairs: M.

   Contact   • Mental Health Counseling: M = Dr. Victoria L. Bacon.; S = NP.
                    • School Counseling: M = Dr. Maxine Rawlins.
                    • Student Affairs: M = Dr. Michael Kocet.

Admission and Graduation Data
Admission
   Requirements   • Mental Health Counseling(M): GPA 2.80; GRE 1000; Interview.
                    • Mental Health Counseling(S): GPA 2.80; GRE 1000; Interview.
                    • School Counseling(M): GPA 2.80; GRE 1000; Interview.
                    • Student Affairs(M): GPA 2.80; GRE 1000; Interview.

   Enrollment   • Mental Health Counseling(M & S): 30 Admitted yearly; 15 Graduated yearly; 50 Female;
                      40 Male.
                    • School Counseling(M): 15 Admitted yearly; 8 Graduated yearly; 10 Male.
                    • Student Affairs(M): 15 Admitted yearly; 8 Graduated yearly; 15 Female; 12 Male.

   Diversity   • African-American; Asian-American; Caucasian; Multiracial.

Graduation
   Requirements   • Mental Health Counseling(M): 60 Class hours; 100 Practicum hours; 900 Internship hours;
                      Comprehensive exam.
                    • Mental Health Counseling(S):
                    • School Counseling(M): 48 Class hours; 100 Practicum hours; 600 Internship hours;
                      Comprehensive exam.
                    • Student Affairs(M): 48 Class hours; 100 Practicum hours; 600 Internship hours;
                      Comprehensive exam.

   Postgraduation activity: Advanced education and employment setting percentages.
                    • Mental Health Counseling(M & S): 2 Advanced education; 90 Managed care.
                    • School Counseling(M): 5 Elementary school; 25 Middle school; 70 Secondary school.
                    • Student Affairs(M): 2 Advanced education; 100 Student affairs.

Planned Program Modifications
   Courses   Drop   Add
                    • NP.   • Adventure Counseling
                                                      • Gender Studies
                                                      • Supervision.

   Other   Decrease   Increase
                    • NP.   • Number of Degree Majors
                                                      • Number of Off-Campus Courses.

Related Programs Clinical Social Workers

Faculty

   nbcc Percent of faculty reported with NCC certification: 0%.   **ncc**

   Percent in professional counseling practice: 100%.

   Research interests Multicultural Issues; Enhancing Counseling through Technology; Counseling Athletes;
                    Childhood Violence

Diversity   •   African-American; Caucasian; Native American.

Name, Degree, Rank, State/National Credentials, % time devoted to program, email
- Bacon, Victoria L; EdD; Assoc.; Licensed Psychologist; >81%; *vbacon@bridgew.edu*
- Calicchia, John; PhD; Assist.; Licensed Psychologist; >81%; *jcalicchia@bridgew.edu*
- Graham, Louise; PhD; Assist.; Licensed Psychologist; >81%; *lgraham@bridgew.edu*
- Kocet, Michael; PhD; Assist.; NCC; >81%; *mkocet@bridgew.edu*
- Rawlins, Maxine; PhD; Full Prof.; Licensed Psychologist; >81%; *mrawlins@bridgew.edu*

MA: Fitchburg State College

160 Pearl St.
Fitchburg, MA 01420-2697
USA

Dean Dorothy Boisvert - Sanders Administration
Administrator Michael Bloomfield & Richard J. Spencer, Co-chairpersons - Graduate Counseling Program
Department   Behavioral Sciences
(978) 665-3349, fax (978) 665-3616, MBLOOMFIELD@fsc.edu or
RSPENCER@fsc.edu

Key See key for Data on Each Department (this section) on page 79.

Program
Accreditation   Regional Accreditation

Uniqueness   The primary goal of the Fitchburg State College Graduate Counseling Program is to develop counselors who can assist clients in the enhancement of their well-being. It is based on a developmental socialization model of intervention, which recognizes that in each developmental stage individuals face tasks that can lead to problems, which may require professional assistance. The program recognizes the profesional counselor as a human developmental teacher or facilitator whose primary function is to help individuals enhance life adjustment, facilitate growth, and expand behavioral competencies so that they can cope more effectively with their environments. The educational program is based on the belief that effective counselors are both personally and professionally integrated. For this reason, a balance betweeen dialogue, didactic and experiential learning is maintained. The Program offers the student the opportunity to apply for Massachusetts licensure as a Mental Health Counselor, Marriage and Family Therapist, or School Guidance Counselor.

Degrees
- Mental Health Counseling: M.
- School Counseling: M.
- Marriage and Family Counseling: M.
- Other: S.

Contact
- Mental Health Counseling: M = Richard J. Spencer.
- School Counseling: M = Carol Globiana.
- Marriage and Family Counseling: M = Michael Bloomfield.
- Other: S = Michael Bloomfield.

Admission and Graduation Data
Admission
Requirements
- Mental Health Counseling(M): GPA 2.80; GRE 1475; MAT 47.
- School Counseling(M): GPA 2.80; GRE 1475; MAT 47.
- Marriage and Family Counseling(M): GPA 2.80; GRE 1475; MAT 47.
- Other(S):

Enrollment
- Mental Health Counseling(M): 10 Admitted yearly; 8 Graduated yearly; 28 Female; 2 Male.
- School Counseling(M): 16 Admitted yearly; 18 Graduated yearly; 7 Male.
- Marriage and Family Counseling(M): 1 Admitted yearly; 1 Graduated yearly; 6 Female.
- Other(S): 2 Admitted yearly; 2 Graduated yearly; 5 Female; 2 Male.

Diversity
- African-American; Asian-American; Caucasian; Hispanic.

Graduation
Requirements
- Mental Health Counseling(M): 60 Class hours; 100 Practicum hours; 600 Internship hours.
- School Counseling(M): 51 Class hours; 100 Practicum hours; 450 Internship hours.
- Marriage and Family Counseling(M): 60 Class hours; 100 Practicum hours; 600 Internship hours.
- Other(S): 21 Class hours; 300 Internship hours.

Postgraduation activity: Advanced education and employment setting percentages.
- Mental Health Counseling(M): 5 Managed care; 20 Private practice; 75 Agency practice.
- School Counseling(M): 15 Elementary school; 10 Middle school; 75 Secondary school.
- Marriage and Family Counseling(M): 100 Agency practice.
- Other(S): 40 Agency practice; 5 Elementary school; 5 Middle school; 50 Secondary school.

Planned Program Modifications
Courses   Drop   Add
- NP.   - NP.

Other   Decrease   Increase
- NP.   - NP.

Related Programs

Faculty

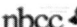 Percent of faculty reported with NCC certification: 5%.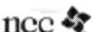

Percent in professional counseling practice: 65%.

Research interests

Diversity • Caucasian.

Name, Degree, Rank, State/National Credentials, % time devoted to program, email
* Bail, Paul; EdD; Lecturer; LPC; <21%;
* Benson, Gorden; PhD; Lecturer; LPC; <21%;
* Bloomfield, Michael; EdD; Assist.; LPC; 22-40%;
* Breen, G. Jefferson; EdD; Full Prof.; LPC; 22-40%;
* Creedon, Chandler; CAGS; Lecturer; LPC; 22-40%;
* Globiana, Carol; PhD; Full Prof.; LPC; <21%;
* Hamolsky, David; MEd; Lecturer; LPC; <21%;
* Hancock, John; PhD; Assoc.; LPC; 22-40%;
* King, Mary; EdD; Full Prof.; LPC; <21%;
* Lawrence, James; MA; Lecturer; LPC; <21%;
* Crosson, Cynthia; EdD; Lecturer; LPC; <21%;
* Spencer, Richard J; PhD; Full Prof.; LPC; 22-40%;
* Wassel, Frederick; EdD; Lecturer; LPC; <21%;
* Haddad, David; EdD; Lecturer; LPC; <21%;
* Okerman, Gail; MEd; Lecturer; LPC; <21%;
* O'Leary, Stephen; MS; Lecturer; <21%;
* Schilling, Thomas; PhD; Assist.; <21%;
* Frye, Robin; PhD; Lecturer; <21%;
* Kellner, Lynne; PhD; Assist.; NCC; <21%;

MA: Lesley University

	29 Everett Street
	Cambridge, MA 02138-2790
	USA
Dean	Dr. Martha Barry McKenna. Cambridge, MA
Administrator	Dr. Lisa Tsoi Hoshmand, Division Director
	Department Counseling and Psychology
	(617) 349-8370 or (800) 999-1959 Ext. 8370, fax (617) 349-8333,
	http://www.lesley.edu/gsass/30cpp.html

Key   See key for Data on Each Department (this section) on page 79.

Program

Accreditation   Regional Accreditation

Uniqueness   Recognition that human development includes mind, body and spirit - Focus on the development of the self of the counselor - Strong emphasis on clinical training and professional development - Curriculum focuses on integration of theory and practice - Coursework grounded on issues of health and resiliency as well as an understanding of mental disorders - Multicultural perspective - Student centered learning environment and a strong sense of community

Degrees
- Community Counseling: M, S.
- Mental Health Counseling: M, S.
- School Counseling: M, S.
- Other: M, S.

Contact
- Community Counseling: M, S = Yishiuan Chin (617) 349-8339; (800) 999-1959 ext. 8339.
- Mental Health Counseling: M, S = Yishiuan Chin (617) 349-8339; (800) 999-1959 ext. 8339.
- School Counseling: M, S = Yishiuan Chin (617) 349-8339; (800) 999-1959 ext. 8339.
- Other: M, S = Yishiuan Chin (617) 349-8339; (800) 999-1959 ext. 8339.

Admission and Graduation Data

Admission

Requirements
- Community Counseling(M): GPA 3.00; MAT 40; Interview.
- Community Counseling(S): GPA 3.00; MAT 40; Interview.
- Mental Health Counseling(M): GPA 3.00; MAT 40; Interview.
- Mental Health Counseling(S): GPA 3.00; MAT 40; Interview.
- School Counseling(M): GPA 3.00; MAT 40; Interview.
- School Counseling(S): GPA 3.00; MAT 40; Interview.
- Other(M): GPA 3.00; MAT 40; Interview.
- Other(S): GPA 3.00; MAT 40; Interview.

Enrollment
- Community Counseling(M & S).
- Mental Health Counseling(M & S).
- School Counseling(M & S).
- Other(M & S).

Diversity
- African-American; Asian-American; Caucasian; Hispanic; Native American; Multiracial.

Graduation

Requirements
- Community Counseling(M): 60 Class hours; 100 Practicum hours; 600/1200 Internship hours.
- Community Counseling(S): 36 Class hours; 600 Internship hours.
- Mental Health Counseling(M): 60 Class hours; 100 Practicum hours; 600/1200 Internship hours.
- Mental Health Counseling(S): 36 Class hours; 600 Internship hours.
- School Counseling(M): 48/60 Class hours; 100 Practicum hours; 600/1200 Internship hours.
- School Counseling(S): indiv. Class hours; 100 Practicum hours; 600 Internship hours.
- Other(M): 48/60 Class hours; 100 Practicum hours; 600/1200 Internship hours.
- Other(S):

Postgraduation activity: Advanced education and employment setting percentages.
- Community Counseling(M & S).
- Mental Health Counseling(M & S).
- School Counseling(M & S).
- Other(M & S).

Planned Program Modifications

Courses	Drop	Add
	• NP.	• Gender Studies
		• Wellness.

Other   <u>Decrease</u>   <u>Increase</u>
- NP.
                    - Diversity Recruiting of Faculty
                    - Diversity Recruiting of Students
                    - National Accreditation.

Related Programs Arts Therapists
        Other

Faculty

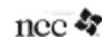 Percent of faculty reported with NCC certification: 0%.

Percent in professional counseling practice: 100%.

Research interests Trauma recovery, spiritual development, cultural issues, gay/lesbian issues, school counseling issues.

Diversity - African-American; Asian-American; Caucasian; Hispanic; Multiracial.

Name, Degree, Rank, State/National Credentials, % time devoted to program, email
- Crowley, Paul; PhD; Full Prof.; Licensed Psychologist; >81%;
- Dass-Brailsford, Priscilla; EdD; Assist.; Licensed Psychologist; 61-80%;
- Gere, Susan; PhD; Assoc.; LICSW; >81%;
- Hoshmand, Lisa; PhD; Full Prof.; Licensed Psychologist; >81%; *lhoshman@mail.lesley.edu*
- Kass, Jared; PhD; Full Prof.; LMHC; >81%;
- Llera, Dalia; EdD; Assoc.; Licensed Psychologist and Licensed School Psychologist; 61-80%;
- Reinkraut, Rick; PhD, EdD; Assoc.; Licensed Psychologist; >81%;
- Roffman, Eleanor; EdD; Full Prof.; Licensed Psychologist and Licensed School Guidance Counselor; >81%;
- Ritchie, Jill; MA; Instructor; LMHC; <21%;

MA: Salem State College

101 Sullivan Building
Salem, MA 01970-5353
USA

Dean   Marc Glasser, Dean of the Graduate School
Administrator   Patrice Marie Miller, Coordinator
                    Department   M.S. in Counseling and Psychological Services
                                    (978) 542-6322, fax (978) 542-7215, patrice.miller@salemstate.edu,
                                    http://www.salemstate.edu/graduate/

Key   See key for Data on Each Department (this section) on page 79.

Program
   Accreditation   Regional Accreditation

   Uniqueness   Salem State College tailors the graduate study of each student to better accommodate their
                      busy working lives and their individual professional interests

   Degrees   • NP.

   Contact   • NP.

Admission and Graduation Data
Admission
   Requirements   • NP.

   Enrollment   • NP.

   Diversity   • NP.

Graduation
   Requirements   • NP.

   Postgraduation activity: Advanced education and employment setting percentages.
                   •

Planned Program Modifications
   Courses   Drop   Add
                      • NP.   • NP.

   Other   Decrease   Increase
                      • NP.   • NP.

Related Programs

Faculty

   nbcc ❦   Percent of faculty reported with NCC certification: 0%.   ncc ❦

   Percent in professional counseling practice: NP.

   Research interests Origins of psychopathology, Dialectical behavioral therapy, cognitive behavior therapy,
                      multiculturalism, marriage and family, organizational and industrial psychology

   Diversity   • Asian-American; Caucasian; Hispanic.

   Name, Degree, Rank, State/National Credentials, % time devoted to program, email
   • NP.

MA: Suffolk University

Beacon Hill
Boston, MA 02114-4280
USA

Dean   Michael R. Ronayne, Boston
Administrator   Glen A. Eskedal, Chair/Professor
     Department   Education & Human Services Department
       (617) 573-8261, fax (617) 722-9440,
       http://www.suffolk.edu/cas/grad-counselingprograms.html

Key   See key for Data on Each Department (this section) on page 79.

Program

Accreditation   Regional Accreditation

Uniqueness   The focus of this program is on the practitioner. Extensive practical experiences, and a full complement of courses, provide a balanced learning experience.

Degrees
- Mental Health Counseling: M, S.
- School Counseling: M, S.
- Other: M.

Contact
- Mental Health Counseling: M = Dr. Glen Eskedal.; S = Dr. Glen Eskedal.
- School Counseling: M = Dr. R. Arthur Winters; S = NP.
- Other: M = NP.

Admission and Graduation Data

Admission

Requirements
- Mental Health Counseling(M): GPA 2.75; GRE R; MAT R.
- Mental Health Counseling(S): GPA 2.75; GRE R; MAT R.
- School Counseling(M): GPA 2.75; GRE R; MAT R.
- School Counseling(S): GPA 2.75; GRE R; MAT R.
- Other(M): GPA 2.75; GRE R; MAT R.

Enrollment
- Mental Health Counseling(M & S): 25 Admitted yearly; 15 Graduated yearly; 20 Female; 5 Male.
- School Counseling(M & S): 12 Admitted yearly; 8 Graduated yearly; 10 Female; 2 Male.
- Other(M): 10 Admitted yearly; 6 Graduated yearly; 9 Female; 1 Male.

Diversity
- African-American; Asian-American; Caucasian; Hispanic.

Graduation

Requirements
- Mental Health Counseling(M): 36 Class hours; 450 Practicum hours.
- Mental Health Counseling(S): 30 Class hours; 600 Internship hours.
- School Counseling(M): 36 Class hours; 450 Practicum hours; Portfolio.
- School Counseling(S): 30 Class hours; 600 Internship hours; Portfolio.
- Other(M): 30 Class hours; 450 Practicum hours.

Postgraduation activity: Advanced education and employment setting percentages.
- Mental Health Counseling(M & S): 5 Advanced education; 60 Managed care; 5 Private practice; 20 Agency practice; 10 Other.
- School Counseling(M & S): 2 Advanced education; 10 Middle school; 84 Secondary school; 5 Other.
- Other(M): 2 Advanced education; 5 Private practice; 75 Agency practice; 18 Other.

Planned Program Modifications

Courses	Drop	Add
	• NP.	• NP.

Other	Decrease	Increase
	• NP.	• Admission Requirements
		• Diversity Recruiting of Faculty
		• Diversity Recruiting of Students
		• Faculty FTE.

Related Programs Psychology

Faculty

 Percent of faculty reported with NCC certification: 10%.

Percent in professional counseling practice: 70%.

Research interests Personality disorders, forensic psychology, infancy/childhood development, school counseling, & mental health counseling services.

Diversity   • African-American; Caucasian.

Name, Degree, Rank, State/National Credentials, % time devoted to program, email
- DiBiase, Rose; PhD; Assoc.; 61-80%; *rdibiase@suffolk.edu*
- Eskedal, Glen A; EdD; Full Prof.; NCC, Psych; >81%; *gesekedal@suffolk.edu*
- Medoff, David; PhD; Assist.; Psych; >81%; *dmedoff@suffolk.edu*
- Winters, R. Arthur; PhD; Assoc.; *awntrs2@aol.com*
- Fahey, Jean; PsyD; Adjunct; Psych; 22-40%;
- Foster, Barry; PsyD; Adjunct; Psych; <21%;
- Helfrich, Barbara; CAGS; Adjunct; School Counselor; <21%;
- Jackson, Kathryn; PhD; Assist.; Psych; <21%; *kjackson@suffolk.edu*
- Martin, Thomas; PhD; Adjunct; Psych; <21%;
- Stryker, David; EdD; Adjunct; <21%;

MD: Frostburg State University

College of Liberal Arts & Sciences
Frostburg, MD 21532
USA

Dean Dr. Fred Yaffe, Library 5th Floor
Administrator Ann R. Bristow, Ph.D., Program Coordinator
Department   Psychology
(301) 687-4446, fax (301) 687-7418, abristow@frostburg.edu,
http://www.frostburg.edu/dept/psyc/graduate/coupsy.htm

Key   See key for Data on Each Department (this section) on page 79.

Program

Accreditation   Regional Accreditation

Uniqueness   Providing training in professional psychology at the Master's level, FSU's program is designed for those pursuing further study in science-based counseling psychology. Our theoretical perspective is integrative, including cognitive-behavioral, family systems, developmental, feminist, multicultural, humanistic and brief therapies. We emphasize training in empirically supported treatments for children, adolescents, families and adults. We offer Graduate Certificates in Addictions Counseling Psychology and Child & Family Counseling Psychology. Two semesters of internship offer extensive, supervised experience. We also offer a 60 credit hour licensure and certification option.

Degrees   • Mental Health Counseling: M.

Contact   • Mental Health Counseling: M = Ann R. Bristow.

Admission and Graduation Data

Admission

Requirements   • Mental Health Counseling(M): GPA 3.00; GRE 1000; MAT 50; 1 Year work experience; Interview.

Enrollment   • Mental Health Counseling(M): 15 Admitted yearly; 12 Graduated yearly; 25 Female; 7 Male.

Diversity   • African-American; Caucasian; Hispanic.

Graduation

Requirements   • Mental Health Counseling(M): 49 Class hours; 450 Internship hours.

Postgraduation activity: Advanced education and employment setting percentages.
• Mental Health Counseling(M): 10 Advanced education; 10 Private practice; 70 Agency practice; 10 Other.

Planned Program Modifications

Courses   Drop   Add
• NP.   • NP.

Other   Decrease   Increase
• NP.   • NP.

Related Programs Other

Faculty

nbcc ❧   Percent of faculty reported with NCC certification: 0%.   ncc ❧
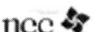

Percent in professional counseling practice: 40%.

Research interests developmental psychopathology; child mental health services (child/adolescent therapy utilization and outcome), ADHD, pediatric headaches, and child trauma; substance abuse treatment; multicultural counselor training

Diversity   • African-American; Caucasian.

Name, Degree, Rank, State/National Credentials, % time devoted to program, email
• Bradley, Megan; PhD; Assist.; 22-40%; *mbradley@frostburg.edu*
• Bristow, Ann R; PhD; Full Prof.; Licensed Psychologist; 61-80%; *abristow@frostburg.edu*
• Edwards, Jason H; PhD; Assoc.; Licensed Psychologist; 41-60%; *jedwards@frostburg.edu*
• Peterson, Kevin H; EdD; Assoc.; Licensed Psychologist; 41-60%; *kpeterson@frostburg.edu*
• Redmond, Trina; PhD; Assist.; 41-60%; *tredmond@frostburg.edu*

MD: Johns Hopkins University

105 Whitehead Hall/3400 N. Charles Street
Baltimore, MD 21218-2692
USA

Dean Dr. Ralph Fessler, Baltimore, MD
Administrator Mary H. Guindon, Ph.D., Associate Professor and Chair
Department   Counseling and Human Services
(410) 516-7928 or (301) 294-7037, fax (301) 294-7106, counseling@jhu.edu,
http://www.spsbe.jhu.edu/programs/grad_edu.cfm

Key   See key for Data on Each Department (this section) on page 79.

Program

Accreditation   Regional Accreditation

Uniqueness   As part of the Johns Hopkins climate, our mission is to develop cutting edge programs such
as our master's degrees in Urban School Counseling and Organizational Counseling and our
many specialized post-master's certificates. We have school partnerships and grant projects
with Baltimore City and Baltimore County. We offer our courses and programs on three
campuses: Homewood-Baltimore, Columbia, and Rockville-Montgomery County.

Degrees
- Community Counseling: M, S.
- School Counseling: M.
- Other: M.

Contact
- Community Counseling: M = Fred Hanna, Mary Guindon.; S = Fred Hanna.
- School Counseling: M = Alan Green, Susan Keys.
- Other: M = Organizationa Counseling = Mary Guindon.

Admission and Graduation Data

Admission

Requirements
- Community Counseling(M): GPA 3.00; Interview.
- Community Counseling(S): GPA 3.00; Interview.
- School Counseling(M): GPA 3.00; Interview.
- Other(M): GPA 3.00; Interview.

Enrollment
- Community Counseling(M & S): 56 Admitted yearly; 42 Graduated yearly.
- School Counseling(M): 50 Admitted yearly; 43 Graduated yearly.
- Other(M): 49 Admitted yearly; 15 Graduated yearly.

Diversity
- African-American; Asian-American; Caucasian; Hispanic; Native American; Multiracial;
Other.

Graduation

Requirements
- Community Counseling(M): 48 Class hours; 500 Internship hours; Oral exam.
- Community Counseling(S): 30 Class hours; 300 Internship hours.
- School Counseling(M): 48 Class hours; 200 Internship hours; Oral exam.
- Other(M): 48 Class hours; 600 Internship hours; Oral exam.

Postgraduation activity: Advanced education and employment setting percentages.
- Community Counseling(M & S).
- School Counseling(M): NP.
- Other(M): NP.

Planned Program Modifications

Courses

Drop	Add
• Career/Life Planning.	• Consultation
	• Experiential Component.

Other

Decrease	Increase
• Course Offerings.	• Diversity Recruiting of Students
	• Faculty FTE
	• Number of Degree Majors
	• Number of Distance Education Courses
	• Number of Off-Campus Courses.

Related Programs Psychology
Psychiatric Nurses
Psychiatrists
Organizational Behaviorists
Communications
International Studies

Faculty

nbcc 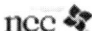   Percent of faculty reported with NCC certification: 62%.   ncc

Percent in professional counseling practice: 80%.

Research interests Collaboration; Youth-at-Risk; Urban Schools; Clinical Treatment Approaches; Oppression Interventions, Self-esteem and many more.

Diversity • African-American; Asian-American; Caucasian; Hispanic; Multiracial.

Name, Degree, Rank, State/National Credentials, % time devoted to program, email
• Hanna, Fred J; PhD; Full Prof.; LPC, NCC; >81%; *fhanna@jhu.edu*
• Keys, Susan G; PhD; Assoc.; LPC, NCC; >81%; *keys@jhu.edu*
• Guindon, Mary H; PhD; Assoc.; LPC, NCC, NCCC,Lic.Psych.; >81%; *mguindon@jhu.edu*
• Green, Alan G; PhD; Assist.; NCC; >81%; *agreen@jhu.edu*
• Rosenberg, Leon; PhD; Instructor; Lic.Psych.; <21%;
• Beil, Elizabeth; PhD; Instructor; Lic.Psych.; <21%;
• Bovard, Kathy; MS; Instructor; NCC, NCCC; <21%;
• Heitt, Michael; PhD; Instructor; Lic.Psych.; <21%;
• Hunt, Wayne; EdD; Instructor; NCSP,Lic.Psych.; <21%;
• Lockhart, Estes; EdD; Instructor; LPC, NCC, CCMHC, NCSP.; <21%;
• Wanda, Mays; EdD; Instructor; LPC, NCC, Lic.Psych.Nurse Prac.; <21%;
• McBrien, Donald; PhD; Instructor; NCC; <21%;
• Savage, Rowland L; MS; Instructor; NCC; <21%;
• Somers, Mary; MS; Instructor; NCC, NCCC; <21%;
• Voit, Ecford; PhD; Instructor; <21%;
• Wechsler, Susan; PhD; Instructor; Lic.Psych.; <21%;
• Wilson, Catherine; PhD; Instructor; NCC, NCSC; <21%;
• Wodiska, Wodiska B; PhD; Instructor; Lic.Psych.; <21%;
• Reile, David; PhD; Instructor; NCC, NCCC, CDF,Lic.Psych.; <21%;
• Suddarth, Barbara; PhD; Instructor; NCC, NCCC,Lic.Psych.; <21%;
• David, Hopkins; PhD; Instructor; Lic.Psych.;

Has CHI SIGMA IOTA (International Counseling Society) chapter.

MD: Loyola College in Maryland

	8890 McGraw Road
	Columbia, MD 21045
	USA
Dean	Dr. James Buckley, Humanities Building
Administrator	Dr. Joseph W. Ciarrocchi, Chair
	Department Pastoral Counseling
	(410) 617-7620, fax (410) 617-7644, AMcDonald@Loyola.edu,
	www.Loyola.edu/pastoral

Key   See key for Data on Each Department (this section) on page 79.

Program

Accreditation   Regional Accreditation, **CACREP:** Community Counseling

CACREP

Uniqueness   The Pastoral Counseling program is an intensive clinical program with an emphasis on the integration of spirituality in the student and in the counseling process.

Degrees
- Community Counseling: M.
- Pastoral Counseling: M, S, PhD.

Contact
- Community Counseling: M = K. Elizabeth Oakes.
- Pastoral Counseling: M = K. Elizabeth Oakes.; D = Ralph Piedmont.

Admission and Graduation Data

Admission

Requirements
- Community Counseling(M): GPA 2.50; Interview.
- Pastoral Counseling(M): GPA same; Interview.
- Pastoral Counseling(S): GPA same; Interview.
- Pastoral Counseling(D): GRE V 500; GRE Q 500; GRE A 500; 2 Years work experience.

Enrollment
- Community Counseling(M): 120 Admitted yearly; 80 Graduated yearly; 250 Female; 150 Male.
- Pastoral Counseling(M & S).
- Pastoral Counseling(D): 12 Admitted yearly; 6-10 Graduated yearly; 25 Female; 15 Male.

Diversity
- African-American; Asian-American; Caucasian; Hispanic; Native American; Pacific Islander; Multiracial.

Graduation

Requirements
- Community Counseling(M): 52 Class hours; 250 Practicum hours; 750 Internship hours; Thesis; Portfolio.
- Pastoral Counseling(M): same Class hours; same Practicum hours; same Internship hours; Thesis; Portfolio.
- Pastoral Counseling(S): same Class hours; same Practicum hours; same Internship hours.
- Pastoral Counseling(D): 60 Class hours; 1500 Internship hours; Comprehensive exam; Dissertation.

Postgraduation activity: Advanced education and employment setting percentages.
- Community Counseling(M): 10 Private practice; 50 Agency practice; 1 Elementary school; 1 Middle school; 3 Secondary school; 10 Student affairs; 10 Other.
- Pastoral Counseling(M & S): 15 Advanced education; 10 Private practice; 50 Agency practice; 1 Elementary school; 1 Middle school; 3 Secondary school; 10 Student affairs; 10 Other.
- Pastoral Counseling(D): 25 Advanced education; 35 Private practice; 15 Agency practice; 2 Secondary school; 3 Student affairs; 20 Other.

Planned Program Modifications

Courses	Drop	Add
	• NP.	• NP.

Other	Decrease	Increase
	• NP.	• Diversity Recruiting of Faculty
		• Financial Aid.

Related Programs

Faculty

nbcc ❖   Percent of faculty reported with NCC certification: 21%.   ncc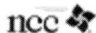

Percent in professional counseling practice: 90%.

Research interests Image of God, Clinical work with Abused Clients, Addictions such as Gambling & Substance Abuse, Scrupulosity, Hope, Forgiveness, Personality, NEO, and many other topics.

Diversity   •   African-American; Caucasian.

Name, Degree, Rank, State/National Credentials, % time devoted to program, email
- Wicks, Robert J; PsyD; Full Prof.; Licensed Psychologist; >81%; *RWicks@Loyola.edu*
- Cheston, Sharon E; EdD; Full Prof.; NCC, LCPC; >81%; *SCheston@Loyola.edu*
- Ciarrocchi, Joseph W; PhD; Full Prof.; Licensed Psychologist; >81%; *JCiarrocchi@Loyola.edu*
- Gillespie, Kevin; PhD; Assist.; NCC, Diplomate in AAPC; >81%; *KGillespie@Loyola.edu*
- Greer, Joanne M; PhD; Full Prof.; Licensed Psychologist; >81%; *JGreer@Loyola.edu*
- Murray, Kelly M; PhD; Assist.; Licensed Psychologist; >81%; *KMurray@Loyola.edu*
- Piedmont, Ralph L; PhD; Assoc.; >81%; *RPiedmont@Loyola.edu*
- Oakes, K. Elizabeth; PhD; Assist.; LCPC; >81%; *KOakes@Loyola.edu*
- Eanes, Beverly E; PhD; Assist.; NCC, LCPC; >81%; *BEanes@Loyola.edu*
- Fialkowski, Geraldine M; PhD; Assist.; NCC, LCPC; >81%; *GFialkowski@Loyola.edu*
- Cook, Donelda; PhD; Assist.; Licensed Psychologist; 22-40%; *DCook@Loyola.edu*
- Ellis, Ronald E; PhD; Assist.; Licensed Psychologist; 22-40%; *REllis@Loyola.edu*
- Hales, Shawn W; PsyD; Assist.; Licensed Psychologist; 22-40%; *SHales@Loyola.edu*
- Hamilton, Eleanor D; PhD; Assist.; Licensed Psychologist; 22-40%; *EHamilton@Loyola.edu*
- Hayes, John M; PhD; Assist.; Licensed Psychologist; 22-40%; *JHayes@Loyola.edu*
- Huss, Gary P; PhD; Assist.; Licensed Clinical Marriage and Family Therapist; 22-40%; *GHuss@Loyola.edu*
- Jeffreys, Shep; EdD; Assist.; Licensed Psycholoist; 22-40%; *JJeffreys@Loyola.edu*
- McLaughlin, John L; PhD; Assist.; Licensed Psychologist; 41-60%; *JMcLaughlin@Loyola.edu*
- Merrick, Mary E; PhD; Assist.; LCPC; 22-40%; *MMerrick@Loyola.edu*

Has CHI SIGMA IOTA (International Counseling Society) chapter.

MD: McDaniel College

2 College Hill
Westminster, MD 21157-4390
USA
Dean   Dr. Ken Pool
Administrator   Dr. Julia L. Orza, Coordinator
Department   Graduate and Professional Studies
(410) 857-2500, fax (410) 857-2515, jorza@wmdc.edu, mcdaniel.edu

Key   See key for Data on Each Department (this section) on page 79.

Program
Accreditation   Regional Accreditation

Uniqueness

Degrees   • Community Counseling: M.
                 • School Counseling: M.

Contact   • Community Counseling: M = Dr. Simeon Schlossberg.
                 • School Counseling: M = Dr. Julia Orza.

Admission and Graduation Data
Admission
Requirements   • Community Counseling(M): GPA 2.50; Interview.
                 • School Counseling(M): GPA 2.50; Interview.

Enrollment   • Community Counseling(M): 15 Admitted yearly; 5 Graduated yearly.
                 • School Counseling(M): 60 Admitted yearly; 25 Graduated yearly.

Diversity   • African-American; Asian-American; Caucasian; Multiracial.

Graduation
Requirements   • Community Counseling(M): 39 Class hours; 200-500 Internship hours; Comprehensive
                   exam.
                 • School Counseling(M): 45 Class hours; 200-500 Internship hours; Comprehensive exam.

Postgraduation activity: Advanced education and employment setting percentages.
                 • Community Counseling(M): 5 Advanced education; 5 Private practice; 40 Agency practice;
                   50 Other.
                 • School Counseling(M): 30 Elementary school; 30 Middle school; 40 Secondary school.

Planned Program Modifications
Courses   Drop   Add
                 • NP.   • Consultation
                                                  • Gender Studies
                                                  • Gerontological Counseling
                                                  • Technology.

Other   Decrease   Increase
                 • NP.   • Admission Requirements
                                                  • Course Offerings
                                                  • Clinical Supervision
                                                  • Diversity Recruiting of Faculty
                                                  • Diversity Recruiting of Students
                                                  • Graduation Requirements
                                                  • Number of Off-Campus Courses.

Related Programs Other

Faculty

nbcc ❖   Percent of faculty reported with NCC certification: 20%.   ncc ❖

Percent in professional counseling practice: 90%.

Research interests Diversity training, oppositional defiant adolescents, gay/lesbian issues

Diversity   • African-American; Caucasian; Multiracial.

Name, Degree, Rank, State/National Credentials, % time devoted to program, email
• Orza, Julia L; PhD; Assoc.; NCC; >81%; *jorza@mcdaniel.edu*
• Schlossberg, Simeon K; PhD; Assist.; LPC; >81%;
• Reichelt, Mary Anne; DMin; Instructor; LPC; 41-60%;
• Redmond, Robert F; EdD; Instructor; 22-40%;
• Bearr, David W; CAGS; Lecturer; 22-40%;

ME: University of Southern Maine

400 Bailey Hall
Gorham, ME 04038-1088
USA
Dean   Betty Lou Whitford, Ph.D., 118 Bailey Hall
Administrator John M. Sutton, Jr., Ed.D., Chair & Professor
      Department Dept. of Human Resource Development
            (207) 780-5316, fax (207) 780-5043,
            www.usm.maine.edu/cehd/academics9.htm

Key See key for Data on Each Department (this section) on page 79.

Program
Accreditation Regional Accreditation, **CACREP:** Mental Health Counseling, **CACREP:** School Counseling,
       CORE: Rehabilitation Counseling

CACREP

Uniqueness   The USM Counselor Education Program is the only one in New England that has both
       CACREP-approved programs in mental health and school counseling and a CORE-approved
       program in rehabilitation counseling. The program also have some unique certificate
       programs. All programs require either the GRE or MAT for admission.

Degrees   • Mental Health Counseling: M.
       • School Counseling: M.
       • Rehabilitation Counseling: M.

Contact   • Mental Health Counseling: M = Reid D. Stevens, Ph.D..
       • School Counseling: M = Marijane Fall, Ed.D..
       • Rehabilitation Counseling: M = Stephen T. Murphy, Ph.D..

Admission and Graduation Data
Admission
Requirements • Mental Health Counseling(M): GPA R; GRE R; MAT R; Interview.
       • School Counseling(M): GPA R; GRE R; MAT R; Interview.
       • Rehabilitation Counseling(M): GRE R; MAT R; Interview.

Enrollment   • Mental Health Counseling(M): 15 Admitted yearly; 15 Graduated yearly; 11 Female;
       4 Male.
       • School Counseling(M): 15 Admitted yearly; 15 Graduated yearly; 11 Female; 4 Male.
       • Rehabilitation Counseling(M): 10 Admitted yearly; 5 Graduated yearly; 9 Female; 1 Male.

Diversity   • African-American; Caucasian; Hispanic.

Graduation
Requirements • Mental Health Counseling(M): 60 Class hours; 100 Practicum hours; 900 Internship hours;
       Comprehensive exam; CPCE.
       • School Counseling(M): 54 Class hours; 100 Practicum hours; 600 Internship hours;
       Comprehensive exam; CPCE; Portfolio.
       • Rehabilitation Counseling(M): 48 Class hours; 100 Practicum hours; 600 Internship hours;
       Comprehensive exam; CPCE.

Postgraduation activity: Advanced education and employment setting percentages.
       • Mental Health Counseling(M): 5 Advanced education; 5 Managed care; 10 Private practice;
       80 Agency practice.
       • School Counseling(M): 5 Advanced education; 35 Elementary school; 30 Middle school;
       35 Secondary school.
       • Rehabilitation Counseling(M): 2 Managed care; 1 Private practice; 96 Agency practice; 1
       Other.

Planned Program Modifications
Courses   <u>Drop</u>   <u>Add</u>
       • NP.   • NP.

Other   <u>Decrease</u>   <u>Increase</u>
       • NP.   • NP.

Related Programs Clinical Social Workers
         Marriage and Family Therapists
         Psychiatric Nurses

Faculty

nbcc ❖   Percent of faculty reported with NCC certification: 83%.   **ncc** ❖

Percent in professional counseling practice: 67%.

Research interests Clinical supervision, child counseling, ethics, counselor regulation, gender issues, abuse & abusers, deinstitutionalization

Diversity   • Caucasian.

Name, Degree, Rank, State/National Credentials, % time devoted to program, email
- Fall, Marijane E; EdD; Full Prof.; NCC, LCTC, ACS, LCPC; >81%; *mjfall@usm.maine.edu*
- Stevens, Reid D; PhD; Assoc.; NCC, LCPC, CRC; >81%; *stevens@usm.maine.edu*
- Katsekas, Bette S; EdD; Assoc.; NCC, ACS, LCPC; >81%; *katsekas@usm.maine.edu*
- Murphy, Stephen T; PhD; Full Prof.; CRC; >81%; *smurphy@usm.maine.edu*
- Sutton, Jr., John M; EdD; Full Prof.; NCC, ACS, LCPC; >81%; *sutton@maine.maine.edu*
- VanZandt, C.(Zark) E; EdD; Full Prof.; NCC; >81%; *zark@usm.maine.edu*

MI: Andrews University

	Berrien Springs, MI 49104
	USA
Dean	Karen Graham, Bell Hall
Administrator	Jerome Thayer, Chair
	Department Educational and Counseling Psychology
	(616) 471-3473, fax (616) 471-6374, ecp@andrews.edu,
	www.educ.andrews.edu/program_ecp0.html

Key   See key for Data on Each Department (this section) on page 79.

Program

Accreditation   Regional Accreditation, **CACREP**: Community Counseling, **CACREP**: School Counseling

Uniqueness   Christian world view

Degrees
- Community Counseling: M.
- Mental Health Counseling: EdD.
- School Counseling: M.

Contact
- Community Counseling: M = Elvin Gabriel.
- Mental Health Counseling: D = NP.
- School Counseling: M = Frederick Kosinski, Jr.

Admission and Graduation Data

Admission

Requirements
- Community Counseling(M): GPA 2.70; Interview.
- Mental Health Counseling(D): NP.
- School Counseling(M): GPA 2.70; Interview.

Enrollment
- Community Counseling(M): 15 Admitted yearly; 12 Graduated yearly; 8 Female; 7 Male.
- Mental Health Counseling(D): NP.
- School Counseling(M): 5 Admitted yearly; 4 Graduated yearly; 2 Male.

Diversity
- African-American; Asian-American; Caucasian; Hispanic.

Graduation

Requirements
- Community Counseling(M): 48 Class hours; 100 Practicum hours; 600 Internship hours; Comprehensive exam.
- Mental Health Counseling(D): NP.
- School Counseling(M): 48 Class hours; 100 Practicum hours; 600 Internship hours; Comprehensive exam.

Postgraduation activity: Advanced education and employment setting percentages.
- Community Counseling(M): 20 Private practice; 60 Agency practice.
- Mental Health Counseling(D):
- School Counseling(M): 10 Advanced education; 30 Elementary school; 30 Middle school; 30 Secondary school.

Planned Program Modifications

Courses	Drop		Add
	• NP.	• NP.	

Other	Decrease		Increase
	• NP.	• Number of On-Line Courses.	

Related Programs Clinical Social Workers
Psychology

Faculty

nbcc ❖   Percent of faculty reported with NCC certification: 0%.   ncc ❖

Percent in professional counseling practice: NP.

Research interests NP.

Diversity
- African-American; Asian-American; Caucasian; Native American.

Name, Degree, Rank, State/National Credentials, % time devoted to program, email
- Bailey, Rudolph D; PhD; Full Prof.; 41-60%; *rbailey@andrews.edu*
- Carbonell, Nancy J; PhD; Assoc.; >81%; *carbonel@andrews.edu*
- Gabriel, Elvin S; PhD; Assoc.; >81%; *gabriel@andrews.edu*
- Kosinski, Jr, Frederick A; PhD; Full Prof.; >81%; *kosinskf@andrews.edu*
- Waite, Dennis; EdD; Assist.; 41-60%; *denwaite@qtm.net*
- Kijai, Jimmy; PhD; Full Prof.; 22-40%; *kijai@andrews.edu*

Has CHI SIGMA IOTA (International Counseling Society) chapter.

MI: Eastern Michigan University

	304 Porter
	Ypsilanti, MI 48197-2706
	United States
Dean	Jerry Robbins
Administrator	Jaclyn C. Tracy, Interim Department Head
	Department Leadership and Counseling
	(734) 487-0255, fax (734) 487-4608

Key   See key for Data on Each Department (this section) on page 79.

Program

Accreditation   Regional Accreditation, **CACREP:** Community Counseling, **CACREP:** School Counseling, **CACREP:** Student Affairs - Counseling

Uniqueness   Faculty in the program maintain and encourage strong participation in professional organizations.

Degrees
- Community Counseling: M.
- School Counseling: M.
- College Counseling: M.

Contact
- Community Counseling: M = Irene Ametrano.
- School Counseling: M = Sue Stickel.
- College Counseling: M = Yvonne Callaway.

Admission and Graduation Data

Admission

Requirements
- Community Counseling(M): GPA 2.75; Interview.
- School Counseling(M): GPA 2.75; Interview.
- College Counseling(M): GPA 2.75; Interview.

Enrollment
- Community Counseling(M): 15 Admitted yearly; 8 Graduated yearly; 6 Female; 2 Male.
- School Counseling(M): 35 Admitted yearly; 29 Graduated yearly; 20 Female; 9 Male.
- College Counseling(M): 10 Admitted yearly; 3 Graduated yearly; 2 Female; 1 Male.

Diversity
- African-American; Asian-American; Caucasian; Hispanic; Multiracial.

Graduation

Requirements
- Community Counseling(M): 48 Class hours; 100 Practicum hours; 600 Internship hours; Portfolio.
- School Counseling(M): 48 Class hours; 100 Practicum hours; 600 Internship hours; Portfolio.
- College Counseling(M): 48 Class hours; 100 Practicum hours; 600 Internship hours; Portfolio.

Postgraduation activity: Advanced education and employment setting percentages.
- Community Counseling(M): 5 Advanced education; 90 Agency practice; 5 Other.
- School Counseling(M): 20 Elementary school; 40 Middle school; 40 Secondary school.
- College Counseling(M): 10 Advanced education; 2 Agency practice; 88 Other.

Planned Program Modifications

Courses	Drop	Add
	• Wellness.	• Crisis/Violence Counseling
		• Diversity
		• Special Needs Populations.

Other	Decrease	Increase
	• NP.	• Course Offerings
		• Diversity Recruiting of Faculty
		• Diversity Recruiting of Students
		• Financial Aid
		• Number of Degree Majors.

Related Programs Clinical Social Workers
Psychology
Arts Therapists
Communications

Faculty

nbcc ❖   Percent of faculty reported with NCC certification: 71%.   ncc ❖

Percent in professional counseling practice: 15%.

Research interests Multicultural competencies

Diversity   •   African-American; Caucasian; Other.

Name, Degree, Rank, State/National Credentials, % time devoted to program, email
- Ametrano, Irene M; EdD; Full Prof.; LPC, NCC; >81%; *irene.ametrano@emich.edu*
- Broughton, Elizabeth A; EdD; Assoc.; LPC; >81%; *elizabeth.broughton@emich.edu*
- Callaway, Yvonne L; PhD; Full Prof.; LPC; >81%; *yvonne.callaway@emich.edu*
- Chaudhuri, Dibya; PhD; Assist.; LPC, NCC; >81%; *dibya.choudhuri@emich.edu*
- Hobson, Suzanne; EdD; Assoc.; LPC, NCC; >81%; *suzanne.hobson@emich.edu*
- Thayer, Louis C; EdD; Full Prof.; LPC, NCC; >81%; *louis.thayer@emich.edu*
- Stickel, Sue A; PhD; Full Prof.; LPC, NCC; >81%; *sue.stickel@emich.edu*

MI: Oakland University

School of Education and Human Services
Rochester, MI 48309
USA
Dean   Mary Otto, Dean, School of Education and Human Services
Administrator   Luellen Ramey, Ph.D., Associate Professor and Chair
        Department   Department of Counseling
               (248) 370-4185 Ext. 4179, fax (248) 370-4141, mhill@oakland.edu,
               www.oakland.edu/sehs/

Key   See key for Data on Each Department (this section) on page 79.

Program
  Accreditation   Regional Accreditation, **CACREP:** Community Counseling, **CACREP:** School Counseling

  Uniqueness   State of the art clinical and classroom facilities, suburban location, growing campus, diverse
              faculty, advanced specializations in Mental Health Counseling, Child and Adolescent
              Counseling, Advanced Career Counseling, Couple and Family Counseling and School
              Counseling

  Degrees
- Community Counseling: M, PhD.
- Mental Health Counseling: PhD.
- School Counseling: M, PhD.
- Career Counseling: PhD.
- Marriage and Family Counseling: PhD.
- Other: PhD.
- Counselor Education: PhD.

  Contact
- Community Counseling: M = ramey@oakland.edu.; D = blume@oakland.edu.
- Mental Health Counseling: D = blume@oakland.edu.
- School Counseling: M = parfitt@oakland.edu.; D = blume@oakland.edu.
- Career Counseling: D = blume@oakland.edu.
- Marriage and Family Counseling: D = blume@oakland.edu.
- Other: D = NP.
- Counselor Education: D = blume@oakland.edu.

Admission and Graduation Data
Admission
  Requirements
- Community Counseling(M): GPA 3.00; Interview.
- Community Counseling(D): Masters and GPA 3.60; GRE R.
- Mental Health Counseling(D): Masters and GPA 3.60; GRE R.
- School Counseling(M): GPA 3.00; Interview.
- School Counseling(D): Masters and GPA 3.60; GRE R.
- Career Counseling(D): Masters and GPA 3.60; GRE R.
- Marriage and Family Counseling(D): Masters and GPA 3.60; GRE R.
- Other(D): NP.
- Counselor Education(D): Masters and GPA 3.60; GRE R.

  Enrollment
- Community Counseling(M): 85 Admitted yearly; 70 Graduated yearly; 61 Female; 9 Male.
- Community Counseling(D): 1 Admitted yearly.
- Mental Health Counseling(D): 2 Admitted yearly; 2 Graduated yearly.
- School Counseling(M): 75 Admitted yearly; 60 Graduated yearly; 8 Male.
- School Counseling(D): NP.
- Career Counseling(D): 1 Admitted yearly.
- Marriage and Family Counseling(D): 1 Admitted yearly; 1 Graduated yearly.
- Other(D): 18 Female; 5 Male.
- Counselor Education(D): 3 Admitted yearly; 3 Graduated yearly.

  Diversity
- African-American; Asian-American; Caucasian; Hispanic; Multiracial.

Graduation
  Requirements
- Community Counseling(M): 48 Class hours; 100 Practicum hours; 600 Internship hours.
- Community Counseling(D): 82 Class hours; 100 Practicum hours; 600 Internship hours;
  Comprehensive exam; Dissertation.
- Mental Health Counseling(D): 82 Class hours; 100 Practicum hours; 600 Internship hours;
  Comprehensive exam; Dissertation.
- School Counseling(M): 48 Class hours; 100 Practicum hours; 600 Internship hours.
- School Counseling(D): 82 Class hours; 100 Practicum hours; 600 Internship hours;
  Dissertation.
- Career Counseling(D): 82 Class hours; 100 Practicum hours; 600 Internship hours;
  Comprehensive exam; Dissertation.

- Marriage and Family Counseling(D): 82 Class hours; 100 Practicum hours; 600 Internship hours; Comprehensive exam; Dissertation.
- Other(D): NP.
- Counselor Education(D): 82 Class hours; 100 Practicum hours; 600 Internship hours; Comprehensive exam; Dissertation.

Postgraduation activity: Advanced education and employment setting percentages.
- Community Counseling(M): 10 Managed care; 10 Private practice; 45 Agency practice; 20 Other.
- Community Counseling(D):
- Mental Health Counseling(D):
- School Counseling(M): 10 Elementary school; 40 Middle school; 40 Secondary school; 10 Student affairs.
- School Counseling(D):
- Career Counseling(D):
- Marriage and Family Counseling(D):
- Other(D):
- Counselor Education(D):

Planned Program Modifications

Courses	Drop	Add
	• NP.	• NP.

Other	Decrease	Increase
	• NP.	• Diversity Recruiting of Faculty
		• Diversity Recruiting of Students
		• Financial Aid
		• National Accreditation.

Related Programs Psychology

Faculty

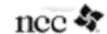 Percent of faculty reported with NCC certification: 45%.

Percent in professional counseling practice: 75%.

Research interests Trauma, group counseling, socioeconomic status in counseling, technology and supervision, couples counseling, integration of psychoanalytic and humanist therapies, adult transition, career and multicultural issues.

Diversity   • African-American; Caucasian.

Name, Degree, Rank, State/National Credentials, % time devoted to program, email
- Anderson, Mary L; MA; Assist.; LPC; >81%; *shaieb@oakland.edu*
- Blume, Thomas W; PhD; Assoc.; LPC, LMFT; >81%; *blume@oakland.edu*
- Cron, Elyce A; PhD; Assoc.; LPC, NCC; >81%; *ecron@oakland.edu*
- Fink, Robert S; PhD; Assoc.; NCC, LP; >81%; *fink@oakland.edu*
- Goodman, Jane S; PhD; Assoc.; LPC, NCC; >81%; *goodman@oakland.edu*
- Hansen, James T; PhD; Assoc.; LPC, NCC, LP; >81%; *jthansen@oakland.edu*
- Hawley, Lisa D; PhD; Assist.; LPC; >81%; *hawley@oakland.edu*
- Junior, Victoria Y; PhD; Assist.; LPC; >81%; *junior@oakland.edu*
- Parfitt, Diane L; MA; Assist.; LPC; >81%; *parfitt@oakland.edu*
- Ramey, Luellen; PhD; Assoc.; LPC, NCC; >81%; *ramey@oakland.edu*
- Surrey, Lynn R; PhD; Assoc.; LP; >81%; *surrey@oakland.edu*

Has CHI SIGMA IOTA (International Counseling Society) chapter.

MI: Siena Heights University

1247E. Siena Heights Drive
Adrian, MI 49221-1796
USA
Dean   Robert Gordon, EdD
Administrator   Linda M. Brewster, Ph.D., Director, Counselor Education
      Department   Graduate College
      (517) 264-7666, fax (517) 264-7714, lbrewste@sienahts.edu

Key   See key for Data on Each Department (this section) on page 79.

Program
Accreditation   Regional Accreditation

Uniqueness

Degrees
- Community Counseling: M.
- School Counseling: M.

Contact
- Community Counseling: M = Linda M. Brewster.
- School Counseling: M = Linda M. Brewster.

Admission and Graduation Data
Admission
Requirements
- Community Counseling(M): GPA 3.00; 2 Years work experience; Interview.
- School Counseling(M): GPA 3.00; 1 Year work experience; Interview.

Enrollment
- Community Counseling(M): 30 Admitted yearly; 20 Graduated yearly.
- School Counseling(M): 7 Admitted yearly; 5 Graduated yearly.

Diversity
- NP.

Graduation
Requirements
- Community Counseling(M): 48 Class hours; 100 Practicum hours; 600 Internship hours.
- School Counseling(M): 48 Class hours; 100 Practicum hours; 600 Internship hours.

Postgraduation activity: Advanced education and employment setting percentages.
- Community Counseling(M): 10 Advanced education; 20 Private practice; 60 Agency practice.
- School Counseling(M): 10 Elementary school; 20 Middle school; 60 Secondary school; 10 Student affairs.

Planned Program Modifications
Courses   Drop   Add
- NP.   • NP.

Other   Decrease   Increase
- NP.   • NP.

Related Programs

Faculty

nbcc ❧   Percent of faculty reported with NCC certification: 0%.   ncc ❧

Percent in professional counseling practice: 66%.

Research interests NP.

Diversity   • NP.

Name, Degree, Rank, State/National Credentials, % time devoted to program, email
- Brady, Robert; EdD; Full Prof.; Psych; 61-80%;
- Brewster, Linda; PhD; Assoc.; Psych; >81%;
- deSouza, Joan; PhD; Adjunct; Psych; <21%;
- Hudson, Sharon; PhD; Adjunct; <21%;
- O'Reilly, Virginia; PhD; Adjunct; Psych; <21%;
- Reinink, Barry; MA; Adjunct; LPC; 41-60%;
- McDonald, Patricia; EdD; Adjunct; LPC; 41-60%;
- Allen, Roxanne; PhD; Adjunct; LPC;
- Sam, James; PhD; Adjunct; LPC; 22-40%;
- Mervak, Thomas; Phd; Adjunct; Psych; 41-60%;
- Day, Mary Rose; PhD; Adjunct; LPC; 22-40%;

Has CHI SIGMA IOTA (International Counseling Society) chapter.

MN: Capella University

222 South 9th Street, 20th Floor
Minneapolis, MN 55402
United States

Dean   Pamela K. S. Patrick

Administrator   Pamela K. S. Patrick, Ph.D., Executive Director

Department   School of Human Services

(386) 673-3619, fax (208) 975-2900, PKSP@aol.com, www.capella.edu

Key   See key for Data on Each Department (this section) on page 79.

Program

Accreditation   Regional Accreditation

Uniqueness   Online Counselor Education programs in Mental Health Counseling, Marital, Couple and Family Counseling/Therapy and Counseling Studies.

Degrees
- Mental Health Counseling: M.
- Marriage and Family Counseling: M.
- Other: M, PhD.

Contact
- Mental Health Counseling: M = Pamela Patrick.
- Marriage and Family Counseling: M = Pamela Patrick.
- Other: M = NP.; D = Pamela Patrick.

Admission and Graduation Data

Admission

Requirements
- Mental Health Counseling(M): GPA 2.70; Interview.
- Marriage and Family Counseling(M): GPA 2.70; Interview.
- Other(M): GPA 2.70; Interview.
- Other(D): Masters and GPA 3.00.

Enrollment
- Mental Health Counseling(M): 40 Admitted yearly; 35 Female; 5 Male.
- Marriage and Family Counseling(M): 20 Admitted yearly; 19 Female; 1 Male.
- Other(M): 20 Admitted yearly; 19 Female; 1 Male.
- Other(D): 20 Admitted yearly; 17 Female; 3 Male.

Diversity
- African-American; Asian-American; Caucasian; Hispanic; Multiracial.

Graduation

Requirements
- Mental Health Counseling(M): 100 Practicum hours; 900 Internship hours; Portfolio.
- Marriage and Family Counseling(M): 100 Practicum hours; 900 Internship hours; Portfolio.
- Other(M): NP.
- Other(D): Oral exam; Dissertation.

Postgraduation activity: Advanced education and employment setting percentages.
- Mental Health Counseling(M): NP.
- Marriage and Family Counseling(M): NP.
- Other(M): NP.
- Other(D):

Planned Program Modifications

Courses	Drop	Add
	• NP.	• NP.

Other	Decrease	Increase
	• NP.	• National Accreditation.

Related Programs

Faculty

nbcc ❖   Percent of faculty reported with NCC certification: 62%.   ncc ❖

Percent in professional counseling practice: NP.

Research interests Online education; faculty interaction variables; learner interaction variables; and outcomes.

Diversity
- African-American; Asian-American; Caucasian; Pacific Islander; Multiracial.

Name, Degree, Rank, State/National Credentials, % time devoted to program, email
- Auxier, C. R; PhD; Assoc.; LPC, NCC; 41-60%; *cauxier3@cableone.net*
- Caron, Janice; EdD; Full Prof.; LPC, LMHC; >81%; *jcaron@springmail.com*

- Johnson, Eric; EdD; Assoc.; LPC, NCC; 41-60%; *drej4u@msn.com*
- Lorbeer, Charles; PhD; Assoc.; LICSW; 41-60%; *lorbeer@attbi.com*
- Muchnick, Sherri; PhD; Assoc.; LPC, MFT/MHC; 41-60%; *docmunch@aol.com*
- Pietrzak, Dale; EdD; LPC, NCC, NCCMHC; 41-60%; *pietrzak7@mchsi.com*
- Raman, Pattabi; EdD; LPC; 41-60%; *praman@ix.netcom.com*
- Muchnick, Ron; PhD; LPC, NCC, MFT; >81%; *docrmunch@aol.com*
- Dahlen, Penelope; EdD; LPC, NCC; >81%; *pdahlen@earthlink.net*
- Costin, Amanda; PhD; LPC, NCC; >81%; *amandacostin@yahoo.com*
- Farley, Lou; PhD; LPC, NCC; 41-60%; *LouFar@msn.com*
- Yick-Flanagan, Alice; PhD; LCSW; >81%; *ayick@videosymphony.com*
- Zimmermann, Sandra; PhD; NCC, LCSW; 41-60%; *sandra.zimmermann@sbcglobal.net*
- Moredock, Randolph; PhD; NCC; 41-60%; *rmoredoc@brockport.edu*
- Clekis, Joanna; PhD; LPC, NCC; 41-60%; *joanna.clekis@verizon.net*
- Lucas, Jeff; PhD; LPC; 41-60%; *ermjeff@hotmail.com*

MN: Minnesota State University Moorhead

1104 7th Ave. S.
Moorhead, MN 56563-0001
USA

Dean   In Transition
Administrator   William T. Packwood, Director, Counseling and Student Affairs
                    Department   Counseling, Educational Leadership, Foundations, and Field Experiences
                                  (218) 236-2297, fax (218) 236-2547, packwood@mnstate.edu,
                                  www.mnstate.edu/cnsa

Key   See key for Data on Each Department (this section) on page 79.

Program

Accreditation   **CACREP:** Student Affairs - Counseling, **CACREP:** Student Affairs - Professional Practice,
                 CACREP: Community Counseling

Uniqueness   Program has a strong emphasis on, and two-year sequence of, skills. Small, quality program
                 with considerable faculty contact. Provides comprehensive K-12 degree.

Degrees   • Community Counseling: M.
                 • School Counseling: M.
                 • Other: M.

Contact   • Community Counseling: M = Wes Erwin.
                 • School Counseling:
                 • Other: M = Bill Packwood.

Admission and Graduation Data

Admission

Requirements   • Community Counseling(M): GPA 3.00; GRE R; MAT R; Interview.
                 • School Counseling(M): GPA 3.00; GRE R; MAT R; Interview.
                 • Other(M): GPA 3.00; GRE R; MAT R; Interview.

Enrollment   • Community Counseling(M): 7 Admitted yearly; 4 Female; 1 Male.
                 • School Counseling(M): 7 Admitted yearly; 4 Graduated yearly.
                 • Other(M): 7 Admitted yearly; 4 Graduated yearly.

Diversity   • Asian-American; Caucasian.

Graduation

Requirements   • Community Counseling(M): 48 Class hours; 100 Practicum hours; 650 Internship hours;
                   Comprehensive exam; CPCE; Oral exam; Thesis.
                 • School Counseling(M): 48 Class hours; 100 Practicum hours; 650 Internship hours;
                   Comprehensive exam; CPCE; Oral exam; Thesis.
                 • Other(M): 48 Class hours; 100 Practicum hours; 650 Internship hours; Comprehensive
                   exam; CPCE; Oral exam; Thesis.

Postgraduation activity: Advanced education and employment setting percentages.
                 • Community Counseling(M): 10 Managed care; 10 Private practice; 80 Agency practice.
                 • School Counseling(M): NP.
                 • Other(M): 100 Student affairs.

Planned Program Modifications

Courses   Drop   Add
                 • NP.   • Ethics.

Other   Decrease   Increase
                 • NP.   • Diversity Recruiting of Students
                                                • Faculty FTE.

Related Programs

Faculty

nbcc ♦   Percent of faculty reported with NCC certification: **100%**.   **ncc** ♦

Percent in professional counseling practice: 0%.

Research interests Current faculty interests and research areas include: emotional maturity and its development in college students; ethics, supervision, and group counseling; eating disorders and women's issues, grief therapies, spirituality.

Diversity • Caucasian.

Name, Degree, Rank, State/National Credentials, % time devoted to program, email
• Erwin, Wesley J; PhD; Assoc.; LPC, NCC; >81%; *erwin@mnstate.edu*
• Neuman, Patricia A; EdS; Full Prof.; NCC; >81%; *neuman@mnstate.edu*
• Packwood, William T; PhD; Full Prof.; NCC; >81%; *packwood@mnstate.edu*

MN: Minnesota State University, Mankato

107 Armstrong Hall
Mankato, MN 56001
USA

Dean   Joanne Brandt, Interim Dean
Administrator Diane H. Coursol, Department Chair
                  Department   Counseling and Student Personnel
                  (507) 389-2423, fax (507) 389-5074, diane.coursol@mnsu.edu,
                  http://www.coled.mnsu.edu/departments/csp/

Key   See key for Data on Each Department (this section) on page 79.

Program
Accreditation   Regional Accreditation, **CACREP:** Community Counseling, **CACREP:** School Counseling,
                CACREP: Student Affairs - Professional Practice

Uniqueness   Department offers 3 CACREP accredited programs. History of accreditation since 1986.
                Department & Faculty are inviting and dedicated to student development and invested in
                cooperative research with students culminating in conference presentations and publications.

Degrees   • Community Counseling: M.
                • School Counseling: M.
                • Student Affairs: M.

Contact   • Community Counseling: M = Diane Coursol & John Seymour.
                • School Counseling: M = Walter Roberts & Richard Auger.
                • Student Affairs: M = Anne Blackhurst & Jacqueline Lewis.

Admission and Graduation Data
Admission
Requirements   • Community Counseling(M): GPA 3.00; GRE 1350; GRE V Minimum 900 Verbal +
                  Quantitative with a Minimum of 500 on either Verbal or Quantitative; MAT 44; Interview.
                • School Counseling(M): GPA 3.00; GRE 1350; GRE V Minimum 900 Verbal + Quantitative
                  with a Minimum of 500 on either Verbal or Quantitative; MAT 44; Interview.
                • Student Affairs(M): GPA 3.00; GRE 1350; GRE V Minimum 900 Verbal + Quantitative with a
                  Minimum of 500 on either Verbal or Quantitative; MAT Interview.

Enrollment   • Community Counseling(M): 15 Admitted yearly; 15 Graduated yearly; 11 Female; 4 Male.
                • School Counseling(M): 15 Admitted yearly; 15 Graduated yearly; 10 Female; 5 Male.
                • Student Affairs(M): 15 Admitted yearly; 15 Graduated yearly; 12 Female; 3 Male.

Diversity   • African-American; Asian-American; Caucasian; Hispanic; Native American; Multiracial.

Graduation
Requirements   • Community Counseling(M): 50 Class hours; 100 Practicum hours; 600 Internship hours;
                  Comprehensive exam; Portfolio.
                • School Counseling(M): 50 Class hours; 100 Practicum hours; 700 Internship hours;
                  Comprehensive exam; Portfolio.
                • Student Affairs(M): 50 Class hours; 100 Practicum hours; 600 Internship hours; Portfolio.

Postgraduation activity: Advanced education and employment setting percentages.
                • Community Counseling(M): 2 Advanced education; 98 Agency practice.
                • School Counseling(M): 20 Elementary school; 20 Middle school; 60 Secondary school.
                • Student Affairs(M): 1 Advanced education; 99 Student affairs.

Planned Program Modifications
Courses   <u>Drop</u>   <u>Add</u>
                  • NP.   • Legal/Ethical Issues.

Other   <u>Decrease</u>   <u>Increase</u>
                  • NP.   • Number of Off-Campus Courses.

Related Programs Clinical Social Workers
                     Psychology

Faculty

nbcc ❖   Percent of faculty reported with NCC certification: 33%.   ncc ❖

Percent in professional counseling practice: NP.

Research interests Faculty research interests include: counseling process, cybercounseling, technology in counseling, bullying, mental health in the schools, career development, women's issues, play therapy, marriage and family research.

Diversity   •   Caucasian; Multiracial.

Name, Degree, Rank, State/National Credentials, % time devoted to program, email
- Coursol, Diane H; PhD; Full Prof.; >81%; *diane.coursol@mnsu.edu*
- Roberts, Walter B; EdD; Full Prof.; LPC, NCC, NCSC, LSC; >81%; *walter.roberts@mnsu.edu*
- Blackhurst, Anne; PhD; Assoc.; >81%; *anne.blackhurst@mnsu.edu*
- Lewis, Jacqueline; PhD; Assoc.; >81%; *jacqueline.lewis@mnsu.edu*
- Auger, Richard; PhD; Assist.; >81%; *richard.auger@mnsu.edu*
- Seymour, John; PhD; Assist.; LPC, NCC, LMFT; >81%; *john.seymour@mnsu.edu*

MN: Winona State University at Rochester

	859 30th Ave. - S.E.
	Rochester, MN 55904
	USA
Dean	Dr. Carol Anderson, Dean - College of Education
Administrator	Dr. Nick Ruiz, Professor and Department Chair
	Department Counselor Education Department
	(800) 366-5418 Ext. 7137, fax (507) 286-7170,
	www.winona.edu, www.winona.msus.edu/counselor education

Key   See key for Data on Each Department (this section) on page 79.

Program

Accreditation   Regional Accreditation, **CACREP:** Community Counseling, **CACREP:** School Counseling

Uniqueness   The goal of the Winona State University Counselor Education Department is to provide students with quality services and educational opprotunities in order to help them meet their unique career goals. The Counselor Education Department is a student friendly program that offers students throughout their program of study. Employment upon graduation is high.

Degrees   • NP.

Contact   • NP.

Admission and Graduation Data

Admission

Requirements   • NP.

Enrollment   • NP.

Diversity   • NP.

Graduation

Requirements   • NP.

Postgraduation activity: Advanced education and employment setting percentages.

Planned Program Modifications

Courses	Drop	Add
• NP.		• NP.

Other	Decrease	Increase
• NP.		• NP.

Related Programs

Faculty

     Percent of faculty reported with NCC certification: 0%.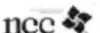

Percent in professional counseling practice: NP.

Research interests Faculty have a variety of research interests including career counseling, play therapy, clinical supervision, counselor credentialing, and stress management.

Diversity   • Caucasian; Hispanic.

Name, Degree, Rank, State/National Credentials, % time devoted to program, email
• NP.

Has CHI SIGMA IOTA (International Counseling Society) chapter.

MN: Winona State University

	132 Gildemeister Hall
	Winona, MN 55987
	USA
Dean	Dr. Carol Anderson, Dean - College of Education
Administrator	Dr. Nick Ruiz, Professor and Department Chair
	Department Counselor Education Department
	(800) 242-8978 Ext. 5335, fax (507) 457-5882,
	www.winona.edu, www.winona.msus.edu/counselor education

Key   See key for Data on Each Department (this section) on page 79.

Program

Accreditation   Regional Accreditation, **CACREP:** Community Counseling, **CACREP:** School Counseling

Uniqueness   The goal of the Winona State University Counselor Education Departmen is to provide students with quality services and educational opprotunities in order to help them meet their unique career goals. The Counselor Education Department is a student friendly program that offers students throughout their program of study. Employment upon graduation is high.

Degrees   •   NP.

Contact   •   NP.

Admission and Graduation Data

Admission

Requirements   •   NP.

Enrollment   •   NP.

Diversity   •   NP.

Graduation

Requirements   •   NP.

Postgraduation activity: Advanced education and employment setting percentages.

Planned Program Modifications

Courses	Drop	Add
	• NP.	• NP.
Other	Decrease	Increase
	• NP.	• NP.

Related Programs

Faculty

    Percent of faculty reported with NCC certification: 0%.   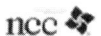

Percent in professional counseling practice: NP.

Research interests   Faculty have a variety of research interests including career counseling, play therapy, clinical supervision, counselor credentialing, and stress management.

Diversity   •   Caucasian; Hispanic.

Name, Degree, Rank, State/National Credentials, % time devoted to program, email
•   NP.

Has CHI SIGMA IOTA (International Counseling Society) chapter.

MO: Northwest Missouri State University

2440 Colder Hall
Maryville, MO 64468
USA

Dean	
Administrator	John K. Bowers, Chairperson
Department	Dept of Psychology, Sociology, Counseling
	(660) 562-1260, fax (660) 562-1731, psysoc@mail.NWMissouri.edu

Key See key for Data on Each Department (this section) on page 79.

Program

Accreditation NP.

Uniqueness Staffed by licensed and experienced faculty, this department involves students with close supervision. The MS Counseling program is on furlough and will no longer accept applications.

Degrees
- Mental Health Counseling: M.
- School Counseling: M.

Contact
- Mental Health Counseling: M = Carla Edwards.
- School Counseling: M = Rochelle Hiatt.

Admission and Graduation Data

Admission

Requirements
- Mental Health Counseling(M): GPA 3.00; GRE ~1500; GRE V 500; GRE Q 500; GRE A 500; Letters.
- School Counseling(M): GPA 2.50; GRE ~1400; GRE V 500; GRE Q 400; GRE A 500; Letters.

Enrollment
- Mental Health Counseling(M): 12 Admitted yearly; 10 Graduated yearly.
- School Counseling(M): 12 Admitted yearly; 12 Graduated yearly.

Diversity
- NP.

Graduation

Requirements
- Mental Health Counseling(M): 51 Class hours; 500 Practicum hours; Comprehensive exam; Thesis.
- School Counseling(M): 44 Class hours; 150 Practicum hours; Comprehensive exam; Portfolio.

Postgraduation activity: Advanced education and employment setting percentages.
- Mental Health Counseling(M): 5 Advanced education; 95 Agency practice.
- School Counseling(M): 30 Elementary school; 20 Middle school; 50 Secondary school.

Planned Program Modifications

Courses	Drop	Add
	• NP.	• NP.

Other	Decrease	Increase
	• NP.	• NP.

Related Programs

Faculty

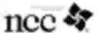 Percent of faculty reported with NCC certification: 0%.

Percent in professional counseling practice: 60%.

Research interests Ranges from research on the learning process to substance abuse

Diversity
- NP.

Name, Degree, Rank, State/National Credentials, % time devoted to program, email
- Barnett, Jerrold; PhD; Full Prof.; 22-40%;
- Edwards, Carla; PhD; Assist.; 22-40%;
- Claflin, Carol; PhD; Assoc.; <21%;
- Riley, Larry; PhD; Full Prof.; <21%;
- Hiatt, Rochelle; EdD; Instructor; <21%;
- Kibler, Jackie; PhD; Assist.; 41-60%;
- Stamp, Melinda; EdS; Assist.; <21%;

Has CHI SIGMA IOTA (International Counseling Society) chapter.

MO: Southeast Missouri State University

One University Plaza/MS 5550
Cape Girardeau, MO 63701-4799
USA

Dean	Dr. I Sue Shepard, College of Education, Scully Building
Administrator	Dr. Verl T. Pope, Counseling Coordinator
	Department Educational Administration and Counseling
	(573) 651-2137, fax (573) 986-6812, vpope@semo.edu, http://www4.semo.edu/counsel

Key   See key for Data on Each Department (this section) on page 79.

Program

Accreditation   **CACREP:** Community Counseling

CACREP

Uniqueness   Low student-faculty ratio; strong scientist-practitioner emphasis; graduates find employment in a wide range of settings

Degrees
- Community Counseling: M.
- School Counseling: M.

Contact
- Community Counseling: M = Dr. Verl Pope.
- School Counseling: M = Dr. Doris Skelton.

Admission and Graduation Data

Admission

Requirements
- Community Counseling(M): GPA 3.00; GRE 1600; GRE V 450; GRE Q 600; GRE A 550; Interview.
- School Counseling(M): GPA 3.00; GRE 1600; GRE V 450; GRE Q 600; GRE A 550; Interview.

Enrollment
- Community Counseling(M): 15 Admitted yearly; 12 Graduated yearly.
- School Counseling(M): 20 Admitted yearly; 18 Graduated yearly.

Diversity
- African-American; Asian-American; Caucasian; Hispanic; Native American.

Graduation

Requirements
- Community Counseling(M): 48 Class hours; 100 Practicum hours; 600 Internship hours; Comprehensive exam; CPCE; Portfolio.
- School Counseling(M): 48 Class hours; 100 Practicum hours; 600 Internship hours; Comprehensive exam; CPCE; Portfolio.

Postgraduation activity: Advanced education and employment setting percentages.
- Community Counseling(M): 20 Advanced education; 80 Agency practice.
- School Counseling(M): 5 Advanced education; 35 Elementary school; 20 Middle school; 30 Secondary school; 10 Student affairs.

Planned Program Modifications

Courses	Drop	Add
	• NP.	• Crisis/Violence Counseling
		• Grief Counseling
		• Teaching.

Other	Decrease	Increase
	• NP.	• Admission Requirements
		• Diversity Recruiting of Faculty
		• Diversity Recruiting of Students
		• Number of Degree Majors
		• Number of Distance Education Courses
		• Number of Off-Campus Courses
		• Number of On-Line Courses.

Related Programs Communications

Faculty

nbcc ❧   Percent of faculty reported with NCC certification: 80%.   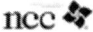

Percent in professional counseling practice: 40%.

Research interests Counselor supervision; skills acquisition, marriage and family, school counseling professionalization issues

Diversity   • Asian-American; Caucasian.

Name, Degree, Rank, State/National Credentials, % time devoted to program, email
• Milde, Cheryl; PhD; Assist.; LPC, NCC; >81%; *cmilde@semo.edu*
• MohdZain, A. Zaidy; PhD; Assoc.; LPC, NCC; >81%; *zmohdzain@semo.edu*
• Monteiro-Leitner, Julieta; PhD; Assist.; *jleitner@semo.edu*
• Pope, Verl; EdD; Assoc.; LPC, NCC; >81%; *vpope@semo.edu*
• Skelton, Doris; EdD; Assoc.; LPC, NCC; >81%; *dskelton@semo.edu*

Has CHI SIGMA IOTA (International Counseling Society) chapter.

MO: Truman State University

100 E. Normal Street
Kirksville, MO 63501
USA
Dean Sam Minner, Head, Division of Education, Violette Hall
Administrator Christopher J. Maglio, Ph.D., Program Director
Department Counselor Preparation Programs/Division of Social Science
(660) 785-4403, fax (660) 785-4383, cjmaglio@truman.edu,
http://counseling.truman.edu

Key See key for Data on Each Department (this section) on page 79.

Program
Accreditation Regional Accreditation, **CACREP:** Community Counseling, **CACREP:** School Counseling, **CACREP:** Student Affairs - Professional Practice

CACREP

Uniqueness The Counselor Preparation Programs at Truman State University are designed to provide students with a strong theoretical and research base, closely supervised clinical experiences, opportunities for personal growth, and the flexibility to meet varied academic and professional goals. Close and frequent interaction between students and faculty is highly valued and emphasized. Graduate assistantships available for all endorsements.

Degrees
- Community Counseling: M.
- School Counseling: M.
- Student Affairs: M.

Contact
- Community Counseling: M = Christopher J. Maglio, Ph.D..
- School Counseling: M = Tricia K. Brown, Ph.D..
- Student Affairs: M = Michael Mann, Ph.D..

Admission and Graduation Data
Admission
Requirements
- Community Counseling(M): GPA 3.00; GRE 50th%; GRE V 50th%; GRE Q 50th%; GRE A 50th%.
- School Counseling(M): GPA 3.00; GRE 50th%; GRE V 50th%; GRE Q 50th%; GRE A 50th%.
- Student Affairs(M): GPA 3.00; GRE 50th%; GRE V 50th%; GRE Q 50th%; GRE A 50th%.

Enrollment
- Community Counseling(M): 7 Admitted yearly; 7 Graduated yearly; 4 Female; 3 Male.
- School Counseling(M): 5 Admitted yearly; 5 Graduated yearly; 4 Female; 1 Male.
- Student Affairs(M): 3 Admitted yearly; 3 Graduated yearly; 1 Female; 2 Male.

Diversity
- Asian-American; Caucasian; Hispanic; Pacific Islander; Multiracial.

Graduation
Requirements
- Community Counseling(M): 48 Class hours; 150 Practicum hours; 600 Internship hours; Comprehensive exam; Thesis.
- School Counseling(M): 48 Class hours; 150 Practicum hours; 600 Internship hours; Comprehensive exam; Thesis; Portfolio.
- Student Affairs(M): 48 Class hours; 150 Practicum hours; 600 Internship hours; Thesis.

Postgraduation activity: Advanced education and employment setting percentages.
- Community Counseling(M): 30 Advanced education; 70 Agency practice.
- School Counseling(M): 10 Advanced education; 50 Elementary school; 40 Secondary school.
- Student Affairs(M): 10 Advanced education; 10 Agency practice; 80 Other.

Planned Program Modifications

Courses	Drop	Add
	• NP.	• Internet Use
		• Play Therapy.

Other	Decrease	Increase
	• NP.	• Diversity Recruiting of Students
		• Number of Degree Majors.

Related Programs

Faculty

nbcc ❧   Percent of faculty reported with NCC certification: **100%**.   ncc ❧

Percent in professional counseling practice: 50%.

Research interests Family life cycles, care giving, work with young children, death education, death fear and anxiety, professional ethics training in counseling and psychology programs, meta-analytic approaches in counseling research, career development, multicultural counseling, student affairs practice, college counseling, supervision, and perfectionism.

Diversity   • Caucasian.

Name, Degree, Rank, State/National Credentials, % time devoted to program, email
- Maglio, Christopher J; PhD; Assoc.; NCC, Licensed Psychologist; >81%; *cjmaglio@truman.edu*
- Brown, Tricia K; PhD; Assist.; LPC, NCC; >81%; *tbrown@truman.edu*
- Mann, Michael; PhD; Assist.; NCC; >81%; *mmann@truman.edu*
- Gilchrist, LouAnn; EdD; Full Prof.; LPC, NCC; <21%; *ad57@truman.edu*

MO: University of Missouri - St. Louis

	8001 Natural Bridge Rd., 469 MH
	Saint Louis, MO 63121-4499
	United States
Dean	Charles Schmitz, PhD/ College of Education
Administrator	Therese Cristiani, EdD, Chair
	Department Division of Counseling & Family Therapy
	(314) 516-5782, fax (314) 516-5784, cristiani@umsl.edu,
	www.umsl.edu/educate

Key   See key for Data on Each Department (this section) on page 79.

Program

Accreditation   Regional Accreditation, **CACREP:** Community Counseling, **CACREP:** Career Counseling, **CACREP:** School Counseling

CACREP

Uniqueness   Only CACREP program in Saint Louis region or in University of Missouri system; stong urban and multicultural orientation

Degrees
- Community Counseling: M.
- School Counseling: M.
- Career Counseling: M.
- Counselor Education: EdD, PhD.

Contact
- Community Counseling: M = Susan Kashubeck-West, PhD.
- School Counseling: M = Therese Cristiani, EdD.
- Career Counseling: M = Mark Pope, EdD.
- Counselor Education: D = R. Rocco Cottone, PhD.

Admission and Graduation Data

Admission

Requirements
- Community Counseling(M): GPA 3.00.
- School Counseling(M): GPA 3.00.
- Career Counseling(M): GPA 3.00.
- Counselor Education(D): Masters and GPA 3.00; GRE 1000.

Enrollment
- Community Counseling(M): 40 Admitted yearly; 30 Graduated yearly; 96 Female; 24 Male.
- School Counseling(M): 50 Admitted yearly; 40 Graduated yearly; 120 Female; 30 Male.
- Career Counseling(M): 10 Admitted yearly; 8 Graduated yearly; 24 Female; 8 Male.
- Counselor Education(D): NP.

Diversity
- African-American; Asian-American; Caucasian; Hispanic; Native American; Pacific Islander; Multiracial.

Graduation

Requirements
- Community Counseling(M): 48 Class hours; 150 Practicum hours; 600 Internship hours; Comprehensive exam; CPCE.
- School Counseling(M): 48 Class hours; 150 Practicum hours; 600 Internship hours; Comprehensive exam; CPCE; Portfolio.
- Career Counseling(M): 48 Class hours; 150 Practicum hours; 600 Internship hours; CPCE.
- Counselor Education(D): 110 Class hours; 150 Practicum hours; 600 Internship hours; Comprehensive exam; Oral exam; Dissertation.

Postgraduation activity: Advanced education and employment setting percentages.
- Community Counseling(M): NP.
- School Counseling(M): NP.
- Career Counseling(M): NP.
- Counselor Education(D):

Planned Program Modifications

Courses	Drop	Add
	• Wellness.	• Advocacy
		• Human Sexuality
		• Social Justice.

Other	Decrease	Increase
	• NP.	• Admission Requirements
		• Diversity Recruiting of Faculty
		• Diversity Recruiting of Students
		• Faculty FTE
		• Financial Aid
		• National Accreditation
		• Number of Degree Majors
		• Number of Distance Education Courses
		• Number of Off-Campus Courses
		• Number of On-Line Courses.

Related Programs Psychology

Faculty

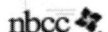 Percent of faculty reported with NCC certification: 29%.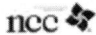

Percent in professional counseling practice: 0%.

Research interests multicultural (including LGBT), ethics, children, history of counseling, eating disorders

Diversity   • African-American; Caucasian; Native American; Multiracial.

Name, Degree, Rank, State/National Credentials, % time devoted to program, email
• Cristiani, Therese; EdD; Full Prof.; LPC, NCC; >81%; *cristiani@umsl.edu*
• Cottone, R. Rocco; PhD; Full Prof.; Psychologist; >81%; *cottone@umsl.edu*
• Pope, Mark; EdD; Assoc.; LPC, NCC, MAC, MCC, NCCC; >81%; *pope@umsl.edu*
• Kashubeck-West, Susan; PhD; Assoc.; Psychologist; >81%;
• Butler, S. Kent; PhD; Assist.; >81%;
• Kosteck-Bunch, Lela; PhD; Assist.; >81%;
• Szymanski, Dawn; PhD; Assist.; >81%;

Has CHI SIGMA IOTA (International Counseling Society) chapter.

MO: University of Missouri-Columbia

16 Hill Hall
Columbia, MO 65211
USA
Dean   Dean Richard Andrews
Administrator   P. Paul Heppner, Professor & Chairperson
               Department   Dept of Educational & Co Psychology
               (573) 882-7731, fax (573) 884-5989, ecpgrad@tiger.coe.missouri.edu,
               http://www.coe.missouri.edu/%7Eecp/

Key   See key for Data on Each Department (this section) on page 79.

Program

Accreditation   Regional Accreditation, CORE: Rehabilitation Counseling

Uniqueness   The graduate program in the Department is designed to meet the specific needs of the student in a particular area of emphasis. Graduates find employment in a wide range of settings.

Degrees
- Community Counseling: M, S.
- School Counseling: M, S.
- Career Counseling: M, S.
- Other: M, S, PhD, D.
- Rehabilitation Counseling: M, S.
- Student Affairs: M, S.

Contact
- Community Counseling: M = Laurie Mintz.; S = NP.
- School Counseling: M = Norman Gysbers or Richard Lapan.; S = NP.
- Career Counseling: M = Mary Heppner or Joe Johnson..; S = NP.
- Other: M = Richard Cox.; S = NP.; D = Laurie Mintz.
- Rehabilitation Counseling: M = David Roberts.; S = NP.
- Student Affairs: M = Glenn Good.; S = NP.

Admission and Graduation Data

Admission

Requirements
- Community Counseling(M): GPA 3.00; GRE 1000; GRE V 500; GRE Q 500; GRE A 500.
- Community Counseling(S): GPA 3.00; GRE 1000; GRE V 500; GRE Q 500; GRE A 500.
- School Counseling(M): GPA 3.00; GRE 1000; GRE V 500; GRE Q 500; GRE A 500.
- School Counseling(S): GPA 3.00; GRE 1000; GRE V 500; GRE Q 500; GRE A 500.
- Career Counseling(M): GPA 3.00; GRE 1000; GRE V 500; GRE Q 500; GRE A 500.
- Career Counseling(S): GPA 3.00; GRE 1000; GRE V 500; GRE Q 500; GRE A 500.
- Other(M): GPA 3.00; GRE 1000; GRE V 500; GRE Q 500; GRE A 500.
- Other(S): GPA 3.00; GRE 1000; GRE V 500; GRE Q 500; GRE A 500.
- Other(D): Masters and GPA 3.00; GRE 1200; GRE V 600; GRE Q 600; GRE A 600.
- Rehabilitation Counseling(M): GPA 3.00; GRE 1000; GRE V 500; GRE Q 500; GRE A 500.
- Rehabilitation Counseling(S): GPA 3.00; GRE 1000; GRE V 500; GRE Q 500; GRE A 500.
- Student Affairs(M): GPA 3.00; GRE 1000; GRE V 500; GRE Q 500; GRE A 500.
- Student Affairs(S): GPA 3.00; GRE 1000; GRE V 500; GRE Q 500; GRE A 500.

Enrollment
- Community Counseling(M & S): 6-10 Admitted yearly; 6-10 Graduated yearly; 15 Female; 10 Male.
- School Counseling(M & S): 6-8 Admitted yearly; 6-8 Graduated yearly; 15 Female; 2 Male.
- Career Counseling(M & S): 6 Admitted yearly; 6 Graduated yearly; 7 Female; 6 Male.
- Other(M & S): 3 Admitted yearly; 3 Graduated yearly; 3 Female; 1 Male.
- Other(D): 8 Admitted yearly; 6 Graduated yearly; 44 Female; 23 Male.
- Rehabilitation Counseling(M & S): 6 Admitted yearly; 5 Graduated yearly; 5 Female; 7 Male.
- Student Affairs(M & S): 1-2 Admitted yearly; 1-2 Graduated yearly; 2 Female; 2 Male.

Diversity
- African-American; Asian-American; Caucasian; Hispanic; Native American; Pacific Islander; Multiracial; Other.

Graduation

Requirements
- Community Counseling(M): 48 Class hours; Comprehensive exam.
- Community Counseling(S): 30 Class hours; one practicum course: specific hours vary and are determined in consultation with advisor Practicum hours; Comprehensive exam.
- School Counseling(M): 48 Class hours; Oral exam; Portfolio.
- School Counseling(S): 30 Class hours; same Practicum hours; Comprehensive exam.
- Career Counseling(M): 48 Class hours.
- Career Counseling(S): 30 Class hours; same Practicum hours; Comprehensive exam.
- Other(M): 48 Class hours.
- Other(S): 30 Class hours; same Practicum hours; Comprehensive exam.
- Other(D): 82 Class hours; 400 Practicum hours; 2000 Internship hours; Oral exam; Dissertation; Portfolio.

- Rehabilitation Counseling(M): 48 Class hours; Comprehensive exam.
- Rehabilitation Counseling(S): 30 Class hours; same Practicum hours; Comprehensive exam.
- Student Affairs(M): 48 Class hours.
- Student Affairs(S): 30 Class hours; same Practicum hours; Comprehensive exam.

Postgraduation activity: Advanced education and employment setting percentages.
- Community Counseling(M & S): 30 Advanced education; 30 Private practice; 40 Agency practice.
- School Counseling(M & S): 50 Elementary school; 25 Middle school; 25 Secondary school.
- Career Counseling(M & S): 25 Advanced education; 25 Agency practice; 50 Other.
- Other(M & S): 100 Other.
- Other(D): 1 Managed care; 1 Private practice; 49 Agency practice; 33 Student affairs; 16 Other.
- Rehabilitation Counseling(M & S): 20 Advanced education; 80 Agency practice.
- Student Affairs(M & S): 50 Advanced education; 50 Other.

Planned Program Modifications

Courses	Drop	Add
• NP.	• NP.

Other	Decrease	Increase
• NP.	• NP.

Related Programs Clinical Social Workers
                   Psychiatrists

Faculty

nbcc ❖   Percent of faculty reported with NCC certification: 0%.   ncc ❖

Percent in professional counseling practice: 43%.

Research interests NP.

Diversity   • African-American; Caucasian; Hispanic; Multiracial.

Name, Degree, Rank, State/National Credentials, % time devoted to program, email
- Boggs, Kathleen A; PhD; Assist.; Licensced psychologist; <21%; *BoggsKA@missouri.edu*
- Cox, Richard H; PhD; Full Prof.; >81%; *CoxRH@missouri.edu*
- Good, Glenn E; PhD; Assoc.; Licensed Psychologist; >81%; *GoodG@missouri.edu*
- Gysbers, Norman; PhD; Full Prof.; >81%; *GysbersN@missouri.edu*
- Heppner, Mary J; PhD; Assoc.; 41-60%; *HeppnerM@missouri.edu*
- Heppner, P. Paul; PhD; Full Prof.; Licensed Psychologist; >81%; *HeppnerP@missouri.edu*
- Johnson, Joseph; PhD; Full Prof.; 41-60%; *JohnstonJ@missouri.edu*
- Flores, Lisa; PhD; Assist.; >81%; *Floresly@missouri.edu*
- Mallinckrodt, Brent; PhD; Assoc.; >81%; *MallinckrodtB@missouri.edu*
- Lapan, Richard T; PhD; Full Prof.; Licensed Pychologist; >81%; *LapanR@missouri.edu*
- Mintz, Laurie B; PhD; Assoc.; Licenced Psychologist; >81%; *MintzL@missouri.edu*
- Mobley, Michael; PhD; Assist.; >81%; *MobleyMi@missouri.edu*
- Multon, Karen D; PhD; Full Prof.; Licenced Psychologist; >81%; *MultonK@missouri.edu*
- Martz, Erin; PhD; Assist.; >81%; *MartzE@missouri.edu*
- Roberts, Dave; PhD; Assoc.; >81%; *RobertsC@missouri.edu*
- Worthington, Roger L; PhD; Assist.; >81%; *WorthingtonR@missouri.edu*

MS: Mississippi College

Box 4013, Mississippi College
Clinton, MS 39058
USA
Dean   Don W. Locke, School of Education
Administrator   Harold W. Wheeler, Jr. Ph.D., Chair
                  Department   Department of Psychology and Counseling
                               (601) 925-3841, fax (601) 925-3951, wheeler@mc.edu,
                               www.mc.edu

Key   See key for Data on Each Department (this section) on page 79.

Program
Accreditation   Regional Accreditation, **CACREP:** Marriage and Family Counseling, **CACREP:** Mental Health Counseling, **CACREP:** School Counseling

Uniqueness   The integration of psychological and counseling knowledge and theory with the Christian faith and an opportunity to perform internships with a variety of client populations.

Degrees
- Mental Health Counseling: M.
- School Counseling: M, S.
- Marriage and Family Counseling: M.

Contact
- Mental Health Counseling: M = Katherine Jones.
- School Counseling: M, S = Edith Carlisle.
- Marriage and Family Counseling: M = Bill Wheeler.

Admission and Graduation Data
Admission
Requirements
- Mental Health Counseling(M): GPA 3.00; GRE 900; GRE V 450; GRE Q 450; Interview.
- School Counseling(M): GPA 2.50; GRE Praxis; 1 Year work experience; Interview.
- School Counseling(S): GPA 2.50; GRE Praxis; 1 Year work experience; Interview.
- Marriage and Family Counseling(M): GPA 3.00; GRE 900; GRE V 450; GRE Q 450; 1 Year work experience; Interview.

Enrollment
- Mental Health Counseling(M): 15 Admitted yearly; 8 Graduated yearly.
- School Counseling(M & S): 10 Admitted yearly; 3 Graduated yearly.
- Marriage and Family Counseling(M): 15 Admitted yearly; 5 Graduated yearly.

Diversity
- African-American; Caucasian; Other.

Graduation
Requirements
- Mental Health Counseling(M): 60 Class hours; 100 Practicum hours; 900 Internship hours; Oral exam.
- School Counseling(M): 48 Class hours; 100 Practicum hours; 600 Internship hours; Oral exam.
- School Counseling(S): 36 Class hours; 100 Practicum hours; 300 Internship hours; Oral exam.
- Marriage and Family Counseling(M): 60 Class hours; 100 Practicum hours; 600 Internship hours; Oral exam.

Postgraduation activity: Advanced education and employment setting percentages.
- Mental Health Counseling(M): 10 Advanced education; 10 Private practice; 50 Agency practice; 30 Other.
- School Counseling(M & S): 10 Advanced education; 20 Elementary school; 30 Middle school; 40 Secondary school.
- Marriage and Family Counseling(M): 10 Advanced education; 10 Private practice; 20 Agency practice; 60 Other.

Planned Program Modifications

Courses	Drop	Add
	• NP.	• Legal/Ethical Issues.

Other	Decrease	Increase
	• NP.	• Clinical Supervision • Diversity Recruiting of Faculty • Diversity Recruiting of Students.

Related Programs

Faculty

nbcc ✿   Percent of faculty reported with NCC certification: 35%.   ncc ✿

Percent in professional counseling practice: 55%.

Research interests Dr. John Jolly is working with Dr. Aaron Beck on the reliability and validity of new measures of child depression, anxiety, and disruptive behavior. Dr. Bill Wheeler is conducting research investigating the validity of the prototypical definition of emotion using the Semantic Structure of Affect Model.

Diversity   • Caucasian; Multiracial.

Name, Degree, Rank, State/National Credentials, % time devoted to program, email
• Carlisle, Edith; EdD; Assoc.; LPC, NCC, LMFT; >81%; *carlisle@mc.edu*
• Fisher, Gloria; PhD; Full Prof.; Lic Psych.; <21%; *fisher@mc.edu*
• Cotton, Randy; PhD; Adjunct; Lic Psych; <21%;
• Jones, Katherine; PhD; Assist.; LPC, NCC; 61-80%; *jones@mc.edu*
• Jolly, John; PsyD; Assoc.; Lic Psych; >81%; *jolly@mc.edu*
• Summerlin, Curtis; PhD; Assoc.; 22-40%; *summerlin@mc.edu*
• Wagner, Buddy; PhD; Assist.; NCC; 41-60%; *wagner@mc.edu*
• Wheeler, Harold W; PhD; Full Prof.; LPC, NCC; 61-80%; *wheeler@mc.edu*
• Wooten, James W; PhD; Full Prof.; NCC; 41-60%; *wooten@mc.edu*
• Clark, David A; PhD; Adjunct; <21%;
• Locke, Don W; EdD; Full Prof.; <21%; *locke@mc.edu*
• Boudreaux, Charles; EdD; Adjunct; LMFT; 22-40%; *cboudreaux@fbcj.org*
• Mumbower, Ronald; EdD; Adjunct; LMFT; 22-40%; *rmumbower@fbcj.org*
• Williams, Tom; EdD; Assoc.; <21%; *williams@mc.edu*
• Jacobson, Barbara J; PhD; Adjunct; LPC, NCC; <21%;
• Nevels, Robert; PhD; Adjunct; Lic Psych; <21%;
• Weisz, John R; PhD; Adjunct; Lic Psych; <21%;

MS: Mississippi State University

	P. O. Box 9727
	Mississippi State University, MS 39762-5740
	USA
Dean	Dr. Roy Ruby, 309 Allen Hall, Mississippi State University, MS 39762
Administrator	Dr. Thomas W. Hosie, Department Head
	Department Counseling, Educational Psychology & Special Education
	(662) 325-3426, fax (662) 325-3263, hosie@colled.msstate.edu,
	www.educ.msstate.edu/CEdEPy/cedepy.html

Key   See key for Data on Each Department (this section) on page 79.

Program
Accreditation   Regional Accreditation, **CACREP:** Community Counseling, **CACREP:** Counselor Education and Supervision, **CACREP:** School Counseling, **CACREP:** Student Affairs - Counseling, CORE: Rehabilitation Counseling; Applied for CACREP: Student Affairs - Professional Practice,

CACREP

Uniqueness   State-of-the-art Counseling/School Psychology lab. Family, group, play therapy & 8 individual counseling rooms. Electronic classroom. Chi Sigma Iota Chapter.

Degrees
- Community Counseling: M, S.
- School Counseling: M, S, EdD, PhD.
- Rehabilitation Counseling: M, S.
- College Counseling: M, S.
- Student Affairs: M, S.
- Counselor Education: EdD, PhD.

Contact
- Community Counseling: M, S = Dr. Joan Looby.
- School Counseling: M, S, D = Dr. Joe Ray Underwood.
- Rehabilitation Counseling: M, S = Dr. Glen Hendren.
- College Counseling: M, S = Dr. Mari Ann Callais.
- Student Affairs: M, S = Dr. Mari Ann Callais.
- Counselor Education: D = Dr. Joan Looby.

Admission and Graduation Data
Admission
Requirements
- Community Counseling(M): GPA 2.75; GRE 1200.
- Community Counseling(S): GPA 2.75; GRE 1400.
- School Counseling(M): GPA 2.75; GRE 1200.
- School Counseling(S): GPA 2.75; GRE 1400.
- School Counseling(D): Masters and GPA 3.50; GRE 1500; 2 Years work experience.
- Rehabilitation Counseling(M): GPA 2.75; GRE 1200.
- Rehabilitation Counseling(S): GPA 2.75; GRE 1400.
- College Counseling(M): GPA 2.75; GRE 1200.
- College Counseling(S): GPA 2.75; GRE 1400.
- Student Affairs(M): GPA 2.75; GRE 1200.
- Student Affairs(S): GPA 2.75; GRE 1400.
- Counselor Education(D): NP.

Enrollment
- Community Counseling(M & S): 16 Admitted yearly; 15 Graduated yearly; 27 Female; 4 Male.
- School Counseling(M & S): 20 Admitted yearly; 18 Graduated yearly; 34 Female; 4 Male.
- School Counseling(D): NP.
- Rehabilitation Counseling(M & S): 16 Admitted yearly; 15 Graduated yearly; 27 Female; 4 Male.
- College Counseling(M & S): 10 Admitted yearly; 8 Graduated yearly; 16 Female; 2 Male.
- Student Affairs(M & S): 16 Admitted yearly; 10 Graduated yearly; 23 Female; 3 Male.
- Counselor Education(D): NP.

Diversity
- African-American; Asian-American; Caucasian; Hispanic.

Graduation
Requirements
- Community Counseling(M): 60 Class hours; 100 Practicum hours; 600 Internship hours; Comprehensive exam; CPCE.
- Community Counseling(S): 90 Class hours; 100 Practicum hours; 600 Internship hours; Comprehensive exam.
- School Counseling(M): 48 Class hours; 100 Practicum hours; 600 Internship hours; Comprehensive exam; CPCE.
- School Counseling(S): 78 Class hours; 100 Practicum hours; 600 Internship hours; Comprehensive exam.

- School Counseling(D): 98 Class hours; 1200 Internship hours; Oral exam; Dissertation.
- Rehabilitation Counseling(M): 48 Class hours; 100 Practicum hours; 600 Internship hours; Comprehensive exam; CPCE.
- Rehabilitation Counseling(S): 78 Class hours; 100 Practicum hours; 600 Internship hours; Comprehensive exam.
- College Counseling(M): 48 Class hours; 100 Practicum hours; 600 Internship hours; Comprehensive exam; CPCE.
- College Counseling(S): 78 Class hours; 100 Practicum hours; 600 Internship hours; Comprehensive exam.
- Student Affairs(M): 48 Class hours; 100 Practicum hours; 600 Internship hours; CPCE.
- Student Affairs(S): 78 Class hours; 100 Practicum hours; 600 Internship hours; Comprehensive exam.
- Counselor Education(D): 98 Class hours; 1200 Internship hours; Oral exam; Dissertation.

Postgraduation activity: Advanced education and employment setting percentages.
- Community Counseling(M & S): 10 Advanced education; 5 Managed care; 5 Private practice; 65 Agency practice; 5 Middle school; 10 Other.
- School Counseling(M & S): 5 Advanced education; 10 Agency practice; 15 Elementary school; 35 Middle school; 35 Secondary school.
- School Counseling(D): 10 Private practice; 90 Other.
- Rehabilitation Counseling(M & S): 10 Advanced education; 5 Managed care; 15 Private practice; 70 Agency practice.
- College Counseling(M & S): 100 Other.
- Student Affairs(M & S): 100 Other.
- Counselor Education(D): 10 Private practice; 90 Student affairs.

Planned Program Modifications

Courses	Drop	Add
	• NP.	• Abuse of Individual
		• Career/Life Planning
		• Diversity
		• Group Work
		• Legal/Ethical Issues
		• Research Methods
		• Supervision
		• Testing, Appraisal, Assessment.

Other	Decrease	Increase
	• NP.	• Course Offerings
		• Clinical Supervision
		• Diversity Recruiting of Faculty
		• Diversity Recruiting of Students
		• Graduation Requirements
		• National Accreditation
		• Number of Distance Education Courses
		• Number of Off-Campus Courses
		• Number of On-Line Courses.

Related Programs

Faculty

 Percent of faculty reported with NCC certification: 35%.

Percent in professional counseling practice: 10%.

Research interests Diversity, spirituality, addictions, supervision, ethics, credentialing, giftedness, deafness, blindness, aging, student development, rehab counseling

Diversity   • African-American; Caucasian; Hispanic.

Name, Degree, Rank, State/National Credentials, % time devoted to program, email
- Abraham, Jimmy; PhD; Assist.; <21%; *jimmy@saffairs.msstate.edu*
- Callais, Mari Ann; PhD; Assist.; >81%; *mcallais@colled.msstate.edu*
- Dooley, Kathy; PhD; Full Prof.; >81%; *kathyd@ra.msstate.edu*
- Hendren, Glen; PhD; Full Prof.; LPC, CRC; >81%; *glen@ra.msstate.edu*
- Hermann, Mary; PhD; Assist.; LPC, NCC; >81%; *mhermann@colled.msstate.e*
- Hosie, Thomas; PhD; Full Prof.; LPC, NCC; >81%; *hosie@colled.msstate.edu*
- Housley, Warren; PhD; Full Prof.; <21%; *warh@ra.msstate.edu*
- Keith, Eddie; PhD; Assist.; <21%; *ekeith@ra.msstate.edu*
- Looby, Joan; PhD; Assoc.; LPC, NCC; >81%; *jlooby@colled.msstate.edu*
- Miller, Jason; MEd; Instructor; NCC; >81%; *jlm495@colled.msstate.edu*
- Moore, Elton; PhD; Full Prof.; CRC; <21%; *jemoore@ra.msstate.edu*
- Palmer, Charles; PhD; Assist.; CRC; >81%; *cpalmer@colled.msstate.edu*
- Porter, Julia; PhD; Assist.; LPC, NCC, NCSC; >81%; *jporter@meridian.msstate.ed*

- Puckett, Frank; PhD; Assist.; CRC; >81%; *fp15@colled.msstate.edu*
- Ruby, Roy; PhD; Full Prof.; <21%; *rhr2@colled.msstate.edu*
- Sheperis, Carl; PhD; Assist.; LPC, NCC; >81%; *csheperis@colled.msstate.ed*
- Thomas, George; PhD; Full Prof.; >81%; *gthomas@meridian.msstate.e*
- Underwood, Joe Ray; PhD; Full Prof.; >81%; *joeray@colled.msstate.edu*
- Wozny, Darren; PhD; Assist.; >81%; *dwozny@meridian.msstate.e*
- Young, Scott; PhD; Assoc.; LPC, NCC; >81%; *jsyoung@colled.msstate.edu*

Has CHI SIGMA IOTA (International Counseling Society) chapter.

MS: William Carey College

498 Tuscan Ave.
Hattiesburg, MS 39401

Dean
Administrator   Dr. Tommy King, Graduate Dean and Director of Graduate Psychology Programs
                      Department   Psychology
                                     (601) 318-6774, fax (601) 318-6488, Gradoff@wmcarey.edu,
                                     www.wmcarey.edu

Key   See key for Data on Each Department (this section) on page 79.

Program
   Accreditation   Regional Accreditation

   Uniqueness   The mission of William Carey College is to provide liberal arts and professional education
                    programs within a caring Christian academic community.

   Degrees   • Community Counseling: M.
                    • School Counseling: M.
                    • Gerontological Counseling: M.
                    • Pastoral Counseling: M.

   Contact   • Community Counseling: M = Dr. Tommy King.
                    • School Counseling: M = Dr. Tommy King.
                    • Gerontological Counseling: M = Dr. Paul Cotten.
                    • Pastoral Counseling: M = Dr. Tommy King.

Admission and Graduation Data
Admission
   Requirements   • Community Counseling(M): GPA 2.50; GRE 900.
                    • School Counseling(M): GPA 2.50; GRE 850.
                    • Gerontological Counseling(M): GPA *; GRE 630+.
                    • Pastoral Counseling(M): GPA *; GRE 630+.

   Enrollment   • Community Counseling(M): 10 Admitted yearly; 10 Graduated yearly; 8 Female; 12 Male.
                    • School Counseling(M): 10 Admitted yearly; 10 Graduated yearly; 8 Male.
                    • Gerontological Counseling(M): 10 Admitted yearly; 10 Graduated yearly; 12 Female;
                      8 Male.
                    • Pastoral Counseling(M): 10 Admitted yearly; 10 Graduated yearly; 4 Female; 16 Male.

   Diversity   • African-American; Caucasian; Native American; Multiracial.

Graduation
   Requirements   • Community Counseling(M): 60 Class hours; 100 Practicum hours; 100 Internship hours;
                      Portfolio.
                    • School Counseling(M): 48 Class hours; 100 Practicum hours; 100 Internship hours;
                      Portfolio.
                    • Gerontological Counseling(M): 54 Class hours; 100 Practicum hours; 100 Internship hours;
                      Portfolio.
                    • Pastoral Counseling(M): 60 Class hours; 100 Practicum hours; 100 Internship hours;
                      Portfolio.

   Postgraduation activity: Advanced education and employment setting percentages.
                    • Community Counseling(M): 80 Agency practice.
                    • School Counseling(M): 100 Agency practice; 20 Elementary school; 20 Middle school; 60
                      Secondary school.
                    • Gerontological Counseling(M): NP.
                    • Pastoral Counseling(M): NP.

Planned Program Modifications
   Courses   Drop   Add
                    • NP.   • Addictions
                                                 • Forensic Counseling
                                                 • Supervision.

   Other   Decrease   Increase
                    • NP.   • Admission Requirements
                                                 • Diversity Recruiting of Faculty
                                                 • National Accreditation
                                                 • Number of Degree Majors.

Related Programs Arts Therapists
                     Other

Faculty

nbcc ✹   Percent of faculty reported with NCC certification: 60%.   ncc ✹

Percent in professional counseling practice: 40%.

Research interests Gerontology research. Second-chance programs for high school dropouts.

Diversity   • African-American; Caucasian.

Name, Degree, Rank, State/National Credentials, % time devoted to program, email
• Cotten, Paul D; PhD; Full Prof.; Licensed Psychologist; 41-60%;
• Burkett, Olivia; PhD; Lecturer; >81%;
• King, Tommy; EdD; Full Prof.; LPC, NCC; >81%;
• Madonna, Steven; PhD; Lecturer; LPC, NCC; 61-80%;
• Crowson, William D; EdD; Lecturer; LPC, NCC; 61-80%;

MT: Montana Sate University - Northern

PO Box 7751
Havre, MT 59501
USA
Dean   Darlene Sellers Ph.D.
Administrator   John Foley, Ph.D., Program Coordinator
                    Department   College of Education and Graduate Programs
                    (406) 265-3738, fax (406) 265-3721, sellersd@msun.edu, www.msun

Key   See key for Data on Each Department (this section) on page 79.

Program
Accreditation   Regional Accreditation

Uniqueness   Faculty hold a variety of counseling specialities and backgrounds with a shared expertise in preparing graduates to work in isolated, rural communities that serve economically disadvantaged populations.

Degrees   • Community Counseling: M.
           • School Counseling: M.

Contact   • Community Counseling: M = John Foley.
           • School Counseling: M = John Foley.

Admission and Graduation Data
Admission
Requirements   • Community Counseling(M): GPA 3.00; GRE 900; GRE V 400; GRE Q 400; GRE A 400; MAT 29; 2 Years work experience.
                • School Counseling(M): GPA 3.00; GRE 900; GRE V 400; GRE Q 400; GRE A 400; MAT 29; 3 Years work experience.

Enrollment   • Community Counseling(M): 5 Admitted yearly; 5 Graduated yearly.
              • School Counseling(M): 15 Admitted yearly; 15 Graduated yearly; 20 Female; 10 Male.

Diversity   • African-American; Caucasian; Hispanic; Multiracial.

Graduation
Requirements   • Community Counseling(M): 60 Class hours; 100 Practicum hours; 600 Internship hours; Comprehensive exam; Oral exam.
                • School Counseling(M): 50 Class hours; 100 Practicum hours; 600 Internship hours; Portfolio.

Postgraduation activity: Advanced education and employment setting percentages.
              • Community Counseling(M): NP.
              • School Counseling(M): NP.

Planned Program Modifications
Courses   Drop   Add
                • NP.   • Grief Counseling
                                         • Play Therapy.

Other   Decrease   Increase
                • NP.   • NP.

Related Programs

Faculty

nbcc ❧   Percent of faculty reported with NCC certification: **100**%.   ncc ❧

Percent in professional counseling practice: 70%.

Research interests Crisis counseling; school counseling; curriculum development

Diversity   • Caucasian; Native American; Multiracial.

Name, Degree, Rank, State/National Credentials, % time devoted to program, email
• Sellers, Darlene; PhD; Assoc.; NCC; 22-40%; *sellersd@msun.edu*
• Foley, John; PhD; Assist.; LPC, NCC; >81%;
• Taylor, William; PhD; Lecturer; NCC, Lic. Psyc.; 41-60%;
• Cecil, Kendrick; PhD; Assist.; LPC, NCC; 41-60%;

MT: Montana State University - Billings

1500 University Drive
Billings, MT 59101
USA

Dean
Administrator George White, Dean
Department College of Education and Human Services
(406) 657-2285, gwhite@msubillings.edu

Key See key for Data on Each Department (this section) on page 79.

Program
Accreditation Regional Accreditation, **CORE:** Rehabilitation Counseling

Uniqueness Only site for the REHAB Counseling degree in MT.

Degrees • School Counseling: M.
• Rehabilitation Counseling: M.

Contact • School Counseling: M = James Nowlin.
• Rehabilitation Counseling: M = Alan Davis.

Admission and Graduation Data
Admission
Requirements • School Counseling(M): GPA 3.00; GRE 1350; GRE V 400; GRE Q 400; GRE A 400.
• Rehabilitation Counseling(M): GPA 3.00; GRE 1371; GRE V 400; GRE Q 400; GRE A 400; Interview.

Enrollment • School Counseling(M): 15-25 Admitted yearly; 10-20 Graduated yearly; 75% Female; 25% Male.
• Rehabilitation Counseling(M): NP.

Diversity • Caucasian; Hispanic; Native American; Multiracial.

Graduation
Requirements • School Counseling(M): 40-60 Class hours; 100 Practicum hours; 600 Internship hours; Portfolio.
• Rehabilitation Counseling(M): 60 Class hours; 600 Internship hours; Comprehensive exam.

Postgraduation activity: Advanced education and employment setting percentages.
• School Counseling(M): 5 Advanced education; 15% Private practice; 26 Elementary school; 26 Middle school; 26 Secondary school; 2 Other.
• Rehabilitation Counseling(M): 5 Advanced education; 5 Private practice; 90 Agency practice.

Planned Program Modifications
Courses
	Drop		Add
•	NP.	•	Addictions.

Other
	Decrease		Increase
•	NP.	•	NP.

Related Programs Psychology

Faculty

 Percent of faculty reported with NCC certification: 0%.

Percent in professional counseling practice: 0%.

Research interests NP.

Diversity • Caucasian.

Name, Degree, Rank, State/National Credentials, % time devoted to program, email
• Davis, Alan H; PhD; LPC, CRC; >81%; *adavis@msubillings.edu*
• Nowlin, James E; PhD; >81%; *jnowlin@msubillings.edu*
• Colling, Kyle K; PhD; >81%; *kcolling@msubillings.edu*
• Yazak, Daniel L; EdD; Assoc.; CRC; 41-60%; *dyazak@msubillings.edu*

Has CHI SIGMA IOTA (International Counseling Society) chapter.

MT: Montana State University - Bozeman

218 Herrick Hall
Bozeman, MT 59717
USA

Dean   Greg Weisenstein
Administrator   Ellen Kreighbaum, Department Head
                Department   Health and Human Development
                              (406) 994-3241, fax (406) 994-2013

Key   See key for Data on Each Department (this section) on page 79.

Program

Accreditation   Regional Accreditation, **CACREP:** Marriage and Family Counseling, **CACREP:** Mental Health Counseling, **CACREP:** School Counseling

Uniqueness   The counseling program offers specialties in marriage and family, mental health, and school counseling. We are located in a diverse department that includes a wide range of faculty.

Degrees
- Mental Health Counseling: M.
- School Counseling: M.
- Marriage and Family Counseling: M.

Contact
- Mental Health Counseling: M = Patrick (Rick) Johnson.
- School Counseling: M = Mark Nelson.
- Marriage and Family Counseling: M = Jill Thorngren.

Admission and Graduation Data

Admission

Requirements
- Mental Health Counseling(M): GPA 3.00; GRE 900; GRE V 450; GRE Q 450; 1 Year work experience; Interview.
- School Counseling(M): GPA 3.00; GRE 900; GRE V 450; GRE Q 450; 1 Year work experience; Interview.
- Marriage and Family Counseling(M): GPA 3.00; GRE 900; GRE V 450; GRE Q 450; 1 Year work experience; Interview.

Enrollment
- Mental Health Counseling(M): 8-9 Admitted yearly; 6-8 Graduated yearly; 6 Female; 2 Male.
- School Counseling(M): 8-9 Admitted yearly; 6-8 Graduated yearly; 6 Female; 2 Male.
- Marriage and Family Counseling(M): 8-96 Admitted yearly; 6-8 Graduated yearly; 6 Female; 2 Male.

Diversity
- Caucasian; Native American.

Graduation

Requirements
- Mental Health Counseling(M): 60 Class hours; 400 Practicum hours; 400 Internship hours; Comprehensive exam.
- School Counseling(M): 48 Class hours; 200 Practicum hours; 600 Internship hours; Comprehensive exam.
- Marriage and Family Counseling(M): 60 Class hours; 400 Practicum hours; 400 Internship hours; Comprehensive exam.

Postgraduation activity: Advanced education and employment setting percentages.
- Mental Health Counseling(M): 10 Advanced education; 20 Managed care; 20 Private practice; 50 Agency practice.
- School Counseling(M): 10 Advanced education; 10 Elementary school; 40 Middle school; 40 Secondary school.
- Marriage and Family Counseling(M): 10 Advanced education; 10 Managed care; 30 Private practice; 50 Agency practice.

Planned Program Modifications

Courses   <u>Drop</u>   <u>Add</u>
- NP.   • Adventure Counseling.

Other   <u>Decrease</u>   <u>Increase</u>
- NP.   • Diversity Recruiting of Students
                                       • Number of Distance Education Courses.

Related Programs Psychology

Faculty

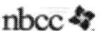 Percent of faculty reported with NCC certification: 38%.

Percent in professional counseling practice: 80%.

Research interests Research interests of faculty members include adventure based counseling, promotion of healthy couple and family relationships, social interest, differentiation among and between different populations, connections between mind/body wellness, and effects of divorce.

Diversity   • Caucasian.

Name, Degree, Rank, State/National Credentials, % time devoted to program, email
- Nelson, Mark D; EdD; Assoc.; LPC; >81%; *markn@montana.edu*
- Johnson, Patrick; PhD; Assoc.; LPC, NCC; >81%; *rjohnson@montana.edu*
- Thorngren, Jill M; PhD; Assist.; LPC, NCC; >81%; *jillt@montana.edu*
- Christopher, John C; PhD; Assoc.; LPC, NCC, Licensed Psychologist; >81%; *jcc@montana.edu*
- Smith, Adina J; PhD; Assist.; licensed psychologist; 41-60%; *adinas@montana.edu*
- Donahoe, Patrick; PhD; Instructor; LPC, licensed psychologist; <21%; *uccpd@montana.edu*
- Blank, Cheryl; PhD; Instructor; LPC, licensed psychologist; <21%; *cblank@montana.edu*
- Lande, Gary; MD; Instructor; LPC; <21%; *glande@montana.edu*

NC: Appalachian State University

Boone, NC 28608
USA

Dean
Administrator   Lee Baruth, Chair
Department   Dept of Counseling & Human Development
(828) 262-2055, fax (828) 262-2128, BaruthLG@appstate.edu

Key   See key for Data on Each Department (this section) on page 79.

Program
  Accreditation   Regional Accreditation, **CACREP:** Community Counseling, **CACREP:** School Counseling,
CACREP: Student Affairs - Counseling

  Uniqueness   High percentage of full-time students. Very student oriented, student/practitioner focus with
emphasis on faculty as professional mentors.

  Degrees   • Community Counseling: M.
• School Counseling: M.
• Marriage and Family Counseling: M.
• Student Affairs: M.

  Contact   • Community Counseling: M = Diana Quealy-Berge.
• School Counseling: M = Laurie Williamson.
• Marriage and Family Counseling: M = Jon Winek.
• Student Affairs: M = Cathy Clark.

Admission and Graduation Data
Admission
  Requirements   • Community Counseling(M): GPA R; GRE R.
• School Counseling(M): GPA R; GRE R; Interview.
• Marriage and Family Counseling(M): GPA R; GRE R; Interview.
• Student Affairs(M): GPA R; GRE R.

  Enrollment   • Community Counseling(M): 25 Admitted yearly; 20 Graduated yearly.
• School Counseling(M): 20 Admitted yearly; 17 Graduated yearly.
• Marriage and Family Counseling(M): 12 Admitted yearly; 11 Graduated yearly.
• Student Affairs(M): 15 Admitted yearly; 13 Graduated yearly.

  Diversity   • African-American; Asian-American; Caucasian; Hispanic; Native American.

Graduation
  Requirements   • Community Counseling(M): 60 Class hours; 100 Practicum hours; 600 Internship hours;
Comprehensive exam; CPCE.
• School Counseling(M): 48 Class hours; 100 Practicum hours; 600 Internship hours;
Comprehensive exam; CPCE.
• Marriage and Family Counseling(M): 48 Class hours; 500 Internship hours.
• Student Affairs(M): 48 Class hours; 100 Practicum hours; 600 Internship hours.

Postgraduation activity: Advanced education and employment setting percentages.
• Community Counseling(M): 5 Advanced education; 5 Private practice; 80 Agency practice;
10 Other.
• School Counseling(M): 5 Advanced education; 55 Elementary school; 20 Middle school; 20
Secondary school.
• Marriage and Family Counseling(M): 3 Advanced education; 25 Managed care; 25 Private
practice; 25 Agency practice; 22 Other.
• Student Affairs(M): 4 Advanced education; 75 Student affairs; 21 Other.

Planned Program Modifications
  Courses   Drop   Add
• NP.   • NP.

  Other   Decrease   Increase
• NP.   • NP.

Related Programs Psychology

Faculty

nbcc ❧   Percent of faculty reported with NCC certification: 16%.   ncc ❧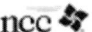

Percent in professional counseling practice: NP.

Research interests

Diversity   •   African-American; Caucasian; Native American.

Name, Degree, Rank, State/National Credentials, % time devoted to program, email
- Alschuler, Al; PhD; Full Prof.; NCC; >81%;
- Atkins, Sally; EdD; Full Prof.; >81%;
- Badders, Fred; PhD; Full Prof.; NCC; >81%;
- Baruth, Lee; EdD; Full Prof.; >81%;
- Blimling, Greg; PhD; Full Prof.; <21%;
- Clark, Cathy; PhD; Assist.; >81%;
- Fleming, Willie; PhD; Assist.; >81%;
- Greene, Al; MSW; Full Prof.; >81%;
- Hubbard, Glenda; PhD; Full Prof.; NCC; <21%;
- Miller, Geri; PhD; Full Prof.; >81%;
- Mulgrew, Jack; PhD; Full Prof.; >81%;
- Sack, Terry; PhD; Full Prof.; >81%;
- Spann, Bunk; PhD; Full Prof.; >81%;
- Williamson, Laurie; PhD; Assist.; >81%;
- Winek, Jon; PhD; Assist.; >81%;
- Davis, Keith; PhD; Assist.; >81%;
- Quealy-Berge, Diana; PhD; Assist.; >81%;
- Lancaster, James; PhD; Assist.; >81%;
- Lambie, Glenn; PhD; Assist.; >81%;

Has CHI SIGMA IOTA (International Counseling Society) chapter.

NC: Campbell University

P.O. Box 369
Buies Creek, NC 27506
United States
Dean   Dean Karen Nery/ School of Education/ Taylor Hall
Administrator   Harriett Enzor, Coordinator/Counselor Education Program
                    Department   School of Education
                                    (910) 893-1630, fax (910) 893-1999,
                                    www.auburn.edu/academic/education/ccp

Key   See key for Data on Each Department (this section) on page 79.

Program
  Accreditation

  Uniqueness   Nontraditional graduate student population with emphasis on preparing students for entry
                   level counseling employment.

  Degrees   • Community Counseling: M.
                   • School Counseling: M.

  Contact   • Community Counseling: M = Wayne Hatcher.
                   • School Counseling: M = Harriet Enzor.

Admission and Graduation Data
Admission
  Requirements   • Community Counseling(M): GPA 3.00; GRE 850; GRE V 425; GRE Q 425; Interview.
                   • School Counseling(M): GPA 3.00; GRE 850; GRE V 425; GRE Q 425; Interview.

  Enrollment   • Community Counseling(M): 10 Admitted yearly; 8-10 Graduated yearly; 20 Female; 10
                     Male.
                   • School Counseling(M): 15 Admitted yearly; 13-15 Graduated yearly; 60 Female; 10 Male.

  Diversity   • African-American; Caucasian; Native American.

Graduation
  Requirements   • Community Counseling(M): 48 Class hours; 100 Practicum hours; 600 Internship hours;
                     Comprehensive exam.
                   • School Counseling(M): 48 Class hours; 100 Practicum hours; 600 Internship hours;
                     Comprehensive exam.

  Postgraduation activity: Advanced education and employment setting percentages.
                   • Community Counseling(M): 5 Advanced education; 5 Private practice; 85 Agency practice;
                     5 Other.
                   • School Counseling(M): 40 Elementary school; 40 Middle school; 20 Secondary school.

Planned Program Modifications
  Courses   Drop   Add
                   • NP.   • Diversity.

  Other   Decrease   Increase
                   • NP.   • Diversity Recruiting of Faculty
                                                    • National Accreditation.

Related Programs Other

Faculty

  nbcc ❧   Percent of faculty reported with NCC certification: **100**%.   ncc ❧

  Percent in professional counseling practice: 100%.

  Research interests

  Diversity   • Caucasian.

  Name, Degree, Rank, State/National Credentials, % time devoted to program, email
  • Enzor, Harriett; EdD; Assoc.; LPC, NCC; >81%; *enzor@mailcenter.campbell.edu*
  • Hatcher, Wayne; EdD; Assoc.; NCC; >81%; *hatcher@mailcenter.cambell.edu*
  • Kendrick, Ron; EdD; Assoc.; LPC, NCC; >81%; *kendrick@mailcenter.campbell.edu*

NC: East Carolina University

School of Allied Health Sciences-Rehab Dept.
Greenville, NC 27858-4353
USA
Dean Stephen Thomas, Ed.D.
Administrator Lloyd Goodwin, Ph.D., LPC, CRC-MAC, Interim Chair
Department   Rehabilitation Studies
(252) 328-4455, fax (252) 328-0725, GoodwinL@mail.ecu.edu,
www.ecu.edu/rehb

Key   See key for Data on Each Department (this section) on page 79.

Program
Accreditation   Regional Accreditation, CORE: Rehabilitation Counseling

Uniqueness   Offers an M.S. degree in Substance Abuse & Clinical Counseling, Vocational Evaluation, and Rehabilitation Counseling. Students usually combine Rehabilitation Counseling with one of the other two programs for a dual-program M.S. degree. Dept. also offers an undergraduate major in Rehabilitation Services and a minor in Alcohol & Drug Studies. Graduates from this major or minor can eliminate one semester from the master's program. ~1/3 of graduate students are older (i.e. 30-50 years old—with oldest being 72 years old) and come from a variety of paraprofessional and professional backgrounds (e.g. education, health care, business) and 2/3 are younger students usually right out of bachelor degree programs with majors in psychology and rehabilitation services. Most graduate courses are offered at night or in a 2-5 pm block once a week for part-time students who work full-time.

Degrees   • Mental Health Counseling: M.
                 • Addictions Counseling: M.
                 • Other: M.
                 • Rehabilitation Counseling: M.

Contact   • Mental Health Counseling: M = Lloyd Goodwin.
                 • Addictions Counseling: M = Lloyd Goodwin.
                 • Other: M = Steve Thomas.
                 • Rehabilitation Counseling: M = Mark Stebnicki.

Admission and Graduation Data
Admission
Requirements   • Mental Health Counseling(M): GPA ~3.00; MAT ~35; Interview.
                 • Addictions Counseling(M): GPA ~3.00; MAT ~35; Interview.
                 • Other(M): GPA ~3.00; MAT ~30; Interview.
                 • Rehabilitation Counseling(M): GPA ~3.00; MAT ~35; Interview.

Enrollment   • Mental Health Counseling(M): 15 Admitted yearly; 15 Graduated yearly; 10 Female; 5 Male.
                 • Addictions Counseling(M): 15 Admitted yearly; 15 Graduated yearly; 10 Female; 5 Male.
                 • Other(M): 10 Admitted yearly; 10 Graduated yearly; 7 Female; 3 Male.
                 • Rehabilitation Counseling(M): 25 Admitted yearly; 25 Graduated yearly; 17 Female; 8 Male.

Diversity   • African-American; Asian-American; Caucasian; Hispanic; Native American; Multiracial.

Graduation
Requirements   • Mental Health Counseling(M): 48 Class hours; 100 Practicum hours; 600 Internship hours; Oral exam; Thesis.
                 • Addictions Counseling(M): 48 Class hours; 100 Practicum hours; 600 Internship hours; Oral exam; Thesis.
                 • Other(M): 45 Class hours; 100 Practicum hours; 600 Internship hours; Oral exam; Thesis.
                 • Rehabilitation Counseling(M): 48 Class hours; 100 Practicum hours; 600 Internship hours; Oral exam; Thesis.

Postgraduation activity: Advanced education and employment setting percentages.
                 • Mental Health Counseling(M): 95 Agency practice; 5 Other.
                 • Addictions Counseling(M): 95 Agency practice; 5 Other.
                 • Other(M): 95 Agency practice; 5 Other.
                 • Rehabilitation Counseling(M): 95 Agency practice; 5 Other.

Planned Program Modifications
Courses   Drop   Add
                 • NP.   • NP.

Other   Decrease   Increase
                 • NP.   • Faculty FTE
                                                • Number of Distance Education Courses
                                                • Number of On-Line Courses.

Related Programs Clinical Social Workers
Marriage and Family Therapists
Psychology
Psychiatric Nurses
Psychiatrists
Communications
International Studies

Faculty

 Percent of faculty reported with NCC certification: 0%.

Percent in professional counseling practice: NP.

Research interests Substance abuse, school violence, cognitive-behavioral therapy (i.e. Button Therapy), counselor education applicant screening, and rehabilitation services education.

Diversity • Caucasian.

Name, Degree, Rank, State/National Credentials, % time devoted to program, email
- Goodwin, Jr., Lloyd R; PhD; Full Prof.; LPC, CRC-MAC; >81%; *goodwinL@mail.ecu.edu*
- Paul, Alston; PhD; Full Prof.; L.HSP-Psy.,CRC; >81%; *alstonp@mail.ecu.edu*
- Stebnicki, Mark; RhD; Assoc.; LPC, CRC, CCM; >81%; *stebnickim@mail.ecu.edu*
- Chapin, Martha H; PhD; Assist.; LPC, CRC, CDMS, NCC; >81%; *chapinm@mail.ecu.edu*
- Thomas, Stephen W; EdD; Full Prof.; CRC, CVE; >81%; *thomass@mail.ecu.edu*
- Shallow, Sharon; MEd; Instructor; LPC, CRC-MAC, LMFT, CTA; 41-60%; *sshallow2001@yahoo.com*
- Lotterhos, Jerry F; MSW; Adjunct; LPC, CRC-MAC; <21%; *lotterhosj@mail.ecu.edu*
- Gentile, Cheryl; MS; Adjunct; LPC, CRC-MAC, CCAS; <21%; *cgentile@pcmh.com*
- Young, Glyn; PhD; Adjunct; <21%; *gyoung@pcmh.com*
- Wong, Henry; RhD; Adjunct; CRC; <21%; *wongh@nccat.org*
- Anema, John; MEd; Adjunct; LPC, CRC; <21%; *skeezik@greenvillenc.com*
- Badger, Nancy; PhD; Adjunct; L.Psy., CRC; <21%; *badgern@mail.ecu.edu*
- Ward-Ross, Lisa; MS; Adjunct; CRC, CVE; <21%; *Lwardross@ecvcinc.com*

NC: East Carolina University

	Speight Building 136
	Greenville, NC 27858
	USA
Dean	Dr. Marilyn Sheerer, School of Education
Administrator	VACANT, Department Chair
	Department Counselor and Adult Education
	(252) 328-6856, fax (252) 328-5114, warrenl@mail.ecu.edu,
	http://www.soe.ecu.edu/coad/

Key   See key for Data on Each Department (this section) on page 79.

Program

Accreditation   Regional Accreditation

Uniqueness   The counselor education program provides a student-friendly curriculum with flexible elective study. Career options include school, agency, and higher education.

Degrees   •   Other: M, S.

Contact   •   Other: M, S = NP.

Admission and Graduation Data

Admission

Requirements
- Other(M): GPA 2.50; GRE 1350; GRE V 450; GRE Q 450; GRE A 450; MAT 40; Interview.
- Other(S): GPA 2.50; GRE 1350; GRE V 450; GRE Q 450; GRE A 450; MAT 40; Interview.

Enrollment
- Other(M & S): 40 Admitted yearly; 28 Graduated yearly; 80% Female; 20% Male.

Diversity
- African-American; Caucasian; Hispanic; Native American.

Graduation

Requirements
- Other(M): 48 Class hours; 90 Practicum hours; 225 minimum Internship hours.
- Other(S): 30 Class hours; Comprehensive exam.

Postgraduation activity: Advanced education and employment setting percentages.
- Other(M & S): 5 Advanced education; 5 Agency practice; 40 Middle school; 20 Secondary school; 15 Student affairs; 15 Other.

Planned Program Modifications

Courses	Drop	Add
	• NP.	• NP.

Other	Decrease	Increase
	• NP.	• NP.

Related Programs Clinical Social Workers
Marriage and Family Therapists
Psychology
Psychiatric Nurses
Psychiatrists
Communications
Other

Faculty

nbcc ❖   Percent of faculty reported with NCC certification: 75%.   ncc ❖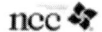

Percent in professional counseling practice: 0%.

Research interests School counseling program evaluation, assessment in counseling.

Diversity   •   Caucasian.

Name, Degree, Rank, State/National Credentials, % time devoted to program, email
- Ciechalski, Joseph C; EdD; Full Prof.; LPC, NCC; >81%; *ciechalskij@mail.ecu.edu*
- Pinkney, James; PhD; Full Prof.; >81%; *pinkneyj@mail.ecu.edu*
- Schmidt, John J; EdD; Full Prof.; LPC, NCC; >81%; *schmidtj@mail.ecu.edu*
- Weaver, Florence S; PhD; Full Prof.; LPC, NCC; >81%; *weaverf@mail.ecu.edu*

Has CHI SIGMA IOTA (International Counseling Society) chapter.

NC: North Carolina A&T State University

212 Hodgin Hall
Greensboro, NC 27411-1066
United States

Dean   Dr. Lelia Vickers, Hodgin Hall, NC A&T State University
Administrator Dr. Wyatt D. Kirk, Chairperson
                   Department   Human Development & Services
                                 (336) 334-7916, fax (336) 334-7280, kirkw@ncat.edu, www.ncat.edu

Key   See key for Data on Each Department (this section) on page 79.

Program
Accreditation   Regional Accreditation, **CACREP:** Community Counseling, **CACREP:** School Counseling

Uniqueness   Counseling Programs accredited by Council for Accreditation of Counseling and Related
                 Programs (CACREP)

Degrees   • Community Counseling: M.
                 • School Counseling: M.

Contact   • Community Counseling: M = Dr. Wyatt D. Kirk.
                 • School Counseling: M = Dr. Wyatt D. Kirk.

Admission and Graduation Data
Admission
Requirements   • Community Counseling(M): GPA R.
                 • School Counseling(M): GPA R.

Enrollment   • Community Counseling(M): NP.
                 • School Counseling(M): NP.

Diversity   • African-American; Caucasian.

Graduation
Requirements   • Community Counseling(M): 48 Class hours; Comprehensive exam; CPCE.
                 • School Counseling(M): 60 Class hours; Comprehensive exam; CPCE.

Postgraduation activity: Advanced education and employment setting percentages.
                 • Community Counseling(M): NP.
                 • School Counseling(M): NP.

Planned Program Modifications
Courses   Drop   Add
                 • NP.   • Addictions
                                                 • Rehabilitation.

Other   Decrease   Increase
                 • NP.   • Course Offerings.

Related Programs Clinical Social Workers
                 Marriage and Family Therapists
                 Psychology
                 Communications
                 International Studies

Faculty

nbcc 🔆   Percent of faculty reported with NCC certification: 80%.   ncc 🔆

Percent in professional counseling practice: NP.

Research interests Grief and loss; divorce; assessment; personality disorders; professional standards and
                 practice in the schools; DSM-IV-TR criteria; Spirituality; School Safety

Diversity   • African-American; Caucasian.

Name, Degree, Rank, State/National Credentials, % time devoted to program, email
• Kirk, Wyatt D; EdD; Full Prof.; NCC; >81%; *kirkw@ncat.edu*
• Bethea-Whitfield, Patricia D; EdD; Assoc.; NCC; >81%; *betheap@ncat.edu*
• Hall, Brenda; EdD; Assist.; NCC; >81%; *hallb@ncat.edu*
• Lundberg, David; PhD; Assist.; NCC; >81%; *lundberg@ncat.edu*
• Wagner, Miriam L; EdD; Assist.; 61-80%; *wagnerm@ncat.edu*

Has CHI SIGMA IOTA (International Counseling Society) chapter.

NC: The University of North Carolina at Chapel Hill

CB# 3500
Chapel Hill, NC 27599-3500
USA

Dean   Madeleine Grumet, Peabody Hall
Administrator   Bob Barrett, Professor and School Program Coordinator
                    Department   Education
                                  (919) 966-1354, fax (919) 962-1533, jgalassi@email.unc.edu, http://
                                  www.unc.edu/depts/ed/counseling/

Key   See key for Data on Each Department (this section) on page 79.

Program
Accreditation   **CACREP:** School Counseling

CACREP

Uniqueness   The Masters Program in School Counseling at the University of North Carolina is predicated
              on a Developmental Advocacy model that asserts that the counselor's primary mission is to
              promote the optimal development of all students. The counselor is a school leader who works
              with students, teachers, administrators, parents, and other members of the community to build
              a supportive learning environment which nurtures the development of academic, career, and
              personal/social competence among students as well as fosters an appreciation of diversity
              and a commitment to social justice. While remediation of deficits and the removal of barriers
              play a role in the model, developmental advocates focus on proactive and preventive
              approaches to help students build skills and to enhance the asset-building capacity of the
              school environment.

Degrees   • School Counseling: M.

Contact   • School Counseling: M = John P. Galassi.

Admission and Graduation Data
Admission
Requirements • School Counseling(M): GPA 3.00; GRE V 50%ile; GRE Q 50%ile; Interview.

Enrollment   • School Counseling(M): 15-20 Admitted yearly; 15-20 Graduated yearly.

Diversity   • African-American; Asian-American; Caucasian; Native American; Multiracial.

Graduation
Requirements • School Counseling(M): 60 Class hours; 100 Practicum hours; 600 min. Internship hours;
              Comprehensive exam.

Postgraduation activity: Advanced education and employment setting percentages.
              • School Counseling(M): 40 Elementary school; 20 Middle school; 40 Secondary school.

Planned Program Modifications
Courses   Drop   Add
                     • NP.   • NP.

Other   Decrease   Increase
                     • NP.   • Clinical Supervision
                                             • Diversity Recruiting of Faculty
                                             • Number of Distance Education Courses
                                             • Number of On-Line Courses.

Related Programs Clinical Social Workers
                     Psychology
                     Other

Faculty
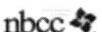   Percent of faculty reported with NCC certification: 20%.   ncc

Percent in professional counseling practice: 20%.

Research interests School transitions, career development, resiliency, positive psychology, and strength-
                   based approaches to counseling

Diversity   • Caucasian.

Name, Degree, Rank, State/National Credentials, % time devoted to program, email
- Galassi, John P; PhD; Full Prof.; >81%; *jgalassi@email.unc.edu*
- Brown, Duane; PhD; Full Prof.; LPC; >81%; *pinnowedna@charter.net*
- Akos, Patrick; PhD; Assist.; NCC; >81%; *pakos@email.unc.edu*
- Perot, Annette; PhD; Assist.; Practicing Psychologist; <21%;
- Petrusa, Jodi; MS; Instructor; Nationally Certified School Psychologist; <21%;

Has CHI SIGMA IOTA (International Counseling Society) chapter.

NC: The University of North Carolina at Greensboro

PO Box 26170
Greensboro, NC 27402-6170
USA
Dean Dean Dale Schunk, School of Education
Administrator L. DiAnne Borders, Professor and Chair
Department   Department of Counseling and Educational Development
(336) 334-3423, fax (336) 334-3433, ced@uncg.edu, www.uncg.edu/ced

Key   See key for Data on Each Department (this section) on page 79.

Program
Accreditation   Regional Accreditation, **CACREP:** Community Counseling, **CACREP:** Gerontological
Counseling, **CACREP:** Counselor Education and Supervision, **CACREP:** Marriage and Family
Counseling, **CACREP:** School Counseling, **CACREP:** Student Affairs - Counseling

Uniqueness   Fulltime cohorts contribute to strong sense of community and shared learning. Supervised
experience with clients throughout the program in state-of-the-art in-house clinic as well as
field-based experiences. Five CACREP-accredited tracks at the master's level with options for
EdS also. CACREP-accredited doctoral program emphasizes advanced clinical skills,
supervised teaching and supervision experiences, as well as strong research training. Faculty
are active researchers, quite involved in professional leadership, and provide active and
deliverate mentoring of leadership skills for students. Program affiliates include NBCC, ERIC/
CASS, and Chi Sigma Iota, and new Pathways Career Resource Center (state-wide, online)
for high school students. Graduate assistantships and waivers are available.

Degrees   • Community Counseling: M, S.
    • School Counseling: M, S.
    • Gerontological Counseling: M, S.
    • Marriage and Family Counseling: S.
    • Student Affairs: M, S.
    • Counselor Education: PhD.

Contact   • Community Counseling: M, S = For all programs in all tracks contact the Departmental
admissions office at ced@uncg.edu or (336) 334-3434.
    • School Counseling: M, S = NP.
    • Gerontological Counseling: M, S = NP.
    • Marriage and Family Counseling: S = NP.
    • Student Affairs: M, S = NP.
    • Counselor Education: D = NP.

Admission and Graduation Data
Admission
Requirements   • Community Counseling(M): GPA 3.00; GRE R.
    • Community Counseling(S): GPA 3.00; GRE R.
    • School Counseling(M): GPA 3.00; GRE R.
    • School Counseling(S): GPA 3.00; GRE R.
    • Gerontological Counseling(M): GPA 3.00; GRE R.
    • Gerontological Counseling(S): GPA 3.00; GRE R.
    • Marriage and Family Counseling(S): GPA 3.00; GRE R.
    • Student Affairs(M): GPA 3.00; GRE R.
    • Student Affairs(S): GPA 3.00; GRE R.
    • Counselor Education(D): Masters and GPA 3.00; GRE R.

Enrollment   • Community Counseling(M & S): 12 Admitted yearly; 12 Graduated yearly; 18 Female;
6 Male.
    • School Counseling(M & S): 12 Admitted yearly; 12 Graduated yearly; 21 Female; 3 Male.
    • Gerontological Counseling(M & S): 2 Admitted yearly; 2 Graduated yearly; 2 Female.
    • Marriage and Family Counseling(S): 8 Admitted yearly; 8 Graduated yearly; 4 Female;
4 Male.
    • Student Affairs(M & S): 5 Admitted yearly; 5 Graduated yearly; 7 Female; 3 Male.
    • Counselor Education(D): 8 Admitted yearly; 8 Graduated yearly; 15 Female; 15 Male.

Diversity   • African-American; Asian-American; Caucasian; Hispanic; Native American; Pacific
Islander; Multiracial.

Graduation
Requirements   • Community Counseling(M): 48 Class hours; 120+ Practicum hours; 600 Internship hours;
Comprehensive exam.
    • Community Counseling(S): 66 Class hours; 120+ Practicum hours; 600 Internship hours;
Comprehensive exam.

- School Counseling(M): 48 Class hours; 120+ Practicum hours; 600 Internship hours; Comprehensive exam.
- School Counseling(S): 66 Class hours; 120+ Practicum hours; 600 Internship hours; Comprehensive exam.
- Gerontological Counseling(M): 48 Class hours; 600 Internship hours.
- Gerontological Counseling(S): 66 Class hours; 120+ Practicum hours; 600 Internship hours; Comprehensive exam.
- Marriage and Family Counseling(S): 66 Class hours; 120+ Practicum hours; 600 Internship hours; Comprehensive exam.
- Student Affairs(M): 48 Class hours; 120+ Practicum hours; 600 Internship hours; Comprehensive exam.
- Student Affairs(S): 66 Class hours; 120+ Practicum hours; 600 Internship hours; Comprehensive exam.
- Counselor Education(D): 60 min Class hours; 100 Practicum hours; 600 Internship hours; Comprehensive exam; Oral exam; Dissertation.

Postgraduation activity: Advanced education and employment setting percentages.
- Community Counseling(M & S): 10 Advanced education; 5 Managed care; 30 Private practice; 45 Agency practice; 10 Other.
- School Counseling(M & S): 10 Advanced education; 30 Elementary school; 30 Middle school; 25 Secondary school; 5 Other.
- Gerontological Counseling(M & S): 30 Agency practice; 70 Other.
- Marriage and Family Counseling(S): 10 Advanced education; 5 Managed care; 35 Private practice; 50 Agency practice.
- Student Affairs(M & S): 100 Other.
- Counselor Education(D):

Planned Program Modifications

Courses	Drop		Add
	• NP.		• NP.

Other	Decrease		Increase
	• NP.		• Diversity Recruiting of Faculty
			• Diversity Recruiting of Students
			• Financial Aid
			• National Accreditation.

Related Programs Psychology
Psychiatric Nurses
Other

Faculty

 Percent of faculty reported with NCC certification: 70%.

Percent in professional counseling practice: 50%.

Research interests Career development/choice of adolescent females, particularly in math, science, and engineering; peer supervision and consultation, clinical supervision process, supervisor training; adopted children and their families, violence prevention in the schools, substance abuse counseling, college student drinking behaviors and effective counseling inverventions, play therapy, spritual development, wellness and assessment of wellness, crisis intervention, cultural influences in academic achievement, professional issues (e.g., counselor credentialing, advocacy, ethics, women in nontraditional careers, gender role conflict, adolescent sex offenders, school counseling.

Diversity   • Caucasian; Hispanic.

Name, Degree, Rank, State/National Credentials, % time devoted to program, email
- Benshoff, James M; PhD; Assoc.; LPC, NCC, NCGS, ACS; >81%; *benshoff@uncg.edeu*
- Borders, L. DiAnne; PhD; Full Prof.; LPC, NCC, ACS; >81%; *borders@uncg.edu*
- Cashwell, Craig S; PhD; Assoc.; LPC, NCC, ACS; >81%; *cscashwell@uncg.edu*
- Juhnke, Gerald A; EdD; Assoc.; LPC, NCC, ACS, MAC, CCAS; >81%; *gajuhnke@uncg.edu*
- Myers, Jane E; PhD; Full Prof.; LPC, NCC, NCGC; >81%; *jemyers@uncg.edu*
- Purkey, William W; EdD; Full Prof.; LPC, NCC; 41-60%; *wwpurkey@uncg.edu*
- Shoffner, Marie F; PhD; Assoc.; NCC, NCC; >81%; *mfshoffn@uncg.edu*
- Lewis, Todd; PhD; Assist.; LPC; >81%; *tflewis@uncg.edu*
- Villalba, Jose A; PhD; Assist.; NCC; >81%; *javilla@uncg.edu*
- Wester, Kelly L; PhD; Assist.; >81%; *klwester@uncg.edu*

Has CHI SIGMA IOTA (International Counseling Society) chapter.

NC: University of North Carolina at Charlotte

9201 University City Blvd.
Charlotte, NC 28223-0001
US
Dean   Dr. Mary Lynne Calhoun, 3049-A Colvard
Administrator Bob Barret, Professor
              Department   Counseling, Special Education, and Child Development
                            (704) 687-2531, fax (704) 687-2916

Key   See key for Data on Each Department (this section) on page 79.

Program

Accreditation   Regional Accreditation, **CACREP:** Community Counseling, **CACREP:** School Counseling

Uniqueness   Our master's program has a focus on group counseling, a certfication in Substance Abuse
                counseling, and an excellent selection of focused electives. Our doctoral program has a focus
                on multiculturalism.

Degrees
- Community Counseling: M, PhD.
- School Counseling: M, PhD.
- Counselor Education: PhD.

Contact
- Community Counseling: M = Phyllis Post.; D = Robert Barret.
- School Counseling: M = Phyllis Post.; D = Robert Barret.
- Counselor Education: D = Robert Barret.

Admission and Graduation Data

Admission
Requirements
- Community Counseling(M): GPA R; GRE R; MAT R; Interview.
- Community Counseling(D): Masters and GPA R; GRE R; MAT yes.
- School Counseling(M): GPA R; GRE R; MAT R.
- School Counseling(D): Masters and GPA R; GRE R; MAT yes.
- Counselor Education(D): Masters and GPA R; GRE R; MAT yes.

Enrollment
- Community Counseling(M): NP.
- Community Counseling(D): NP.
- School Counseling(M): NP.
- School Counseling(D): NP.
- Counselor Education(D): NP.

Diversity
- African-American; Asian-American; Caucasian; Hispanic; Native American.

Graduation
Requirements
- Community Counseling(M): 60 Class hours; 150 Practicum hours; 600 Internship hours;
  Comprehensive exam.
- Community Counseling(D): 57 Class hours; 150 Practicum hours; 600 Internship hours;
  Comprehensive exam; Oral exam; Dissertation.
- School Counseling(M): 60 Class hours; 150 Practicum hours; 600 Internship hours;
  Comprehensive exam.
- School Counseling(D): 57 Class hours; 150 Practicum hours; 600 Internship hours; Oral
  exam; Dissertation.
- Counselor Education(D): 57 Class hours; 150 Practicum hours; 600 Internship hours;
  Comprehensive exam; Oral exam; Dissertation.

Postgraduation activity: Advanced education and employment setting percentages.
- Community Counseling(M): NP.
- Community Counseling(D):
- School Counseling(M): NP.
- School Counseling(D):
- Counselor Education(D):

Planned Program Modifications

Courses	Drop	Add
	• NP.	• Marriage and Family Counseling • School Counseling.

Other	Decrease	Increase
	• NP.	• Diversity Recruiting of Faculty • Diversity Recruiting of Students • Number of Degree Majors • Number of Distance Education Courses • Number of On-Line Courses.

Related Programs Clinical Social Workers
Psychology
Organizational Behaviorists
Communications
International Studies

Faculty

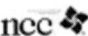 Percent of faculty reported with NCC certification: 88%.

Percent in professional counseling practice: 20%.

Research interests NP.

Diversity   • African-American; Caucasian; Other.

Name, Degree, Rank, State/National Credentials, % time devoted to program, email
• Abrams, Lyndon; PhD; Assist.; LPC, NCC; >81%; *lpabrams@email.uncc.edu*
• Barret, Robert; PhD; Full Prof.; LPP, CMFT; >81%; *rlbarret@email.uncc.edu*
• Carroll, Jane; PhD; Assoc.; LPC, NCC; >81%; *jacarrol@email.uncc.edu*
• Furr, Susan; PhD; Assoc.; LPC, NCC; >81%; *srfurr@email.uncc.edu*
• Post, Phyllis; PhD; Full Prof.; LPC, NCC; >81%; *ppost@email.uncc.edu*
• Wiersalis, Ed; PhD; Assist.; LPC, NCC; >81%;
• Ng, Kokmun; PhD; Assist.; LPC, NCC; >81%;

Has CHI SIGMA IOTA (International Counseling Society) chapter.

NC: Wake Forest University

Dean
Administrator

Box 7406
Winston-Salem, NC 27109-7266
Forsyth
Paul Escott, School of Arts and Sciences
Samuel T. Gladding, Chair, Department of Counseling
Department   Counseling Department
336) 758-4932, fax (336) 758-4591, karrpr@wfu.edu, www.wfu.edu/cep

Key   See key for Data on Each Department (this section) on page 79.

Program

Accreditation   Regional Accreditation, **CACREP:** Community Counseling, **CACREP:** School Counseling

Uniqueness   Small size allows much faculty/student interaction and strong cohort support. Full tuition
scholarships available to most students

Degrees   • Community Counseling: M.
                   • School Counseling: M.

Contact   • Community Counseling: M = Laura Veach.
                   • School Counseling: M = Donna Henderson.

Admission and Graduation Data

Admission

Requirements   • Community Counseling(M): GPA 3.00; GRE 1000; Interview.
                   • School Counseling(M): GPA 3.00; GRE 1000; Interview.

Enrollment   • Community Counseling(M): 8 Admitted yearly; 8 Graduated yearly; 6 Female; 2 Male.
                   • School Counseling(M): 7 Admitted yearly; 7 Graduated yearly; 1 Male; 6 Female.

Diversity   • African-American; Asian-American; Caucasian; Hispanic; Multiracial; Other.

Graduation

Requirements   • Community Counseling(M): 60 Class hours; 135 Practicum hours; 600 Internship hours.
                   • School Counseling(M): 60 Class hours; 135 Practicum hours; 600 Internship hours.

Postgraduation activity: Advanced education and employment setting percentages.
                   • Community Counseling(M): 12.5 Advanced education; 25 Managed care; 12.5 Private
                     practice; 37.5 Agency practice; 12.5 Other.
                   • School Counseling(M): 16 Advanced education; 28 Elementary school; 28 Middle school;
                     28 Secondary school.

Planned Program Modifications

Courses   Drop   Add
                   • NP.   • Advocacy
                                                  • Crisis/Violence Counseling
                                                  • Experiential Component.

Other   Decrease   Increase
                   • NP.   • Diversity Recruiting of Faculty
                                                  • Diversity Recruiting of Students.

Related Programs

Faculty

nbcc ❦.   Percent of faculty reported with NCC certification: **100**%.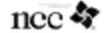

Percent in professional counseling practice: 80%.

Research interests Gladding: Creative Arts & Counseling, Impact of Lyrics; Group Counseling; Counselors
                   who worked with victims of 911. Henderson: School Counseling; Counseling Children;
                   Family Counseling in schools. Anderson: Executive coaching and REBT; attachment
                   theory; data mining. Newsome: Girl's career-related interests in science, math and
                   technology; expressive arts in counseling and supervision; counseling with children and
                   adolescents. Veach: addiction counseling; outcome measurement; advocacy; community
                   counseling

Diversity   • NP.

Name, Degree, Rank, State/National Credentials, % time devoted to program, email
- Gladding, Samuel T; PhD; Full Prof.; LPC, NCC, NCMHC; 41-60%; *stg@wfu.edu*
- Henderson, Donna A; PhD; Assoc.; LPC, NCC, NCSC; >81%; *henderda@wfu.edu*
- Newsome, Debbie; PhD; Assist.; LPC, NCC, NCSC; >81%; *newsomdw@wfu.edu*
- Veach, Laura; PhD; Assist.; LPC, NCC, NCSC; >81%; *veachlj@wfu.edu*
- Anderson, John P; PhD; Full Prof.; NCC; 22-40%; *jpa@wfu.edu*

Has CHI SIGMA IOTA (International Counseling Society) chapter.

ND: North Dakota State University

Family Life Center, Room 210
Fargo, ND 58105-5057
United States
Dean Dr. Virginia Clark Johnson
Administrator Dr. James V. Wigtil, Chair, School of Education
Department School of Education
(701) 231-7202, fax (701) 231-7416,
www.ndsu.nodak.edu/school of education

Key See key for Data on Each Department (this section) on page 79.

Program
Accreditation **CACREP:** Community Counseling, **CACREP:** School Counseling; Applied for CACREP:
Counselor Education and Supervision,

Uniqueness Only CACREP program in North Dakota

Degrees
- Community Counseling: M.
- School Counseling: M.
- Counselor Education: PhD.

Contact
- Community Counseling: M = Dr. Lee Covington Rush.
- School Counseling: NP.
- Counselor Education: D = Dr. Robert Nielsen.

Admission and Graduation Data
Admission
Requirements
- Community Counseling(M): GPA 3.00; Interview.
- School Counseling(M): GPA 3.00; Interview.
- Counselor Education(D): NP.

Enrollment
- Community Counseling(M): 7 Admitted yearly; 4 Graduated yearly; 27 Female; 3 Male.
- School Counseling(M): 19 Admitted yearly; 11 Graduated yearly; 34 Female; 6 Male.
- Counselor Education(D): 8 Admitted yearly; 5 Female; 3 Male.

Diversity
- Asian-American; Caucasian; Hispanic; Native American.

Graduation
Requirements
- Community Counseling(M): 48 Class hours; 40 Practicum hours; 600/900 Internship hours; Comprehensive exam; CPCE.
- School Counseling(M): 48 Class hours; 40 Practicum hours; 600/900 Internship hours; Comprehensive exam; CPCE.
- Counselor Education(D): 71+ Masters Class hours; 600 Internship hours; Comprehensive exam; Oral exam; Dissertation.

Postgraduation activity: Advanced education and employment setting percentages.
- Community Counseling(M): 3 Advanced education; 1 Private practice; 70 Agency practice; 23 Other.
- School Counseling(M): 5 Advanced education; 25 Elementary school; 15 Middle school; 40 Secondary school; 15 Other.
- Counselor Education(D): 5 Managed care; 10 Private practice; 10 Agency practice; 75 Other.

Planned Program Modifications

Courses	Drop	Add
	• NP.	• NP.

Other	Decrease	Increase
	• NP.	• Course Offerings
		• Clinical Supervision
		• Diversity Recruiting of Faculty
		• Diversity Recruiting of Students
		• National Accreditation
		• Number of Distance Education Courses
		• Number of On-Line Courses.

Related Programs Marriage and Family Therapists
Psychology

Faculty

nbcc ❧   Percent of faculty reported with NCC certification: 86%.   ncc ❧

Percent in professional counseling practice: NP.

Research interests   The Person-Centered Approach; School Counseling; Group Work; Stress Management;
Cognitive Counseling; Community; Substance Abuse; Group; Multicultural Counseling;
Professional Ethics; Research; Public Policy; Multiculural Orientation to Supervision;
Critical and Feminist Perspectives; Qualitative Research; Supervision; Special Education &
Sec. 504; Existentialist Approach; Life Span Career Development

Diversity   • African-American; Caucasian; Native American.

Name, Degree, Rank, State/National Credentials, % time devoted to program, email
• Hannon, J. W; EdD; Assoc.; NCC; >81%; *Wade.Hannon@ndsu.nodak.edu*
• Hundley, Steven F; PhD; Assist.; NCC, ACS, NCSC; >81%; *Steven.Hundley@ndsu.nodak.edu*
• Nielsen, Robert C; EdD; Full Prof.; LPC, NCC, LPCC; >81%; *Robert.Nielsen@ndsu.nodak.edu*
• Pennymon, Waulene; PhD; Assist.; NCC; >81%; *W.Pennymon@ndsu.nodak.edu*
• Rush, Lee Covington; PhD; Assist.; >81%; *Lee.Rush@ndsu.nodak.edu*
• Wigtil, James V; EdD; Full Prof.; LPC, NCC, LPCC; 41-60%; *Jim.Wigtil@ndsu.nodak.edu*
• Rogne, Carol; PhD; Adjunct; LPC, NCC; <21%; *crogne@dgf.k12.mn.us*

NE: Chadron State College

	1000 Main
	Chadron, NE 69337
	USA
Dean	Dr. David Welch
Administrator	Loren Froehlich, Professor
	Department Dept of Counseling/Psychology/Social Work
	(308) 432-6333, fax (308) 432-6429

Key   See key for Data on Each Department (this section) on page 79.

Program

Accreditation   Regional Accreditation

Uniqueness   Small, rural, considerable individual attention given to students.

Degrees
- Community Counseling: M.
- School Counseling: M.

Contact
- Community Counseling: M = Linda Brockbank, PhD.
- School Counseling: M = Laura Gaudet, PhD.

Admission and Graduation Data

Admission

Requirements
- Community Counseling(M): NP.
- School Counseling(M): NP.

Enrollment
- Community Counseling(M): 15 Admitted yearly; 10 Graduated yearly.
- School Counseling(M): 7 Admitted yearly; 5 Graduated yearly.

Diversity
- NP.

Graduation

Requirements
- Community Counseling(M): 48 Class hours; 40 Practicum hours; 600 Internship hours.
- School Counseling(M): 39 Class hours; 20 Practicum hours; 300 Internship hours.

Postgraduation activity: Advanced education and employment setting percentages.
- Community Counseling(M): NP.
- School Counseling(M): NP.

Planned Program Modifications

Courses	Drop		Add
	• NP.	• NP.	

Other	Decrease		Increase
	• NP.	• NP.	

Related Programs

Faculty

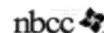 Percent of faculty reported with NCC certification: 0%.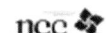

Percent in professional counseling practice: 50%.

Research interests Graduate studies, brain trauma, cognition, Native American health.

Diversity
- Hispanic.

Name, Degree, Rank, State/National Credentials, % time devoted to program, email
- Froehlich, Loren H; PhD; Full Prof.; 61-80%; *lfroehlich@csc.edu*
- Gaudet, Laura; PhD; Assist.; 61-80%; *lgaudet@csc.edu*
- Brockbank, Linda; PhD; Assist.; *lbrockbank@csc.edu*
- Hinesley, Gail; Assist.; *ghinesly@csc.edu*

Has CHI SIGMA IOTA (International Counseling Society) chapter.

NE: University of Nebraska-Omaha

60th & Dodge, Kayser Hall 421
Omaha, NE 68182-0167
USA

Dean
Administrator   Dr. Jeannette Seaberry, Chairperson
Department   Dept of Counseling
(402) 554-2727, fax (402) 554-3684, jseaberry@mail.unomaha.edu

Key   See key for Data on Each Department (this section) on page 79.

Program

Accreditation   Regional Accreditation, **CACREP:** Community Counseling, **CACREP:** School Counseling

Uniqueness   Metropolitan university in urban area.

Degrees   • Community Counseling: M.
• School Counseling: M.
• Student Affairs: M.

Contact   • Community Counseling: M = Dept. Chair.
• School Counseling: M = Dept. Chair.
• Student Affairs: M = Dept. Chair.

Admission and Graduation Data

Admission
Requirements   • Community Counseling(M): GPA 3.00; MAT 35; Interview.
• School Counseling(M): GPA 3.00; MAT 35; 2 Years work experience; Interview.
• Student Affairs(M): GPA 3.00; MAT 35; Interview.

Enrollment   • Community Counseling(M): 40 Admitted yearly; 38 Graduated yearly.
• School Counseling(M): 10 Admitted yearly; 9 Graduated yearly.
• Student Affairs(M): 5 Admitted yearly; 4 Graduated yearly.

Diversity   • African-American; Asian-American; Caucasian; Hispanic; Multiracial.

Graduation
Requirements   • Community Counseling(M): 48 Class hours; 170 Practicum hours; 130 Internship hours.
• School Counseling(M): 51 Class hours; 100 Practicum hours; 500 Internship hours.
• Student Affairs(M): 48 Class hours; 600 Internship hours.

Postgraduation activity: Advanced education and employment setting percentages.
• Community Counseling(M): 5 Advanced education; 30 Managed care; 5 Private practice; 60 Agency practice.
• School Counseling(M): 90 Secondary school.
• Student Affairs(M): 100 Other.

Planned Program Modifications

Courses   Drop   Add
• NP.   • Crisis/Violence Counseling
• Internet Use
• Play Therapy
• Special Needs Populations
• Gambling/Addiction.

Other   Decrease   Increase
• NP.   • Diversity Recruiting of Students.

Related Programs Clinical Social Workers
Psychology
Organizational Behaviorists

Faculty

   Percent of faculty reported with NCC certification: 33%.   ncc

Percent in professional counseling practice: NP.

Research interests Multicultural issues, custody and grandparent issues, capstone portfolio as exit competency, childhood guidance, case studies, case writing,

Diversity   •   African-American; Asian-American; Caucasian.

Name, Degree, Rank, State/National Credentials, % time devoted to program, email
- Bertinetti, Joseph F; PhD; Assoc.; >81%;
- Carter, David J; PhD; Assist.; NCC; >81%;
- Barnes, Paul E; PhD; Assist.; >81%;
- Harrington, Scott A; PhD; Assoc.; >81%;
- Seaberry, Jeannette S; PhD; Assoc.; >81%;
- Radd, Tommie R; PhD; Full Prof.; NCC; >81%;

Has CHI SIGMA IOTA (International Counseling Society) chapter.

NE: Wayne State College

School of Education and Counseling
Wayne, NE 68787
USA

Dean   Paul Theobald
Administrator   Keith Willis, Chair
Department   Dept of Counseling and Special Education
              (402) 375-7210, fax (402) 375-7414, kewilli1@wsc.edu,
              http://www.wsc.edu/schools/edc/clsp/

Key   See key for Data on Each Department (this section) on page 79.

Program
Accreditation   Regional Accreditation

Uniqueness   Highly respected regional program delivered with a rural picturesque setting. Noted for
              personalized attention to students and service to schools and community agencies.

Degrees   • Community Counseling: M.
           • School Counseling: M.
           • Student Affairs: M.

Contact   • Community Counseling: M = Keith Willis.
           • School Counseling: M = NP.
           • Student Affairs: M = Keith Willis.

Admission and Graduation Data
Admission
Requirements   • Community Counseling(M): GRE 1050; GRE W 3.0; Interview.
                • School Counseling(M): GRE 1050; GRE W 3.0; Interview.
                • Student Affairs(M): GRE 1050; GRE W 3.0; Interview.

Enrollment   • Community Counseling(M): 12 Admitted yearly; 8 Graduated yearly.
              • School Counseling(M): 15 Admitted yearly; 10 Graduated yearly.
              • Student Affairs(M): 1 Admitted yearly; 1 Graduated yearly.

Diversity   • African-American; Asian-American; Caucasian; Hispanic; Native American; Multiracial.

Graduation
Requirements   • Community Counseling(M): 48 Class hours; 100 Practicum hours; 600 Internship hours;
                  Portfolio.
                • School Counseling(M): 48 Class hours; 100 Practicum hours; 450 Internship hours;
                  Portfolio.
                • Student Affairs(M): 36 Class hours; 100 Practicum hours; 600 Internship hours; Portfolio.

Postgraduation activity: Advanced education and employment setting percentages.
                • Community Counseling(M): 10 Private practice; 90 Agency practice.
                • School Counseling(M): 50 Elementary school; 50 Middle school; 50 Secondary school.
                • Student Affairs(M): 100 Other.

Planned Program Modifications
Courses   Drop   Add
                    • NP.   • Diversity.

Other   Decrease   Increase
                    • NP.   • Course Offerings
                                                  • Diversity Recruiting of Faculty
                                                  • Diversity Recruiting of Students
                                                  • Graduation Requirements
                                                  • National Accreditation
                                                  • Number of Distance Education Courses.

Related Programs

Faculty

nbcc ❧   Percent of faculty reported with NCC certification: 0%.   ncc ❧

Percent in professional counseling practice: 25%.

Research interests Math education program for Winnebago Tribal Schools, Narrative therapy approaches,
                   empathy training activities, authentic assessment, supervision, role of hope in counseling,
                   psychopharmacology

Diversity   • Caucasian.

Name, Degree, Rank, State/National Credentials, % time devoted to program, email
- Conway, Kathleen L; PhD; Full Prof.; LMHP, CPC; 61-80%; *kaconwa1@wsc.edu*
- Dinsmore, Steven C; EdD; Full Prof.; 61-80%; *stdinsm1@wsc.edu*
- Wingett, Terry J; PhD; Full Prof.; LMHP, CPC; 61-80%; *tewinge1@wsc.edu*
- Willis, Keith A; PhD; Assoc.; LP CADAC; 61-80%; *kewilli1@wsc.edu*

NH: Plymouth State College

17 High Street, MSC 38
Plymouth, NH 03264
United States
Dean   Dr. Dennise Bartelo, Associate Vice President
Administrator   Dr. Gary Goodnough, Coordinator of Counselor Education
                    Department   Division of Graduate Studies, Continuing Education & Outreach
                                  (603) 535-2821, fax (603) 535-2572, forgrad@mail.plymouth.edu,
                                  www.plymouth.edu/psc/graded

Key   See key for Data on Each Department (this section) on page 79.

Program
Accreditation   NP.

Uniqueness   The counselor education program at Plymouth State College has several unique aspects to it.
                 In addition to School and Mental Health Counseling programs, the department offers content
                 strands in therapeutic adventure, conflict in families and parenting education. Opportunities
                 also exist for students looking to combine interests in counseling and theatre, as the graduate
                 programs in counseling and integrated arts have teamed up to create a professional touring
                 theatre company. As of fall 2002, the company is touring schools presenting shows,
                 workshops, and professional development credits on bullying and prevention.

Degrees   • Mental Health Counseling: M.
                 • School Counseling: M.

Contact   • Mental Health Counseling: M = Dr. Gail Mears.
                 • School Counseling: M = Dr. Gary Goodnough.

Admission and Graduation Data
Admission
Requirements   • Mental Health Counseling(M): GPA 3.00; Interview.
                 • School Counseling(M): GPA 3.00; Interview.

Enrollment   • Mental Health Counseling(M): 10 Admitted yearly; 8 Graduated yearly; 4 Female; 4 Male.
                 • School Counseling(M): 25 Admitted yearly; 15 Graduated yearly; 9 Female; 6 Male.

Diversity   • African-American; Asian-American; Caucasian; Hispanic.

Graduation
Requirements   • Mental Health Counseling(M): 60 Class hours; 100 Practicum hours; 900 Internship hours.
                 • School Counseling(M): 48 Class hours; 100 Practicum hours; 600 Internship hours.

Postgraduation activity: Advanced education and employment setting percentages.
                 • Mental Health Counseling(M): 25 Managed care; 75 Agency practice.
                 • School Counseling(M): 2 Advanced education; 38 Elementary school; 30 Middle school; 30
                   Secondary school.

Planned Program Modifications

Courses	Drop		Add	
	• NP.		• NP.	
Other	Decrease		Increase	
	• NP.		• NP.	

Related Programs

Faculty

nbcc ❧   Percent of faculty reported with NCC certification: 12%.   ncc ❧

Percent in professional counseling practice: 63%.

Research interests Gary Goodnough: School counseling national standards, group counseling in schools, and
                    principals' perspectives on school counseling. Gail Mears: Cognitive complexity and
                    relational aspects of supervision; substance abuse. Leo Sandy: Service learning, peace
                    education, and faculty development. Gary Richey: Assessment, cognitive behavioral
                    approaches, and disability. Michael Fischler: Multiculturalism and diversity issues. Susan
                    Walsh: Narrative therapy and critical issues in counseling. Linda Hassan: ADD and adult
                    women. Linda Navelski: Play therapy.

Diversity   • Caucasian.

Name, Degree, Rank, State/National Credentials, % time devoted to program, email
- Goodnough, Gary E; PhD; Assoc.; LPC, NCC; >81%; *ggoodno@mail.plymouth.edu*
- Mears, Gail; PhD; Assist.; LPC; >81%; *gmears@mail.plymouth.edu*
- Sandy, Leo R; EdD; Assoc.; >81%; *lsandy@mail.plymouth.edu*
- Fischler, Michael L; EdD; Full Prof.; 41-60%; *mfischle@mail.plymouth.edu*
- Richey, Gary K; PhD; Assoc.; 41-60%; *grichet@mail.plymouth.edu*
- Walsh, Susan; MSW; Instructor; 22-40%; *swalsh@mail.plymouth.edu*
- Hassan, Linda; PhD; Instructor; Psychologist; 22-40%;
- Navelski, Linda; CAGS; Lecturer; LPC, RPT; 22-40%

NJ: The College of New Jersey

P.O. Box 7718
Ewing, NJ 08628-0718
USA
Dean   Terrence O'Connor, Ph.D.
Administrator   Mark S. Kiselica, Ph.D., HSPP, NCC, LPC, Chairperson
                    Department   Department of Counselor Education - 337 Forcina Hall
                    (609) 771-2119, fax (609) 637-5166, counsel@tcnj.edu,
                    http://www.tcnj.edu/~educat/cpsindex.htm

Key   See key for Data on Each Department (this section) on page 79.

Program

Accreditation   Regional Accreditation, **CACREP:** Community Counseling, **CACREP:** School Counseling

CACREP

Uniqueness   The department has the first and the longest running CACREP-accredited programs in school and community counseling in New Jersey. The department is consistently ranked among the top 15 schools in the nation in terms of the total number of students ever inducted into Chi Sigma Iota, the Counseling Academic and Professional Honor Society International. The faculty of the Department of Counselor Education are national leaders in the profession and take pride in helping students to feel at home in the department.

Degrees
- Community Counseling: M.
- School Counseling: M.
- Addictions Counseling: M.
- Marriage and Family Counseling: S.

Contact
- Community Counseling: M = Dr. Mark Woodford.
- School Counseling: M = Dr. MaryLou Ramsey.
- Addictions Counseling: M = Dr. Mark Woodford.
- Marriage and Family Counseling: S = Dr. Charleen Alderfer.

Admission and Graduation Data

Admission
Requirements
- Community Counseling(M): GPA R; GRE V R; Letters; Interview.
- School Counseling(M): GPA R; GRE V R; Letters; Interview.
- Addictions Counseling(M): GPA R; GRE V R; Letters; Interview.
- Marriage and Family Counseling(S): GPA R; Letters; Interview.

Enrollment
- Community Counseling(M): 20 Admitted yearly; 20 Graduated yearly.
- School Counseling(M): 20 Admitted yearly; 20 Graduated yearly.
- Addictions Counseling(M): 10 Admitted yearly; 10 Graduated yearly.
- Marriage and Family Counseling(S): 20 Admitted yearly; 20 Graduated yearly.

Diversity
- African-American; Asian-American; Caucasian; Hispanic; Native American; Pacific Islander; Multiracial.

Graduation
Requirements
- Community Counseling(M): 48 Class hours; 100 Practicum hours; 600 Internship hours; Comprehensive exam.
- School Counseling(M): 48 Class hours; 100 Practicum hours; 600 Internship hours; Comprehensive exam.
- Addictions Counseling(M): 48 Class hours; 100 Practicum hours; 600 Internship hours.
- Marriage and Family Counseling(S): 24 Class hours; 100 Practicum hours; 200 Internship hours.

Postgraduation activity: Advanced education and employment setting percentages.
- Community Counseling(M): 5 Advanced education; 40 Agency practice; 35 Other.
- School Counseling(M): 5 Advanced education; 33 Middle school; 33 Secondary school.
- Addictions Counseling(M): 5 Advanced education; 50 Agency practice; 45 Other.
- Marriage and Family Counseling(S): 5 Advanced education; 25 Private practice; 20 Agency practice; 50 Other.

Planned Program Modifications

Courses	Drop		Add
	• NP.		• NP.

Other	Decrease		Increase
	• NP.		• Number of Degree Majors.

Related Programs NP.

Faculty

nbcc ❧ Percent of faculty reported with NCC certification: 83%. ncc ❧

Percent in professional counseling practice: NP.

Research interests Our faculty have won numerous national awards for their scholarly projects, which include the topics of confronting racisism, multicultural counseling and training, scholarship in counselor education, supervision in family therapy, ethical issues in supervision, counseling boys and teenage fathers, addictions screening and therapy, and family therapy.

Diversity   • African-American; Caucasian.

Name, Degree, Rank, State/National Credentials, % time devoted to program, email
• Ramsey, MaryLou; EdD; Full Prof.; LPC, NCC; >81%; *ramsey@tcnj.edu*
• Cavallaro, Marion; PhD; Assoc.; LPC, NCC; >81%; *cavallar@tcnj.edu*
• Kiselica, Mark; PhD; Full Prof.; LPC, NCC, Licensed Psychologist; >81%; *kiselica@tcnj.edu*
• Alderfer, Charleen; EdD; Assoc.; Licensed Marriage and Family Therapist; >81%; *alderfer@tcnj.edu*
• Woodford, Mark; PhD; Assist.; LPC, NCC, MAC; >81%; *woodford@tcnj.edu*
• Bordeau, Wendy; PhD; Assist.; LPC, NCC; >81%; *bordeau@tcnj.edu*

Has CHI SIGMA IOTA (International Counseling Society) chapter.

NJ: William Paterson University

300 Pompton Rd.
Wayne, NJ 07470
USA
Dean   Dr. Leslie Agard-Jones, College of Education
Administrator Dr. Mathilda Catarina, Director, Counseling Services Program
              Department   Special Education and Counseling
                        (973) 720-2118, www.wpunj.edu/coe

Key   See key for Data on Each Department (this section) on page 79.

Program
    Accreditation   Regional Accreditation, **CACREP:** Community Counseling, **CACREP:** School Counseling

CACREP

    Uniqueness   This counseling program offers the student a strong background in multicultural counseling.

    Degrees   • Community Counseling: M.
                    • School Counseling: M.

    Contact   • Community Counseling: M = Paula R. Danzinger, Ph.D., LPC, CCMHC.
                    • School Counseling: M = Mathilda Catarina, Ph.D., LPC.

Admission and Graduation Data
Admission
    Requirements   • Community Counseling(M): GPA 2.75; MAT 42; Interview.
                    • School Counseling(M): GPA 2.75; MAT 42; Interview.

    Enrollment   • Community Counseling(M): 6 Admitted yearly; 5 Graduated yearly; 12 Female; 3 Male.
                    • School Counseling(M): 24 Admitted yearly; 15 Graduated yearly; 10 Male.

    Diversity   • African-American; Asian-American; Caucasian; Hispanic.

Graduation
    Requirements   • Community Counseling(M): 48 Class hours; 100 Practicum hours; 600 Internship hours;
                      Comprehensive exam; Thesis; Portfolio.
                    • School Counseling(M): 48 Class hours; 100 Practicum hours; 600 Internship hours;
                      Comprehensive exam; Thesis; Portfolio.

    Postgraduation activity: Advanced education and employment setting percentages.
                    • Community Counseling(M): 85 Agency practice; 15 Other.
                    • School Counseling(M): 32 Elementary school; 32 Middle school; 32 Secondary school; 3
                      Other.

Planned Program Modifications
    Courses   Drop   Add
                    • NP.   • Crisis/Violence Counseling.

    Other   Decrease   Increase
                    • NP.   • National Accreditation.

Related Programs Psychology

Faculty

nbcc ❖   Percent of faculty reported with NCC certification: 33%.   ncc ❖

    Percent in professional counseling practice: 33%.

    Research interests Faculty research interests include: Suicide in adolescents, crisis intervention, violence in
                    the schools, grandparents raising grandchildren with AIDS, ethical implications of
                    managed mental health care, counselor licensure issues, ageism in mental health
                    professionals

    Diversity   • Asian-American; Caucasian.

    Name, Degree, Rank, State/National Credentials, % time devoted to program, email
    • Danzinger, Paula R; PhD; Assist.; LPC, NCC, CCMHC, ACS, NCGC; >81%; *danzingerp@wpunj.edu*
    • Heluk, Jr., Henry; PhD; Assist.; CSC; >81%; *helukh@wpunj.edu*
    • Catarina, Mathilda; PhD; Assoc.; LPC, Licensed Psychologist; >81%; *catarinam@wpunj.ed*

Has CHI SIGMA IOTA (International Counseling Society) chapter.

NM: University of Phoenix - Albuquerque, NM Campus

	7471 Pan American Freeway, NE
	Albuquerque, NM 87109-4645
	USA
Dean	Patrick Romine, Ph.D. - Phoenix, AZ
Administrator	Darren Adamson, Ph.D., Director of Academic Affairs
	Department College of Social and Behavioral Sciences
	(505) 821-4800, fax (505) 821-5551, darren.adamson@phoenix.edu,
	www.phoenix.edu

Key   See key for Data on Each Department (this section) on page 79.

Program
Accreditation   Regional Accreditation

Uniqueness   Our department focuses on one primiary mission - to prepare graduates for clinical practice and licensure in the State of New Mexico. The program offered here is very comprehensive as it relates to requirements for licensure in New Mexico and in other states that offer licensure. Our faculty is multidisciplinary, with representation from Marriage and Family Therapy, Social Work, Educational Counseling, Professional Psychology, Alcohol and Drug Abuse Counseling, and Psychiatry. Our model is founded in facilitation of adult learning. The University of Phoenix is considered the leader in providing educational services to working adults.

Degrees
- Community Counseling: M.
- Mental Health Counseling: M.
- Marriage and Family Counseling: M.

Contact
- Community Counseling: M = Darren Adamson, Ph.D..
- Mental Health Counseling: M = Darren Adamson, Ph.D..
- Marriage and Family Counseling: M = Darren Adamson, Ph.D..

Admission and Graduation Data
Admission
Requirements
- Community Counseling(M): GPA 2.50; 3 Years work experience; Interview.
- Mental Health Counseling(M): GPA 2.50; 3 Years work experience; Interview.
- Marriage and Family Counseling(M): GPA 2.50; 3 Years work experience; Interview.

Enrollment
- Community Counseling(M): NP.
- Mental Health Counseling(M): NP.
- Marriage and Family Counseling(M): 20 Admitted yearly; 18 Graduated yearly; 36 Female; 6 Male.

Diversity
- African-American; Caucasian; Hispanic; Native American; Multiracial.

Graduation
Requirements
- Community Counseling(M): NP.
- Mental Health Counseling(M): NP.
- Marriage and Family Counseling(M): 60 Class hours; 900 Internship hours; Portfolio.

Postgraduation activity: Advanced education and employment setting percentages.
- Community Counseling(M): NP.
- Mental Health Counseling(M): NP.
- Marriage and Family Counseling(M): 14 Advanced education; 4 Managed care; 21 Private practice; 39 Agency practice; 4 Middle school; 4 Secondary school; 14 Other.

Planned Program Modifications
Courses

Drop	Add
• Career/Life Planning.	• Crisis/Violence Counseling
	• Grief Counseling
	• School Counseling.

Other

Decrease	Increase
• NP.	• Course Offerings
	• National Accreditation
	• Number of Degree Majors.

Related Programs Marriage and Family Therapists
Organizational Behaviorists

Faculty

nbcc ❖   Percent of faculty reported with NCC certification: 0%.   ncc ❖

Percent in professional counseling practice: 91%.

Research interests   All of our faculty are practitioner faculty—working full time in the areas in which they facilitate courses. Many are conducting various projects in their private practices, however, their emphasis is on practice of the skills and concepts that they facilitate in the classroom.

Diversity   •   Caucasian; Hispanic; Multiracial.

Name, Degree, Rank, State/National Credentials, % time devoted to program, email
- Beverage, Pamela L; EdD; Assoc.; LPC; >81%; *procdyn@abq.com*
- Andrade, Joseph J; MS; Assoc.; LPC; 41-60%; *jandrade@salud.unm.edu*
- Fate, Suzanne L; MSW; Instructor; LISW; 41-60%;
- Garcia, Melinda; PhD; Assoc.; LPC; >81%;
- Ghammachi-Bennett, Maryrose; PhD; Assoc.; Clinical Psychologist; >81%; *axis@cnsp.com*
- Gerstein, Jaclyn S; EdD; Assoc.; LPC; 22-40%; *jgerst1111@aol.com*
- Hammond, Ann E; PsyD; Full Prof.; LPC; >81%; *hammondae@aol.com*
- Adamson, Darren W; PhD; Full Prof.; LMFT; >81%; *darren.adamson@phoenix.edu*
- Okon, Deborah M; PhD; Full Prof.; Clinical Pshychologist; >81%; *dmokon@highstream.net*
- Salomone, Linda S; PhD; Assoc.; LPC; >81%; *lslpcc@zianet.com*
- Smith, Richard M; EdD; Full Prof.; LPC, LMFT; >81%; *richs@unm.edu*
- Barber, Andrew; PhD; Full Prof.; clinical psychologist; >81%; *andrew.barber@phoenix.edu*

NV: University of Nevada

Department of Counseling and Educational Psychology/281
Reno, NV 89557-0213
Washoe
Dean   William Sparkman, College of Education
Administrator   Marlowe H. Smaby, Professor and Chair
Department   Counseling and Educational Psychology
(775) 784-6637, fax (775) 784-1990, herzig@unr.edu,
http://www.unr.edu/educ/cep/cepindex.html

Key   See key for Data on Each Department (this section) on page 79.

Program
Accreditation   Regional Accreditation, **CACREP:** Community Counseling, **CACREP:** Counselor Education
and Supervision, **CACREP:** School Counseling, **CACREP:** Student Affairs - Counseling

Uniqueness   The Counseling and Educational Psychology Department includes the Counseling Program
and Educational Psychology Program. The Department includes nationally recognized faculty
scholars in counseling, educational psychology, information technology and research and
statistics. Faculty members are prolific researchers and publishers. Faculty members are also
excellent teachers. Doctoral students collaborate with faculty in terms of research,
publications, teaching and service activities. Master's students are also engaged in research
acitivities.

Degrees
- Community Counseling: M, S, EdD, PhD.
- School Counseling: M, S, EdD, PhD.
- Addictions Counseling: M, EdD, PhD.
- Student Affairs: M, S, EdD, PhD.
- Counselor Education: EdD, PhD.

Contact
- Community Counseling: M, S, D = Thomas Harrison.
- School Counseling: M, S = Jill Packman.; D = Marlowe Smaby.
- Addictions Counseling: M, D = Thomas Harrison.
- Student Affairs: M, S, D = Mary Maples.
- Counselor Education: D = Marlowe Smaby.

Admission and Graduation Data
Admission
Requirements
- Community Counseling(M): GPA 3.00; GRE 750; GRE V 375; GRE Q 375; 2 Years work experience.
- Community Counseling(S): GPA 3.00; GRE 750; GRE V 375; GRE Q 375; 2 Years experience.
- Community Counseling(D): Masters and GPA 3.50; GRE 1000; GRE V 500; GRE Q 500; 2 Years work experience.
- School Counseling(M): GPA 3.00; GRE 750; GRE V 375; GRE Q 375; 2 Years work experience.
- School Counseling(S): GPA 3.00; GRE 750; GRE V 375; GRE Q 375; 2 Years work experience.
- School Counseling(D): Masters and GPA 3.50; GRE 1000; GRE V 500; GRE Q 500; 2 Years work experience.
- Addictions Counseling(M): GPA 3.00; GRE 750; GRE V 375; GRE Q 375; 2 Years work experience.
- Addictions Counseling(D): Masters and GPA 3.50; GRE 1000; GRE V 500; GRE Q 500; 2 Years work experience.
- Student Affairs(M): GPA 3.00; GRE 750; GRE V 375; GRE Q 375; 2 Years work experience.
- Student Affairs(S): GPA 3.00; GRE 750; GRE V 375; GRE Q 375; 2 Years work experience.
- Student Affairs(D): Masters and GPA 3.50; GRE 1000; GRE V 500; GRE Q 500; 2 Years work experience.
- Counselor Education(D): NP.

Enrollment
- Community Counseling(M & S): 15 Admitted yearly; 12 Graduated yearly; 35 Female; 20 Male.
- Community Counseling(D): 2 Admitted yearly; 1 Graduated yearly; 12 Female; 2 Male.
- School Counseling(M & S): 15 Admitted yearly; 12 Graduated yearly; 35 Female; 20 Male.
- School Counseling(D): 2 Admitted yearly; 1 Graduated yearly; 12 Female; 2 Male.
- Addictions Counseling(M): 5 Admitted yearly; 3 Graduated yearly; 8 Female; 2 Male.
- Addictions Counseling(D): 1 Admitted yearly; 1 Graduated yearly; 4 Female; 1 Male.
- Student Affairs(M & S): 5 Admitted yearly; 3 Graduated yearly; 8 Female; 2 Male.
- Student Affairs(D): 1 Admitted yearly; 1 Graduated yearly; 4 Female; 1 Male.
- Counselor Education(D): NP.

Diversity • African-American; Asian-American; Caucasian; Hispanic; Native American; Multiracial.

Graduation
Requirements • Community Counseling(M): 60 Class hours; 100 Practicum hours; 600 Internship hours; Comprehensive exam; CPCE.
• Community Counseling(S): MA+35 Class hours; 600 Internship hours; Comprehensive exam; CPCE; Thesis.
• Community Counseling(D): 100 Class hours; 600 Internship hours; Comprehensive exam; CPCE; Oral exam; Dissertation.
• School Counseling(M): 60 Class hours; 100 Practicum hours; 600 Internship hours; Comprehensive exam; CPCE.
• School Counseling(S): MA+35 Class hours; 600 Internship hours; Comprehensive exam; CPCE; Thesis.
• School Counseling(D): 100 Class hours; 600 Internship hours; Comprehensive exam; Oral exam; Dissertation.
• Addictions Counseling(M): 60 Class hours; 100 Practicum hours; 600 Internship hours; Comprehensive exam; CPCE.
• Addictions Counseling(D): 100 Class hours; 600 Internship hours; Comprehensive exam; CPCE; Oral exam; Dissertation.
• Student Affairs(M): 60 Class hours; 100 Practicum hours; 600 Internship hours; CPCE.
• Student Affairs(S): MA+35 Class hours; 600 Internship hours; Comprehensive exam; CPCE; Thesis.
• Student Affairs(D): 100 Class hours; 600 Internship hours; Comprehensive exam; CPCE; Oral exam; Dissertation.
• Counselor Education(D): 100 Class hours; 600 Internship hours; Comprehensive exam; CPCE; Oral exam; Dissertation.

Postgraduation activity: Advanced education and employment setting percentages.
• Community Counseling(M & S): 20 Advanced education; 80 Agency practice.
• Community Counseling(D): 20 Advanced education; 30 Managed care; 20 Private practice; 30 Agency practice.
• School Counseling(M & S): 20 Advanced education; 40 Elementary school; 40 Middle school; 20 Secondary school; 20 Student affairs.
• School Counseling(D): 20 Advanced education; 40 Middle school; 20 Secondary school; 20 Student affairs.
• Addictions Counseling(M): 20 Advanced education; 30 Managed care; 20 Private practice; 30 Agency practice.
• Addictions Counseling(D): 20 Advanced education; 30 Managed care; 20 Private practice; 30 Agency practice.
• Student Affairs(M & S): 20 Advanced education; 80 Other.
• Student Affairs(D): 20 Advanced education; 80 Other.
• Counselor Education(D): 10 Advanced education; 90 Other.

Planned Program Modifications
Courses   Drop   Add
• Technology.   • Marriage and Family Counseling.

Other   Decrease   Increase
• NP.   • Admission Requirements
                                      • Diversity Recruiting of Faculty
                                      • Diversity Recruiting of Students
                                      • Faculty FTE
                                      • Number of Off-Campus Courses.

Related Programs Clinical Social Workers
Psychology
Psychiatric Nurses
Psychiatrists
Communications
International Studies

Faculty

nbcc Percent of faculty reported with NCC certification: 43%.   ncc

Percent in professional counseling practice: 40%.

Research interests During the 2001-2002 academic year nine CEP faculty members published 21 articles in nationally refereed journals, two books, and seven book chapters, and they presented 22 papers at national conferences. Many of these publications and presentations were jointly authored with current graduate students and recent graduates. In addition, these same faculty members were editors of six nationally referred journals (Counselor Education and Supervision, Computers in the Schools, Educational Technology and Computers in the Schools, Monograph of the Society for Teacher Education and Technology, Journal of Technology and Teacher Education, and Diagnostique), and editorial board members of eight nationally refereed journals (Computers in the Schools-3, Counselor Education and Supervision-2, Psychology Corporation Revision of WISC-III-1, Rural Special Education Quarterly-1, The Turkish Online Journal of Distant Education-1). Thus, each CEP faculty member averaged about three publications, two presentations, and almost 2 editorships and editorial board memberships for last year alone. This record of prolific and distinguished publications has been sustained over the past five years. Also, data collected from students reflect a strong recognition of scholarly activities in the Department. In the last academic year, four faculty members have also received professional awards and recognition for scholarly contributions (Research Article of the Year from the Association for Specialists in Group Work-3, and Research Fellow in the Association for Specialist in Group Work-1). A 1998-99 study conducted by the Department with 45 current students and 30 graduates indicated that they rated the Departmental achievement in teaching, research and service as 4.44 and 4.28 respectively on a five-point scale (1=extremely poor to 5=excellent). Obviously, the CEP faculty members are excellent teachers, prolific scholars, and quality contributors to their respective professional associations.

Diversity • Asian-American; Caucasian; Hispanic.

Name, Degree, Rank, State/National Credentials, % time devoted to program, email
• Abney, Paul; PhD; Assist.; NCC; >81%; *abney@unr.edu*
• D'Andrea, Livia; PhD; Assoc.; 61-80%; *livia@unr.edu*
• Harrison, Thomas; PhD; Assoc.; >81%; *tch@unr.edu*
• Maples, Mary; PhD; Full Prof.; >81%; *maples@unr.edu*
• Packman, Jill; PhD; Assist.; NCC; >81%; *packman@unr.edu*
• Smaby, Marlowe; PhD; Full Prof.; NCC, Licensed Psychologist; >81%; *smaby@unr.edu*
• Torres-Rivera, Edil; PhD; Assoc.; >81%; *torre_e@unr.edu*

NY: Canisius College

2001 Main Street
Buffalo, NY 14208-1098
USA
Dean   Keith Burich, School of Ed and Human Services
Administrator   David Farrugia, Department Chairperson
          Department   Dept. of Counseling and Human Services
                    (716) 888-3298, fax (716) 888-3299, farrugia@canisius.edu,
                    www.canisius.edu

Key   See key for Data on Each Department (this section) on page 79.

Program
    Accreditation   Regional Accreditation

    Uniqueness   Students able to prepare for school or agency counseling in a student friendly atmosphere. Specialty work toward substance abuse and rehabilitation counseling

    Degrees
- Community Counseling: M.
- School Counseling: M.
- Student Affairs: M.

    Contact
- Community Counseling: M = David Farrugia.
- School Counseling: M = David Farrugia.
- Student Affairs: M = Sandra Estanek.

Admission and Graduation Data
Admission
    Requirements
- Community Counseling(M): GPA 2.50; GRE 1300; Interview.
- School Counseling(M): GPA 2.50; GRE 1300; Interview.
- Student Affairs(M): GPA 2.50; GRE 1300; Interview.

    Enrollment
- Community Counseling(M): 10 Admitted yearly; 10 Graduated yearly.
- School Counseling(M): 50 Admitted yearly; 50 Graduated yearly.
- Student Affairs(M): 25 Admitted yearly; 25 Graduated yearly.

    Diversity
- African-American; Caucasian; Hispanic; Other.

Graduation
    Requirements
- Community Counseling(M): 42 Class hours; 160 Practicum hours; 340 Internship hours.
- School Counseling(M): 42 Class hours; 160 Practicum hours; 340 Internship hours.
- Student Affairs(M): 36 Class hours; 500 Internship hours.

    Postgraduation activity: Advanced education and employment setting percentages.
- Community Counseling(M): 10 Advanced education; 10 Managed care; 10 Private practice; 50 Agency practice; 10 Other.
- School Counseling(M): 10 Advanced education; 20 Elementary school; 20 Middle school; 30 Secondary school; 20 Other.
- Student Affairs(M): 10 Advanced education; 30 Student affairs; 20 Other.

Planned Program Modifications

Courses	Drop	Add
	• NP.	• NP.

Other	Decrease	Increase
	• NP.	• NP.

Related Programs

Faculty

nbcc ❖   Percent of faculty reported with NCC certification: 60%.   ncc ❖

Percent in professional counseling practice: NP.

Research interests   Spirituality, school violence and school safety, supervision of counselors, technology, learned optimism, bereavement

    Diversity
- Caucasian.

Name, Degree, Rank, State/National Credentials, % time devoted to program, email
- Burke, Joseph; Other; Assist.; >81%; *burke2@canisius.edu*
- Farrugia, David; EdD; Full Prof.; NCC; >81%; *Farriguia@canisius.edu*
- Lenhardt, Ann Marie; PhD; Full Prof.; NCC; >81%; *lenharda@canisius.edu*
- Moll, Christine E; PhD; Assoc.; NCC; >81%; *moll@canisius.edu*
- Rutter, Michael; PhD; Assist.; >81%; *rutter@canisius.edu*

Has CHI SIGMA IOTA (International Counseling Society) chapter.

NY: College at Oswego SUNY

	321 Mahar Hall
	Oswego, NY 13126
	USA
Dean	Dean Linda Rae Markert
Administrator	Dr. Betsy Waterman, Chairperson
	Department Dept of Counseling & Psyc Services
	(315) 312-4051, fax (315) 312-3198, www.oswego.edu/cps

Key   See key for Data on Each Department (this section) on page 79.

Program

Accreditation   Regional Accreditation; Applied for **CACREP:** Community Counseling, **CACREP:** School Counseling

Uniqueness   Prepares individuals from diverse and representative backgrounds to practice as counselors in a variety of roles including certified school counselors in elementary and secondary schools.

Degrees
- Community Counseling: M.
- School Counseling: M, S.

Contact
- Community Counseling: M = Dr. Jodi Mullen.
- School Counseling: M, S = Dr. Jean Casey.

Admission and Graduation Data

Admission

Requirements
- Community Counseling(M): GPA 3.00; 2 Years work experience; Interview.
- School Counseling(M): GPA 3.00; GRE 1000; Interview.
- School Counseling(S): GPA 3.00; GRE 1000; Interview.

Enrollment
- Community Counseling(M): 30 Admitted yearly; 25 Graduated yearly; 60 Female; 20 Male.
- School Counseling(M & S): 20 Admitted yearly; 25 Graduated yearly; 75 Female; 10 Male.

Diversity
- African-American; Caucasian; Hispanic.

Graduation

Requirements
- Community Counseling(M): 48 Class hours; 100 Practicum hours; 300 Internship hours; Comprehensive exam; CPCE.
- School Counseling(M): 48 Class hours; 100 Practicum hours; 300 Internship hours; Comprehensive exam; CPCE.
- School Counseling(S): 60 Class hours; 200 Practicum hours; 300 Internship hours; Comprehensive exam; CPCE; Thesis.

Postgraduation activity: Advanced education and employment setting percentages.
- Community Counseling(M): 2 Advanced education; 2 Private practice; 85 Agency practice; 9 Other.
- School Counseling(M & S): 10 Advanced education; 10 Agency practice; 10 Elementary school; 30 Middle school; 40 Secondary school.

Planned Program Modifications

Courses	Drop	Add
	• NP.	• Computer and Related Technology
		• Crisis/Violence Counseling.

Other	Decrease	Increase
	• NP.	• Diversity Recruiting of Faculty
		• Diversity Recruiting of Students
		• Graduation Requirements
		• National Accreditation.

Related Programs NP.

Faculty

nbcc ❖   Percent of faculty reported with NCC certification: 75%.   ncc ❖

Percent in professional counseling practice: 25%.

Research interests   Low-aspiration rural students, play therapy, comprehensive guidance programs, family history, students with disabilities

Diversity
- African-American; Caucasian.

Name, Degree, Rank, State/National Credentials, % time devoted to program, email
- Casey, Jean M; PhD; Assoc.; NCC; >81%; *casey@oswego.edu*
- Gibson, Joan M; PhD; Assoc.; NCC; >81%; *jgibson2@oswego.edu*
- LeBlanc, Michael J; PhD; Assist.; >81%; *leblanc@oswego.edu*
- Fiorini, Jody; PhD; Assist.; NCC; >81%; *jfiorini@oswego.edu*

NY: Lehman College of the City University of New York

	Carman Hall B-20
	Bronx, NY 10801
	USA
Dean	Annette Digby, Carman Hall B-33
Administrator	Stuart F. Chen-Hayes, Coordinator, Counselor Education
	Department Specialized Services in Education
	(718) 960-7304 or (718) 960-8173, fax (718) 960-8364,
	stuartc@lehman.cuny.edu,
	www.lehman.cuny.edu or edu38.lehman.cuny.edu:151

Key   See key for Data on Each Department (this section) on page 79.

Program

Accreditation   Regional Accreditation

Uniqueness   The program has many first-generation and/or bilingual immigrant students from Latin America, the Carribean, Africa, and Asia. We are a companion institution with the Education Trust's Transforming School Counseling Initiative. We are involved in the Bronx Educational Alliance's GEAR-UP grant. We are the only CUNY campus to offer an extension in family counseling.

Degrees
- School Counseling: M.
- Marriage and Family Counseling: S.
- Other: S.

Contact
- School Counseling: M = Stuart Chen-Hayes.
- Marriage and Family Counseling: S = Stuart Chen-Hayes.
- Other: S = (bilingual school) Stuart Chen-Hayes.

Admission and Graduation Data

Admission

Requirements
- School Counseling(M): GPA 3.00; GRE R; GRE V No cutoff; GRE Q No cutoff; GRE A No cutoff; Interview.
- Marriage and Family Counseling(S):
- Other(S):

Enrollment
- School Counseling(M): 30 Admitted yearly; 25 Graduated yearly; 20 Male.
- Marriage and Family Counseling(S).
- Other(S).

Diversity
- African-American; Asian-American; Caucasian; Hispanic; Native American; Pacific Islander; Multiracial; Other.

Graduation

Requirements
- School Counseling(M): 48 Class hours; 100 Practicum hours; 600 Internship hours; Portfolio.
- Marriage and Family Counseling(S): 15 Class hours; 100 Practicum hours; Portfolio.
- Other(S): 15 Class hours; 100 Practicum hours; Portfolio.

Postgraduation activity: Advanced education and employment setting percentages.
- School Counseling(M): 10 Agency practice; 10 Elementary school; 10 Middle school; 60 Secondary school; 10 Student affairs.
- Marriage and Family Counseling(S).
- Other(S).

Planned Program Modifications

Courses	Drop	Add
	• NP.	• Grief Counseling
		• Human Sexuality
		• Supervision
		• Technology
		• Child and Adolescent Counseling.

Other	Decrease	Increase
	• NP.	• Course Offerings
		• Clinical Supervision
		• Diversity Recruiting of Faculty
		• Faculty FTE
		• National Accreditation.

Related Programs

Faculty

nbcc ❧   Percent of faculty reported with NCC certification: 25%.   ncc ❧

Percent in professional counseling practice: 85%.

Research interests Transforming School Counseling, Bronx Educational Alliance GEAR-UP School, Counseling Services, LBGTQQ counseling and development, family counseling and development, women's studies and feminism, multicultural and social justice counseling, technology in education and counseling.

Diversity   • Asian-American; Caucasian; Hispanic; Multiracial; Other.

Name, Degree, Rank, State/National Credentials, % time devoted to program, email
- Chen-Hayes, Stuart F; PhD; Assist.; NCC, IL LCPC; >81%; *stuartc@lehman.cuny.edu*
- Deveaux, Faith; PhD; Assoc.; NY Psych. license; >81%; *deveauxmail@aol.com*
- Fazal, Minaz; PhD; Assist.; <21%; *mfazal@att.net*
- Thompson, Patricia; PhD; Full Prof.; 61-80%; *thompson@lehman.cuny.edu*
- Benson, Adam; PsyD; Instructor; NY Psy. license; 41-60%; *doctoradambenson@yahoo.com*
- Dziekan, Kathryn; PhD cand.; Instructor; LPC, MT LPC; 41-60%; *kdziekan@lehman.cuny.edu*
- Wood, Barb; PhD; Instructor; NCC; 22-40%;
- Crespo, Nancy; MEd; Instructor; CSC (NY); *ncrespo@yahoo.com*

Has CHI SIGMA IOTA (International Counseling Society) chapter.

NY: Marist College

North Road
Poughkeepsie, NY 12601
USA

Dean   Margaret Calista
Administrator John Scileppi, Ph.D., Director, MA Psychology Program
Department   School of Social and Behavioral Sciences
(845) 575-3960, fax (845) 575-3965, John.Scileppi@Marist.edu,
www.Marist.edu

Key   See key for Data on Each Department (this section) on page 79.

Program

Accreditation   Regional Accreditation

Uniqueness   Our program utilizes a life span developmental approach.Students are given an orientation to counseling from a community approach and are taught relevant clinical, testing, program evaluation and survey research skills.Students receive hands-on experience in many courses and in the two semester externship. The programn is CAMPP approved.

Degrees   • Community Counseling: M.
              • School Counseling: M.

Contact   • Community Counseling: M = John Scileppi Ph.D..
              • School Counseling: M = Paul Egan Ph.D..

Admission and Graduation Data

Admission

Requirements • Community Counseling(M): GPA 3.00; GRE 1500; GRE V 500; GRE Q 500; GRE A 500; Interview.
              • School Counseling(M): GPA 3.00; GRE 1500; GRE V 500; GRE Q 500; GRE A 500; Interview.

Enrollment   • Community Counseling(M): 46 Admitted yearly; 41 Graduated yearly; 65 Female; 27 Male.
              • School Counseling(M): 30 Admitted yearly; 23 Graduated yearly; 30 Female; 22 Male.

Diversity   • African-American; Asian-American; Caucasian; Hispanic; Native American; Pacific Islander.

Graduation

Requirements • Community Counseling(M): 45 Class hours; 360 Internship hours.
              • School Counseling(M): 62 Class hours; 100 Practicum hours; 600 Internship hours.

Postgraduation activity: Advanced education and employment setting percentages.
              • Community Counseling(M): 10 Advanced education; 70 Agency practice; 10 Other.
              • School Counseling(M): 10 Advanced education; 30 Elementary school; 30 Middle school; 30 Secondary school.

Planned Program Modifications

Courses	Drop	Add
	• NP.	• Addictions
		• Consultation
		• Forensic Counseling
		• Legal/Ethical Issues.

Other	Decrease	Increase
	• Course Offerings.	• Course Offerings
		• Clinical Supervision
		• Diversity Recruiting of Faculty
		• Faculty FTE
		• Graduation Requirements.

Related Programs

Faculty

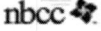   Percent of faculty reported with NCC certification: 5%.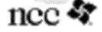

Percent in professional counseling practice: 57%.

Research interests program evaluation, forgiveness and spirituality in counseling, counseling those with multi-cultural identity, preventing violence in the schools, investigating the effects of community based psychosocial rehabilitation programs, neuro-psychological research.

Diversity • Asian-American; Caucasian; Native American; Pacific Islander.

Name, Degree, Rank, State/National Credentials, % time devoted to program, email
* Beneway, Douglas; MA; Adjunct; 22-40%;
* Calabro, Louis; PhD; Adjunct; Psycholog; <21%;
* Canale, Joseph; EdD; Assoc.; Psycholog; 22-40%; *Joseph.Canale@Marist.edu*
* Crispi, Lori; PhD; Assist.; Psycholog; 22-40%; *Lori.Crispi@Marist.edu*
* del Rosario, Peter; PhD; Assist.; Psycholog; 41-60%; *Peter.DelRosario@Marist.edu*
* Dingman, Sherry; PhD; Assist.; <21%; *Sherry.Dingman@Marist.edu*
* Kulaga, Thomas; MA; Adjunct; School Psycholog; <21%;
* Massa, Salvatore; PhD; Adjunct; School Psycholog; <21%;
* Montalto, Mary Jane; PhD; Adjunct; School Psycholog; <21%;
* O'Keefe, Edward; PhD; Full Prof.; Psycholog; 22-40%; *Edward.OKeefe@Marist.edu*
* Pisacano, John; MA; Adjunct; School Psycholog; <21%;
* Regan, James; PhD; Adjunct; Psycholog; <21%;
* Scileppi, John; PhD; Full Prof.; Psycholog; 61-80%; *John.Scileppi@Marist.edu*
* Simon, Matthew; PsyD; Adjunct; Psycholog; <21%;
* Skojec, William; PsyD; Adjunct; Psycholog; <21%;
* Spross, Suzanne; PhD; Adjunct; Psycholog; <21%;
* Teed, Elizabeth; PhD; Assist.; Psycholog; 22-40%; *Elizabeth.Teed@Marist.edu*
* Tsoubris, Gus; PhD; Adjunct; Psycholog;
* VanOrnum, William; PhD; Full Prof.; Psycholog; 22-40%; *William.VanOrnum@Marist.edu*
* Whitley, Cheryl; PhD; Assist.; CSW; <21%; *Cheryl.Whitley@Marist.edu*
* Highley, Tonda; MS; Adjunct; NCC; <21%;

NY: NEW YORK UNIVERSITY

Steinhardt School of Education
239 Greene Street
4th and 5th floors
New York, NY 10003-6674
USA
Dean   Ann Marcus
Administrator   Shefali Patel, Graduate Assistant
     Department   Applied Psychology
     (212) 998-5555, fax (212) 995-4358, www.nyu.edu/education/appsych

Key   See key for Data on Each Department (this section) on page 79.

Program
    Accreditation   CORE: Rehabilitation Counseling; Applied for CORE: Rehabilitation Counseling

    Uniqueness   Diverse faculty and student body. Urban setting, many choices for field placements. Intensive weekend graduate study program.

    Degrees
- Community Counseling: M, S.
- School Counseling: M, S.
- Other: PhD, D.
- Rehabilitation Counseling: M.
- College Counseling: M, S.

    Contact
- Community Counseling: M, S = Samuel Juni.
- School Counseling: M, S = Samuel Juni.
- Other: D = Lisa Suzuki.
- Rehabilitation Counseling: M = David Peterson.
- College Counseling: M = Samuel Juni; S = Samuel Juni.

Admission and Graduation Data
Admission
    Requirements
- Community Counseling(M): GPA 3.00.
- Community Counseling(S): GPA 3.00.
- School Counseling(M): GPA 3.00.
- School Counseling(S): GPA 3.00.
- Other(D): GRE 800; GRE V 400; GRE Q 400.
- Rehabilitation Counseling(M): GPA 2.50; Interview.
- College Counseling(M): GPA 3.00.
- College Counseling(S): GPA 3.00.

    Enrollment
- Community Counseling(M & S).
- School Counseling(M & S).
- Other(D): 4 Admitted yearly.
- Rehabilitation Counseling(M): NP.
- College Counseling(M & S).

    Diversity
- African-American; Asian-American; Caucasian; Hispanic; Native American; Pacific Islander; Multiracial.

Graduation
    Requirements
- Community Counseling(M): 48 Class hours; 84 Practicum hours; 84 Internship hours.
- Community Counseling(S): 30 Class hours; Portfolio.
- School Counseling(M): 48 Class hours; 84 Practicum hours; 84 Internship hours.
- School Counseling(S): 30 Class hours; Portfolio.
- Other(D): 96 Class hours; Oral exam; Dissertation.
- Rehabilitation Counseling(M): 54 Class hours; 100 Practicum hours; 600 Internship hours; Comprehensive exam.
- College Counseling(M): 48 Class hours; 84 Practicum hours; 84 Internship hours.
- College Counseling(S): 30 Class hours; Portfolio.

Postgraduation activity: Advanced education and employment setting percentages.
- Community Counseling(M & S): 20 Advanced education; 26.7 Agency practice; 30.7 Elementary school; 8 Student affairs; 14.7 Other.
- School Counseling(M & S): 13.8 Agency practice; 9.9 Elementary school; 33 Middle school; 33 Secondary school; 8.6 Other.
- Other(D):
- Rehabilitation Counseling(M): 1 Advanced education; 2 Managed care; 3 Private practice; 84 Agency practice; 10 Other.
- College Counseling(M & S): 20 Advanced education; 26.7 Agency practice; 30.7 Elementary school; 8 Student affairs; 14.7 Other.

Planned Program Modifications

Courses	Drop	Add
	• NP.	• NP.

Other	Decrease	Increase
	• NP.	• NP.

Related Programs Clinical Social Workers
Arts Therapists
Psychiatrists
Organizational Behaviorists
Communications
International Studies

Faculty

nbcc ❧.   Percent of faculty reported with NCC certification: 0%.   ncc 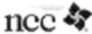 ❧

Percent in professional counseling practice: 35%.

Research interests Multicultural counseling; group dynamics; women's issues; religion and spirituality; work in people's lives; defense mechanisms.

Diversity   • African-American; Asian-American; Caucasian; Hispanic; Native American; Pacific Islander; Multiracial.

Name, Degree, Rank, State/National Credentials, % time devoted to program, email
• Ale, Alisha; PhD; Assist.; 41-60%; *alisha.ali@nyu.edu*
• Katz, Bernard; PhD; Full Prof.; 41-60%; *bk1@nyu.edu*
• Peterson, David; PhD; Assist.; 41-60%; *david.peterson@nyu.edu*
• Mattis, Jacqueline; PhD; Assist.; 41-60%; *jsm2015@nyu.edu*
• Suzuki, Lisa; PhD; Assoc.; 41-60%; *las1@nyu.edu*
• McRae, Mary; EdD; Assoc.; 41-60%; *mary.mcrae@nyu.edu*
• Richardson, Mary Sue; PhD; Full Prof.; 41-60%; *msr1@nyu.edu*
• Juni, Samuel; PhD; Full Prof.; 41-60%; *sam.juni@nyu.edu*

NY: Niagara University

Niagara University, NY
14109-2042
Dean   Dr. Debra Colley O'Shea B-9
Administrator   Morgan Brocks Conway, Coordinator of Counseling Program
             Department   Dept. of Educational Leadership & Counseling
                   (716) 286-8550, fax (716) 286-8561, mkinney@niagara.edu

Key   See key for Data on Each Department (this section) on page 79.

Program
  Accreditation   Regional Accreditation

  Uniqueness   Program has a masters in School Psychology

  Degrees   • Mental Health Counseling: M.
         • School Counseling: M.
         • Other: M.

  Contact   • Mental Health Counseling: M = Dr.Shannon Hodges.
         • School Counseling: M = Dr. Morgan Brocks Conway.
         • Other: M = Dr. Kristine Augustyniak.

Admission and Graduation Data
Admission
  Requirements   • Mental Health Counseling(M): GPA 2.75; GRE 880; GRE V 440; GRE Q 440; GRE A R;
              MAT 40; Interview.
          • School Counseling(M): GPA 2.75; GRE 880; GRE V 440; GRE Q 440; GRE A R; MAT 40;
              Interview.
          • Other (M): GPA 3.00; GRE 1000; GRE V 500; GRE Q 500; GRE A R; MAT 40; Interview.

  Enrollment   • Mental Health Counseling(M): 5 Admitted yearly; 5 Graduated yearly.
          • School Counseling(M): 25 Admitted yearly; 25 Graduated yearly.
          • Other (M): Admitted yearly.

  Diversity   • African-American; Asian-American; Caucasian; Hispanic; Native American; Multiracial.

Graduation
  Requirements   • Mental Health Counseling(M): 60 Class hours; 100 Practicum hours; 900 Internship hours;
              Comprehensive exam; Portfolio.
          • School Counseling(M): 36 Class hours; 100 Practicum hours; 100 Internship hours;
              Comprehensive exam; Portfolio.
          • Other (M): 61 Class hours; 400 Practicum hours; 1200 Internship hours; Comprehensive
              exam; Portfolio.

  Postgraduation activity: Advanced education and employment setting percentages.
          • Mental Health Counseling(M): 100 Agency practice.
          • School Counseling(M): 10 Elementary school; 45 Middle school; 45 Secondary school.
          • Other (M): NP.

Planned Program Modifications
  Courses   Drop   Add
              • NP.   • NP.

  Other   Decrease   Increase
              • NP.   • Graduation Requirements
                                   • National Accreditation
                                   • Course Offerings.

Related Programs Other

Faculty

nbcc ❧   Percent of faculty reported with NCC certification: 33%.   ncc ❧

Percent in professional counseling practice: 0%.

Research interests Grief and loss; divorce assessment; personality disorders; professional standards and
            practice in the schools; DSM-IV-TR criteria; spirituality; school safety.

  Diversity   • Caucasian.

Name, Degree, Rank, State/National Credentials, % time devoted to program, email
  • Hodges, Shannon; PhD; Assist.; >81%; *sjp@niagara.edu*
  • Augustyniak, Kristine; PhD; Assist.; >81%;
  • Conway, Morgan B; PhD; Assist.; NCC; >81%; *mcc@niagara.edu*

NY: Plattsburgh State University

101 Broad Street
Plattsburgh, NY 12901
USA

Dean   Betty Taylor - Faculty of Professional Studies
Administrator   Dr. Donald A. Haight, Department Chairperson
         Department   Counselor Education
                  (518) 564-2164, fax (518) 564-4161, jean.leclair@plattsburgh.edu,
                  www.plattsburgh.edu

Key   See key for Data on Each Department (this section) on page 79.

Program

Accreditation   Regional Accreditation, **CACREP:** Community Counseling, **CACREP:** School Counseling, **CACREP:** Student Affairs - Counseling

CACREP

Uniqueness   The department is small enough that students really get a chance to know their professors, and their professors get a good chance to know them. However, the department is large enough to offer quality education.

Degrees
- Community Counseling: M.
- School Counseling: M, S.
- College Counseling: M.

Contact
- Community Counseling: M = Dr. Stephen Saiz.
- School Counseling: M, S = Dr. Rachelle Perusse.
- College Counseling: M = Dr. Beverly Burnell.

Admission and Graduation Data

Admission

Requirements
- Community Counseling(M): GPA 2.80; GRE 25th%tile; GRE V 25th%tile; GRE Q 25th%tile; GRE A 25th%tile; MAT 25th%tile; Interview.
- School Counseling(M): GPA 2.80; GRE 25th%tile; GRE V 25th%tile; GRE Q 25th%tile; GRE A 25th%tile; MAT 25th%tile; Interview.
- School Counseling(S): GPA 2.80; GRE 25th%tile; GRE V 25th%tile; GRE Q 25th%tile; GRE A 25th%tile; MAT 25th%tile; Interview.
- College Counseling(M): GPA 2.80; GRE 25th%tile; GRE V 25th%tile; GRE Q 25th%tile; GRE A 25th%tile; MAT 25th%tile; Interview.

Enrollment
- Community Counseling(M): 12 Admitted yearly; 11 Graduated yearly; 6 Female; 5 Male.
- School Counseling(M & S): 20 Admitted yearly; 16 Graduated yearly; 16 Female; 4 Male.
- College Counseling(M): 2 Admitted yearly; 2 Graduated yearly; 1 Female; 1 Male.

Diversity
- African-American; Caucasian; Native American; Other.

Graduation

Requirements
- Community Counseling(M): 48 Class hours; 115 Practicum hours; 600 Internship hours; Comprehensive exam; CPCE.
- School Counseling(M): 60 Class hours; 115 Practicum hours; 600 Internship hours; Comprehensive exam; CPCE.
- School Counseling(S): 60 Class hours; 115 Practicum hours; 600 Internship hours; Comprehensive exam; CPCE.
- College Counseling(M): 48 Class hours; 115 Practicum hours; 600 Internship hours; Comprehensive exam; CPCE.

Postgraduation activity: Advanced education and employment setting percentages.
- Community Counseling(M): 5 Managed care; 70 Agency practice; 20 Other.
- School Counseling(M & S): 5 Advanced education; 30 Elementary school; 30 Middle school; 30 Secondary school; 5 Other.
- College Counseling(M): 5 Advanced education; 90 Student affairs; 5 Other.

Planned Program Modifications

Courses   Drop   Add
- Consultation.   • Life span Development.

Other   Decrease   Increase
- NP.   • Diversity Recruiting of Students.

Related Programs Psychology
                         Communications

Faculty

nbcc ✥   Percent of faculty reported with NCC certification: 80%.   ncc ✥

Percent in professional counseling practice: 33%.

Research interests Currently, the faculty members are pursuing research interests in the following areas: school counseling and school counselor education, counselor education accreditation, prevention programs in counseling, the needs of adoptive children and their parents, career development in counseling, multiculturalism in counseling, and emotional/behavioral disorders of children.

Diversity   • Caucasian; Native American; Other.

Name, Degree, Rank, State/National Credentials, % time devoted to program, email
- Haight, Donald A; EdD; Full Prof.; >81%; *donald.haight@plattsburgh.edu*
- Perusse, Rachelle; PhD; Assist.; NCC; >81%; *rachelle.perusse@plattsburgh.edu*
- Burnell, Beverly A; PhD; Assist.; NCC; >81%; *beverly.burnell@plattsburgh.edu*
- Saiz, Stephen; EdD; Assist.; NCC, ACS; >81%; *stephen.saiz@plattsburgh.edu*
- Schnell, Richard; EdD; Full Prof.; NCC, CCMHC; >81%; *richard.schnell@plattsburgh.edu*

Has CHI SIGMA IOTA (International Counseling Society) chapter.

NY: Queens College, City University of New York

	65-30 Kissena Blvd
	Flushing, NY 11367
	USA
Dean	Marian Fish, ECP
Administrator	John Pellitteri, Ph.D., Program Director
	Department Educational & Community Programs
	(718) 997-5250, fax (718) 997-5248, JPellitt@qc1.qc.edu, www.qc.edu

Key   See key for Data on Each Department (this section) on page 79.

Program
Accreditation   Regional Accreditation

Uniqueness   The program offers an integrated training sequence in applied psychological counseling that couples small group experiential labs with rigorous theory courses. There is an emphasis on self awareness, opportunities to be involved in research and/or clinical work with faculty, and flexibility in accommodating professional development. The student body is supportive and cohesive.

Degrees
- Mental Health Counseling: M.
- School Counseling: M.
- Addictions Counseling: M.

Contact
- Mental Health Counseling: M = Dr. Lynn Howell.
- School Counseling: M = Dr. John Pellitteri.
- Addictions Counseling: M = NP.

Admission and Graduation Data
Admission
Requirements
- Mental Health Counseling(M): GPA 3.00; Interview.
- School Counseling(M): GPA 3.00; Interview.
- Addictions Counseling(M): NP.

Enrollment
- Mental Health Counseling(M): NP.
- School Counseling(M): 35 Admitted yearly; 30 - 40 Graduated yearly; 85 Female; 10 Male.
- Addictions Counseling(M): NP.

Diversity
- African-American; Asian-American; Caucasian; Hispanic; Multiracial.

Graduation
Requirements
- Mental Health Counseling(M): 60 Class hours; 100 Practicum hours; 600 Internship hours; Comprehensive exam; Thesis.
- School Counseling(M): 60 Class hours; 100 Practicum hours; 600 Internship hours; Comprehensive exam; Thesis.
- Addictions Counseling(M): NP.

Postgraduation activity: Advanced education and employment setting percentages.
- Mental Health Counseling(M): NP.
- School Counseling(M): 1 Advanced education; 14 Elementary school; 30 Middle school; 50 Secondary school; 5 Other.
- Addictions Counseling(M): NP.

Planned Program Modifications

Courses	Drop	Add
	• NP.	• Consultation
		• Marriage and Family Counseling.

Other	Decrease	Increase
	• NP.	• Diversity Recruiting of Faculty
		• National Accreditation.

Related Programs Organizational Behaviorists

Faculty

nbcc ♣   Percent of faculty reported with NCC certification: 25%.   **ncc** ♣

Percent in professional counseling practice: NP.

Research interests Emotional intelligence, personality, adult development, music therapy, counselor training, multiculturalism, school counseling

Diversity
- African-American; Asian-American; Caucasian; Hispanic.

Name, Degree, Rank, State/National Credentials, % time devoted to program, email
- Pellitteri, John S; PhD; Assist.; Licensed Psychologist; >81%; *Jpellitter@aol.com*
- Vazquez, Jesse M; PhD; Full Prof.; NCC; 22-40%;
- Howell, Lynn; PhD; Assist.; LPC, NCC; 61-80%;
- Woods, Patricia; EdD; Assoc.; LPC, NCC; <21%;
- Schwartz, Lester; PhD; Full Prof.; Lic. Psych; <21%;
- Katz, Robert; PhD; Adjunct; Lic. Psych; <21%;
- Berkson, Nancy; PhD; Adjunct; Lic. Psych; 22-40%;
- Merladet, John; PhD; Adjunct; Lic. Psych; <21%;
- Galette, Fritz; PhD; Adjunct; Lic Psych; <21%;
- Don, Anthony; MS; Adjunct; CSC; <21%;
- Grassel, Ed; MS; Adjunct; CSC; <21%;
- Warden, Ken; MS; Adjunct; CSC; <21%;

Has CHI SIGMA IOTA (International Counseling Society) chapter.

NY: State University of New York at Oneonta

	211 Fitzelle Hall
	Oneonta, NY 13820
	USA
Dean	Richard Couch, Netzer Admin Bldg.
Administrator	Dr. Anuradhaa Shastri, Chairperson
	Department Dept of Ed Psych & Counseling
	(607) 436-3554, fax (607) 436-3799, ryanca@oneonta.edu, oneonta.edu

Key   See key for Data on Each Department (this section) on page 79.

Program

Accreditation   Regional Accreditation

Uniqueness   NP.

Degrees   • School Counseling: M, S.

Contact   • School Counseling: M, S = Emily Phillips.

Admission and Graduation Data
Admission
Requirements   • School Counseling(M): GPA 2.80; Interview.
   • School Counseling(S): Interview.

Enrollment   • School Counseling(M & S): 30 Admitted yearly; 30 Graduated yearly.

Diversity   • African-American; Asian-American; Caucasian; Hispanic; Native American; Multiracial.

Graduation
Requirements   • School Counseling(M): 33/will be 60 by 2005, Class hours; 180 Practicum hours; 600
   Internship hours; Comprehensive exam; Portfolio.
   • School Counseling(S): 27 Class hours; 600 Internship hours.

Postgraduation activity: Advanced education and employment setting percentages.
   • School Counseling(M & S): 35 Elementary school; 30 Middle school; 35 Secondary school;
   2.5 Other.

Planned Program Modifications

Courses	Drop	Add
	• NP.	• Consultation
		• Diversity
		• Grief Counseling
		• Play Therapy
		• Special Needs Populations.

Other	Decrease	Increase
	• NP.	• Course Offerings
		• Clinical Supervision
		• Diversity Recruiting of Faculty
		• Diversity Recruiting of Students
		• Graduation Requirements
		• Number of On-Line Courses.

Related Programs

Faculty

nbcc ❧   Percent of faculty reported with NCC certification: 11%.   ncc ❧
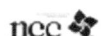

Percent in professional counseling practice: 10%.

Research interests school counselor supervison, special needs children

Diversity   • African-American; Asian-American.

Name, Degree, Rank, State/National Credentials, % time devoted to program, email
• Bakari, Rosenna; PhD; Assist.; <21%; *bakirir@oneonta.edu*
• Curran, Joanne; PhD; Assoc.; <21%; *curranjm@oneonta.edu*
• LaFrance, Ron; EdD; Assoc.; >81%; *lafranrc@oneonta.edu*
• Li, Daqi; PhD; Assist.; <21%; *lid@oneonta.edu*
• Marshall, Joan; PhD; Assoc.; >81%; *marshajh@oneonta.edu*
• Phillips, Emily; PhD; Assist.; NCC; >81%; *phillie@oneonta.edu*
• Shastri, Anuradhaa; PhD; Assoc.; <21%; *shastra@oneonta.edu*
• Staley, Richard; EdD; Assoc.; <21%; *statleyrk@oneonta.edu*
• VanValkenburg, John; PhD; Assoc.; <21%; *vanvalj@oneonta.edu*

NY: SUNY College of Brockport

350 New Campus Drive
Brockport, NY 14420-2953
United States
Dean   Joseph R. Mason, School of Professions
Administrator   Muhyi Shakoor, Chairperson
     Department   Department of Counselor Education
                   (585) 395-2258, fax (585) 395-2366, dreed@po.brockport.edu,
                   www.brockport.edu/~counsele/CE

Key   See key for Data on Each Department (this section) on page 79.

Program
Accreditation   **CACREP:** Community Counseling, **CACREP:** School Counseling, **CACREP:** Student Affairs - Counseling

Uniqueness   The department emphasizes experiential education throughout its programs.

Degrees
- Community Counseling: M.
- School Counseling: M.
- College Counseling: M.

Contact
- Community Counseling: M = S. R. Seem.
- School Counseling: M = J. Cochran.
- College Counseling: M = T. Hernandez.

Admission and Graduation Data
Admission
Requirements
- Community Counseling(M): GPA 2.50; Interview.
- School Counseling(M): GPA 2.50; Interview.
- College Counseling(M): GPA 2.50.

Enrollment
- Community Counseling(M): 10 Admitted yearly; 10 Graduated yearly; 3 Female; 7 Male.
- School Counseling(M): 30 Admitted yearly; 30 Graduated yearly; 20 Female; 10 Male.
- College Counseling(M): 5 Admitted yearly; 5 Graduated yearly; 4 Female; 1 Male.

Diversity
- African-American; Asian-American; Caucasian; Hispanic; Multiracial.

Graduation
Requirements
- Community Counseling(M): 48 Class hours; 100 Practicum hours; 600 Internship hours.
- School Counseling(M): 48 Class hours; 100 Practicum hours; 600 Internship hours.
- College Counseling(M): 48 Class hours; 100 Practicum hours; 600 Internship hours.

Postgraduation activity: Advanced education and employment setting percentages.
- Community Counseling(M): 5 Private practice; 95 Agency practice.
- School Counseling(M): 30 Elementary school; 30 Middle school; 40 Secondary school.
- College Counseling(M): NP.

Planned Program Modifications
Courses   <u>Drop</u>   <u>Add</u>
- NP.   • NP.

Other   <u>Decrease</u>   <u>Increase</u>
- NP.   • Graduation Requirements.

Related Programs Clinical Social Workers
                      Psychology

Faculty

nbcc   Percent of faculty reported with NCC certification: 83%.   **ncc**

Percent in professional counseling practice: 0%.

Research interests Counseling outcomes, career counseling, play therapy, conduct disorder, psychological aspects of large scale human crisis, gender, culture & sexual orientation issues, feminist therapy

Diversity
- African-American; Caucasian; Hispanic.

Name, Degree, Rank, State/National Credentials, % time devoted to program, email
- Shakoor, Muhyi A; PhD; Full Prof.; NCC; >81%; *mshakoor@brockport.edu*
- Hernandez, Thomas J; EdD; Assist.; >81%; *thernandez@brockport.edu*
- Cochran, Jeff L; PhD; Assist.; NCC; >81%; *jcochran@brockport.edu*
- Seem, Susan R; PhD; Assoc.; NCC; >81%; *sseem@brockport.edu*
- McCulloch, Leslie A; PhD; Assist.; NCC; >81%;
- Goodspeed, Patricia; PhD; Assist.; NCC; >81%; *pgoodspeed@brockport.edu*

Has CHI SIGMA IOTA (International Counseling Society) chapter.

NY: SUNY University at Buffalo

409 Baldy Hall
Buffalo, NY 14260-1000
USA

Dean   Mary Gresham, 367 Baldy Hall
Administrator   Thomas T. Frantz, Chairperson
Department   Dept of Counseling & Educational Psychology
                (716) 645-2484, fax (716) 645-2479

Key   See key for Data on Each Department (this section) on page 79.

Program
Accreditation   Regional Accreditation, CORE: Rehabilitation Counseling

Uniqueness   Fairly intense blend of practical, theoretical and research knowledge that provides each student with specific job skills and a depth of knowledge to underlie the skills. Program also has a doctorate in Counseling Psychology.

Degrees   • School Counseling: M.
                • Other: PhD, D.
                • Rehabilitation Counseling: M.
                • Counselor Education: PhD.

Contact   • School Counseling: M = Dr. Janis DeLucia-Waack.
                • Other: D = Dr. Scott Meier.
                • Rehabilitation Counseling: M = Dr. Tim Janikowski.
                • Counselor Education: D = Dr. T.T. Frantz.

Admission and Graduation Data
Admission
Requirements   • School Counseling(M): Interview.
                • Other(D): Interview.
                • Rehabilitation Counseling(M): Interview.
                • Counselor Education(D): 1 Year work experience.

Enrollment   • School Counseling(M): 30 Admitted yearly; 27 Graduated yearly; 24 Female; 6 Male.
                • Other(D): 10 Admitted yearly; 10 Graduated yearly; 7 Female; 3 Male.
                • Rehabilitation Counseling(M): 10 Admitted yearly; 10 Graduated yearly; 6 Female; 4 Male.
                • Counselor Education(D): 6 Admitted yearly; 5 Graduated yearly; 3 Female; 3 Male.

Diversity   • African-American; Asian-American; Caucasian; Hispanic; Native American; Multiracial.

Graduation
Requirements   • School Counseling(M): 36 Class hours; 150 Practicum hours; Comprehensive exam.
                • Other(D): 90 Class hours; 1000 Practicum hours; 2000 Internship hours; Comprehensive exam; Dissertation.
                • Rehabilitation Counseling(M): 48 Class hours; 300 Practicum hours; 300 Internship hours; Thesis.
                • Counselor Education(D): 90 Class hours; 500 Practicum hours; Comprehensive exam; Dissertation.

Postgraduation activity: Advanced education and employment setting percentages.
                • School Counseling(M): 15 Advanced education; 5 Agency practice; 80 Secondary school.
                • Other(D): 60 Managed care; 30 Private practice; 10 Agency practice.
                • Rehabilitation Counseling(M): 20 Advanced education; 10 Private practice; 70 Agency practice.
                • Counselor Education(D): 35 Agency practice; 60 Student affairs; 5 Other.

Planned Program Modifications
Courses   Drop   Add
                • NP.   • Teaching
                                            • Wellness.

Other   Decrease   Increase
                • NP.   • Faculty FTE.

Related Programs Clinical Social Workers
                Psychology
                Psychiatric Nurses
                Psychiatrists
                Communications
                International Studies

Faculty

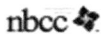 Percent of faculty reported with NCC certification: 0%.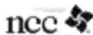

Percent in professional counseling practice: 18%.

Research interests Group work, assessment, grief and death, abuse, addictions, qualify of life, wellness, class size, counseling

Diversity   • African-American; Asian-American; Caucasian; Hispanic.

Name, Degree, Rank, State/National Credentials, % time devoted to program, email
- DeLucia-Waack, Janice; PhD; Assoc.; 22-40%; *jdeluci@acsu.buffalo.edu*
- Finn, Jeremy; PhD; Full Prof.; <21%; *finn@acsu.buffalo.edu*
- Frantz, Thomas T; PhD; Assoc.; >81%; *ttfrantz@acsu.buffalo.edu*
- Gentile, Ronald J; PhD; Full Prof.; <21%; *gentile@acsu.buffalo.edu*
- Meier, Scott; PhD; Full Prof.; <21%; *stmeier@acsu.buffalo.edu*
- Phelps, LeAdelle; PhD; Full Prof.; <21%; *phelps@acsu.buffalo.edu*
- Shuell, Thomas; PhD; Full Prof.; <21%; *shuell@acsu.buffalo.edu*
- Truscott, Stephen; PhD; Assist.; <21%; *sdt55@acsu.buffalo.edu*
- Donnelly, Jim; PhD; Assist.; 22-40%;
- Gerrity, Deb; PhD; Assist.; <21%;
- Cook-Cotone, Cathy; PhD; Assist.; <21%;
- Volker, Marty; PhD; Assist.; <21%;
- Robinson, Cecil; PhD; Assist.; <21%;
- Lee, Jaek; PhD; Assoc.; <21%;
- Torres-Rivera, Edil; PhD; Assoc.; <21%;
- Janikowski, Tim; PhD; Assoc.

NY: Syracuse University

259 Huntington Hall
Syracuse, NY 13244-2340
USA

Dean	Louise Wilkinson
Administrator	Janine M. Bernard, Professor and Chair
	Department Counseling and Human Services
	(315) 443-2266, fax (315) 443-5732, sklord@syr.edu or bernard@syr.edu, http://soeweb.syr.edu/chs/counhumserv.html

Key   See key for Data on Each Department (this section) on page 79.

Program

Accreditation   Regional Accreditation, **CACREP:** Counselor Education and Supervision, **CACREP:** School Counseling, **CACREP:** Student Affairs - Counseling, **CORE:** Rehabilitation Counseling

Uniqueness   Student-centered doctoral program with particular emphasis on clincal supervision and leadership development. Combination of CACREP and CORE programs.

Degrees
- Community Counseling: M, S.
- School Counseling: M, S.
- Rehabilitation Counseling: M.
- Student Affairs: M, S.
- Counselor Education: PhD.

Contact
- Community Counseling: M, S = Janine Bernard.
- School Counseling: M, S = Janna Scarborough.
- Rehabilitation Counseling: M = Dennis Gilbride.
- Student Affairs: M, S = Janine Bernard.
- Counselor Education: D = Harold (Dick) Hackney.

Admission and Graduation Data

Admission

Requirements
- Community Counseling(M): GPA 3.00; GRE NA; GRE V NA; 1 Year work experience; Interview.
- Community Counseling(S): GPA 3.00; GRE NA; GRE V NA; 1 Year work experience; Interview.
- School Counseling(M): GPA 3.00; GRE NA; GRE V NA; 1 Year work experience; Interview.
- School Counseling(S): GPA 3.00; GRE NA; GRE V NA; 1 Year work experience; Interview.
- Rehabilitation Counseling(M): GPA 3.00; GRE NA; GRE V NA; 1 Year work experience; Interview.
- Student Affairs(M): GPA 3.00; GRE NA; GRE V NA; 1 Year work experience; Interview.
- Student Affairs(S): GPA 3.00; GRE NA; GRE V NA; 1 Year work experience; Interview.
- Counselor Education(D): Masters and GPA 3.50; GRE V 500; GRE Q 500; GRE A 500; 1 Year work experience.

Enrollment
- Community Counseling(M & S): 10 Admitted yearly; 8 Graduated yearly; 8 Female; 2 Male.
- School Counseling(M & S): 20 Admitted yearly; 20 Graduated yearly; 50 Female; 10 Male.
- Rehabilitation Counseling(M): 10 Admitted yearly; 8 Graduated yearly; 15 Female; 8 Male.
- Student Affairs(M & S): 5 Admitted yearly; 5 Graduated yearly; 5 Female; 5 Male.
- Counselor Education(D): 4-6 Admitted yearly; 4-6 Graduated yearly; 13 Female; 8 Male.

Diversity
- African-American; Asian-American; Caucasian; Hispanic; Other.

Graduation

Requirements
- Community Counseling(M): 48 Class hours; 100 Practicum hours; 600 Internship hours; Comprehensive exam; CPCE; Portfolio.
- Community Counseling(S): 60 to include M.A. Class hours.
- School Counseling(M): 48 Class hours; 100 Practicum hours; 600 Internship hours; Comprehensive exam; CPCE; Portfolio.
- School Counseling(S): 60 Class hours.
- Rehabilitation Counseling(M): 48 Class hours; 100 Practicum hours; 600 Internship hours; Comprehensive exam.
- Student Affairs(M): 48 Class hours; 100 Practicum hours; 600 Internship hours; CPCE; Portfolio.
- Student Affairs(S): 60 Class hours.
- Counselor Education(D): 102 Class hours; 100 Practicum hours; 600 Internship hours; Comprehensive exam; Oral exam; Dissertation.

Postgraduation activity: Advanced education and employment setting percentages.
- Community Counseling(M & S).
- School Counseling(M & S): 10 Advanced education; 10 Elementary school; 30 Middle school; 30 Secondary school.
- Rehabilitation Counseling(M): 10 Advanced education; 90 Agency practice.
- Student Affairs(M & S): 10 Advanced education; 90 Student affairs.
- Counselor Education(D): 10 Private practice; 20 Agency practice; 70 Other.

Planned Program Modifications

Courses	Drop	Add
	• NP.	• Internet Use.

Other	Decrease	Increase
	• NP.	• Diversity Recruiting of Faculty
		• Diversity Recruiting of Students
		• National Accreditation.

Related Programs Clinical Social Workers
Marriage and Family Therapists
Psychology
Psychiatric Nurses

Faculty

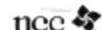 Percent of faculty reported with NCC certification: 71%. ncc

Percent in professional counseling practice: 12.5%.

Research interests Clinical supervision, counseling process analysis, professional identity of school counselors, transition to work for persons with disabilities, sexual abuse, spirituality.

Diversity • Caucasian.

Name, Degree, Rank, State/National Credentials, % time devoted to program, email
- Bernard, Janine M; PhD; Full Prof.; LPC, NCC, LMFT, ACS; >81%; *bernard@syr.edu*
- Bellini, James L; PhD; Assoc.; CRC; >81%; *jlbellin@syr.edu*
- Gilbride, Dennis D; PhD; Assoc.; CRC; >81%; *ddgilbri@syr.edu*
- Goldberg, Alan D; PhD; Assoc.; NCC; <21%; *adgoldbe@syr.edu*
- Hackney, Harold L; PhD; Full Prof.; LPC, NCC, ACS; >81%; *hackney@syr.edu*
- Pearson, Richard E; PhD; Full Prof.; NCC; <21%; *repearso@syr.edu*
- Scarborough, Janna L; PhD; Assist.; LPC, NCC, ACS; >81%; *scarboro@syr.edu*

NY: University of Rochester

Warner Graduate School of Education and Human Development
Rochester, NY 14627-0425
USA

Dean   Raffaella Borasi, Dean, Warner Grad. School of Education and Human Dev.
Administrator   Howard Kirschenbaum, Chair
                    Department   Counseling and Human Development
                                    (585) 273-1764, fax (585) 273-1196, Howard.Kirschenbaum@rochester.edu,
                                    www.rochester.edu/warner

Key   See key for Data on Each Department (this section) on page 79.

Program
Accreditation   Regional Accreditation, **CACREP:** Community Counseling, **CACREP:** Counselor Education
                and Supervision, **CACREP:** School Counseling

CACREP

Uniqueness   An ecological, social context approach to counseling; a sense of community among students
                and faculty; excellent relationships with local schools and community.

Degrees   • Community Counseling: M, S.
                • School Counseling: M, S.
                • Counselor Education: EdD, PhD.

Contact   • Community Counseling: M = Kathryn Douthit.; S = NP.
                • School Counseling: M = Howard Kirschenbaum.; S = NP.
                • Counselor Education: D = Howard Kirschenbaum.

Admission and Graduation Data
Admission
Requirements   • Community Counseling(M): GPA no spec; GRE NR; Interview.
                • Community Counseling(S): GPA no spec; GRE NR; Interview.
                • School Counseling(M): GPA no spec; GRE NR; Interview.
                • School Counseling(S): GPA no spec; GRE NR; Interview.
                • Counselor Education(D): Masters and GPA no spec.; GRE NR; MAT not req.; 2 Years work
                  experience.

Enrollment   • Community Counseling(M & S): 8 Admitted yearly; 6 Graduated yearly; 11 Female; 3 Male.
                • School Counseling(M & S): 25 Admitted yearly; 23 Graduated yearly; 36 Female; 10 Male.
                • Counselor Education(D): 5 recently Admitted yearly; 2 in past Graduated yearly; 13
                  Female; 11 Male.

Diversity   • African-American; Asian-American; Caucasian; Hispanic; Pacific Islander; Multiracial.

Graduation
Requirements   • Community Counseling(M): 51 Class hours; 120 Practicum hours; 600 Internship hours;
                  Thesis.
                • Community Counseling(S): at least 12 Class hours.
                • School Counseling(M): 48 Class hours; 120 Practicum hours; 600 Internship hours; Thesis.
                • School Counseling(S): at least 12 Class hours.
                • Counselor Education(D): 96 Class hours; 100 Practicum hours; 600 Internship hours;
                  Comprehensive exam; Dissertation.

Postgraduation activity: Advanced education and employment setting percentages.
                • Community Counseling(M & S): 25 Managed care; 75 Agency practice.
                • School Counseling(M & S): 5 Agency practice; 15 Elementary school; 30 Middle school; 45
                  Secondary school; 5 Other.
                • Counselor Education(D): 40 Advanced education; 15 Managed care; 15 Private practice;
                  15 Agency practice; 5 Middle school; 5 Secondary school; 5 Student affairs.

Planned Program Modifications
Courses   Drop   Add
                • NP.   • Advocacy
                                               • Testing, Appraisal, Assessment
                                               • Wellness.

Other   Decrease   Increase
                • NP.   • Course Offerings
                                               • Clinical Supervision
                                               • National Accreditation.

Related Programs Marriage and Family Therapists
Psychology
Psychiatric Nurses
Psychiatrists

Faculty

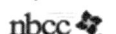 Percent of faculty reported with NCC certification: 25%.

Percent in professional counseling practice: NP.

Research interests Carl Rogers and the Person-Centered Apporach; ADHD and new directions in mental health; African-American students' adjustment to college; gerontology; values and character development; body-mind connections; comprehensive school counseling

Diversity   • African-American; Caucasian.

Name, Degree, Rank, State/National Credentials, % time devoted to program, email
• Kirschenbaum, Howard; EdD; Assoc.; >81%; *Howard.Kirschenbaum@rochester.edu*
• Barclay, Craig R; PhD; Assoc.; 41-60%; *crba@troi.cc.rochester.edu*
• Dannefer, Dale; PhD; Full Prof.; 41-60%; *dane@troi.cc.rochester.edu*
• Douthit, Kathryn Z; PhD; Assist.; NY School Couns.; >81%; *duth@troi.cc.rochester.edu*
• Guiffrida, Doug; PhD; Assist.; NCC; >81%; *douglas.guiffrida@rochester.edu*
• Rubenstein, Bonnie J; EdD; Assist.; NY School Couns.; 41-60%; *brubenstein@rcsdk12.org*
• Rubenstein, Gerald; EdD; Assoc.; 41-60%; *grubens1@rochester.rr.com*
• Mackie, Karen L; PhD; Instructor; NCC, NY School Couns.; 41-60%; *makk@troi.cc.rochester.edu*
• Jefferson, Jr., Frederick C; EdD; Full Prof.; <21%; *jeff8366@aol.com*
• Gray, Susan; PhD; Adjunct; Lic.Psych; <21%; *susan_gray@penfield.monroe.edu*
• Stein, Paul; PhD; Adjunct; <21%; *pstn@troi.cc.rochester.edu*
• Linnenberg, Dan M; EdD; Adjunct; LPC, NCC, Lic. Social Worker; <21%; *DMCGL1772@aol.com*

Has CHI SIGMA IOTA (International Counseling Society) chapter.

OH: Cleveland State University

RT 1419, 2121 Euclid Ave.
Cleveland, OH 44115-2214
USA

Dean   James McLoughlin, College of Education
Administrator   Elliott Ingersoll, Chairperson
                    Department   CASAL
                                  (216) 687-4612, fax (216) 687-5378

Key   See key for Data on Each Department (this section) on page 79.

Program

Accreditation   Regional Accreditation, **CACREP:** Community Counseling, **CACREP:** School Counseling

Uniqueness   The program prepares school and agency counselors for work in an urban setting. The faculty
                 are well published and adhere to high standards in teaching.

Degrees   • Community Counseling: M.
                 • School Counseling: M.

Contact   • Community Counseling: M = Kathy MacCluskie.
                 • School Counseling: M = Elliott Ingersoll.

Admission and Graduation Data

Admission
Requirements   • Community Counseling(M): GPA 2.75; GRE V no cutoff; MAT R.
                 • School Counseling(M): GPA 2.75; GRE V No cutoff; MAT R.

Enrollment   • Community Counseling(M): 30 Admitted yearly; 26 Graduated yearly.
                 • School Counseling(M): 30 Admitted yearly; 26 Graduated yearly.

Diversity   • African-American; Caucasian; Hispanic; Multiracial.

Graduation
Requirements   • Community Counseling(M): 60 Class hours; 100 Practicum hours; 600 Internship hours;
                   Comprehensive exam.
                 • School Counseling(M): 48 Class hours; 100 Practicum hours; 600 Internship hours;
                   Comprehensive exam.

Postgraduation activity: Advanced education and employment setting percentages.
                 • Community Counseling(M): NP.
                 • School Counseling(M): NP.

Planned Program Modifications

Courses   Drop   Add
                 • NP.   • NP.

Other   Decrease   Increase
                 • NP.   • NP.

Related Programs

Faculty

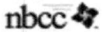   Percent of faculty reported with NCC certification: 50%.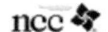

Percent in professional counseling practice: 30%.

Research interests Psychopharmacology, Ethics, Counseling and Spirituality, Psychodynamic approaches to
                   counseling, Gestalt therapy, Career Development, Multicultural counseling, and
                   Community Crisis Response.

Diversity   • Caucasian; Hispanic.

Name, Degree, Rank, State/National Credentials, % time devoted to program, email
• Bauer, Ann; PhD; Assist.; School Counseling; >81%; *a.l.bauer@csuohio.edu*
• Ingersoll, Elliott; PhD; Assoc.; NCC, PCC, psychologist; 41-60%; *r.ingersoll@csuohio.edu*
• MacCluskie, Kathryn; PhD; Assoc.; Psychologist; >81%; *k.maccluskie@csuohio.edu*
• Quinones-Delvalle, Rose; PhD; Assist.; NCC, PCC; >81%; *r.quinonesdelvalle@csuohio.edu*
• Rak, Carl; PhD; Assoc.; PCC; 41-60%; *c.rak@csuohio.edu*
• Schultheiss, Donna; PhD; Assist.; NCC, School Psychologist; >81%; *d.schultheiss@csuohio.edu*
• Toman, Sarah; PhD; Assoc.; NCC, psychologist; *s.toman@csuohio.edu*
• Welfel, Elizabeth; PhD; Full Prof.; psychologist; >81%; *e.welfel@csuohio.edu*

Has CHI SIGMA IOTA (International Counseling Society) chapter.

OH: John Carroll University

20700 North Park Blvd.
Cleveland, OH 44118-4581
USA
Dean   Mary Beadle, PhD, Graduate School
Administrator   Christopher M. Faiver, PhD, Coordinator, Counselor Education Program
    Department   Education and Allied Studies
        (216) 397-4331, fax (216) 397-3045, Faiver@JCU.EDU,
        WWW.JCU.EDU/Graduate

Key   See key for Data on Each Department (this section) on page 79.

Program

Accreditation   Regional Accreditation, **CACREP:** Community Counseling

CACREP

Uniqueness   John Carroll University is a Jesuit institution which follows the precept of "persons for others." Thus, the Counselor Education program endeavors to train professional community and school counselors who embody this essence. The University is located in University Heights, a lovely suburb of Cleveland.

Degrees
- Community Counseling: M.
- School Counseling: M.

Contact
- Community Counseling: M = Christopher M. Faiver, PhD.
- School Counseling: M = David C. Helsel, PhD.

Admission and Graduation Data

Admission

Requirements
- Community Counseling(M): GPA 2.75; GRE 1000; MAT 50; Interview.
- School Counseling(M): GPA 2.75; GRE 1000; MAT 50; 2 Years work experience; Interview.

Enrollment
- Community Counseling(M): 35 Admitted yearly; 35 Graduated yearly; 75 Female; 25 Male.
- School Counseling(M): 20 Admitted yearly; 15 Graduated yearly; 5 Male.

Diversity
- African-American; Asian-American; Caucasian; Hispanic.

Graduation

Requirements
- Community Counseling(M): 60 Class hours; 150 Practicum hours; 600 Internship hours; Comprehensive exam; CPCE.
- School Counseling(M): 48 Class hours; 150 Practicum hours; 600 Internship hours; Comprehensive exam.

Postgraduation activity: Advanced education and employment setting percentages.
- Community Counseling(M): 10 Managed care; 10 Private practice; 75 Agency practice.
- School Counseling(M): 20 Elementary school; 20 Middle school; 60 Secondary school.

Planned Program Modifications

Courses	Drop	Add
	• NP.	• NP.

Other	Decrease	Increase
	• NP.	• Diversity Recruiting of Faculty
		• Diversity Recruiting of Students
		• Financial Aid
		• National Accreditation
		• Number of Degree Majors
		• Number of Distance Education Courses.

Related Programs

Faculty

nbcc   Percent of faculty reported with NCC certification: 30%.   **ncc**

Percent in professional counseling practice: 50%.

Research interests   Women's issues, diversity issues, HIV and AIDs, Clinical Hypnosis, Sports Counseling, ADHD, Forgiveness, Wellness, Spirituality and Counseling, Victimology, Grief issues, Internship, Consultation and Supervision, Ethics, Stress Management, Testing, Eating Disorders, among others

Diversity
- African-American; Asian-American; Caucasian.

Name, Degree, Rank, State/National Credentials, % time devoted to program, email

- Britton, Paula J; PhD; Assoc.; LPC, NCC, Psych OH; >81%; *PBritton@EDU*
- Faiver, Christopher M; PhD; Full Prof.; LPC, NCC, ASCH Clinical Consultant, NRHSPP, Psych OH; >81%; *Faiver@JCU.EDU*
- Helsel, David C; PhD; Assist.; LPC, NCC; >81%; *DHelsel@JCU.EDU*
- Taylor, Nancy P; PhD; Assist.; LPC, Psych OH; >81%; *NTaylor@JCU.EDU*
- Guidubaldi, John; EdD; Full Prof.; LPC, Psych OH; 61-80%; *JGuidubaldi@JCU.EDU*
- Jenkins, Jeanne E; PhD; Assoc.; Sch Psych OH; 61-80%; *JJenkins@JCU.EDU*
- Harsch, Dawn; MA; Assist.; LPC; 61-80%; *DHarsch@JCU.EDU*
- Rausch, John; PhD; Assist.; 61-80%; *JRausch@JCU.EDU*
- Harris, Phyllis B; PhD; Full Prof.; LISW; <21%; *PHarris@JCU.EDU*
- Ropar, John; PhD; Instructor; LPC; <21%; *JRopar@JCU.EDU*

Has CHI SIGMA IOTA (International Counseling Society) chapter.

OH: Kent State University

	P.O. Box 5190
	Kent, OH 44242-0001
	USA
Dean	Dean David England, College and Graduate School of Education
Administrator	Dr. Donald Bubenzer, Department Chairperson
	Department ACHVE
	(330) 672-2692, fax (330) 672-3063

Key   See key for Data on Each Department (this section) on page 79.

Program

Accreditation   Regional Accreditation, **CACREP:** Community Counseling, **CACREP:** Counselor Education and Supervision, **CACREP:** School Counseling

Uniqueness   NP.

Degrees
- Community Counseling: M.
- School Counseling: M.
- Other: S.
- Counselor Education: PhD.

Contact
- Community Counseling: M = Dr. Jason McGlothlin.
- School Counseling: M = Dr. Jason McGlothlin.
- Other: S = NP.
- Counselor Education: D = Dr. John West.

Admission and Graduation Data

Admission

Requirements
- Community Counseling(M): GPA 2.75; Interview.
- School Counseling(M): GPA 2.75; Interview.
- Other(S): GPA 2.75; Interview.
- Counselor Education(D): Masters and GPA 3.50; GRE V 550; Interview.

Enrollment
- Community Counseling(M): 40 Admitted yearly; 34 Graduated yearly; 90 Female; 30 Male.
- School Counseling(M): 32 Admitted yearly; 25 Graduated yearly; 52 Female; 5 Male.
- Other(S): 7 Admitted yearly; 4 Graduated yearly; 9 Female; 1 Male.
- Counselor Education(D): 14 Admitted yearly; 10 Graduated yearly; 62 Female; 18 Male.

Diversity
- African-American; Asian-American; Caucasian; Hispanic; Multiracial; Other.

Graduation

Requirements
- Community Counseling(M): 60 Class hours; 100 Practicum hours; 600 Internship hours.
- School Counseling(M): 49 Class hours; 100 Practicum hours; 600 Internship hours.
- Other(S):
- Counselor Education(D): 110 Class hours; 600 Internship hours; Comprehensive exam; Oral exam; Dissertation.

Postgraduation activity: Advanced education and employment setting percentages.
- Community Counseling(M): 12 Advanced education; 5 Managed care; 75 Agency practice; 8 Other.
- School Counseling(M): 35 Elementary school; 25 Middle school; 40 Secondary school.
- Other(S).
- Counselor Education(D): 4 Managed care; 10 Private practice; 35 Agency practice; 2 Elementary school; 2 Middle school; 2 Secondary school; 45 Student affairs.

Planned Program Modifications

Courses	Drop	Add
	• NP.	• NP.

Other	Decrease	Increase
	• NP.	• Faculty FTE
		• Financial Aid.

Related Programs NP.

Faculty

 Percent of faculty reported with NCC certification: 9%.

Percent in professional counseling practice: 0%.

Research interests Research interests include: group work, supervision of counseling, crisis intervention, school counselor preparation, multicultrual counseling skill training, CACREP standards, substance abuse, family counseling, and integration of technology in counseling and counselor education

Diversity • Caucasian.

Name, Degree, Rank, State/National Credentials, % time devoted to program, email
• Bubenzer, Donald; PhD; Full Prof.; LPC; >81%; *dbubenze@kent.edu*
• Jencius, Marty J; PhD; Assist.; >81%; *mjencius@kent.edu*
• McGlothlin, Jason M; PhD; Assist.; LPC; >81%; *jmcgloth@kent.edu*
• Osborn, Cynthia J; PhD; Assoc.; >81%; *cosborn@kent.edu*
• Page, Betsy J; EdD; Assoc.; NCC, LPCC; Supervising Counselor OH; ACS (NBCC); >81%; *bpage@kent.edu*
• Rainey, John S; PhD; Assist.; >81%; *jrainey@kent.edu*
• Silverberg, Robert A; PhD; Assoc.; >81%; *rsilverb@kent.edu*
• West, John D; EdD; Full Prof.; LPC; >81%; *jwest@kent.edu*
• Savickas, Mark L; PhD; Adjunct; LPC; <21%; *msavakas@kent.edu*
• Nemec, William; PhD; LPC; <21%; *wnemec@kent.edu*
• Guillot-Miller, Lynne; PhD; Assist.

Has CHI SIGMA IOTA (International Counseling Society) chapter.

OH: Malone College

Dean
Administrator

515 25th Street, NW
Canton, OH 44709-3897
USA
Dr. Marietta Dalton
Kenneth G. McCurdy, Ph.D., Director of the Graduate Program in Counselor Education
Department   Counselor Education
(330) 471-8224, fax (330) 471-8343, www.malone.edu

Key   See key for Data on Each Department (this section) on page 79.

Program
Accreditation   Regional Accreditation

Uniqueness   Malone College Counselor Education Program prepares professional counselors through a
Christian foundation.

Degrees   • Community Counseling: M.
• School Counseling: M.

Contact   • Community Counseling: M = Dr. Dan Merz.
• School Counseling: M = Dr. Ken McCurdy.

Admission and Graduation Data
Admission
Requirements   • Community Counseling(M): GPA 3.00; Interview.
• School Counseling(M): GPA 3.00; Interview.

Enrollment   • Community Counseling(M): 15-20 Admitted yearly; 10-15 Graduated yearly; 90% Female;
10% Male.
• School Counseling(M): 15-20 Admitted yearly; 10-15 Graduated yearly; 80% Female;
20% Male.

Diversity   • African-American; Asian-American; Caucasian; Multiracial.

Graduation
Requirements   • Community Counseling(M): 48+12 Class hours; 100 Practicum hours; 600 Internship
hours.
• School Counseling(M): 48 Class hours; 100 Practicum hours; 600 Internship hours.

Postgraduation activity: Advanced education and employment setting percentages.
• Community Counseling(M): 5 Advanced education; 85 Agency practice; 10 Other.
• School Counseling(M): 10 Advanced education; 25 Elementary school; 25 Middle school;
40 Secondary school.

Planned Program Modifications
Courses   Drop   Add
• NP.   • Supervision.

Other   Decrease   Increase
• NP.   • Admission Requirements
• Clinical Supervision
• Diversity Recruiting of Faculty
• Diversity Recruiting of Students
• Faculty FTE.

Related Programs

Faculty

nbcc ❧   Percent of faculty reported with NCC certification: 50%.   ncc ❧

Percent in professional counseling practice: 0%.

Research interests

Diversity   • Caucasian.

Name, Degree, Rank, State/National Credentials, % time devoted to program, email
• Merz, Daniel R; PhD; Assoc.; LPCC; >81%; *dmerz@malone.edu*
• McCurdy, Kenneth G; PhD; Assist.; NCC, LPCC, ACS; >81%; *kmccurdy@malone.edu*

OH: Ohio University

201 McCracken Hall
Athens, OH 45701-2979
USA

Dean   James Heap
Administrator   Thomas Davis Ph.D. PCC, Chair
                    Department   Dept of Counseling & Higher Education
                    (740) 593-4440, http://www.ohiou.edu/education/index.html

Key   See key for Data on Each Department (this section) on page 79.

Program

Accreditation   **CACREP:** Community Counseling, **CACREP:** Counselor Education and Supervision,
                 CACREP: School Counseling, **CORE:** Rehabilitation Counseling

Uniqueness   Close Faculty-student interaction. Aid in the design of one's program to fit own personal goal.

Degrees   • Community Counseling: M.
                 • School Counseling: M.
                 • Rehabilitation Counseling: M.
                 • Counselor Education: PhD.

Contact   • Community Counseling: M = Pat Beamish.
                 • School Counseling: M = Tracy Leinbaugh.
                 • Rehabilitation Counseling: M = Jerry Olsheski.
                 • Counselor Education: D = Tom Davis.

Admission and Graduation Data

Admission

Requirements   • Community Counseling(M): GPA 3.00; GRE 900.
                 • School Counseling(M): GPA 3.00; GRE 900.
                 • Rehabilitation Counseling(M): GPA 3.00; GRE 900.
                 • Counselor Education(D): GRE 1000; GRE V 500; GRE Q 500.

Enrollment   • Community Counseling(M): 30 Admitted yearly; 25 Graduated yearly; 20 Female; 10 Male.
                 • School Counseling(M): 8 Admitted yearly; 8 Graduated yearly.
                 • Rehabilitation Counseling(M): 7 Admitted yearly; 7 Graduated yearly.
                 • Counselor Education(D): 12 Admitted yearly; 12 Graduated yearly.

Diversity   • African-American; Asian-American; Caucasian; Hispanic; Native American; Multiracial.

Graduation

Requirements   • Community Counseling(M): NP.
                 • School Counseling(M): NP.
                 • Rehabilitation Counseling(M): NP.
                 • Counselor Education(D): 720 Internship hours; Comprehensive exam; Dissertation.

Postgraduation activity: Advanced education and employment setting percentages.
                 • Community Counseling(M): NP.
                 • School Counseling(M): NP.
                 • Rehabilitation Counseling(M): NP.
                 • Counselor Education(D):

Planned Program Modifications

Courses   Drop   Add
                 • NP.   • NP.

Other   Decrease   Increase
                 • NP.   • NP.

Related Programs

Faculty

nbcc ❖   Percent of faculty reported with NCC certification: 30%.   **ncc** ❖

Percent in professional counseling practice: NP.

Research interests NP.

Diversity   •   African-American; Caucasian; Multiracial.

Name, Degree, Rank, State/National Credentials, % time devoted to program, email
- Beamish, Patricia; EdD; Assoc.; LPC; >81%; *beamish@ohio.edu*
- Davis, Thomas; PhD; Full Prof.; LPC; >81%; *davist@ohio.edu*
- Doston, Glenn; PhD; Full Prof.; >81%; *doston@ohio.edu*
- Hazler, Richard; EdD; Full Prof.; LPC, NCC; >81%; *hazler@ohio.edu*
- Leinbaugh, Tracy; PhD; Assist.; LPC, NCC; >81%; *leinbaug@ohio.edu*
- Sweeney, Thomas; PhD; Adjunct; 22-40%;
- Levitt, Dana; PhD; Assist.; >81%; *levitt@ohio.edu*
- Stump, Earl; PhD; Instructor; LPC; *Stump@ohio.edu*
- Olsheski, Jerry; PhD; Assoc.; LPC; >81%; *olsheski@ohio.edu*
- Kline, Bill; PhD; Full Prof.; LPC; NCC; CCMHO; *klineb@ohio.edu*

Has CHI SIGMA IOTA (International Counseling Society) chapter.

OH: The University of Toledo

Mail Stop 119
Toledo, OH 43606-3390
U.S.A.
Dean   Jerome Sullivan Health & Human Services Bldg
Administrator   Nick J. Piazza, Chairperson
            Department   Counseling and Mental Health Services
                          (419) 530-2718, fax (419) 530-7879, sue.martin@utoledo.edu,
                          http://cmhs.utoledo.edu

Key   See key for Data on Each Department (this section) on page 79.

Program

Accreditation   **CACREP:** Counselor Education and Supervision, **CACREP:** School Counseling, **CACREP:**
                 Community Counseling

Uniqueness   All programs are accredited and meet licensure requirements in Ohio and Michigan.
                 Opportunities for international students and for international experiences for students.

Degrees   • Community Counseling: M, PhD.
                 • School Counseling: M, PhD.

Contact   • Community Counseling: M = Paula Dupuy.; D = Nick Piazza.
                 • School Counseling: M = Martin Ritchie.; D = Nick Piazza.

Admission and Graduation Data

Admission
Requirements   • Community Counseling(M): GPA 3.00; GRE 800; Interview.
                 • Community Counseling(D): Masters and GPA 3.00; GRE 1040; 2 Years work experience.
                 • School Counseling(M): GPA 3.00; GRE 800; Interview.
                 • School Counseling(D): Masters and GPA 3.00; GRE 1040; 2 Years work experience.

Enrollment   • Community Counseling(M): 20 Admitted yearly; 18 Graduated yearly; 13 Female; 7 Male.
                 • Community Counseling(D): 10 Admitted yearly; 8 Graduated yearly; 5 Female; 5 Male.
                 • School Counseling(M): 20 Admitted yearly; 18 Graduated yearly; 8 Male.
                 • School Counseling(D): 4 Admitted yearly; 3 Graduated yearly; 3 Female; 1 Male.

Diversity   • African-American; Asian-American; Caucasian; Hispanic; Native American; Multiracial.

Graduation
Requirements   • Community Counseling(M): 48 Class hours; 100 Practicum hours; 600 Internship hours.
                 • Community Counseling(D): 96 Class hours; 100 Practicum hours; 600 Internship hours;
                   Comprehensive exam; Oral exam; Dissertation.
                 • School Counseling(M): 48 Class hours; 100 Practicum hours; 600 Internship hours.
                 • School Counseling(D): 96 Class hours; 100 Practicum hours; 600 Internship hours; Oral
                   exam; Dissertation.

Postgraduation activity: Advanced education and employment setting percentages.
                 • Community Counseling(M): 5 Advanced education; 20 Managed care; 5 Private practice;
                   70 Agency practice.
                 • Community Counseling(D): 10 Managed care; 70 Private practice; 20 Agency practice.
                 • School Counseling(M): 2 Advanced education; 40 Elementary school; 18 Middle school; 40
                   Secondary school.
                 • School Counseling(D): 20 Private practice; 80 Agency practice.

Planned Program Modifications

Courses   Drop   Add
                 • NP.   • Addictions
                                                    • Marriage and Family Counseling.

Other   Decrease   Increase
                 • NP.   • Course Offerings
                                                    • Diversity Recruiting of Faculty
                                                    • Diversity Recruiting of Students
                                                    • Financial Aid
                                                    • Number of Distance Education Courses
                                                    • Number of On-Line Courses.

Related Programs Clinical Social Workers
                     Psychology

Faculty

   Percent of faculty reported with NCC certification: 11%.

Percent in professional counseling practice: NP.

Research interests Multicultural and gender issues; Legal and ethical issues; Substance abuse; Assessing counseling effectiveness

Diversity   • Caucasian.

Name, Degree, Rank, State/National Credentials, % time devoted to program, email
- Dupuy, Paula; EdD; Full Prof.; LPC, PCC; >81%; *paula.dupuy@utoledo.edu*
- Laux, John; PhD; Assist.; LPC, PCC; >81%; *john.laux@utoledo.edu*
- Lewton, John; PhD; Full Prof.; LPC, PCC; >81%; *john.lewton@utoledo.edu*
- Piazza, Nick; EdD; Full Prof.; LPC, PCC; >81%; *nick.piazza@utoledo.edu*
- Ritchie, Martin; PhD; Full Prof.; LPC, NCC; >81%; *martin.ritchie@utoledo.edu*
- Salyers, Kathleen; PhD; Assist.; LPC, PCC; >81%; *kathleen.salyers@utoledo.edu*
- Seamon, Dan; PhD; Instructor; 22-40%; *dan.seamon@utoledo.edu*
- Wakelin, Cheryl; MA; Instructor; 41-60%; *cheryl.wakelin@utoledo.edu*
- Zake, Jerome; PhD; Instructor; >81%; *jerome.zake@utoledo.edu*

Has CHI SIGMA IOTA (International Counseling Society) chapter.

OH: University of Cincinnati

Teachers College 526
Cincinnati, OH 45221-0002
USA
Dean   Lawrence J. Johnson, College of Education
Administrator   Robert K. Conyne, Professor and Program Director
                      Department   Counseling Program in the Division of Human Services
                                      (513) 055-6333 Ext. 5, fax (513) 556-3898, conynerk@email.uc.edu,
                                      http://homepages.uc.edu/counseling/

Key   See key for Data on Each Department (this section) on page 79.

Program

Accreditation   Regional Accreditation, **CACREP:** Counselor Education and Supervision, **CACREP:** Mental
                 Health Counseling, **CACREP:** School Counseling

Uniqueness   Our accredited programs in School, Mental Health, and Counselor Education and Supervision
                 (Doctoral) emphasize an ecological orientation with a focus on diversity and the underserved.

Degrees   • Mental Health Counseling: M.
                 • School Counseling: M.
                 • Counselor Education: EdD.

Contact   • Mental Health Counseling: M = F. Robert Wilson, Ph.D.
                 • School Counseling: M = Mei Tang, Ph.D.
                 • Counselor Education: D = Ellen Cook, Ph.D.

Admission and Graduation Data

Admission

Requirements   • Mental Health Counseling(M): GPA 2.80; GRE 1500; GRE V 500; GRE Q 500; GRE A 500;
                   Interview.
                 • School Counseling(M): GPA 2.80; GRE 1500; GRE V 500; GRE Q 500; GRE A 500;
                   Interview.
                 • Counselor Education(D): Masters and GPA 3.20; GRE 1500; GRE V 500; GRE Q 500;
                   GRE A 500; 1 Year work experience.

Enrollment   • Mental Health Counseling(M): 20 Admitted yearly; 15 Graduated yearly; 40 Female; 5
                   Male.
                 • School Counseling(M): 20 Admitted yearly; 8 Graduated yearly; 14 Female; 4 Male.
                 • Counselor Education(D): 8 Admitted yearly; 3 Graduated yearly; 19 Female; 10 Male.

Diversity   • African-American; Caucasian; Hispanic; Native American; Multiracial.

Graduation

Requirements   • Mental Health Counseling(M): 100 Practicum hours; 900 Internship hours; Comprehensive
                   exam; CPCE.
                 • School Counseling(M): 100 Practicum hours; 600 Internship hours; Comprehensive exam;
                   CPCE.
                 • Counselor Education(D): 1000 Practicum hours; 600 Internship hours; Comprehensive
                   exam; Oral exam; Dissertation; Portfolio.

Postgraduation activity: Advanced education and employment setting percentages.
                 • Mental Health Counseling(M): 25 Advanced education; 5 Managed care; 5 Private practice;
                   55 Agency practice; 10 Other.
                 • School Counseling(M): 33 Elementary school; 33 Middle school; 33 Secondary school.
                 • Counselor Education(D): 10 Managed care; 25 Private practice; 40 Agency practice; 25
                   Student affairs.

Planned Program Modifications

Courses	Drop	Add
	• NP.	• NP.

Other	Decrease	Increase
	• NP.	• Diversity Recruiting of Faculty
		• Diversity Recruiting of Students
		• Number of Distance Education Courses
		• Number of On-Line Courses.

Related Programs Clinical Social Workers
Psychology
Psychiatric Nurses
Psychiatrists
Communications

Faculty

 Percent of faculty reported with NCC certification: 43%.

Percent in professional counseling practice: 50%.

Research interests Ecological counseling, Supervision, Problem-based learning, Mental Health Services to the Underserved, Career Development, Group Work, Prevention.

Diversity • African-American; Asian-American; Caucasian.

Name, Degree, Rank, State/National Credentials, % time devoted to program, email
• Conyne, Robert K; PhD; Full Prof.; LPC, NCC, ACS; Psy.; >81%; *robert.conyne@uc.edu*
• Cook, Ellen P; PhD; Full Prof.; LPC, Psy.; >81%; *ellen.cook@uc.edu*
• Tang, Mei; PhD; Assist.; >81%; *mei.tang@uc.edu*
• Watson, Albert L; PhD; Assoc.; LPC; >81%; *albert.l.watson@uc.edu*
• Wilson, F. Robert; PhD; Full Prof.; LPC, NCC, ACS; >81%; *wilsonfr@email.uc.edu*
• Yager, Geoffrey G; PhD; Full Prof.; LPC, NCC, ACS; Psy.; >81%; *geof.yager@uc.edu*
• Rapin, Lynn S; PhD; Lecturer; LPC, Psy.; <21%; *rapinls@email.uc.edu*

Has CHI SIGMA IOTA (International Counseling Society) chapter.

OH: Walsh University

2020 Easton Street N.W.
North Canton, OH 44720-3396
USA

Dean
Administrator   Linda L. Barclay Ph.D., Coordinator, CHD Program
Department   Dept of Graduate Studies
(330) 490-7231, fax (330) 490-7165, lbarclay@walsh.edu, www.walsh.edu

Key   See key for Data on Each Department (this section) on page 79.

Program
Accreditation

Uniqueness   A program designed for evening study on a half-time basis. Small student to teacher ratio. Master's level program for mental health counselor training and school counseling.

Degrees   • Mental Health Counseling: M.
            • School Counseling: M.

Contact   • Mental Health Counseling: M = Linda L. Barclay Ph.D.
            • School Counseling: M = Judy Green Ph.D.

Admission and Graduation Data
Admission
Requirements   • Mental Health Counseling(M): GPA 3.00; GRE 900; GRE V 450; GRE Q 450; GRE A 0; MAT 40; Interview.
            • School Counseling(M): GPA 3.00; GRE 900; GRE V 450; GRE Q 450; GRE A 0; MAT 40; Interview.

Enrollment   • Mental Health Counseling(M): 10-15 Admitted yearly; 8-10 Graduated yearly.
            • School Counseling(M): 12 Admitted yearly; 10-12 Graduated yearly.

Diversity   • African-American; Caucasian.

Graduation
Requirements   • Mental Health Counseling(M): 60 Class hours; 100 Practicum hours; 600 Internship hours; Comprehensive exam; CPCE.
            • School Counseling(M): 48 Class hours; 100 Practicum hours; 600 Internship hours; Comprehensive exam; CPCE.

Postgraduation activity: Advanced education and employment setting percentages.
            • Mental Health Counseling(M): 10 Advanced education; 5 Managed care; 5 Private practice; 80 Agency practice.
            • School Counseling(M): 20 Elementary school; 20 Middle school; 60 Secondary school.

Planned Program Modifications
Courses   Drop   Add
            • NP.   • NP.

Other   Decrease   Increase
            • NP.   • Diversity Recruiting of Faculty
                  • Diversity Recruiting of Students
                  • National Accreditation
                  • Number of Distance Education Courses.

Related Programs

Faculty

 Percent of faculty reported with NCC certification: 22%.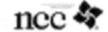

Percent in professional counseling practice: 90%.

Research interests Book under contract: Mental Health Counseling: An Introduction to Clinical Practice

Diversity   • Caucasian.

Name, Degree, Rank, State/National Credentials, % time devoted to program, email
• Barclay, Linda; Other; LPC, NCC; 61-80%; *lbarclay@walsh.edu*
• Humphrey, Robert; PhD; Lic. Psych.; <21%; *bhumphrey@walsh.edu*
• Humphries, Gerry; PhD; <21%;
• Green, Judy; PhD; LPC, NCC; >81%; *jgreen@walsh.edu*

- Roberts Martin, Rebecca; PhD (Cand.); LPC; >81%; *rrobertsmartin@walsh.edu*
- Putt, Geoffrey; PsyD; Lic. Psych.; <21%;
- Willcoxson, Milli; PhD; Lic. Psych.; <21%;
- Parvinbenam, Daryush; Other; LPC; <21%;
- Wroblewski, David; Other; <21%;

Has CHI SIGMA IOTA (International Counseling Society) chapter.

OH: Xavier University

3800 Victory Parkway
Cincinnati, OH 45207-6612
United States
Dean   Dr. Neil Heighberger
Administrator   Lon S. Kriner, PhD, Director, Graduate Counseling Programs
                      Department   Education
                                     (513) 745-3822, fax (513) 745-2920, kriner@xavier.edu, www.xu.edu

Key   See key for Data on Each Department (this section) on page 79.

Program
Accreditation   Regional Accreditation; Applied for **CACREP:** Community Counseling, **CACREP:** School
                 Counseling

Uniqueness   Programs in both M.Ed. In School Counseling and M.A. in Community Counseling are tailored
                 for the part-time student.

Degrees   • Community Counseling: M.
                 • School Counseling: M.

Contact   • Community Counseling: M = Lon S. Kriner, PhD.
                 • School Counseling: M = Lon S. Kriner, PhD.

Admission and Graduation Data
Admission
Requirements   • Community Counseling(M): GPA 2.7+; GRE A 500 or; MAT 35; Interview.
                 • School Counseling(M): GPA 2.7+; GRE A 500 or; MAT 35; Interview.

Enrollment   • Community Counseling(M): 75 Admitted yearly; 30 Graduated yearly; 70% Female; 30%
                   Male.
                 • School Counseling(M): 75 Admitted yearly; 30 Graduated yearly; 70% Female; 30% Male.

Diversity   • African-American; Asian-American; Caucasian; Hispanic.

Graduation
Requirements   • Community Counseling(M): 60 Class hours; 100 Practicum hours; 600 Internship hours.
                 • School Counseling(M): 48 Class hours; 100 Practicum hours; 600 Internship hours.

Postgraduation activity: Advanced education and employment setting percentages.
                 • Community Counseling(M): 10 Advanced education; 10 Managed care; 5 Private practice;
                   70 Agency practice; 5 Other.
                 • School Counseling(M): 10 Advanced education; 20 Elementary school; 20 Middle school;
                   25 Secondary school; 20 Other.

Planned Program Modifications
Courses   Drop   Add
                 • NP.   • NP.

Other   Decrease   Increase
                 • NP.   • Admission Requirements
                                                   • Clinical Supervision
                                                   • National Accreditation.

Related Programs Psychology

Faculty

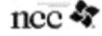 Percent of faculty reported with NCC certification: **100%**.

Percent in professional counseling practice: 100%.

Research interests Counseling challenging youth, supervision in counseling, counseling chronically ill children
                   and families

Diversity   • African-American; Caucasian.

Name, Degree, Rank, State/National Credentials, % time devoted to program, email
• Kriner, Lon S; PhD; Assoc.; PCC; >81%; *kriner@xavier.edu*
• Richardson, Brent G; EdD; Assoc.; PCC; >81%; *richardb@xavier.edu*
• Shupe, Margery; EdD; Assist.; PCC; >81%; *shupe@xavier.edu*
• O'Connell, Silliam P; EdD; Assist.; LPC, PCC; >81%; *o'connell@xavier.edu*
• Norman, Rhonda; EdD; PCC

Has CHI SIGMA IOTA (International Counseling Society) chapter.

OH: Youngstown State University

	1 University Plaza
	Youngstown, OH 44555
	USA
Dean	Dr. Phil Ginnetti, College of Education
Administrator	Dr. Don Martin, Chairperson
	Department Counseling
	(330) 941-3257, fax (330) 941-2369, dmartin@ysu.edu,
	www.cc.ysu.edu/counseling

Key   See key for Data on Each Department (this section) on page 79.

Program

Accreditation   Regional Accreditation, **CACREP:** Community Counseling, **CACREP:** School Counseling

Uniqueness   Our program is focused on issues of poverty particularly related to both urban and rural poor. We have an active community clinic and a large number of assistantships.

Degrees
- Community Counseling: M.
- School Counseling: M.
- Student Affairs: M.

Contact
- Community Counseling: M = Dr. Don Martin.
- School Counseling: M = NP.
- Student Affairs: M = NP.

Admission and Graduation Data

Admission

Requirements
- Community Counseling(M): GPA 3.00; GRE 450; GRE V 450; GRE Q 450; GRE A 450; MAT 40; Interview.
- School Counseling(M): GRE same; Interview.
- Student Affairs(M): GRE same; Interview.

Enrollment
- Community Counseling(M): 50 Admitted yearly; 25 Graduated yearly; 70 Female; 20 Male.
- School Counseling(M): 20 Admitted yearly; 10 Graduated yearly.
- Student Affairs(M): NP.

Diversity
- African-American; Asian-American; Caucasian; Hispanic; Native American; Pacific Islander; Multiracial.

Graduation

Requirements
- Community Counseling(M): 60-64 Class hours; 200 Practicum hours; 600 Internship hours; Comprehensive exam.
- School Counseling(M): 51 Class hours; 200 Practicum hours; 600 Internship hours; Comprehensive exam.
- Student Affairs(M): 36 Class hours; 200 Practicum hours; 600 Internship hours.

Postgraduation activity: Advanced education and employment setting percentages.
- Community Counseling(M): 5 Advanced education; 95 Agency practice; 30 Middle school; 40 Secondary school; 40 Student affairs; 100 Other.
- School Counseling(M): 5 Advanced education; 95 Elementary school.
- Student Affairs(M): 5 Advanced education; 95 Elementary school.

Planned Program Modifications

Courses	Drop	Add
	• NP.	• Abuse of Individual
		• Crisis/Violence Counseling
		• Gerontological Counseling
		• Play Therapy
		• Sports Counseling
		• Theory Component.

Other	Decrease	Increase
	• NP.	• Admission Requirements
		• Diversity Recruiting of Faculty
		• Diversity Recruiting of Students
		• Faculty FTE
		• Number of Degree Majors.

Related Programs

Faculty

nbcc ♣   Percent of faculty reported with NCC certification: 57%.   ncc ♣

Percent in professional counseling practice: 80%.

Research interests character education, multicultural issues, domestic abuse, self mutilation, school violence and bullying, CFS

Diversity • African-American; Caucasian; Multiracial.

Name, Degree, Rank, State/National Credentials, % time devoted to program, email
- Carney, JoLynn; PhD; Assoc.; LPC, NCC; >81%; *jlcarney@ysu.edu*
- Ford, Stephanie; PhD; Assist.; LPC, NCC; >81%; *sjford@ysu.edu*
- Gill-Wigal, Jan; PhD; Full Prof.; LPC; >81%; *gawa@ysu.edu*
- Gallagher-Warden, Jherry; PhD; Full Prof.; LPC; *sagallag.ysu.edu*
- Miller, Jenneth; PhD; Assist.; LPC, NCC; *klmiller@ysu.edu*
- Martin, Don; PhD; Assoc.; LPC; *vewhite@ysu.edu*
- White, Vicki; PhD; Assist.; LPC, NCC; *ncrespo1@aol.com*

Has CHI SIGMA IOTA (International Counseling Society) chapter.

OR: George Fox University

12753 SW 68th Avenue
Portland, OR 97223
USA
Dean   James Foster
Administrator   Karin Jordan, Ph.D., Department Chair, Director
                    Department   Graduate Department of Counseling
                                      (503) 554-6104, fax (503) 554-6111, jfreitag@georgefox.edu,
                                      www.georgefox.edu/academics/graduate/counseling

Key   See key for Data on Each Department (this section) on page 79.

Program

Accreditation   Regional Accreditation

Uniqueness   Faculty are active clinicians and eductors; Integrative focus on the best counselor education in an atmosphere of Christian faith.

Degrees   • Mental Health Counseling: M.
                 • School Counseling: M.
                 • Marriage and Family Counseling: M.

Contact   • Mental Health Counseling: M = Karin Jordan, Director.
                 • School Counseling: M = Karin Jordan, Director.
                 • Marriage and Family Counseling: M = Karin Jordan, Director.

Admission and Graduation Data
Admission

Requirements   • Mental Health Counseling(M): GPA 2.70; Interview.
                 • School Counseling(M): GPA 2.70; Interview.
                 • Marriage and Family Counseling(M): GPA 2.70; Interview.

Enrollment   • Mental Health Counseling(M): 47 Admitted yearly; 25 Graduated yearly; 99 Female; 24 Male.
                 • School Counseling(M): 25 Admitted yearly; 7 Male.
                 • Marriage and Family Counseling(M): 40 Admitted yearly; 25 Graduated yearly; 73 Female; 22 Male.

Diversity   • African-American; Asian-American; Caucasian; Hispanic; Native American; Pacific Islander; Multiracial.

Graduation

Requirements   • Mental Health Counseling(M): 64 Class hours; 600 Internship hours.
                 • School Counseling(M): 60 Class hours; 200 Practicum hours; 600 Internship hours.
                 • Marriage and Family Counseling(M): 79 Class hours; 700 Internship hours.

Postgraduation activity: Advanced education and employment setting percentages.
                 • Mental Health Counseling(M): 1 Advanced education; 20 Private practice; 75 Agency practice; 21 Elementary school; 2 Other.
                 • School Counseling(M): NP.
                 • Marriage and Family Counseling(M): 1 Advanced education; 20 Private practice; 75 Agency practice; 2 Middle school; 2 Secondary school.

Planned Program Modifications

Courses   <u>Drop</u>   <u>Add</u>
                 • NP.   • NP.

Other   <u>Decrease</u>   <u>Increase</u>
                 • NP.   • National Accreditation.

Related Programs Psychology

Faculty

nbcc ❖   Percent of faculty reported with NCC certification: 0%.   ncc ❖
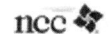

Percent in professional counseling practice: 70%.

Research interests Trauma (PTSD), Play Therapy, Spirituality Issues, Supervision, Program Distance Writing

Diversity   • African-American; Asian-American; Caucasian; Hispanic; Native American; Pacific Islander; Multiracial.

Name, Degree, Rank, State/National Credentials, % time devoted to program, email
- Bearden, Steve; PhD; Assist.; >81%;
- Maher, Anita B; PhD; Assist.; >81%;
- Michael, Rand; DMin; Assoc.; >81%;
- Shaw, Richard; DMFT; Assist.; LMHC; >81%;
- Jordan, Karin; PhD; Assist.; LMFT; >81%;
- Kelly, William; PhD; >81%;
- DeKruyf, Lorraine; MEd; >81%;

OR: Oregon State University

	Education Hall #210
	Corvallis, OR 97331-8536
	USA
Dean	Sam Stern - School of Education
Administrator	Gene Eakin, Ph.D., Program Coordinator
	Department Counselor Education & Supervision
	(541) 737-9215, fax (541) 737-2040, gene.eakin@orst.edu,
	http://oregonstate.edu/education/programs/counselorEd.html

Key   See key for Data on Each Department (this section) on page 79.

Program

Accreditation   Regional Accreditation, **CACREP:** Community Counseling, **CACREP:** School Counseling, **CACREP:** Counselor Education and Supervision

Uniqueness   The faculty and students honor lived experiences of all individuals and affirm the concepts of D.R.I.V.E: Dignity, Respect, Integrity, Value, and Equality.

Degrees
- Community Counseling: M.
- School Counseling: M.
- College Counseling: M.
- Counselor Education: PhD.

Contact
- Community Counseling: M = Gene Eakin.
- School Counseling: M = Gene Eakin.
- College Counseling: M = Gene Eakin.
- Counselor Education: D = Cass Dykeman.

Admission and Graduation Data
Admission
Requirements
- Community Counseling(M): GPA 3.00; Interview.
- School Counseling(M): GPA 3.00; Interview.
- College Counseling(M): GPA 3.00; Interview.
- Counselor Education(D): Masters and GPA 3.00.

Enrollment
- Community Counseling(M): 3 Admitted yearly; 3 Graduated yearly; 3 Female.
- School Counseling(M): 20 Admitted yearly; 20 Graduated yearly; 15 Female; 5 Male.
- College Counseling(M): 3 Admitted yearly; 3 Graduated yearly; 2 Female; 1 Male.
- Counselor Education(D): 4 Admitted yearly; 4 Graduated yearly; 12 Female.

Diversity
- Asian-American; Caucasian; Native American; Multiracial.

Graduation
Requirements
- Community Counseling(M): 100 Practicum hours; 600 Internship hours; Oral exam; Portfolio.
- School Counseling(M): 100 Practicum hours; 600 Internship hours; Oral exam; Portfolio.
- College Counseling(M): 100 Practicum hours; 600 Internship hours; Oral exam; Portfolio.
- Counselor Education(D): 600 Internship hours; Comprehensive exam; Oral exam; Dissertation.

Postgraduation activity: Advanced education and employment setting percentages.
- Community Counseling(M): 50 Agency practice; 50 Other.
- School Counseling(M): 30 Elementary school; 20 Middle school; 50 Secondary school.
- College Counseling(M): 100 Other.
- Counselor Education(D): 50 Private practice; 50 Student affairs.

Planned Program Modifications

Courses	Drop	Add
	• NP.	• Psychopharmacology.

Other	Decrease	Increase
	• NP.	• Clinical Supervision
		• Diversity Recruiting of Students.

Related Programs

Faculty

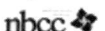   Percent of faculty reported with NCC certification: 60%.   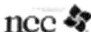

Percent in professional counseling practice: 0%.

Research interests School Counseling, Addictive Behavior, Career Counseling, Multi-Cultural Issues, Play Therapy, Group Process, Poetry Therapy

Diversity   • African-American; Caucasian; Multiracial.

Name, Degree, Rank, State/National Credentials, % time devoted to program, email
- Dykeman, C; PhD; Assoc.; NCC, MAC, NCSC; >81%; *dykemanc@onid.orst.edu*
- Eakin, Gene A; PhD; Instructor; TSPC; >81%; *gene.eakin@orst.edu*
- Ingram, Michael A; PhD; Assist.; >81%; *ingramm@orst.edu*
- Pehrsson, Dale E; PhD; Assist.; LPC, NCC, ACS, RN, RPTS; >81%; *dale.pehrsson@orst.edu*
- Rubel, Deborah J; PhD; Assist.; LPC, NCC; >81%; *deborah.rubel@oregonstate.edu*

Has CHI SIGMA IOTA (International Counseling Society) chapter.

OR: Portland State University

Graduate School of Education, PO Box 751
Portland, OR 97207
USA

Dean   Phyllis Edmundson, Portland, OR
Administrator   David Capuzzi, Ph.D., LPC, NCC, Coordinator, Counselor Education
       Department   Special and Counselor Education
                (503) 725-4619, fax (503) 725-5599, capuzzida@pdx.edu

Key   See key for Data on Each Department (this section) on page 79.

Program

Accreditation   Regional Accreditation, **CACREP:** Community Counseling, **CACREP:** School Counseling

CACREP

Uniqueness   The Counselor Education program offers specializations in school, community, rehabilitation and couples, marriage and family counseling. It is accredited by CACREP and CORE and in good standing with the licensure board. The in-house practicum clinic provides excellent supervision and receives referrals from schools and agencies from every sector of the city and surrounding areas. Internship placements abound and classes are formated for evenings and weekends. Faculty are personable and bring diverse life experiences and teaching styles to our students.

Degrees
- Community Counseling: M.
- School Counseling: M.
- Marriage and Family Counseling: M.
- Rehabilitation Counseling: M.

Contact
- Community Counseling: M = Capuzzi.
- School Counseling: M = Lewis, Halverson.
- Marriage and Family Counseling: M = Halverson, Capuzzi.
- Rehabilitation Counseling: M = Livneh.

Admission and Graduation Data

Admission

Requirements
- Community Counseling(M): GPA points assigned; GRE R; MAT same; Interview.
- School Counseling(M): GPA points assigned; GRE R; MAT same; Interview.
- Marriage and Family Counseling(M): GPA points assigned; GRE R; MAT same; Interview.
- Rehabilitation Counseling(M): GPA points assigned; GRE R; MAT same; Interview.

Enrollment
- Community Counseling(M): 14 Admitted yearly; 14-28 Graduated yearly; 75% Female; 25% Male.
- School Counseling(M): 14 Admitted yearly.
- Marriage and Family Counseling(M): 14 Admitted yearly.
- Rehabilitation Counseling(M): 14 Admitted yearly.

Diversity
- African-American; Asian-American; Caucasian; Hispanic; Native American; Pacific Islander; Multiracial.

Graduation

Requirements
- Community Counseling(M): 100 Practicum hours; 600 Internship hours; Comprehensive exam.
- School Counseling(M): 100 Practicum hours; 600 Internship hours; Comprehensive exam; Portfolio.
- Marriage and Family Counseling(M): 100 Practicum hours; 600 Internship hours; Comprehensive exam.
- Rehabilitation Counseling(M): 100 Practicum hours; 600 Internship hours; Comprehensive exam.

Postgraduation activity: Advanced education and employment setting percentages.
- Community Counseling(M): 10 Advanced education; 10 Managed care; 10 Private practice; 70 Agency practice.
- School Counseling(M): 20 Elementary school; 20 Middle school; 60 Secondary school.
- Marriage and Family Counseling(M): 10 Advanced education; 10 Managed care; 10 Private practice; 70 Agency practice.
- Rehabilitation Counseling(M): 10 Advanced education; 10 Managed care; 10 Private practice; 70 Agency practice.

Planned Program Modifications

Courses	Drop	Add
	• NP.	• NP.

Other	Decrease	Increase
	• NP.	• Financial Aid
		• Number of On-Line Courses.

Related Programs Clinical Social Workers

Faculty

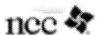 Percent of faculty reported with NCC certification: 25%.

Percent in professional counseling practice: 25%.

Research interests Psychosocial aspects of disability, youth at risk, grief and loss, suicide prevention, ethical decision-making, group work, theories of counseling and psychotherapy.

Diversity   • African-American; Asian-American; Caucasian; Native American; Other.

Name, Degree, Rank, State/National Credentials, % time devoted to program, email
• Halverson, Susan; PhD; Assist.; LPC; >81%; *halversons@pdx.edu*
• Capuzzi, David; PhD; Full Prof.; LPC, NCC; >81%; *capuzzida@pdx.edu*
• Lewis, Rolla; EdD; Assoc.; >81%; *lewisr@pdx.edu*
• Livneh, Hanoch; PhD; Full Prof.; LPC; >81%; *livnehh@pdx.edu*
• Miars, Russ; PhD; Assoc.; Lic. Psych; >81%; *miarsr@pdx.edu*
• Wosley-George, Liz; PhD; Assoc.; LPC, NCC; >81%; *wosleygeorgee@pdx.edu*
• Wilson, Lisa; PhD; Assist.; >81%; *wilsonlm@pdx.edu*
• Maynard, Glenn; MEd; Instructor; LPC; 41-60%; *maynardg@pdx.edu*

Has CHI SIGMA IOTA (International Counseling Society) chapter.

PA: Arcadia University

	450 South Easton Road Glenside, PA 19038 USA
Dean	Dr. Mark Curchack, Office of Graduate and Professional Studies
Administrator	Carol Lyman, MA., Administrator, M.A. in Counseling Program
	Department Psychology Department (215) 572-2988, fax (215) 572-8758, lyman@arcadia.edu, http://gargoyle.arcadia.edu/psychology

Key   See key for Data on Each Department (this section) on page 79.

Program

Accreditation   Regional Accreditation

Uniqueness   The Master of Arts in Counseling Program prepares students for jobs as community health specialists, mental health counselors, marriage and family counselors, crisis counselors, college counselors, employee-assistance counselors, staff developers or trainers, and school counselors.

Degrees
- Community Counseling: M, S.
- School Counseling: M.

Contact
- Community Counseling: M, S = Mrs. Carol Lyman.
- School Counseling: M = Mrs. Carol Lyman.

Admission and Graduation Data

Admission

Requirements
- Community Counseling(M): GPA 3.00; GRE R; MAT R; Interview.
- Community Counseling(S): GPA 3.00; GRE R; MAT R; Interview.
- School Counseling(M): GPA 3.00; GRE R; MAT R; Interview.

Enrollment
- Community Counseling(M & S): 14 (2001) Admitted yearly; 13 (2001) Graduated yearly; 30 Female; 5 Male.
- School Counseling(M): 17 (2001) Admitted yearly; 1 (2001) Graduated yearly; 5 Male.

Diversity
- African-American; Asian-American; Caucasian; Hispanic.

Graduation

Requirements
- Community Counseling(M): 48-60 Class hours; 100 Practicum hours; 300-600 Internship hours.
- Community Counseling(S): 12 Class hours.
- School Counseling(M): 54-57 Class hours; 100 Practicum hours; 300-600 Internship hours.

Postgraduation activity: Advanced education and employment setting percentages.
- Community Counseling(M & S): 10 Advanced education; 10 Managed care; 80 Agency practice.
- School Counseling(M): 60 Elementary school; 40 Secondary school.

Planned Program Modifications

Courses	Drop	Add
	• NP.	• Diversity.

Other	Decrease	Increase
	• NP.	• Number of Degree Majors.

Related Programs

Faculty

nbcc ❖   Percent of faculty reported with NCC certification: 0%.   ncc ❖

Percent in professional counseling practice: 50%.

Research interests NP.

Diversity
- African-American; Asian-American; Caucasian.

Name, Degree, Rank, State/National Credentials, % time devoted to program, email
- Blustein, Joshua; PhD; Assoc.; <21%; *blustein@arcadia.edu*
- Bowlan, Veronica; MSW; Lecturer; 22-40%; *Veronica.Bowlan@drexel.edu*
- Cameron, Samuel; PhD; Full Prof.; 41-60%; *cameron@arcadia.edu*
- Dickson, Dean; MS; Lecturer; <21%; *deanmarg@yahoo.com*
- Gallagher, Dennis; PhD; Assist.; <21%;

- Gillem, Angela; PhD; Assoc.; 41-60%; *gillem@arcadia.edu*
- Johnston, Scott; MEd; Lecturer; <21%; *sjonstonus@hotmail.com*
- Keithley, Kathryn; PsyD; Lecturer; <21%; *KdkPsyD@aol.com*
- Miller, Judith; PhD; Lecturer; 41-60%; *dovelane@aol.com*
- Minkoff, Hilda; EdD; Lecturer; 41-60%;
- Nicholls, Greg; PhD; Lecturer; <21%; *gnicholl@sju.edu*
- Rosenthal, Robert; PhD; Lecturer; <21%; *robertrosenthal@abington.k12.pa.us*
- Schwartz, Lisa; PhD; Lecturer; <21%; *lisabschwartz@mindspring.com*
- Sdorow, Lester; PhD; Lecturer; <21%; *lsdorow@aol.com*
- Snyder, Matthew; PhD; Lecturer; 41-60%; *snyder@sju.edu*
- Wadley, James; PhD; Lecturer; <21%; *phdcorby@msn.com*
- Whitehouse, Wayne; PhD; Lecturer; 22-40%; *whitehou@fast.net*
- Winn, Mary; MA; Lecturer; <21%; *mmrwinn@aol.com*

PA: California University of Pennsylvania

250 University Avenue, Box 13
California, PA 15419-1394
USA
Dean   Gerri Jones
Administrator   Gloria Cataldo Brusoski, Ph.D., Chairperson
            Department   Dept of Counselor Education
                           (724) 938-4123, fax (724) 938-4314, Brusoski@cup.edu,
                           http://www.cup.edu/graduate/counsed

Key   See key for Data on Each Department (this section) on page 79.

Program

Accreditation   Regional Accreditation; Applied for **CACREP:** Community Counseling

Uniqueness   1. Program emphasis on self-awareness. We require students to participate in a personal growth group, for credit, that is facilitated by a faculty member outside the department. This sets the tone, in which experiential activities are infused throughout the curriculum. 2. Program prepares students for PA professional counseling license.

Degrees   •   Community Counseling: M.
               •   School Counseling: M.

Contact   •   Community Counseling: M = Gloria C. Brusoski, PhD.
               •   School Counseling: M = Gloria C. Brusoski, PhD.

Admission and Graduation Data

Admission

Requirements   •   Community Counseling(M): GPA 3.00; MAT 45; Interview.
                •   School Counseling(M): GPA 3.00; MAT 45; Interview.

Enrollment   •   Community Counseling(M): 15 Admitted yearly; 15 Graduated yearly; 38 Female; 9 Male.
              •   School Counseling(M): 18 Admitted yearly; 13 Graduated yearly; 31 Female; 8 Male.

Diversity   •   African-American; Asian-American; Caucasian; Hispanic; Native American; Multiracial.

Graduation

Requirements   •   Community Counseling(M): 48 Class hours; 150 Practicum hours; 600 Internship hours; Comprehensive exam; CPCE.
                •   School Counseling(M): 48 Class hours; 300 Practicum hours; Comprehensive exam; CPCE.

Postgraduation activity: Advanced education and employment setting percentages.
                •   Community Counseling(M): 2 Advanced education; 80 Agency practice; 18 Other.
                •   School Counseling(M): 25 Agency practice; 20 Elementary school; 10 Middle school; 20 Secondary school; 20 Other.

Planned Program Modifications

Courses	Drop	Add
	• NP.	• NP.

Other	Decrease	Increase
	• Faculty FTE.	• Diversity Recruiting of Students
		• National Accreditation.

Related Programs Clinical Social Workers
                       Psychology
                       Communications

Faculty

nbcc ❖   Percent of faculty reported with NCC certification: **100%**.   **ncc** ❖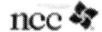

Percent in professional counseling practice: 25%.

Research interests Career counseling, college counseling, theoretical and practical aspects of empathy, use of technology in counseling.

Diversity   •   African-American; Caucasian; Native American; Multiracial.

Name, Degree, Rank, State/National Credentials, % time devoted to program, email
•   Brusoski, Gloria C; PhD; Full Prof.; NCC, CSC;Licensed Psychologist; >81%; *Brusoski@cup.edu*
•   Powe, Alton N; PhD; Full Prof.; LPC, NCC; >81%; *powe@cup.edu*
•   Walsh, Jacqueline A; PhD; Assist.; LPC, NCC; >81%; *walsh@cup.edu*
•   John, Patrick; EdD; Assist.; LPC, NCC, CRC; >81%; *patrick@cup.edu*

Has CHI SIGMA IOTA (International Counseling Society) chapter.

PA: Duquesne University

School of Education
Pittsburgh, PA 15282
USA

Dean   Dr. James E. Henderson
Administrator Nicholas Hanna, Ph.D., Coordinator
              Department   Dept of Counseling Psychology & Special Educ
                            (412) 396-5567, fax (412) 396-5585, CESEDD@DUQ.EDU,
                            www.education.duq.edu/counselored

Key   See key for Data on Each Department (this section) on page 79.

Program

Accreditation   Regional Accreditation, **CACREP:** Community Counseling, **CACREP:** Counselor Education
                 and Supervision, **CACREP:** Marriage and Family Counseling, **CACREP:** School Counseling

CACREP

Uniqueness   Students are exposed to various philosophical approaches and learn the value of accepting
                 differences.

Degrees   • Community Counseling: M, S.
                 • School Counseling: M, S.
                 • Marriage and Family Counseling: M, S.
                 • Counselor Education: EdD.

Contact   • Community Counseling: M, S = Nicholas Hanna.
                 • School Counseling: M, S = William J. Casile.
                 • Marriage and Family Counseling: M, S = Paul M. Bernstein.
                 • Counselor Education: D = Joseph F. Maola.

Admission and Graduation Data

Admission

Requirements   • Community Counseling(M): GPA 3.00; MAT 40.
                 • Community Counseling(S): GPA 3.00; MAT 40.
                 • School Counseling(M): GPA 3.00; MAT 40.
                 • School Counseling(S): GPA 3.00; MAT 40.
                 • Marriage and Family Counseling(M): GPA 3.00; MAT 40.
                 • Marriage and Family Counseling(S): GPA 3.00; MAT 40.
                 • Counselor Education(D): Masters and GPA 3.25; GRE 1800; 2 Years work experience.

Enrollment   • Community Counseling(M & S): 25 Admitted yearly; 16 Graduated yearly.
                 • School Counseling(M & S): 25 Admitted yearly; 15 Graduated yearly.
                 • Marriage and Family Counseling(M & S): 10 Admitted yearly; 4 Graduated yearly.
                 • Counselor Education(D): 11 Admitted yearly; 4 Graduated yearly; 15 Female; 15 Male.

Diversity   • African-American; Asian-American; Caucasian; Hispanic; Native American; Multiracial.

Graduation

Requirements   • Community Counseling(M): 60 Class hours; 125 Practicum hours; 600 Internship hours;
                   Oral exam; Portfolio.
                 • Community Counseling(S): 78 Class hours; 125 Practicum hours; 600 Internship hours;
                   Oral exam; Portfolio.
                 • School Counseling(M): 60 Class hours; 125 Practicum hours; 600 Internship hours; Oral
                   exam; Portfolio.
                 • School Counseling(S): 78 Class hours; 125 Practicum hours; 600 Internship hours; Oral
                   exam; Portfolio.
                 • Marriage and Family Counseling(M): 60 Class hours; 125 Practicum hours; 600 Internship
                   hours; Oral exam; Portfolio.
                 • Marriage and Family Counseling(S): 78 Class hours; 125 Practicum hours; 600 Internship
                   hours; Oral exam; Portfolio.
                 • Counselor Education(D): 67 Class hours; 150 Practicum hours; 600 Internship hours;
                   Comprehensive exam; Oral exam; Dissertation.

Postgraduation activity: Advanced education and employment setting percentages.
                 • Community Counseling(M & S): 10 Advanced education; 5 Private practice; 75 Agency
                   practice; 10 Other.
                 • School Counseling(M & S): 6 Advanced education; 38 Elementary school; 23 Middle
                   school; 33 Secondary school.
                 • Marriage and Family Counseling(M & S): 10 Advanced education; 15 Managed care; 5
                   Private practice; 70 Agency practice.
                 • Counselor Education(D): 10 Managed care; 20 Private practice; 25 Agency practice; 5
                   Middle school; 5 Secondary school; 5 Student affairs; 30 Other.

Planned Program Modifications

Courses	Drop	Add
	• NP.	• Crisis/Violence Counseling
		• Gerontological Counseling
		• Technology.

Other	Decrease	Increase
	• NP.	• NP.

Related Programs Psychology
Communications
Other

Faculty

 nbcc   Percent of faculty reported with NCC certification: **100**%.   ncc

Percent in professional counseling practice: 80%.

Research interests NP.

Diversity   • African-American; Caucasian; Hispanic; Native American; Multiracial; Other.

Name, Degree, Rank, State/National Credentials, % time devoted to program, email
• Bernstein, Paul M; PhD; Assoc.; LPC, NCC; >81%; *BernsteinP@duq.edu*
• Casile, William J; PhD; Assoc.; LPC, NCC; >81%; *Casile@duq.edu*
• Delmonico, David; PhD; Assist.; LPC, NCC; >81%; *Delmonico@duq.edu*
• Hanna, Nicholas; PhD; Full Prof.; LPC, NCC; >81%; *Hannan@duq.edu*
• Krushinski, Maura; Other; Instructor; LPC, NCC; >81%; *krushinski@duq.edu*
• Maola, Joseph F; PhD; Full Prof.; LPC, NCC; 61-80%; *maola@duq.edu*
• Mosley, Emma C; PhD; Assist.; NCC; 41-60%; *mosley@duq.edu*
• Myer, Rick; PhD; Assoc.; LPC, NCC; >81%; *myerra@duq.edu*
• Gregoire, Jocelyn; EdD; Assist.; NCC; 41-60%; *gregoire@duq.edu*
• Lopez-Levers, Lisa; PhD; Assist.; LPC, NCC; >81%; *levers@duq.edu*

Has CHI SIGMA IOTA (International Counseling Society) chapter.

PA: Geneva College

3200 College Avenue
Beaver Falls, PA 15010
USA
Dean   Dr. Philip VanBruggen, PHD, Geneva College
Administrator   Dr. Carol Luce, PHD, Director of the MA in Counseling Program
                    Department   Psychology, Counseling, and Human Services
                    (724) 847-6622, fax (724) 847-6101, cbluce@geneva.edu

Key   See key for Data on Each Department (this section) on page 79.

Program
Accreditation   Regional Accreditation

Uniqueness   MA in Counseling with Programs in School Counseling, Marriage and Family Counseling, and
                 Mental Health Counseling. A Christian faith-based approach to professional counseling
                 training.

Degrees   • Mental Health Counseling: M.
                 • School Counseling: M.
                 • Marriage and Family Counseling: M.

Contact   • Mental Health Counseling: M = Dr. Joseph Peters.
                 • School Counseling: M = Dr. David Harvey.
                 • Marriage and Family Counseling: M = Dr. Ronald Moslener.

Admission and Graduation Data
Admission
Requirements   • Mental Health Counseling(M): GPA 3.00; GRE 1000.
                 • School Counseling(M): GPA 3.00; GRE 1000.
                 • Marriage and Family Counseling(M): GPA 3.00; GRE 1000.

Enrollment   • Mental Health Counseling(M): 7 Admitted yearly; 6 Graduated yearly.
                 • School Counseling(M): 7 Admitted yearly; 6 Graduated yearly.
                 • Marriage and Family Counseling(M): 7 Admitted yearly; 6 Graduated yearly.

Diversity   • African-American; Caucasian.

Graduation
Requirements   • Mental Health Counseling(M): 60 Class hours; 100 Practicum hours; 900 Internship hours;
                   Comprehensive exam.
                 • School Counseling(M): 51 Class hours; 100 Practicum hours; 600 Internship hours;
                   Comprehensive exam.
                 • Marriage and Family Counseling(M): 60 Class hours; 100 Practicum hours; 600 Internship
                   hours; Comprehensive exam.

Postgraduation activity: Advanced education and employment setting percentages.
                 • Mental Health Counseling(M): NP.
                 • School Counseling(M): NP.
                 • Marriage and Family Counseling(M): NP.

Planned Program Modifications
Courses   Drop   Add
                 • NP.   • NP.

Other   Decrease   Increase
                 • NP.   • NP.

Related Programs

Faculty

nbcc ❧   Percent of faculty reported with NCC certification: 50%.   ncc ❧

Percent in professional counseling practice: 67%.

Research interests Christian counseling, community-based counseling interventions, marriage and family
                   counseling, counseling with chronically ill patients, eating disorders, school interventions

Diversity   • African-American; Caucasian.

Name, Degree, Rank, State/National Credentials, % time devoted to program, email
- Luce, Carol B; PhD; Assoc.; LPC, NCC, Licensed Psychologist; 41-60%; *cbluce@geneva.edu*
- Harvey, David; PhD; Full Prof.; NCC; 61-80%; *dharvey@geneva.edu*
- Moslener, Ronald; PhD; Assoc.; LMFT; >81%; *rwmoslener@geneva.edu*
- Peters, Joseph E; PhD; Assoc.; Licensed Psychologist; >81%; *jepeters@geneva.edu*
- Sigmund, Cathy; PhD; Assoc.; Licensed Psychologist; 22-40%; *csigmund@geneva.edu*
- Sartor, Dan; PhD; Assist.; LPC, NCC; 41-60%; *dsartor@geneva.edu*

PA: Indiana University of Pennsylvania

	206 Stouffer Hall
	Indiana, PA 15705-1087
	USA
Dean	Dean John W. Butzow, College of Education and Educational Technology
Administrator	Dr. Claire J. Dandeneau, Chairperson
	Department Counseling Department
	(724) 357-2306, fax (724) 357-7821, cdanden@iup.edu,
	http://www.coe.iup.edu/ce

Key   See key for Data on Each Department (this section) on page 79.

Program
   Accreditation   Regional Accreditation

   Uniqueness   • NP.

   Degrees   • Community Counseling: M.
         • School Counseling: M.

   Contact   • Community Counseling: M = Dr. Claire Dandeneau.
         • School Counseling: M = Dr. Claire Dandeneau.

Admission and Graduation Data
Admission
   Requirements   • Community Counseling(M): GPA 2.80; Interview.
         • School Counseling(M): GPA 3.00; Interview.

   Enrollment   • Community Counseling(M): 50 Admitted yearly.
         • School Counseling(M): 45 Admitted yearly.

   Diversity   • African-American; Asian-American; Caucasian.

Graduation
   Requirements   • Community Counseling(M): 48 Class hours; 90 Practicum hours; 300-600 Internship hours.
         • School Counseling(M): 48 Class hours; 90 Practicum hours; 300 Internship hours.

   Postgraduation activity: Advanced education and employment setting percentages.
         • Community Counseling(M): NP.
         • School Counseling(M): NP.

Planned Program Modifications

Courses	Drop	Add
	• NP.	• Human Sexuality
		• Psychodiagnosis
		• Rehabilitation
		• Supervision
		• Marriage and Family Counseling
		• Wellness.

Other	Decrease	Increase
	• NP.	• Admission Requirements
		• Faculty FTE
		• Number of Distance Education Courses
		• Number of Off-Campus Courses.

Related Programs Psychology

Faculty

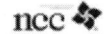 Percent of faculty reported with NCC certification: 89%.

Percent in professional counseling practice: 30%.

Research interests NP.

   Diversity   • Caucasian.

Name, Degree, Rank, State/National Credentials, % time devoted to program, email
• Dandeneau, Claire J; PhD; Assoc.; LPC, NCC; >81%; *cdanden@iup.edu*
• Fontaine, Janet H; PhD; Assoc.; LPC, NCC, NCCC; >81%; *fontaine@iup.edu*
• Guth, Lorraine J; PhD; Assoc.; LPC, NCC; >81%; *lguth@iup.edu*
• L'Amoreaux, Nadene; PhD; Assist.; LPC, NCC, CRC; >81%; *nlamoro@iup.edu*

- McCarthy, John; PhD; Assist.; LPC; >81%; *jmccarth@iup.edu*
- Rishel, Robin; PhD; Assist.; LPC, NCC; >81%; *rrishel@iup.edu*
- Utay, Joseph; PhD; Assist.; LPC, NCC; 41-60%; *joe@totallearningcenter.com*
- Witchel, Robert I; EdD; Full Prof.; NCC; >81%; *bwitchel@iup.edu*
- Worzbyt, John C; EdD; Full Prof.; LPC, NCC; >81%; *jcworz@iup.edul*

Has CHI SIGMA IOTA (International Counseling Society) chapter.

PA: Kutztown University

Graduate Center
Kutztown, PA 19530-0730
USA

Dean	Dr. Charles Cullum, College of Graduate Studies
Administrator	Margaret A. Herrick, Ph.D., Chairperson
	Department Dept of Counseling & Human Services
	(610) 683-4204, fax (610) 683-1585, herrick@kutztown.edu,
	www.kutztown.edu

Key   See key for Data on Each Department (this section) on page 79.

Program

Accreditation   NP.

Uniqueness   All programs offer PA Counselor Licensure option. Faculty members utilize a variety of teaching methods, are on campus on a full-time basis, and encourage special projects to enhance student learning and professional growth.

Degrees
- Community Counseling: M.
- School Counseling: M.
- Marriage and Family Counseling: M.
- Student Affairs: M.

Contact
- Community Counseling: M = Jo Cohen.
- School Counseling: M = Deborah Barlieb, Sandra McSwain.
- Marriage and Family Counseling: M = Thomas Seay.
- Student Affairs: M = Kelley Kenney.

Admission and Graduation Data

Admission

Requirements
- Community Counseling(M): GPA 3.00; GRE 1200; GRE V 400; GRE Q 400; GRE A 400.
- School Counseling(M): GPA 3.00; GRE 1200; GRE V 400; GRE Q 400; GRE A 400; Interview.
- Marriage and Family Counseling(M): GPA 3.00; GRE 1200; GRE V 400; GRE Q 400; GRE A 400; Interview.
- Student Affairs(M): GPA 3.00; GRE 1200; GRE V 400; GRE Q 400; GRE A 400; Interview.

Enrollment
- Community Counseling(M): 20 Admitted yearly; 10 Graduated yearly.
- School Counseling(M): 29 Admitted yearly; 18 Graduated yearly.
- Marriage and Family Counseling(M): 14 Admitted yearly; 7 Graduated yearly.
- Student Affairs(M): 7 Admitted yearly; 7 Graduated yearly.

Diversity
- African-American; Caucasian.

Graduation

Requirements
- Community Counseling(M): 60 Class hours; 100 Practicum hours; 700 Internship hours; Comprehensive exam.
- School Counseling(M): 51 Class hours; 100 Practicum hours; 700 Internship hours; Comprehensive exam.
- Marriage and Family Counseling(M): 60 Class hours; 100 Practicum hours; 700 Internship hours.
- Student Affairs(M): 48 Class hours; 500 Internship hours.

Postgraduation activity: Advanced education and employment setting percentages.
- Community Counseling(M): 2 Advanced education; 10 Managed care; 2 Private practice; 86 Agency practice.
- School Counseling(M): 5 Advanced education; 5 Agency practice; 17 Elementary school; 18 Middle school; 55 Secondary school.
- Marriage and Family Counseling(M): 5 Advanced education; 10 Managed care; 5 Private practice; 80 Agency practice.
- Student Affairs(M): 5 Advanced education; 95 Other.

Planned Program Modifications

Courses	Drop	Add
	• NP.	• NP.

Other	Decrease	Increase
	• NP.	• Course Offerings
		• Number of Degree Majors.

Related Programs NP.

Faculty

nbcc ❧.   Percent of faculty reported with NCC certification: **100%**.   ncc ❧

Percent in professional counseling practice: NP.

Research interests Intercultural Issues, Multicultural Counseling Competencies, School Counseling Services
and Ethics, Marital and Family Therapy Issues, Critical Thinking

Diversity   •   African-American; Caucasian.

Name, Degree, Rank, State/National Credentials, % time devoted to program, email
• Barlieb, Deborah; PhD; Assoc.; NCC; >81%; *barlieb@kutztown.edu*
• Kenney, Kelley R; PhD; Full Prof.; NCC; >81%; *kenney@kutztown.edu*
• Cohen, Jo; PhD; Assoc.; NCC; >81%; *cohen@kutztown.edu*
• Herrick, Margaret A; PhD; Assoc.; NCC; >81%; *herrick@kutztown.edu*
• McSwain, Sandra J; EdD; Full Prof.; NCC; >81%; *mcswain@kutztown.edu*
• Seay, Thomas A; PhD; Full Prof.; NCC; >81%; *seay@kutztown.edu*

PA: Penn State University

307 CEDAR Building
University Park, PA 16802
USA
Dean   David Monk
Administrator   Spencer G. Niles, D.Ed., LPC (VA & PA), NCC, Professor-in-charge
Department   Counselor Education
(814) 865-3427, fax (814) 863-7750, paa2@psu.edu,
http://www.ed.psu.edu/cned/ced.asp

Key   See key for Data on Each Department (this section) on page 79.

Program
Accreditation   Regional Accreditation, **CACREP:** School Counseling, **CACREP:** Counselor Education and
Supervision

Uniqueness   Most students in the program are full-time. Faculty take a mentoring approach to working with
students. Students are actively involved in program development and program activities. The
program has a rich history of leadership in the profession and the faculty are committed to
continual program development. Currently, the program is ranked #7 in the United States.

Degrees   • School Counseling: M.
• College Counseling: M.
• Rehabilitation Counseling: M.
• Counselor Education: PhD.

Contact   • School Counseling:
• College Counseling:
• Rehabilitation Counseling:
• Counselor Education:

Admission and Graduation Data
Admission
Requirements   • School Counseling(M): GRE R.
• College Counseling(M): GRE R.
• Rehabilitation Counseling(M): GRE R.
• Counselor Education(D): GRE R.

Enrollment   • School Counseling(M): 9 Admitted yearly.
• College Counseling(M): 9 Admitted yearly.
• Rehabilitation Counseling(M): 9 Admitted yearly.
• Counselor Education(D): 9 Admitted yearly.

Diversity   • NP.

Graduation
Requirements   • School Counseling(M): NP.
• College Counseling(M): NP.
• Rehabilitation Counseling(M): NP.
• Counselor Education(D): NP.

Postgraduation activity: Advanced education and employment setting percentages.
• School Counseling(M): NP.
• College Counseling(M): NP.
• Rehabilitation Counseling(M): NP.
• Counselor Education(D):

Planned Program Modifications
Courses   Drop   Add
• NP.   • NP.

Other   Decrease   Increase
• NP.   • NP.

Related Programs

Faculty

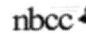 Percent of faculty reported with NCC certification: 20%.

Percent in professional counseling practice: NP.

Research interests Several faculty are leading career development researchers; other faculty interests include: school counseling, multicultural topics and rehabilitation topics

Diversity   • African-American; Caucasian; Asian.

Name, Degree, Rank, State/National Credentials, % time devoted to program, email
- Niles, Spencer G; EdD; LPC, NCC; >81%
- Carney, Jolynn; PhD; >81%
- Crissman, Jennifer; EdD; >81%
- Hazler, Richard; PhD; >81%
- Herr, Edwin L; EdD; LPC; >81%
- Matthews, Connie; PhD; LPC, NCC; >81%
- Salter, Daniel; >81%
- Trusty, Jerry; PhD; LPC, NCC; >81%
- Bie Schke, Kathleen; PhD
- Herbert, James; PhD; LPC
- Hunt, Brandon; PhD; LPC
- Mpofu, Elias; PhD
- Vandiver, Beverly; PhD
- Wilson, Keith; PhD
- Hayes, Jeffrey; PhD

Has CHI SIGMA IOTA (International Counseling Society) chapter.

PA: Shippensburg University of PA

1871 Old Main Drive
Shippensburg, PA 17257-2299
USA
Dean   Robert Bartos, Ed.D.
Administrator   Thomas L. Hozman, Ph.D., Chairperson
Department   Counseling Department
(717) 477-1668, fax (717) 477-4056, tlhozm@ship.edu,
www.ship.edu/~counsel

Key   See key for Data on Each Department (this section) on page 79.

Program
Accreditation   Regional Accreditation, **CACREP:** College Counseling, **CACREP:** Community Counseling, **CACREP:** Mental Health Counseling, **CACREP:** School Counseling, **CACREP:** Student Affairs.

CACREP

Uniqueness   All teaching faculty have extensive experience as practitioners. Our informal interaction with students is a collaborative approach that encourages cooperation, respect, and ethical responsibility.

Degrees
- Community Counseling: M.
- Mental Health Counseling: M.
- School Counseling: M.
- College Counseling: M.
- Student Affairs: M.

Contact
- Community Counseling: M = Thomas Hozman.
- Mental Health Counseling: M = Thomas Hozman.
- School Counseling: M = Thomas Hozman.
- College Counseling: M = Thomas Hozman.
- Student Affairs: M = Thomas Hozman.

Admission and Graduation Data
Admission
Requirements
- Community Counseling(M): GPA 2.75; GRE 800; GRE V 400; GRE Q 400; GRE A 0; 1 Year work experience; Interview.
- Mental Health Counseling(M): GPA 2.75; GRE 800; GRE V 400; GRE Q 400; GRE A 0; 1 Year work experience; Interview.
- School Counseling(M): GPA 3.00; GRE 800; GRE V 400; GRE Q 400; GRE A 0; 1 Year work experience; Interview.
- College Counseling(M): GPA 2.75; GRE 800; GRE V 400; GRE Q 400; GRE A 0; 1 Year work experience; Interview.
- Student Affairs(M): GPA 2.75; GRE 800; GRE V 400; GRE Q 400; GRE A 0; 1 Year work experience; Interview.

Enrollment
- Community Counseling(M): 15 Admitted yearly; 8 Graduated yearly; 13 Female; 4 Male.
- Mental Health Counseling(M): 4 Admitted yearly; 3 Graduated yearly; 31 Female; 5 Male.
- School Counseling(M): 29 Admitted yearly; 20 Graduated yearly; 83 Female; 15 Male.
- College Counseling(M): 1 Admitted yearly; 1 Graduated yearly; 1 Female; 3 Male.
- Student Affairs(M): 10 Admitted yearly; 7 Graduated yearly; 24 Female; 9 Male.

Diversity
- African-American; Asian-American; Caucasian; Hispanic; Native American; Pacific Islander; Multiracial.

Graduation
Requirements
- Community Counseling(M): 48 Class hours; 150 Practicum hours; 600 Internship hours; Portfolio.
- Mental Health Counseling(M): 60 Class hours; 150 Practicum hours; 900 Internship hours; Portfolio.
- School Counseling(M): 48 Class hours; 150 Practicum hours; 600 Internship hours; Portfolio.
- College Counseling(M): 48 Class hours; 150 Practicum hours; 600 Internship hours; Portfolio.
- Student Affairs(M): 48 Class hours; 150 Practicum hours; 600 Internship hours; Portfolio.

Postgraduation activity: Advanced education and employment setting percentages.

- Community Counseling(M): 10 Advanced education; 10 Managed care; 5 Private practice; 75 Agency practice.
- Mental Health Counseling(M): 10 Advanced education; 10 Managed care; 5 Private practice; 75 Agency practice.
- School Counseling(M): 2 Advanced education; 2 Managed care; 1 Agency practice; 30 Elementary school; 30 Middle school; 35 Secondary school.
- College Counseling(M): 15 Advanced education; 5 Managed care; 80 Other.
- Student Affairs(M): 10 Advanced education; 90 Other.

Planned Program Modifications

Courses	Drop	Add
	• NP.	• NP.

Other	Decrease	Increase
	• NP.	• Diversity Recruiting of Faculty
		• Diversity Recruiting of Students
		• Number of Distance Education Courses
		• Number of On-Line Courses.

Related Programs NP.

Faculty

 Percent of faculty reported with NCC certification: 89%.

Percent in professional counseling practice: 50%.

Research interests Adolescence, substance abuse, group counseling

Diversity   • African-American; Caucasian.

Name, Degree, Rank, State/National Credentials, % time devoted to program, email
- Arminio, Jan L; PhD; Assoc.; >81%; *jlarmi@ship.edu*
- Brooks, Clifford W; EdD; Assoc.; LPC, NCC, CAC; >81%; *cwbroo@ship.edu*
- Carey, Andrew L; PhD; Assist.; NCC; >81%; *alcare@ship.edu*
- Hozman, Thomas L; PhD; Full Prof.; NCC, LIC. PSY; >81%; *tlhozm@ship.edu*
- Kraus, Kurt L; EdD; Assist.; LPC, NCC; >81%; *klkrau@ship.edu*
- Kurdt, Kathryn A; PhD; Assist.; LPC, NCC; <21%; *kakurd@ship.edu*
- LaFountain, Rebecca M; EdD; Full Prof.; LPC, NCC, CCMHCLIC. PSY; >81%; *rmlafo@ship.edu*
- Hess, Shirley A; PhD; Assist.; LPC, NCC, LIC. PSY; >81%; *sahess@ship.edu*
- Mustaine, Beverly L; EdD; Full Prof.; LPC, NCC, CCMHCLIC. PSY; >81%; *blmust@ship.edu*

Has CHI SIGMA IOTA (International Counseling Society) chapter.

PA: West Chester University

Department of Counseling and Educational Psychology
West Chester, PA 19383
USA

Dean
Administrator   Angelo F. Gadaleto, Ph.D., Department Chair
                       Department   Dept of Counseling and Educational Psychology
                       (610) 436-2559, agadaleto@wcupda.edu, WCUPA.EDU

Key   See key for Data on Each Department (this section) on page 79.

Program
Accreditation   Regional Accreditation

Uniqueness   27 credit common core of counselor education. Programs allow students to change specialty
                   after additional information obtained. School certification can be added to MS with 12
                   additional hours.

Degrees   • Community Counseling: M.
                   • School Counseling: M.
                   • Student Affairs: M.

Contact   • Community Counseling: M = NP.
                   • School Counseling: M = Dr. Angelo Gadaleto.
                   • Student Affairs: M = Dr. Angelo Gadaleto.

Admission and Graduation Data
Admission
Requirements   • Community Counseling(M): GPA 3.00.
                   • School Counseling(M): GPA 3.00.
                   • Student Affairs(M): GPA 3.00.

Enrollment   • Community Counseling(M): 10 Admitted yearly; 5 Graduated yearly.
                   • School Counseling(M): 80 Admitted yearly; 40 Graduated yearly.
                   • Student Affairs(M): 40 Admitted yearly; 20 Graduated yearly.

Diversity   • African-American; Asian-American; Caucasian; Hispanic; Pacific Islander; Multiracial.

Graduation
Requirements   • Community Counseling(M): 48 Class hours; 360 Practicum hours; Comprehensive exam;
                     Portfolio.
                   • School Counseling(M): 48 Class hours; 360 Practicum hours; Comprehensive exam;
                     Portfolio.
                   • Student Affairs(M): 48 Class hours; 360 Practicum hours; Portfolio.

Postgraduation activity: Advanced education and employment setting percentages.
                   • Community Counseling(M): NP.
                   • School Counseling(M): 30 Elementary school; 20 Middle school; 50 Secondary school.
                   • Student Affairs(M): 20 Advanced education; 10 Managed care; 10 Secondary school; 10
                     Student affairs; 50 Other.

Planned Program Modifications
Courses   Drop   Add
                   • NP.   • NP.

Other   Decrease   Increase
                   • NP.   • NP.

Related Programs NP.

Faculty

nbcc ✿   Percent of faculty reported with NCC certification: 33%.   ncc ✿

Percent in professional counseling practice: NP.

Research interests

Diversity   • African-American; Asian-American.

Name, Degree, Rank, State/National Credentials, % time devoted to program, email
• Broderick, Trish; PhD; Assoc.; LPC; 61-80%; *tbroderick@wcupa.edu*
• Brown, Deborah; PhD; Full Prof.; <21%; *Dbrown@wcupa.edu*

- Gadaleto, Angelo F; PhD; Full Prof.; LPC, NCC; >81%; *Agadaleto@wcupa.edu*
- Hinson, Stephanie; EdD; Assoc.; <21%; *Shinson@wcupa.edu*
- Kahn, Wally; PhD; Full Prof.; >81%; *Wkohn@wcupa.edu*
- Napierkowski, Carol M; PhD; Assoc.; LPC, NCC; >81%; *cnapierkowski@wcupa.edu*
- Parsons, Richard; PhD; Full Prof.; >81%; *Rporsun@wcupa.edu*
- Spradlin, Lynn; EdD; Assoc.; LPC, NCC; >81%; *lspodlin@wcupa.edu*
- Zhang, Naijian; PhD; Assist.; 61-80%;

Has CHI SIGMA IOTA (International Counseling Society) chapter.

PA: Westminster College

313 Old Main
New Wilmington, PA 16172
USA
Dean   Jess Mann, Westminster College, New Wilmington
Administrator   William J. Evans Ph.D., Program Coordinator
     Department   Education
     (724) 946-7184, fax (724) 946-6180, evanswj@westminster.edu,
     www.westminster.edu

Key   See key for Data on Each Department (this section) on page 79.

Program
Accreditation   Regional Accreditation

Uniqueness   Small, intimate learning community, limited to school counseling, curriculum structured on ASCA model program guidelines and CACREP standards, PA Dept. of Education approved, 18 semester-hour post-master's program for Ohio students and 6 semester hour post-master's program for Pennsylvania certification/licensure. Small liberal arts college situated in beautiful pastoral Amish area accessible to Pittsburgh, Youngstown and surrounding area.

Degrees   • School Counseling: M.

Contact   • School Counseling: M = William J. Evans Ph.D.

Admission and Graduation Data
Admission
Requirements   • School Counseling(M): GPA 3.00.

Enrollment   • School Counseling(M): 30 Admitted yearly; 30 Graduated yearly; 70 Female; 30 Male.

Diversity   • African-American; Asian-American; Caucasian; Native American; Multiracial.

Graduation
Requirements   • School Counseling(M): 30 Class hours; 100 Practicum hours; 300/600 Internship hours; Comprehensive exam.

Postgraduation activity: Advanced education and employment setting percentages.
     • School Counseling(M): 15 Elementary school; 70 Middle school; 70 Secondary school.

Planned Program Modifications

Courses	Drop	Add
	• NP.	• Adventure Counseling • Sports Counseling • Wellness.

Other	Decrease	Increase
	• NP.	• Course Offerings • Diversity Recruiting of Students • Financial Aid.

Related Programs

Faculty

nbcc ❖   Percent of faculty reported with NCC certification: 12%.   ncc ❖

Percent in professional counseling practice: 25%.

Research interests Counselor supervision, brief models of counseling, psychometrics, pedagogy

Diversity   • Caucasian.

Name, Degree, Rank, State/National Credentials, % time devoted to program, email
• Evans, William J; PhD; Assoc.; LPC, NCC; >81%; *evanswj@westminster.edu*
• Bookhamer, Judy; PhD; Adjunct; CSC; 22-40%; *jbookhamer@attbi.com*
• Huey, Darwin W; EdD; Assoc.; 41-60%; *hueydw@westminster.edu*
• Domanski, Linda P; EdD; Assist.; <21%; *domanslp@westminster.edu*
• DeCaro, John J; EdD; Adjunct; 22-40%; *decarojj@westminster.edu*
• Santillo, Richard W; EdD; Adjunct; CSC; <21%; *santilrw@westminster.edu*
• Quincy, Barbara I.; MEd; Adjunct; <21%; *quincybi@westminster.edu*
• Garrett, Charles A; MEd; Adjunct; CSC; <21%; *garretca@westminster.edu*

Has CHI SIGMA IOTA (International Counseling Society) chapter.

PR: University of Phoenix, Puerto Rico Campus

PRC Address: Box 3870, Rd 177 KM 2.0 (Les Filtros)
Guaynabo, PR 00970-3870
USA

**Dean
Administrator**   Patrick B. Romine, Dean
Department   College of Social and Behavioral Sciences
(602) 966-9577, fax (602) 929-7164

Key   See key for Data on Each Department (this section) on page 79.

Program
Accreditation   Regional Accreditation

Uniqueness   This is a program for working adults. Courses are at night and on weekends.

Degrees
- Mental Health Counseling: M.
- Marriage and Family Counseling: M.

Contact
- Mental Health Counseling: M = Ana M. Rodriguez, Ed.D.
- Marriage and Family Counseling: M = Ana M. Rodriguez, Ed.D.

Admission and Graduation Data
Admission
Requirements
- Mental Health Counseling(M): GPA 2.50; 2 Years work experience; Interview.
- Marriage and Family Counseling(M): GPA 2.50; 2 Years work experience; Interview.

Enrollment
- Mental Health Counseling(M): 50 Admitted yearly; 50 Graduated yearly; 35 Female; 15 Male.
- Marriage and Family Counseling(M): 50 Admitted yearly; 50 Graduated yearly; 37 Female; 13 Male.

Diversity
- Caucasian; Hispanic.

Graduation
Requirements
- Mental Health Counseling(M): 60 Class hours; 100 Practicum hours; 900 Internship hours; Comprehensive exam; Portfolio.
- Marriage and Family Counseling(M): 60 Class hours; 100 Practicum hours; 900 Internship hours; Portfolio.

Postgraduation activity: Advanced education and employment setting percentages.
- Mental Health Counseling(M): 10 Advanced education; 15 Managed care; 5 Private practice; 60 Agency practice; 10 Other.
- Marriage and Family Counseling(M): 5 Advanced education; 15 Managed care; 5 Private practice; 65 Agency practice; 10 Other.

Planned Program Modifications

Courses	Drop	Add
	• NP.	• Consultation • Marriage and Family Counseling.

Other	Decrease	Increase
	• NP.	• NP.

Related Programs

Faculty

 Percent of faculty reported with NCC certification: 14%.

Percent in professional counseling practice: 40%.

Research interests varied

Diversity
- Hispanic.

Name, Degree, Rank, State/National Credentials, % time devoted to program, email
- Batista, Norma; EdD; Instructor; NCC; 61-80%;
- Velez, Magali; PhD; Instructor; <21%;
- DeLeon-Fuentes, Jose; PhD; Instructor; 61-80%;
- Claudio, Hector; PhD; Instructor; <21%;
- Marrero, Carmen; PhD; Instructor; NCC; 61-80%;
- Negron, Priscilla; EdD; Instructor; 61-80%;

- Rinaldi Jovet, Roberto; PhD; Instructor; 61-80%;
- Nunez, Emma; EdD; Instructor; 61-80%;
- Pedrosa, Idalia; EdD; Instructor; 61-80%;
- Perez de Alejo, Lourdes; EdD; Instructor; 61-80%;
- Rodriguez, Elba; EdD; Full Prof.; >81%;
- Rodriguez, Maria; PhD; Full Prof.; >81%;
- Rodriguez, Ana M.; EdD; Full Prof.; 61-80%;
- Sanchez, Elba; Other; Adjunct; 41-60%;

RI: Rhode Island College

600 Mt. Pleasant Ave. Adams Library
Providence, RI 02908
United States

Dean Dr. John Bucci, Feinstein School of Education and Human Development
Administrator Murray H. Finley, PhD, Director of Counselor Education
    Department Counseling & Educational Psychology
    (401) 456-8023, fax (401) 456-9628, MFinley@RIC.EDU, www.ric.edu/cep

Key See key for Data on Each Department (this section) on page 79.

Program

Accreditation Regional Accreditation

Uniqueness We have three MA programs in counseling and 2 Certificate of Advanced Graduate Studies (CAGS) programs in counseling. Some programs lead to either state certifications or licensing with third party reimbursement.

Degrees
- Mental Health Counseling: M, S.
- School Counseling: M, S.
- Addictions Counseling: M.

Contact
- Mental Health Counseling: M = M. Finely; S = M. Finley.
- School Counseling: M, S = M. Finley.
- Addictions Counseling: M = M. Finley.

Admission and Graduation Data

Admission

Requirements
- Mental Health Counseling(M): GPA 3.00; GRE 900; GRE V 450; GRE Q 450; GRE A 500; MAT 45; 2 Years work experience.
- Mental Health Counseling(S): GPA 3.00; GRE 900; GRE V 450; GRE Q 450; GRE A 500; MAT 45; 2 Years work experience.
- School Counseling(M): GPA 3.00; GRE 900; GRE V 450; GRE Q 450; GRE A 500; MAT 45; 2 Years work experience.
- School Counseling(S): GPA 3.00; GRE 900; GRE V 450; GRE Q 450; GRE A 500; MAT 45; 2 Years work experience.
- Addictions Counseling(M): GPA 3.00; GRE 900; GRE V 450; GRE Q 450; GRE A 500; MAT 45; 2 Years work experience.

Enrollment
- Mental Health Counseling(M & S): 42 Admitted yearly; 22 Graduated yearly; 65 Female; 15 Male.
- School Counseling(M & S): 25 Admitted yearly; 15 Graduated yearly; 30 Female; 10 Male.
- Addictions Counseling(M): 10 Admitted yearly; 5 Graduated yearly; 6 Female; 5 Male.

Diversity
- African-American; Asian-American; Caucasian; Hispanic; Pacific Islander; Multiracial.

Graduation

Requirements
- Mental Health Counseling(M): 36 Class hours; 90 Practicum hours; Comprehensive exam.
- Mental Health Counseling(S): 36 Class hours; 225 Practicum hours; 600 Internship hours; Thesis.
- School Counseling(M): 36 Class hours; 90 Practicum hours; 600 Internship hours; Comprehensive exam.
- School Counseling(S): 36 Class hours; 225 Practicum hours; 600 Internship hours; Thesis.
- Addictions Counseling(M): 36 Class hours; 90 Practicum hours.

Postgraduation activity: Advanced education and employment setting percentages.
- Mental Health Counseling(M & S): 50 Advanced education; 50 Managed care; 25 Private practice; 25 Agency practice.
- School Counseling(M & S): 40 Elementary school; 30 Middle school; 30 Secondary school.
- Addictions Counseling(M): 65 Managed care; 35 Agency practice.

Planned Program Modifications

Courses	Drop	Add
	• NP.	• NP.

Other	Decrease	Increase
	• NP.	• NP.

Related Programs

Faculty

 Percent of faculty reported with NCC certification: 0%.

Percent in professional counseling practice: NP.

Research interests Cognitive Development; School Counselors meeting national standards; portfolio creation with teachers for keeping lower socioeconomic students in school.

Diversity   • Caucasian; Pacific Islander.

Name, Degree, Rank, State/National Credentials, % time devoted to program, email
* Boisvert, Charles; PhD; Assist.; >81%; *CBoisvert@RIC.EDU*
* Finley, Murray H; PhD; Assoc.; >81%; *MFinley@RIC.EDU*
* Obach, Mifrando; PhD; Assoc.; >81%; *MObach@RIC.EDU*
* Perkins, John; PhD; Full Prof.; >81%; *JPerkins@RIC.EDU*
* Reyland, Susan; PhD; Assist.; >81%; *SReyland@RIC.EDU*
* Robertson, Krista; PhD; Assist.; >81%; *KRobertson@RIC.EDU*

SC: Clemson University

	313 Tillman Hall, Box 340710
	Clemson, SC 29634-0710
	United States
Dean	Interim Dean Larry Allen, College of HEHD
Administrator	Tony W. Cawthon, Associate Professor & Unit Coordinator
	Department Counselor Education
	(864) 656-3484, fax (864) 656-1332, cowthot@clemson.edu

Key   See key for Data on Each Department (this section) on page 79.

Program

Accreditation   Regional Accreditation, **CACREP:** Community Counseling, **CACREP:** School Counseling, **CACREP:** Student Affairs - Counseling, **CACREP:** Student Affairs - Professional Practice

CACREP

Uniqueness   Link theory to practice, part-time/full-time students, commitment to multicultural issues, field experience

Degrees
- Community Counseling: M.
- School Counseling: M.
- College Counseling: M.
- Student Affairs: M.

Contact
- Community Counseling: M = NP.
- School Counseling: M = NP.
- College Counseling: M = NP.
- Student Affairs: M = NP.

Admission and Graduation Data

Admission

Requirements
- Community Counseling(M): GPA 3.00; GRE 1250.
- School Counseling(M): GPA 3.00; GRE 1250.
- College Counseling(M): GPA 3.00; GRE 1250.
- Student Affairs(M): GPA 3.00; GRE 1250.

Enrollment
- Community Counseling(M): 60 Admitted yearly; 30 Graduated yearly; 50 Female; 10 Male.
- School Counseling(M): 60 Admitted yearly; 30 Graduated yearly; 50 Female; 10 Male.
- College Counseling(M): 5 Admitted yearly; 2 Graduated yearly; 4 Female; 1 Male.
- Student Affairs(M): 30 Admitted yearly; 20 Graduated yearly; 20 Female; 10 Male.

Diversity
- African-American; Caucasian; Hispanic; Multiracial.

Graduation

Requirements
- Community Counseling(M): 48 Class hours; 100 Practicum hours; 600 Internship hours; Comprehensive exam; CPCE.
- School Counseling(M): 51 Class hours; 100 Practicum hours; 600 Internship hours; Comprehensive exam; CPCE.
- College Counseling(M): 48 Class hours; 100 Practicum hours; 600 Internship hours; Comprehensive exam; CPCE.
- Student Affairs(M): 48 Class hours; 100 Practicum hours; 600 Internship hours; CPCE.

Postgraduation activity: Advanced education and employment setting percentages.
- Community Counseling(M): 10 Advanced education; 20 Private practice; 70 Agency practice.
- School Counseling(M): 50 Elementary school; 50 Secondary school.
- College Counseling(M): NP.
- Student Affairs(M): 10 Advanced education; 90 Other.

Planned Program Modifications

Courses	Drop	Add
	• NP.	• Legal/Ethical Issues
		• Psychodiagnosis.

Other	Decrease	Increase
	• NP.	• Admission Requirements
		• Diversity Recruiting of Faculty
		• Diversity Recruiting of Students
		• Number of Distance Education Courses
		• Number of Off-Campus Courses.

Related Programs Psychology

Faculty

nbcc ❧   Percent of faculty reported with NCC certification: 0%.   ncc ❧

Percent in professional counseling practice: NP.

Research interests Career Development, Supervision, Multicultural, Technology, Administration

Diversity   • African-American; Caucasian; Other.

Name, Degree, Rank, State/National Credentials, % time devoted to program, email
- Cawthon, Tony; PhD; >81%; *cawthot@clemson.edu*
- Griffin, Barbara; D; LPC; >81%; *griffib@clemson.edu*
- Lewis, Jennifer; D; >81%; *lewis3@clemson.edu*
- Brown, Lori; D; >81%; *loribr@clemson.edu*
- Havice, Pamela; PhD; >81%; *havicc@clemson.edu*
- Furkner, Cheryl; D; >81%; *cforkne@clemson.edu*
- Keller, Don; EdD; >81%; *kdon@clemson.edu*
- Jeromen, Neal; EdD; >81%; *jeromen@clemson.edu*
- Abernathy, Larry; M; >81%; *alarry@clemson.edu*

Has CHI SIGMA IOTA (International Counseling Society) chapter.

SC: University of South Carolina

Counselor Education, Wardlaw 266
Columbia, SC 29208
United States
Dean Lee Sternberg, PhD
Administrator Joshua M. Gold, PhD, NCC, Program Coordinator
Department   Educational Psychology
(803) 777-3053, fax (803) 777-3045, slane@gwm.sc.edu

Key   See key for Data on Each Department (this section) on page 79.

Program

Accreditation **CACREP:** Counselor Education and Supervision, **CACREP:** Marriage and Family Counseling, **CACREP:** School Counseling

Uniqueness The counselor education program offers programs in School Counseling (K-12), Marriage and Family Counseling (Ed.S), and the Ph.D. in Counselor Education.

Degrees
- School Counseling: S.
- Marriage and Family Counseling: S.
- Counselor Education: PhD.

Contact
- School Counseling: S = Josh Gold, PhD.
- Marriage and Family Counseling: S = Josh Gold, PhD.
- Counselor Education: D = Josh Gold, PhD.

Admission and Graduation Data

Admission

Requirements
- School Counseling(S): GPA 3.00; GRE V 375; GRE Q 375; GRE A 0; MAT 35; 2 Years work experience; Interview.
- Marriage and Family Counseling(S): GPA 3.00; GRE V 375; GRE Q 375; GRE A 0; MAT 35; 2 Years work experience; Interview.
- Counselor Education(D): Masters and GPA 3.00; GRE 800; GRE V 400; GRE Q 400; GRE A 0; 2 Years work experience.

Enrollment
- School Counseling(S): 40 Admitted yearly; 15 Graduated yearly; 108 Female; 19 Male.
- Marriage and Family Counseling(S): 15 Admitted yearly; 7 Graduated yearly; 35 Female; 4 Male.
- Counselor Education(D): 9 Admitted yearly; 3 Graduated yearly; 16 Female; 7 Male.

Diversity
- African-American; Caucasian; Hispanic; Native American.

Graduation

Requirements
- School Counseling(S): 66 Class hours; 150 Practicum hours; 600 Internship hours; Comprehensive exam.
- Marriage and Family Counseling(S): 66 Class hours; 150 Practicum hours; 600 Internship hours; Comprehensive exam; Oral exam.
- Counselor Education(D): 96 Class hours; 300 Practicum hours; 900 Internship hours; Oral exam; Dissertation.

Postgraduation activity: Advanced education and employment setting percentages.
- School Counseling(S): 40 Elementary school; 20 Middle school; 40 Secondary school.
- Marriage and Family Counseling(S): 100 Managed care.
- Counselor Education(D): 100 Student affairs.

Planned Program Modifications

Courses

	Drop		Add
• NP.		• NP.	

Other

	Decrease		Increase
• NP.		• NP.	

Related Programs Clinical Social Workers

Faculty

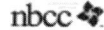 Percent of faculty reported with NCC certification: 17%.

Percent in professional counseling practice: NP.

Research interests NP.

Diversity   • African-American; Caucasian.

Name, Degree, Rank, State/National Credentials, % time devoted to program, email
- Burggraf, Margaret; PhD; Assoc.; >81%; *mburggra@gwm.sc.edu*
- Evans, Kathy; PhD; Assoc.; >81%; *kevans@gwm.sc.edu*
- Gold, Joshua; PhD; Assoc.; NCC; >81%; *josgold@gwm.sc.edu*
- McFadden, John; PhD; Full Prof.; >81%; *jmcfadden@gwm.sc.edu*
- Miller, Gary; PhD; Assoc.; >81%; *gmiller@gwm.sc.edu*
- Rotter, Joseph; EdD; Full Prof.; >81%; *jrotter@gwm.sc.edu*

Has CHI SIGMA IOTA (International Counseling Society) chapter.

SC: Winthrop University

143 Withers Bldg.
Rock Hill, SC 29733
U.S.A.
Dean Dr. Patricia Graham/106 Withers Bldg.
Administrator Dr. Johnny Sanders, Jr., Professor and Unit Head
Department Counseling and Leadership
(803) 323-4725, fax (803) 323-4755,
http://coe.winthrop.edu/graduate/default.htm

Key See key for Data on Each Department (this section) on page 79.

Program
Accreditation Regional Accreditation, **CACREP:** Community Counseling, **CACREP:** School Counseling

CACREP

Uniqueness • NP.

Degrees • Community Counseling: M.
• School Counseling: M.

Contact • Community Counseling: M = Dr. Johnny Sanders, Jr..
• School Counseling: M = Dr. Johnny Sanders, Jr..

Admission and Graduation Data
Admission
Requirements • Community Counseling(M): GPA 2.00; GRE 800; MAT 40; Interview.
• School Counseling(M): GPA 2.00; GRE 800; MAT 40; Interview.

Enrollment • Community Counseling(M): 12 Admitted yearly; 10 Graduated yearly; 10 Female; 2 Male.
• School Counseling(M): 12 Admitted yearly; 14 Graduated yearly; 22 Female; 3 Male.

Diversity • African-American; Caucasian; Hispanic.

Graduation
Requirements • Community Counseling(M): 51 Class hours; 100 Practicum hours; 600 Internship hours; Comprehensive exam.
• School Counseling(M): 51 Class hours; 100 Practicum hours; 600 Internship hours; Comprehensive exam.

Postgraduation activity: Advanced education and employment setting percentages.
• Community Counseling(M): 1 Advanced education; 80 Agency practice; 19% Elementary school.
• School Counseling(M): 40 Elementary school; 30 Middle school; 30 Secondary school.

Planned Program Modifications
Courses	Drop	Add
	• NP.	• Addictions
		• Computer and Related Technology
		• Marriage and Family Counseling
		• Psychodiagnosis
		• Psychopharmacology
		• Supervision
		• Technology.
Other	Decrease	Increase
	• NP.	• Course Offerings
		• Diversity Recruiting of Faculty
		• Diversity Recruiting of Students.

Related Programs Clinical Social Workers
Psychology

Faculty

nbcc ❖. Percent of faculty reported with NCC certification: **100**%. **ncc** ❖.

Percent in professional counseling practice: 0%.

Research interests Loss and grief issues, diversity, group counseling, lifespan development

Diversity   • African-American; Caucasian.

Name, Degree, Rank, State/National Credentials, % time devoted to program, email
• Sanders, Jr., Johnny; PhD; Full Prof.; LPC, NCC; >81%; *sandersj@winthrop.edu*
• Whiting, Peggy P; EdD; Full Prof.; LPC, NCC; >81%; *whitingp@winthrop.edu*

Has CHI SIGMA IOTA (International Counseling Society) chapter.

SD: South Dakota State University

	Box 507 Wenona Hall Brookings, SD 57007-0095 USA
Dean	
Administrator	Jay Trenhaile, Interim Department Head
	Department Dept of Counseling & Human Res. Development (605) 688-4190, fax (605) 688-5929

Key   See key for Data on Each Department (this section) on page 79.

Program

Accreditation   **CACREP:** Community Counseling, **CACREP:** School Counseling, **CACREP:** Student Affairs - Counseling

CACREP

Uniqueness   Cohort group in Mission, SD, on the Rosebud Reservation

Degrees
- Community Counseling: M.
- School Counseling: M.
- Student Affairs: M.

Contact
- Community Counseling: M = Marla Muxen.
- School Counseling: M = Jay Trenhaile.
- Student Affairs: M = Ruth Harper.

Admission and Graduation Data

Admission

Requirements
- Community Counseling(M): GPA 3.00; Interview.
- School Counseling(M): GPA 3.00; Interview.
- Student Affairs(M): GPA 3.00; Interview.

Enrollment
- Community Counseling(M): 25 Admitted yearly; 25 Graduated yearly.
- School Counseling(M): 25 Admitted yearly; 25 Graduated yearly.
- Student Affairs(M): 10 Admitted yearly; 10 Graduated yearly.

Diversity
- African-American; Caucasian; Native American; Multiracial.

Graduation

Requirements
- Community Counseling(M): 48 Class hours; 100 Practicum hours; 600 Internship hours; Comprehensive exam; Oral exam.
- School Counseling(M): 48 Class hours; 100 Practicum hours; 600 Internship hours; Comprehensive exam; Oral exam.
- Student Affairs(M): 48 Class hours; 100 Practicum hours; 600 Internship hours; Oral exam.

Postgraduation activity: Advanced education and employment setting percentages.
- Community Counseling(M): NP.
- School Counseling(M): NP.
- Student Affairs(M): NP.

Planned Program Modifications

Courses

Drop	Add
• Abuse of Individual.	• Diversity • Play Therapy.

Other

Decrease	Increase
• NP.	• Diversity Recruiting of Faculty • Diversity Recruiting of Students • Number of Off-Campus Courses.

Related Programs •   NP.

Faculty

 Percent of faculty reported with NCC certification: 33%.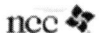

Percent in professional counseling practice: NP.

Research interests Solution Focused Therapy (school and student affairs applications), working with Native American clients and students, grief counseling

Diversity
- Caucasian.

Name, Degree, Rank, State/National Credentials, % time devoted to program, email
- Briddick, William; PhD; Assist.; >81%; *William_Briddick@sdstate.edu*
- Harper, Ruth; PhD; Assoc.; NCC; >81%; *Ruth_Harper@sdstate.edu*
- Martin, Francis; PhD; Full Prof.; NCC; <21%; *Francis_Martin@sdstate.edu*
- Briddick, Hande; PhD; Adjunct; LPC; >81%; *Hande_Briddick@sdstate.edu*
- Muxen, Marla; PhD; Assoc.; >81%; *Marla_Muxen@sdstate.edu*
- Britzman, Mark; EdD; Assoc.; >81%; *Mark_Britzman@sdstate.edu*

Has CHI SIGMA IOTA (International Counseling Society) chapter.

SD: The University of South Dakota

414 East Clark St
Vermillion, SD 57069
USA

Dean   Dr. Hank Rubin, Joint Dean, The University of South Dakota, Vermillion
Administrator Frank Main, Chair, Division of Counseling & Psychology in Education
                   Department   Division of Counseling & Psychology in Education
                   (605) 677-5250, fax (605) 677-5438, fmain@usd.edu, www.usd.edu/cpe/

Key   See key for Data on Each Department (this section) on page 79.

Program

Accreditation   Regional Accreditation, **CACREP:** Community Counseling, **CACREP:** Counselor Education
                 and Supervision, **CACREP:** School Counseling, **CACREP:** Student Affairs - Counseling

Uniqueness   The Division delivers the M.A., Ed.S. and Ph.D. degree in Counseling, School Pychology, and
                 Educational Psychology. The clinical programs are nationally accredited (Counseling,
                 CACREP and School Psychology, NASP). The University of South Dakota has been identified
                 as one of the best buys for Midsized Universities in the country (US News and World Report).

Degrees   • Community Counseling: M.
                 • Mental Health Counseling: S.
                 • School Counseling: M.
                 • Marriage and Family Counseling: S.
                 • Student Affairs: M.
                 • Counselor Education: PhD.

Contact   • Community Counseling: M = Frank Main.
                 • Mental Health Counseling: S = Frank Main.
                 • School Counseling: M = Frank Main.
                 • Marriage and Family Counseling: S = Frank Main.
                 • Student Affairs: M = Frank Main.
                 • Counselor Education: D = Frank Main, Chair CPE.

Admission and Graduation Data

Admission

Requirements   • Community Counseling(M): GPA 3.00; GRE 900; GRE V 450; GRE Q 450; GRE A 450;
                   MAT NA.
                 • Mental Health Counseling(S): GPA 3.00; GRE 900; GRE V 450; GRE Q 450; GRE A 450.
                 • School Counseling(M): GPA 3.00; GRE 900; GRE V 450; GRE Q 450; GRE A 450.
                 • Marriage and Family Counseling(S): GPA 3.00; GRE 900; GRE V 450; GRE Q 450;
                   GRE A 450.
                 • Student Affairs(M): GPA 3.00; GRE 900; GRE V 450; GRE Q 450; GRE A 450.
                 • Counselor Education(D): Masters and GPA 3.40; GRE 1500; GRE V 500; GRE Q 500;
                   GRE A 500.

Enrollment   • Community Counseling(M): 12 Admitted yearly; 75% Female; 25% Male.
                 • Mental Health Counseling(S): 5 Admitted yearly.
                 • School Counseling(M): 12 Admitted yearly; 75% Female; 25% Male.
                 • Marriage and Family Counseling(S).
                 • Student Affairs(M): 5 Admitted yearly; 75% Female; 25% Male.
                 • Counselor Education(D): 8 Admitted yearly; 3 Graduated yearly; 50% Female; 50% Male.

Diversity   • African-American; Asian-American; Caucasian; Native American.

Graduation

Requirements   • Community Counseling(M): 51 Class hours; 45 Practicum hours; 600 Internship hours;
                   Comprehensive exam.
                 • Mental Health Counseling(S): 45 Practicum hours; 600 Internship hours; Comprehensive
                   exam.
                 • School Counseling(M): 51 Class hours; 45 Practicum hours; 600 Internship hours;
                   Comprehensive exam.
                 • Marriage and Family Counseling(S): 45 Practicum hours; 600 Internship hours;
                   Comprehensive exam.
                 • Student Affairs(M): 51 Class hours; 45 Practicum hours; 600 Internship hours;
                   Comprehensive exam.
                 • Counselor Education(D): 90 Practicum hours; 600 Internship hours; Comprehensive exam;
                   Oral exam; Dissertation.

Postgraduation activity: Advanced education and employment setting percentages.
- Community Counseling(M): 100 Advanced education; 25 Managed care; 25 Private practice; 50 Agency practice.
- Mental Health Counseling(S): 100 Advanced education; 25 Managed care; 25 Private practice; 50 Agency practice.
- School Counseling(M): 100 Advanced education; 25 Elementary school; 25 Middle school; 50 Secondary school.
- Marriage and Family Counseling(S): 100 Advanced education; 25 Managed care; 25 Private practice; 50 Agency practice.
- Student Affairs(M): 100 Advanced education.
- Counselor Education(D): 75 Advanced education; 12 Managed care; 12 Private practice.

Planned Program Modifications

Courses	Drop	Add
	• NP.	• Addictions
		• Diversity
		• Legal/Ethical Issues.

Other	Decrease	Increase
	• NP.	• NP.

Related Programs Psychology

Faculty

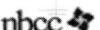 Percent of faculty reported with NCC certification: **100**%.

Percent in professional counseling practice: 75%.

Research interests Family Therapy, Play Therapy, Agency Counseling, Student Affairs Practice, School Counseling and Counselor Education, Diversity training in Secondary schools,

Diversity • Asian-American; Caucasian; Multiracial.

Name, Degree, Rank, State/National Credentials, % time devoted to program, email
- Mims, Grace; PhD; Full Prof.; LPC, NCC, CCMHC; >81%; *gmims@usd.edu*
- Korcuska, Jim; PhD; Assist.; LPC, NCC; >81%; *jkorcusk@usd.edu*
- Pietrzak, Dale; EdD; Assoc.; LPC, NCC; >81%; *dpietrza@usd.edu*
- Logan, Janet; PhD; Assoc.; LPC, NCC, Approved Play Therapy Supervisor; >81%; *jlogan@usd.edu*
- Main, Frank; EdD; Full Prof.; LPC, NCC, AAMFT Approved Supervisor; >81%; *fmain@usd.edu*

Has CHI SIGMA IOTA (International Counseling Society) chapter.

TN: East Tennessee State University

	Box 70548
	Johnson City, TN 37604
	USA
Dean	Dr. Collins, College of Education
Administrator	Clifton Mitchell, Ph.D., Associate Professor
	Department Human Development & Learning Dept.
	(423) 439-7688, fax (423) 439-7688, Mitchelc@etsu.edu,
	coe.etsu.edu/counseling/index.htm

Key   See key for Data on Each Department (this section) on page 79.

Program

Accreditation   Regional Accreditation, **CACREP:** Community Counseling, **CACREP:** School Counseling

Uniqueness   Community Agency and School tracks are CACREP accredited. Program emphasizes training of counselors. There is significant faculty-student contact.

Degrees
- Community Counseling: M.
- School Counseling: M.
- Marriage and Family Counseling: M.

Contact
- Community Counseling: M = Clifton Mitchell.
- School Counseling: M = Patricia Robertson.
- Marriage and Family Counseling: M = Brent Morrow.

Admission and Graduation Data

Admission

Requirements
- Community Counseling(M): GRE R; Interview.
- School Counseling(M): GRE R; Interview.
- Marriage and Family Counseling(M): GRE R; Interview.

Enrollment
- Community Counseling(M): 10 Admitted yearly; 9 Graduated yearly.
- School Counseling(M): 10 Admitted yearly; 9 Graduated yearly.
- Marriage and Family Counseling(M): 10 Admitted yearly; 9 Graduated yearly.

Diversity
- African-American; Asian-American; Caucasian; Hispanic.

Graduation

Requirements
- Community Counseling(M): 48 Class hours; 100 Practicum hours; 600 Internship hours; Comprehensive exam.
- School Counseling(M): 48 Class hours; 100 Practicum hours; 600 Internship hours; Comprehensive exam.
- Marriage and Family Counseling(M): 48 Class hours.

Postgraduation activity: Advanced education and employment setting percentages.
- Community Counseling(M): 2 Advanced education; 5 Private practice; 85 Agency practice; 8 Other.
- School Counseling(M): 2 Advanced education; 30 Elementary school; 30 Middle school; 30 Secondary school; 8 Other.
- Marriage and Family Counseling(M): 2 Advanced education; 5 Private practice; 85 Agency practice; 8 Other.

Planned Program Modifications

Courses	Drop	Add
	• NP.	• NP.

Other	Decrease	Increase
	• NP.	• NP.

Related Programs Clinical Social Workers
Psychology

Faculty

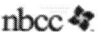   Percent of faculty reported with NCC certification: 67%.   ncc ❖

Percent in professional counseling practice: NP.

Research interests Resistance, mind-body approaches to therapy, family therapy, multicultural issues.

Diversity   •   Caucasian.

Name, Degree, Rank, State/National Credentials, % time devoted to program, email
- Bitter, James R; EdD; Full Prof.; LPC, NCC; >81%; *BitterJ@etsu.edu*
- Disque, J. Graham; PhD; Assoc.; NCC, LMFT; >81%; *Disque@etsu.edu*
- Mitchell, Clifton W; PhD; Assoc.; Lic. Psychologist; >81%; *Mitchelc@etsu.edu*
- Morrow, Brent; PhD; Assoc.; LMFT; >81%; *MorrowB@etsu.edu*
- Robertson, Patricia E; EdD; Assoc.; LPC, NCC; 61-80%; *RobertPE@etsu.edu*
- Whitmore, Harold L; EdD; Full Prof.; LPC, NCC; 41-60%; *Whitmore@etsu.edu*

Has CHI SIGMA IOTA (International Counseling Society) chapter.

TN: Lee University

	1120 North Ocoee Street Cleveland, TN 37311-4475 USA
Dean	Dewayne Thompson, Ph.D., Dean of Arts and Sciences
Administrator	Doyle Goff, Ph.D., Director of Graduate Counseling Programs
	Department Graduate Counseling (423) 614-8124, fax (423) 614-8129, mspsych@leeuniversity.edu, http://www.leeuniversity.edu/acad/graduate/

Key   See key for Data on Each Department (this section) on page 79.

Program

Accreditation   Regional Accreditation

Uniqueness   The purpose of the Lee University Counseling Programs is to train students in the discipline of professional counseling from a Christian perspective.

Degrees
- Mental Health Counseling: M.
- School Counseling: M.

Contact
- Mental Health Counseling: M = Doyle Goff, Ph.D.
- School Counseling: M = Susan Carter, Ph.D.

Admission and Graduation Data
Admission

Requirements
- Mental Health Counseling(M): GPA 3.00; GRE ~1000 V+Q; Interview.
- School Counseling(M): GPA 3.00; GRE ~1000 V+Q; Interview.

Enrollment
- Mental Health Counseling(M): 18 Admitted yearly; 15 Graduated yearly; 40 Female; 11 Male.
- School Counseling(M): 15 Admitted yearly.

Diversity
- African-American; Asian-American; Caucasian; Hispanic; Native American.

Graduation

Requirements
- Mental Health Counseling(M): 60 Class hours; 150 Practicum hours; 500 Internship hours; Comprehensive exam; CPCE; Oral exam.
- School Counseling(M): 48 Class hours; 150 Practicum hours; 600 Internship hours; Comprehensive exam.

Postgraduation activity: Advanced education and employment setting percentages.
- Mental Health Counseling(M): 12 Advanced education; 35 Private practice; 48 Agency practice; 5 Other.
- School Counseling(M): NP.

Planned Program Modifications

Courses	Drop	Add
	• Intelligence Testing.	• Addictions • Psychopharmacology.

Other	Decrease	Increase
	• NP.	• Admission Requirements • Course Offerings • Clinical Supervision • Diversity Recruiting of Faculty • Diversity Recruiting of Students • Faculty FTE • Financial Aid • Graduation Requirements • National Accreditation.

Related Programs •   NP.

Faculty

nbcc ❧   Percent of faculty reported with NCC certification: 17%.   **ncc** ❧

Percent in professional counseling practice: 83%.

Research interests Diagnosis and treatment of attention deficit disorder within a school setting. Use of spiritual resources within professional counseling.

Diversity   •   Caucasian; Multiracial.

Name, Degree, Rank, State/National Credentials, % time devoted to program, email
*   Milliron, Trevor; PhD; Assist.; Licensed Psychologist; >81%; *tmilliron@leeuniversity.edu*
*   Stone, Edward; PhD; Assist.; LPC, NCC; >81%; *estone@leeuniversity.edu*
*   Goff, Doyle; PhD; Full Prof.; MFT; >81%; *drgoff@leeuniversity.edu*
*   Carter, Susan; PhD; Assist.; LPC, CSC; 22-40%; *scarter@leeuniversity.edu*
*   Fisher, Robert; PhD; Assoc.; <21%; *rfisher@leeuniversity.edu*
*   Eckert, Kim; PsyD; Assist.; Licensed Psychologist; <21%; *keckert@leeuniversity.edu*

TN: Middle Tennessee State University

P. O. Box 87
Murfreesboro, TN 37132-0087
USA

Dean   Dr. Gloria Bonner, Education
Administrator   Larry Morris, Ph.D., Chair
    Department   Psychology
    (615) 898-2607, fax (615) 898-5027, lmorris@mtsu.edu

Key   See key for Data on Each Department (this section) on page 79.

Program

Accreditation   **CACREP:** School Counseling

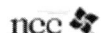
CACREP

Uniqueness   The School Counseling Program is housed in the Department of Psychology which allows students to be exposed to faculty from a variety of disciplines in Psychology. All School Counseling faculty have school Counseling experience. The Program also offers a School Psychology Program.

Degrees   • School Counseling: M.
   • Other: M, S.

Contact   • School Counseling: M = Virginia S. Dansby.
   • Other: M, S = James O. Rust.

Admission and Graduation Data

Admission

Requirements   • School Counseling(M): GPA 3.00; GRE 900; GRE V None speci; GRE Q None speci; GRE A None speci; Interview.
   • Other(M): GPA 3.00; GRE 900; GRE V None speci; GRE Q None speci.
   • Other(S): GPA 3.00; GRE 900; GRE V None speci; GRE Q None speci.

Enrollment   • School Counseling(M): 20 Admitted yearly; 16 Graduated yearly; 2 Male.
   • Other(M & S): 20 Admitted yearly; 16 Graduated yearly; 12 Female; 8 Male.

Diversity   • African-American; Asian-American; Caucasian.

Graduation

Requirements   • School Counseling(M): 49 Class hours; 100 Practicum hours; 600 Internship hours; Comprehensive exam.
   • Other(M): 45 Class hours; 100 Practicum hours; 600 Internship hours; Comprehensive exam; Thesis.
   • Other(S): 30 Class hours; 100 Practicum hours; 1200 Internship hours; Comprehensive exam; Thesis.

Postgraduation activity: Advanced education and employment setting percentages.
   • School Counseling(M): 60 Elementary school; 10 Middle school; 30 Secondary school.
   • Other(M & S): 10 Advanced education; 90 Agency practice.

Planned Program Modifications

Courses   <u>Drop</u>   <u>Add</u>
      • NP.   • Play Therapy.

Other   <u>Decrease</u>   <u>Increase</u>
      • Number of Degree Majors   • Diversity Recruiting of Faculty
      • Number of On-Line Courses.   • Diversity Recruiting of Students
            • National Accreditation.

Related Programs Psychology
       Other

Faculty

nbcc   Percent of faculty reported with NCC certification: 60%.   ncc

Percent in professional counseling practice: NP.

Research interests Group counseling, counselor effectiveness, developmental issues, program evaluation, gender issues, parenting, marriage, divorce issues, and child abuse.

Diversity • African-American; Asian-American; Caucasian; Multiracial.

Name, Degree, Rank, State/National Credentials, % time devoted to program, email
- Dansby, Virginia S; EdD; Full Prof.; NCC, PSY; >81%; *vdansby@mtsu.edu*
- Quarto, Christopher J; PhD; Assoc.; PSY; 61-80%; *cquarto@mtsu.edu*
- Slicker, Ellen K; PhD; Assoc.; NCC, PSY; 61-80%; *eslicker@mtsu.edu*
- West, William B; EdD; Full Prof.; LPC, NCC, LMFT; 22-40%; *wbwest@mtsu.edu*
- Rambo, Brenda C; PhD; Assist.; PSY; 61-80%; *brambo@mtsu.edu*

TN: Peabody College, Vanderbilt University

Box 90, GPC
Nashville, TN 37203
USA

Dean
Administrator   Gina Frieden, Program Director
                    Department   Human Developmental Counseling
                                (615) 322-8484, fax (615) 343-2661, hdc@vanderbilt.edu,
                                http://peabody.vanderbilt.edu/depts/hod/hodweb/grad/hdc.html

Key   See key for Data on Each Department (this section) on page 79.

Program
Accreditation   Regional Accreditation, **CACREP:** Community Counseling, **CACREP:** School Counseling

CACREP

Uniqueness   Program has emphasis on human cognitive development, constructivism, multiculturalism,
                  school counseling

Degrees   • Community Counseling: M.
                  • School Counseling: M.

Contact   • Community Counseling: M = Gina Frieden.
                  • School Counseling: M = H. Lori Schnieders.

Admission and Graduation Data
Admission
Requirements   • Community Counseling(M): GPA 3.00; GRE 1000; MAT 50; Interview.
                  • School Counseling(M): GPA 3.00; GRE 1000; MAT 50; Interview.

Enrollment   • Community Counseling(M): 12 Admitted yearly; 12 Graduated yearly; 90% Female;
                    10% Male.
                  • School Counseling(M): 12 Admitted yearly; 12 Graduated yearly; 90% Female; 10% Male.

Diversity   • African-American; Asian-American; Caucasian; Pacific Islander.

Graduation
Requirements   • Community Counseling(M): 48 Class hours; 100 Practicum hours; 600 Internship hours;
                    Comprehensive exam; Oral exam.
                  • School Counseling(M): 48 Class hours; 100 Practicum hours; 600 Internship hours;
Comprehensive exam; Oral exam; Portfolio.

Postgraduation activity: Advanced education and employment setting percentages.
                  • Community Counseling(M): 10 Advanced education; 10 Managed care; 15 Private practice;
                    45 Agency practice; 2 Student affairs; 18 Other.
                  • School Counseling(M): 5 Advanced education; 25 Elementary school; 30 Middle school; 30
                    Secondary school; 10 Other.

Planned Program Modifications
Courses   Drop   Add
                  • Consultation.   • Legal/Ethical Issues
                                                     • Play Therapy.

Other   Decrease   Increase
                  • NP.   • Course Offerings
                                                     • Diversity Recruiting of Faculty
                                                     • Diversity Recruiting of Students
                                                     • Faculty FTE
                                                     • Financial Aid.

Related Programs Psychology
                    Psychiatrists
                    Organizational Behaviorists

Faculty

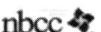   Percent of faculty reported with NCC certification: 0%.   ncc ❧

Percent in professional counseling practice: 75%.

Research interests Development of college students, school counseling/prevention programs, community development, race relations & diversity, adult development/transitions

Diversity   • African-American; Asian-American; Caucasian.

Name, Degree, Rank, State/National Credentials, % time devoted to program, email
• Frieden, Gina L; PhD; Assist.; >81%; *gina.frieden@vanderbilt.edu*
• Nation, Maury; PhD; Assist.; >81%; *maury.nation@vanderbilt.edu*
• Schnieders, H. Lori; EdD; Assist.; >81%; *lori.schnieders@vanderbilt.edu*
• Griffith, Brian A; PhD; Lecturer; 41-60%; *brian.griffith@vanderbilt.edu*
• Freudenthal, Judy; EdD; Adjunct; <21%; *jfreudenthal@oasiscenter.org*
• Barkley, William M; PhD; Adjunct; 22-40%; *william.m.barkley@vanderbilt.edu*
• Speer, Paul W; PhD; Assoc.; <21%; *paul.w.speer@vanderbilt.edu*
• Ota Wang, Vivian; PhD; Assist.; 22-40%; *ota.wang@vanderbilt.edu*
• Prilleltensky, Ora; PhD; Adjunct; 22-40%; *ora.prilleltensky@vanderbilt.edu*

Has CHI SIGMA IOTA (International Counseling Society) chapter.

TN: The University of Tennessee at Knoxville

526 Claxton Addition
Knoxville, TN 37996-3452
USA

Dean
Administrator Steve McCallum, Department Head
Department   Dept. of Educational Psychology and Counseling
(865) 974-8145, fax (865) 974-0135

Key   See key for Data on Each Department (this section) on page 79.

Program
Accreditation   Regional Accreditation, **CACREP:** Mental Health Counseling, **CACREP:** School Counseling,
CORE: Rehabilitation Counseling

Uniqueness   From the national counselor education perspective, the University of Tennessee has oversight
of the International Counselor Network, one faculty member has received the AMCHA
Counselor Educator of the Year Award, one faculty member has received an ASCA Writer of
the Year award, and our graduates are taking leadership roles in both AMCHA and ASCA. Our
faculty have published numerous books and articles on counseling. From the state
perspective, our faculty and students are taking leadership roles in the profession serving on
a state committee for developing standards for school counseling programs. Regionally, we
address issues related to providing counseling services and education to meet the unique
needs of an Appalachian culture. There is a shortage of counselor educators with doctorates
in the areas of school counseling and rehabilitation. We are working to address these
shortages.

Degrees   • Mental Health Counseling: M.
• School Counseling: M, S.
• Rehabilitation Counseling: M.
• Counselor Education: PhD.

Contact   • Mental Health Counseling: M = Dr. Charles Thompson.
• School Counseling: M = Dr. William Poppen.; S = NP.
• Rehabilitation Counseling: M = NP.
• Counselor Education: D = NP.

Admission and Graduation Data
Admission
Requirements   • Mental Health Counseling(M): GPA 3.00; GRE 1000.
• School Counseling(M): GPA 2.70; GRE 1000.
• School Counseling(S): GPA 2.70; GRE 1000.
• Rehabilitation Counseling(M): GPA 2.70; GRE 1000; Interview.
• Counselor Education(D): Masters and GPA 3.50; GRE 1100; GRE V 500; GRE Q 550; 2
Years work experience.

Enrollment   • Mental Health Counseling(M): 20 Admitted yearly; 20 Graduated yearly.
• School Counseling(M & S): 13 Admitted yearly; 11 Graduated yearly.
• Rehabilitation Counseling(M): 15 Admitted yearly; 11 Graduated yearly.
• Counselor Education(D): 5 Admitted yearly; 3 Female; 2 Male.

Diversity   • African-American; Caucasian; Hispanic; Native American; Pacific Islander; Multiracial.

Graduation
Requirements   • Mental Health Counseling(M): 60 Class hours; 100 Practicum hours; 900 Internship hours;
Comprehensive exam.
• School Counseling(M): 48 Class hours; 100 Practicum hours; 600 Internship hours;
Comprehensive exam.
• School Counseling(S): 70 Class hours.
• Rehabilitation Counseling(M): 54 Class hours; 150 Practicum hours; 600 Internship hours;
Comprehensive exam.
• Counselor Education(D): 110 Class hours.

Postgraduation activity: Advanced education and employment setting percentages.
• Mental Health Counseling(M): 25 Advanced education; 20 Private practice; 55 Agency
practice.
• School Counseling(M & S): 10 Advanced education; 40 Elementary school; 20 Middle
school; 30 Secondary school.
• Rehabilitation Counseling(M): 10 Advanced education; 5 Managed care; 10 Private
practice; 75 Agency practice.
• Counselor Education(D):

Planned Program Modifications

Courses	Drop	Add
	• NP.	• NP.

Other	Decrease	Increase
	• NP.	• Course Offerings
		• Diversity Recruiting of Students
		• Financial Aid
		• National Accreditation.

Related Programs Clinical Social Workers
Psychology
Organizational Behaviorists

Faculty

nbcc ❧   Percent of faculty reported with NCC certification: 64%.   ncc ❧

Percent in professional counseling practice: NP.

Research interests Research interests and projects of the counseling faculty include: the study of the interface between counselor and client; investigation of how systems of privilege and oppression affect treatment theory and practice; study of the practice of case management; investigation of the professional development of students; study of international counseling and human services; investigation of evaluating counseling outcomes of Reality Therapy and Solution-focused Counseling; phenomenological study of life events; investigation of the quality of academic life and the locus of control of college students with disabilities; oversight of the International Counselor Network; investigation of student experiences through internship stages; study of efficacy of peer advising and mentoring; study of the use of technology in supervision; and investigation of counselor ego development; the development and study of full service schools.

Diversity   • African-American; Caucasian.

Name, Degree, Rank, State/National Credentials, % time devoted to program, email
• Conwill, William; PhD; Assist.; NCC; >81%; *wconwill@utk.edu*
• Diambra, Joel; EdD; Assist.; LPC, NCC, MHSP; <21%; *jdiambra@utk.edu*
• Kronick, Robert F; PhD; Full Prof.; 22-40%; *rkronick@utk.edu*
• McClam, Tricia; PhD; Full Prof.; NCC; 61-80%; *mcclam@utk.edu*
• Peterson, Marla; PhD; Full Prof.; LPC, NCC; >81%; *peterson@utk.edu*
• Poppen, William A; PhD; Full Prof.; LPC; >81%; *poppen@utk.edu*
• Skinner, Amy; PhD; Assist.; LPC, NCC, CRC; <21%; *askinner@utk.edu*
• Thompson, Charles L; PhD; Full Prof.; LPC, NCC; >81%; *cthomps5@utk.edu*
• Woodside, Marianne; EdD; Full Prof.; LPC, NCC; >81%; *mwoodsid@utk.edu*
• Cassell, Jack; PhD; Assoc.; CRC; 22-40%; *jcassell@utk.edu*
• Colvin, Craig; EdD; Assoc.; CRC; 22-40%; *ccolvin@utk.edu*

TN: Travecca Nazarene University

	333 Murfreesboro Road
	Nashville, TN 37210
	United States
Dean	Henry Spaulding
Administrator	Peter F. Wilson, Director of Graduate Psychology Program
	Department Division of Social & Behavioral Sciences
	(615) 248-1417, fax (615) 248-1366, admissions_psych@trevecca.edu,
	www.trevecca.edu

Key   See key for Data on Each Department (this section) on page 79.

Program

Accreditation   Regional Accreditation

Uniqueness   Traditional program offered in a non-traditional format - Saturday classes available.

Degrees
- Mental Health Counseling: M.
- Marriage and Family Counseling: M.
- Other: M.

Contact
- Mental Health Counseling: M = Peter Wilson.
- Marriage and Family Counseling: M = Don Harvey.
- Other: M = Peter Wilson.

Admission and Graduation Data

Admission

Requirements
- Mental Health Counseling(M): GPA 2.70; GRE 800; MAT 30.
- Marriage and Family Counseling(M): GPA 2.70; GRE 800; MAT 30.
- Other(M): GPA 2.70; GRE 800; MAT 30.

Enrollment
- Mental Health Counseling(M): NP.
- Marriage and Family Counseling(M): NP.
- Other(M): NP.

Diversity
- African-American; Asian-American; Caucasian; Hispanic.

Graduation

Requirements
- Mental Health Counseling(M): 48 Class hours; 300 Practicum hours; 200 Internship hours; Comprehensive exam.
- Marriage and Family Counseling(M): 51 Class hours; 300 Practicum hours.
- Other(M): 54 Class hours; 300 Practicum hours; Comprehensive exam; Thesis.

Postgraduation activity: Advanced education and employment setting percentages.
- Mental Health Counseling(M): NP.
- Marriage and Family Counseling(M): NP.
- Other(M): NP.

Planned Program Modifications

Courses	Drop	Add
	• NP.	• NP.

Other	Decrease	Increase
	• NP.	• Admission Requirements
		• Diversity Recruiting of Faculty.

Related Programs

Faculty

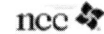 Percent of faculty reported with NCC certification: 11%.

Percent in professional counseling practice: 83.3%.

Research interests

Diversity
- African-American; Caucasian.

Name, Degree, Rank, State/National Credentials, % time devoted to program, email
- Wilson, Peter F; EdD; Psychologist; >81%; *pwilson@trevecca.edu*
- Harvey, Donald R; PhD; LPC, LMFT; >81%; *dharvey@trevecca.edu*
- Pruitt, Terry; EdD; LPC, LPE; 22-40%; *tpruitt@trevecca.edu*
- Anderson, William; EdD; Psychologist; <21%; *williamanderson@worldnett.att.net*

- Carden, Randy L; EdD; <21%; *rlcarden@comcast.net*
- Ericson, Scott; EdD; NCC, Psychologist; <21%; *slericson@juno.com*
- Fox, Bryce E; PhD; <21%; *bfox@trevecca.com*
- Gibson, Carol; PhD; LPC; <21%; *cargip@aol.com*
- Goodyear-Brown, Paris; MSSW; <21%; *parisgb@aol.com*
- Gordon, Sharon M; PsyD; Psychologist; <21%; *sharon.gordon@med.va.gov*
- Hamley, Roy W; EdD; LPC; <21%; *hamleyrw@dlu.edu*
- Jackson, James C; PsyD; Psychologist; <21%; *jm2jacksons@yahoo.com*
- Joslin, Rebecca; EdD; Psychologist; <21%; *cjoslin@bellsouth.net*
- Land, Rebakah; PhD; LPC, LMFT; <21%;
- McCurdy, Bruce E; EdD; Psychologist; <21%; *brucemccurdy@christcommunity.org*
- Slay, Patrick; MA; NCC; <21%; *patrickslay@aol.com*
- Turner, Paul; PhD; <21%; *paul.turner@lispcomb.edu*
- Webb, Carole; MS; LPC, LMFT; <21%; *cackw@mindspring.com*

TX: Angelo State University

	Box 10893, ASU Station
	San Angelo, TX 76909
	USA
Dean	Dr. John Miazga, San Angelo, Texas
Administrator	Dr. David J. Tarver, Assistant Professor
	Department School of Education
	(325) 942-2052, fax (325) 942-2039, david.tarver@angelo.edu, www.angelo.edu

Key   See key for Data on Each Department (this section) on page 79.

Program

Accreditation   Regional Accreditation

Uniqueness   Public School (K-12) Guidance and Counseling Masters' Program

Degrees   •   NP.

Contact   •   NP.

Admission and Graduation Data

Admission

Requirements   •   NP.

Enrollment   •   NP.

Diversity   •   NP.

Graduation

Requirements   •   NP.

Postgraduation activity: Advanced education and employment setting percentages.
    •   NP.

Planned Program Modifications

Courses	Drop		Add
• NP.		• NP.	

Other	Decrease		Increase
• NP.		• NP.	

Related Programs

Faculty

nbcc   Percent of faculty reported with NCC certification: 0%.   ncc

Percent in professional counseling practice: NP.

Research interests Learned optimism, self-efficacy and locus of control

Diversity   •   Caucasian.

Name, Degree, Rank, State/National Credentials, % time devoted to program, email
•   NP.

TX: Dallas Baptist University

3000 Mountain Creek Pkwy
Dallas, TX 75211-9299
USA
Dean Dr. Mike Williams
Administrator Mary Becerril, Ph.D., Director, M. A. in Counseling Program
Department   Humanities and Social Sciences
(214) 333-5265, fax (214) 333-6819, maryb@dbu.edu,
www.dbu.edu/graduate/mac.html

Key   See key for Data on Each Department (this section) on page 79.

Program
Accreditation   Regional Accreditation

Uniqueness   Program offers Christian counseling.

Degrees   • Mental Health Counseling: M.

Contact   • Mental Health Counseling: M = Mary Becerril.

Admission and Graduation Data
Admission
Requirements   • Mental Health Counseling(M): GPA 3.00; GRE 850; GRE V 400; GRE Q NA; GRE W 3.5.

Enrollment   • Mental Health Counseling(M): 95 Admitted yearly; 30 Graduated yearly; 75 Female; 22 Male.

Diversity   • African-American; Asian-American; Caucasian; Hispanic.

Graduation
Requirements   • Mental Health Counseling(M): 48 Class hours; 300 Practicum hours.

Postgraduation activity: Advanced education and employment setting percentages.
• Mental Health Counseling(M): NP.

Planned Program Modifications
Courses   Drop   Add
• NP.   • NP.

Other   Decrease   Increase
• NP.   • NP.

Related Programs

Faculty

 Percent of faculty reported with NCC certification: 0%.

Percent in professional counseling practice: 100%.

Research interests Play therapy certification

Diversity   • African-American; Caucasian.

Name, Degree, Rank, State/National Credentials, % time devoted to program, email
• Becerril, Mary; PhD; Full Prof.; LPC, LMFT; >81%;
• Brownlee, Ernest; MD; Instructor; Psychiatrist; <21%;
• Brunner, Brenda; MA; Instructor; LPC; <21%;
• Cobern, Keith; PhD; Instructor; LPC, LMFT; <21%;
• Colton, Robert; PhD; Full Prof.; Texas Licensed Psychologist; 22-40%;
• Hemminger, Wade; EdD; Assist.; LPC, LMFT, LCDC; >81%;
• Linder, Todd; MA; Instructor; LPC; <21%;
• Mahoney, Sondra; MEd; Instructor; LPC, LMFT; <21%;
• Mungadze, Jerry; PhD; Instructor; <21%;
• Sharp, Kenneth; MS; Instructor; LPC, LMFT; <21%;
• Moon-Hogan, Chery; MA; Instructor; <21%

TX: Houston Baptist University

7502 Fondren Road
Houston, TX 77074-3298
USA

Dean

Administrator Ann Owen, Ph.D., Chair

Department Dept. of Behavioral Science
(281) 649-3240, fax (281) 493-3361, gowen@hbu.edu

Key See key for Data on Each Department (this section) on page 79.

Program

Accreditation • NP.

Uniqueness Small classes; face to face interaction with professors, Christian atmosphere, constructivist approach.

Degrees
- Mental Health Counseling: M.
- School Counseling: M.
- Addictions Counseling: M.
- Career Counseling: M.
- Marriage and Family Counseling: M.
- Pastoral Counseling: M.

Contact
- Mental Health Counseling: M = NP.
- School Counseling: M = NP.
- Addictions Counseling: M = NP.
- Career Counseling: M = NP.
- Marriage and Family Counseling: M = NP.
- Pastoral Counseling: M = NP.

Admission and Graduation Data

Admission

Requirements
- Mental Health Counseling(M): GRE 850; GRE V 400; GRE Q 0; GRE A 0.
- School Counseling(M): NP.
- Addictions Counseling(M): GRE 850; GRE V 400; GRE Q 0; GRE A 0.
- Career Counseling(M): 3 Years work experience.
- Marriage and Family Counseling(M): GRE 400; GRE V 0; GRE Q 0; Interview.
- Pastoral Counseling(M): NP.

Enrollment
- Mental Health Counseling(M): 17 Graduated yearly.
- School Counseling(M): NP.
- Addictions Counseling(M): NP.
- Career Counseling(M): NP.
- Marriage and Family Counseling(M): NP.
- Pastoral Counseling(M): 6 Admitted yearly.

Diversity
- Pacific Islander.

Graduation

Requirements
- Mental Health Counseling(M): 48 Class hours; 450 Practicum hours.
- School Counseling(M): NP.
- Addictions Counseling(M): NP.
- Career Counseling(M): 450 Class hours.
- Marriage and Family Counseling(M): NP.
- Pastoral Counseling(M): NP.

Postgraduation activity: Advanced education and employment setting percentages.
- Mental Health Counseling(M): NP.
- School Counseling(M): NP.
- Addictions Counseling(M): NP.
- Career Counseling(M): NP.
- Marriage and Family Counseling(M): NP.
- Pastoral Counseling(M): NP.

Planned Program Modifications

Courses	Drop	Add
	• NP.	• NP.

Other	Decrease	Increase
	• NP.	• NP.

Related Programs

Faculty

nbcc 🔸   Percent of faculty reported with NCC certification: 0%.   ncc 🔸

Percent in professional counseling practice: NP.

Research interests • NP.

Diversity   • NP.

Name, Degree, Rank, State/National Credentials, % time devoted to program, email
- Alexander, T. John; PhD; Full Prof.; <21%; *tjalex@hbu.edu*
- Ballering, Lawrence; PhD; Adjunct; <21%;
- Borgers, Bill; PhD; <21%; *bborgers@hbu.edu*
- Clay, Gary; EdD; Assist.; <21%; *gclay@hbu.edu*
- Cummins, David; EdD; Adjunct; <21%;
- Fitzgerald, Doug; PhD; Assoc.; 41-60%; *dfitzgerald@hbu.edu*
- Hughes, Eloise; EdD; Assist.; <21%; *ehughes@hbu.edu*
- Lonnecker, Cecilia; PhD; Adjunct; <21%;
- Lutjeemeier, John; EdD; Full Prof.; 22-40%; *jlutjemeier@hbu.edu*
- Maddox, Martha; PhD; Assist.; 22-40%; *mmaddox@hbu.edu*
- Nero, Renata; PhD; Assoc.; 41-60%; *mero@hbu.edu*
- Owen, Ann; PhD; Assoc.; <21%; *aowen@hbu.edu*
- Roff, Linda; EdD; Full Prof.; <21%; *Lroff@hbu.du*
- Smoote, Stanley; PhD; Adjunct; <21%;

TX: Lamar University

4400 Martin Luther King Drive, P.O. Box 10034
Beaumont, TX 77710
USA

Dean
Administrator   Carolyn Crawford, Department Head
Department   Dept of Educational Leadership
                  (409) 880-8689, fax (409) 880-8685, IDS-PAB@hal.lamar.edu

Key   See key for Data on Each Department (this section) on page 79.

Program

Accreditation   • NP.

Uniqueness   Prepares school and community counselors as well as vocational counseling certification; opportunities for placement in correctional, clinical, mental health, and children's residential settings.

Degrees   • Community Counseling: M.
            • School Counseling: M.

Contact   • Community Counseling: M = NP.
            • School Counseling: M = NP.

Admission and Graduation Data

Admission

Requirements   • Community Counseling(M): NP.
                • School Counseling(M): NP.

Enrollment   • Community Counseling(M): 15 Graduated yearly.
              • School Counseling(M): 25 Graduated yearly.

Diversity   • NP.

Graduation

Requirements   • Community Counseling(M): 45 Class hours; 300 Practicum hours.
                • School Counseling(M): 45 Class hours; 300 Practicum hours.

Postgraduation activity: Advanced education and employment setting percentages.
                • Community Counseling(M): NP.
                • School Counseling(M): NP.

Planned Program Modifications

Courses   Drop   Add
                   • NP.   • NP.

Other   Decrease   Increase
                   • NP.   • NP.

Related Programs

Faculty

Percent of faculty reported with NCC certification: 0%.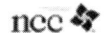

Percent in professional counseling practice: 50%.

Research interests • NP.

Diversity   • NP.

Name, Degree, Rank, State/National Credentials, % time devoted to program, email
• Crawford, Carolyn H; PhD; Assoc.; 41-60%; *crawfordch@hallamar.edu*
• Holmes, William; PhD; Assoc.; >81%; *holmeswr@hal.lamar.edu*
• McLaughlin, George; PhD; Full Prof.; >81%; *george@rocketmail.com*
• Wills, Curtis; EdD; Assoc.; 22-40%;

TX: Our Lady of the Lake University

411 S.W. 24th
San Antonio, TX 78207
USA
Dean   Dr. Robert DeVillar, School of Education and Clinical Studies
Administrator Dr. Joan Bierer, Chairperson
                  Department   Dept of Psychology
                                (210) 431-3914, fax (210) 436-0824, www.ollusa.edu

Key   See key for Data on Each Department (this section) on page 79.

Program
Accreditation   Regional Accreditation

Uniqueness   Focus on brief, systemic approaches and multiculturalism. Offer specialization in providing
                 services to Spanish speaking clients.

Degrees   • Mental Health Counseling: M.
                 • School Counseling: M.
                 • Marriage and Family Counseling: M.

Contact   • Mental Health Counseling: M = Joan Biever.
                 • School Counseling: M = Nadene Peterson.
                 • Marriage and Family Counseling: M = Joan Biever.

Admission and Graduation Data
Admission
Requirements   • Mental Health Counseling(M): GPA 2.50; GRE R; MAT R; Interview.
                 • School Counseling(M): GPA 2.75; GRE R; MAT R; Interview.
                 • Marriage and Family Counseling(M): GPA 2.50; GRE R; MAT R; Interview.

Enrollment   • Mental Health Counseling(M): 10 Admitted yearly; 10 Graduated yearly.
                 • School Counseling(M): 7 Admitted yearly; 7 Graduated yearly.
                 • Marriage and Family Counseling(M): 10 Admitted yearly; 10 Graduated yearly.

Diversity   • African-American; Asian-American; Caucasian; Hispanic; Native American; Multiracial.

Graduation
Requirements   • Mental Health Counseling(M): 60 Class hours; 500 Practicum hours; Comprehensive
                   exam.
                 • School Counseling(M): 48 Class hours; 300 Practicum hours; Comprehensive exam.
                 • Marriage and Family Counseling(M): 60 Class hours; 500 Practicum hours.

Postgraduation activity: Advanced education and employment setting percentages.
                 • Mental Health Counseling(M): 10 Advanced education; 10 Private practice; 70 Agency
                   practice; 10 Other.
                 • School Counseling(M): 30 Elementary school; 40 Middle school; 40 Secondary school.
                 • Marriage and Family Counseling(M): 10 Advanced education; 10 Private practice; 70
                   Agency practice; 10 Other.

Planned Program Modifications
Courses   Drop   Add
                 • NP.   • NP.

Other   Decrease   Increase
                 • NP.   • NP.

Related Programs Clinical Social Workers
                     Psychology

Faculty

nbcc ❖   Percent of faculty reported with NCC certification: 0%.   ncc ❖

Percent in professional counseling practice: 75%.

Research interests Multiculturalism, career development, process and effectiveness of brief therapies

Diversity   • Caucasian; Hispanic.

Name, Degree, Rank, State/National Credentials, % time devoted to program, email

- Bierer, Joan L; PhD; Full Prof.; Pscyhologist; 22-40%;
- Bobele, Monte; PhD; Full Prof.; Psychologist; 41-60%;
- Gardner, Glen T; PhD; Full Prof.; Psychologist; 61-80%;
- de las Fuentes, Cynthia; PhD; Assoc.; Psychologist; 61-80%;
- González, Cynthia; PhD; Assoc.; LSSP; >81%;
- Martinez, Isaac; PhD; Assist.; Psychologist; >81%;
- Peterson, Nadene; Full Prof.; LPC; >81%;

TX: Southwest Texas State University

601 S. University Drive
San Marcos, TX 78666
USA

Dean Mike Willoughby, Dean of Education
Administrator Thelma Duffey, Program Coordinator
Department Educational Administration and Psychological Services
(512) 245-2575, fax (512) 245-8872, www.eaps.swt.edu

Key See key for Data on Each Department (this section) on page 79.

Program

Accreditation **CACREP:** Marriage and Family Counseling, **CACREP:** School Counseling, **CACREP:** Student Affairs - Counseling, **CACREP:** Community Counseling

CACREP

Uniqueness Our program has a very strong clinical skill component. We also beleive in the importance of mentoring students. We have a strong expressive arts offering (play therapy, sandtray, psychodrama).

Degrees
- Community Counseling: M.
- School Counseling: M.
- Marriage and Family Counseling: M.
- Other: M.

Contact
- Community Counseling: M = John Garcia.
- School Counseling: M = JoLynne Reynolds.
- Marriage and Family Counseling: M = Mike Carns.
- Other: M = Jim Studer - Student Affairs.

Admission and Graduation Data

Admission

Requirements
- Community Counseling(M): GRE see below.
- School Counseling(M): NP.
- Marriage and Family Counseling(M): NP.
- Other(M): NP.

Enrollment
- Community Counseling(M): NP.
- School Counseling(M): NP.
- Marriage and Family Counseling(M): NP.
- Other(M): NP.

Diversity
- African-American; Asian-American; Caucasian; Hispanic; Native American; Multiracial.

Graduation

Requirements
- Community Counseling(M): NP.
- School Counseling(M): NP.
- Marriage and Family Counseling(M): NP.
- Other(M): NP.

Postgraduation activity: Advanced education and employment setting percentages.
- Community Counseling(M): NP.
- School Counseling(M): NP.
- Marriage and Family Counseling(M): NP.
- Other(M): NP.

Planned Program Modifications

Courses | Drop | | Add
- NP. | | • NP.

Other | Decrease | | Increase
- NP. | | • NP.

Related Programs Clinical Social Workers
Psychology
Arts Therapists

Faculty

nbcc Percent of faculty reported with NCC certification: 21%. ncc

Percent in professional counseling practice: 100%.

Research interests • NP.

Diversity • African-American; Caucasian; Hispanic; Multiracial.

Name, Degree, Rank, State/National Credentials, % time devoted to program, email
* Homeyer, Linda E; PhD; Assoc.; LPC, NCC, RPT; >81%; *lh12@swt.edu*
* Carns, Mike R; PhD; Assoc.; LPC, NCC, LMFT; TX cert. school counselor; >81%; *mc17@swt.edu*
* Brown, Christopher; PhD; Assist.; LPC, RPT; >81%; *cb29@swt.edu*
* Connolly, Colleen; PhD; Assist.; LPC, LMFT; >81%; *cc32@swt.edu*
* Duffey, Thelma; PhD; Assoc.; LPC, LMFT; >81%; *td05@swt.edu*
* Garcia, John L; PhD; Assoc.; LPC, NCC; >81%; *jg12@swt.edu*
* Garrison, John; PhD; Assist.; <21%;
* Jones, Lesley; PhD; Assoc.; LPC, Psychologist; >81%;
* Kerl, Stella; PhD; Assoc.; Psychologist; >81%; *sk08@swt.edu*
* Moore, Pamela; PhD; Assist.; Psychologist; 22-40%; *pm08@swt.edu*
* Schmidt, Eric; PhD; Assist.; LPC; >81%; *es17@swt.edu*
* Studer, James; PhD; Assoc.; <21%; *js10@swt.edu*
* Wyatt, Carl V; PhD; Assist.; LPC; <21%; *cw23@swt.edu*
* Reynolds, JoLynne; PhD; Assist.; LPC, CSC (TX); *jr36@swt.edu*

Has CHI SIGMA IOTA (International Counseling Society) chapter.

TX: Stephen F. Austin State University

P.O. Box 13019, SFA Station
Nacogdoches, TX 75962-3019
USA
Dean   Dr. John Jacobson
Administrator   Dr. Robert O. Choate, Counseling Program Director
                    Department   Human Services
                              (936) 468-2906, fax (936) 468-1342, rchoate@sfasu.edu, www.sfasu.edu/hs

Key   See key for Data on Each Department (this section) on page 79.

Program

Accreditation   **CACREP:** School Counseling, CORE: Rehabilitation Counseling, **CACREP:** Community Counseling

Uniqueness   Three counseling degrees, community, school and rehabilitation

Degrees
- Community Counseling: M.
- School Counseling: M.
- Rehabilitation Counseling: M.

Contact
- Community Counseling: M = Dr. Tom Caffery.
- School Counseling: M = Dr. Jan Stalling.
- Rehabilitation Counseling: M = Dr. Robert Choate.

Admission and Graduation Data

Admission

Requirements
- Community Counseling(M): Interview.
- School Counseling(M): Interview.
- Rehabilitation Counseling(M): Interview.

Enrollment
- Community Counseling(M): 15 Admitted yearly; 15 Graduated yearly; 13 Female; 2 Male.
- School Counseling(M): 10 Admitted yearly; 10 Graduated yearly; 1 Male.
- Rehabilitation Counseling(M): 8 Admitted yearly; 6 Graduated yearly; 4 Female; 4 Male.

Diversity
- African-American; Caucasian; Hispanic; Multiracial.

Graduation

Requirements
- Community Counseling(M): 48 Class hours; 150 Practicum hours; 600 Internship hours; Comprehensive exam; Oral exam.
- School Counseling(M): 48 Class hours; 150 Practicum hours; 600 Internship hours; Comprehensive exam; Oral exam.
- Rehabilitation Counseling(M): 48 Class hours; 150 Practicum hours; 600 Internship hours; Comprehensive exam; Oral exam.

Postgraduation activity: Advanced education and employment setting percentages.
- Community Counseling(M): 10 Advanced education; 10 Managed care; 10 Private practice; 70 Agency practice.
- School Counseling(M): 50 Elementary school; 30 Middle school; 20 Secondary school.
- Rehabilitation Counseling(M): 10 Advanced education; 60 Agency practice.

Planned Program Modifications

Courses   Drop   Add
- NP.   - Addictions
                                 - Experiential Component
                                 - Marriage and Family Counseling
                                 - Psychodiagnosis
                                 - Psychopharmacology.

Other   Decrease   Increase
- NP.   - Course Offerings
                                 - Faculty FTE
                                 - Number of Distance Education Courses
                                 - Number of Off-Campus Courses.

Related Programs Communications

Faculty

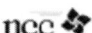 Percent of faculty reported with NCC certification: 50%.

Percent in professional counseling practice: 50%.

Research interests Adjustment Disorder, ethics and decision making

Diversity   • Caucasian; Native American.

Name, Degree, Rank, State/National Credentials, % time devoted to program, email
• Choate, Robert O; EdD; Full Prof.; LPC, NCC, CRC; >81%; *rchoate@sfasu.edu*
• Holland, Jane A; PhD; Assoc.; LPC; >81%; *jholland@sfasu.edu*
• Caffery, Tom E; EdD; Assist.; LPC, NCC; >81%; *tcaffery@sfasu.edu*
• Stalling, Jan; EdD; Assoc.; LPC, NCC; >81%; *jstalling@sfasu.edu*
• Weber, Bill F; EdD; Full Prof.; LPC, CRC, CVE; >81%; *bweber@sfasu.edu*
• Fish, Dale A; EdD; Full Prof.; LPC; >81%; *dfish@sfasu.edu*

Has CHI SIGMA IOTA (International Counseling Society) chapter.

TX: Tarleton State University

T-O820
Stephenville, TX 76402
USA
Dean   Jill Burk, Ph. D.
Administrator Linda Duncan, Ed.D., Coordinator
                   Department   Dept of ED Administration Counseling & Psychology
                                 (254) 968-9090, fax (254) 968-9947, duncan@tarleton.edu,
                                 www.tarleton.edu

Key   See key for Data on Each Department (this section) on page 79.

Program

Accreditation   Regional Accreditation

Uniqueness   The counseling program began with the purpose of preparing school counselors. The program
                now offers both M. Ed. and M. S. degrees in counseling psychology, marriage and family
                counseling, and educational psychology.

Degrees   • Mental Health Counseling: M.
                • School Counseling: M.
                • Marriage and Family Counseling: M.
                • Other: NP.

Contact   • Mental Health Counseling: M = All faculty.
                • School Counseling: M = Albrecht, Duncan, Weissenberger.
                • Marriage and Family Counseling: M = Bill LaBauve, Gary Mauldin.
                • Other: Weissenberger, LaPierre.

Admission and Graduation Data

Admission

Requirements   • Mental Health Counseling(M): GPA 3.00; GRE 850.
                • School Counseling(M): GPA 3.00; GRE 850.
                • Marriage and Family Counseling(M): GPA 3.00; GRE 850.
                • Other (M): GPA 3.00; GRE 850.

Enrollment   • Mental Health Counseling(M): 20 Admitted yearly; 20 Graduated yearly.
                • School Counseling(M): 40 Admitted yearly; 40 Graduated yearly.
                • Marriage and Family Counseling(M): 30 Admitted yearly; 30 Graduated yearly.
                • Other (M): NP.

Diversity   • African-American; Asian-American; Caucasian; Hispanic; Native American; Multiracial.

Graduation

Requirements   • Mental Health Counseling(M): 48 Class hours; 6 Practicum hours; 300 Internship hours;
                  Comprehensive exam.
                • School Counseling(M): 48 Class hours; 6 Practicum hours; 300 Internship hours;
                  Comprehensive exam.
                • Marriage and Family Counseling(M): 48 Class hours; 9 Practicum hours; 500 Internship
                  hours; Comprehensive exam.
                • Other (M): 48 Class hours; 9 Practicum hours; 500 Internship hours; Comprehensive exam.

Postgraduation activity: Advanced education and employment setting percentages.
                • Mental Health Counseling(M): 10 Advanced education; 90 Agency practice.
                • School Counseling(M): 73 Elementary school; 15 Middle school; 15 Secondary school.
                • Marriage and Family Counseling(M): 10 Advanced education; 90 Agency practice.

Planned Program Modifications

Courses   Drop   Add
                       • NP.   • Internet Use
                                                      • Supervision.

Other   Decrease   Increase
                       • NP.   • Admission Requirements
                                                      • Diversity Recruiting of Faculty
                                                      • Diversity Recruiting of Students
                                                      • National Accreditation
                                                      • Number of On-Line Courses.

Related Programs

Faculty

nbcc   Percent of faculty reported with NCC certification: 29%.   ncc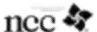

Percent in professional counseling practice: 50%.

Research interests Research includes school counseling and guidance, resiliency in marriage, counseling theory, and spirituality and counseling.

Diversity • Caucasian.

Name, Degree, Rank, State/National Credentials, % time devoted to program, email
- Albrecht, Annette; PhD; Assoc.; LPC, NCC; >81%; *albrech@tarleton.edu*
- Duncan, Linda; EdD; Full Prof.; LPC, NCC, LMFT; >81%; *duncan@tarleton.edu*
- LaBauve, Bill; PhD; LMFT; >81%; *labauve@tarleton.edu*
- LaPierre, Coady; PhD; >81%; *lapierre@tarleton.edu*
- Mauldin, Gary; PhD; LPC, LMFT; >81%; *mauldin@tarleton.edu*
- Moseley, Pauline; EdD; >81%; *moseley@tarleton.edu*
- Weissenberger, David; PhD; >81%; *weissenberg@tarleton.edu*

TX: Texas A & M University - Commerce

202 Ed North
Commerce, TX 75429-3011
USA
Dean   Jerry Hutton, Ph.D., Ed North 203
Administrator   Phyllis Erdman, Department Head
                      Department   Dept of Counseling
                                    (903) 886-5637, fax (903) 886-5780, http://www7.tamu-commerce.edu/

Key   See key for Data on Each Department (this section) on page 79.

Program
Accreditation   Regional Accreditation, **CACREP:** Community Counseling, **CACREP:** Counselor Education
                 and Supervision, **CACREP:** School Counseling, **CACREP:** Student Affairs - Counseling

Uniqueness   TAMU-C offers large, personalized CACREP accredited programs in a small community near
                 Dallas. Doctoral teaching assistantships are available in our undergraduate counseling degree
                 program.

Degrees   • Community Counseling: M.
                 • School Counseling: M.
                 • Student Affairs: M.
                 • Counselor Education: PhD.

Contact   • Community Counseling: M = Dr. Linda Ball.
                 • School Counseling: M = Dr. Richard Lampe.
                 • Student Affairs: M = Dr. Chester Robinson.
                 • Counselor Education: D = Dr. Richard Lampe.

Admission and Graduation Data
Admission
Requirements   • Community Counseling(M): GRE V R; GRE Q Yes; GRE A NA.
                 • School Counseling(M): GRE V R; GRE Q Yes; GRE A NA.
                 • Student Affairs(M): GRE V R; GRE Q Yes; GRE A NA.
                 • Counselor Education(D): Masters and GPA 3.50; GRE V R; GRE Q R; GRE A NA.

Enrollment   • Community Counseling(M): 37 Admitted yearly; 34 Graduated yearly.
                 • School Counseling(M): 43 Admitted yearly; 40 Graduated yearly.
                 • Student Affairs(M): 5 Admitted yearly; 2 Graduated yearly.
                 • Counselor Education(D): 11 Admitted yearly; 8 Graduated yearly.

Diversity   • African-American; Asian-American; Caucasian; Hispanic; Multiracial.

Graduation
Requirements   • Community Counseling(M): 48 Class hours; 100 Practicum hours; 600 Internship hours;
                   Comprehensive exam.
                 • School Counseling(M): 48 Class hours; 100 Practicum hours; 600 Internship hours;
                   Comprehensive exam.
                 • Student Affairs(M): 48 Class hours; 100 Practicum hours; 600 Internship hours.
                 • Counselor Education(D): 69 Class hours; 300 Practicum hours; 600 Internship hours;
                   Comprehensive exam; Oral exam; Dissertation.

Postgraduation activity: Advanced education and employment setting percentages.
                 • Community Counseling(M): 10 Advanced education; 40 Managed care; 10 Private practice;
                   40 Agency practice.
                 • School Counseling(M): 5 Advanced education; 45 Elementary school; 15 Middle school; 35
                   Secondary school.
                 • Student Affairs(M): 10 Advanced education; 90 Other.
                 • Counselor Education(D): 10 Managed care; 10 Private practice; 10 Agency practice; 2
                   Elementary school; 1 Middle school; 2 Secondary school; 65 Other.

Planned Program Modifications
Courses   Drop   Add
                 • NP.   • Group Work.

Other   Decrease   Increase
                 • NP.   • NP.

Related Programs

Faculty

nbcc ❧   Percent of faculty reported with NCC certification: 53%.   ncc ❧

Percent in professional counseling practice: 20%.

Research interests • NP.

Diversity   • African-American; Caucasian; Hispanic; Other.

Name, Degree, Rank, State/National Credentials, % time devoted to program, email
- Ball, Linda; EdD; Assist.; LPC, LMFT; >81%; *linda_ball@tamu-commerce.edu*
- Humphrey, Keren; EdD; Assoc.; LPC, NCC; >81%; *km_humphrey@tamu-commerce.edu*
- Erdman, Phyllis; PhD; Full Prof.; LPC, NCC, LMFT; *Phyllis_Erdman@tamu-commerce.edu*
- Abbassi, Amir; PhD; Assist.; LPC, NCC, LMFT; >81%; *Amir_abbassi@tamu-commerce.edu*
- Harris, Morag; PhD; Assoc.; NCC; >81%; *Morag_.Harris@tamu-commerce.edu*
- Armstrong, Stephen; PhD; Assist.; LPC; >81%; *Steve_armstrong@tamu-commerce.edu*
- Corrigan, Angela; EdD; Assist.; LPC, LMFT; 41-60%; *acorrigan@neto.com*
- Lampe, Richard; EdD; Full Prof.; NCC; >81%; *Richard_lampe@tamu-commerce.edu*
- Francis, Perry; EdD; Assist.; LPC, NCC; >81%; *Perry_francis@tamu-commerce.edu*
- Robinson, Chester; PhD; Assoc.; NCC; >81%; *Chester_Robinson@tamu-commerce.edu*
- Hendricks, LaVelle; EdD; Assist.; >81%; *Lavelle_hendricks@tamu-commerce.edu*
- White, Ruth Ann; PhD; Full Prof.; LPC; >81%; *Ruth_white@tamu-commerce.edu*
- Davis, Vicki; PhD; Full Prof.; 22-40%; *vicki_davis@tamu-commerce.edu*
- Leddick, George; PhD; Assoc.; LPC, NCC; >81%; *george_leddick@tamu-commerce.edu*
- Stacks, James; PhD; Assist.; >81%; *James_Stacks@tamu-commerce.edu*

Has CHI SIGMA IOTA (International Counseling Society) chapter.

TX: Texas Southern University

3100 Cleburne Ave.
Houston, TX 77004
USA

Dean   Dr. Jay Cummings, College of Education
Administrator   Dr. Joyce Jones, Department Chair
                    Department   Department of Counseling
                    (713) 313-7018, fax (713) 313-7481, jones_jk@tsu.edu,
                    www.tsu.edu/education

Key See key for Data on Each Department (this section) on page 79.

Program

Accreditation   Regional Accreditation

Uniqueness   Urban State Supported Historically Black University offering MEd & EdD programs in Counselor Education

Degrees   • Community Counseling: M.
          • School Counseling: M.
          • Counselor Education: EdD.

Contact   • Community Counseling: M = Dr. Joyce K. Jones.
          • School Counseling: M = Dr. Joyce K. Jones.
          • Counselor Education: D = Dr. Joyce Jones.

Admission and Graduation Data

Admission
Requirements   • Community Counseling(M): GPA 2.50; GRE 700.
               • School Counseling(M): GPA 2.50; GRE 700.
               • Counselor Education(D): Masters and GPA 3.25; GRE 750.

Enrollment   • Community Counseling(M): 35 Admitted yearly; 20 Graduated yearly; 75 Female; 30 Male.
             • School Counseling(M): 20 Admitted yearly; 10 Graduated yearly; 15 Male.
             • Counselor Education(D): 15 Admitted yearly; 10 Graduated yearly; 30 Female; 30 Male.

Diversity   • African-American; Asian-American; Caucasian; Hispanic; Multiracial; Other.

Graduation
Requirements   • Community Counseling(M): 48 Class hours; 50 Practicum hours; 600 Internship hours; Comprehensive exam.
               • School Counseling(M): 48 Class hours; 50 Practicum hours; 600 Internship hours; Comprehensive exam.
               • Counselor Education(D): 60 Class hours; 100 Practicum hours; 600 Internship hours; Comprehensive exam; Oral exam; Dissertation.

Postgraduation activity: Advanced education and employment setting percentages.
   • Community Counseling(M): 10 Managed care; 10 Private practice; 75 Agency practice.
   • School Counseling(M): 5 Advanced education; 20 Elementary school; 35 Middle school; 39 Secondary school; 1 Student affairs.
   • Counselor Education(D): 5 Managed care; 5 Private practice; 10 Agency practice; 10 Elementary school; 20 Middle school; 20 Secondary school; 15 Student affairs; 15 Other.

Planned Program Modifications

Courses	Drop	Add
	• NP.	• Addictions • Consultation • Psychodiagnosis • Supervision.

Other	Decrease	Increase
	• NP.	• Clinical Supervision • Diversity Recruiting of Faculty • Faculty FTE • National Accreditation • Number of Distance Education Courses.

Related Programs Clinical Social Workers

Faculty

nbcc   Percent of faculty reported with NCC certification: 43%.   ncc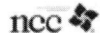

Percent in professional counseling practice: NP.

Research interests Multicultural Counseling, Adolescent and School Counseling, Substance Abuse

Diversity • African-American; Caucasian; Multiracial.

Name, Degree, Rank, State/National Credentials, % time devoted to program, email
• Jones, Joyce K; EdD; Assoc.; LPC, NCC; >81%; *Jones_JK@tsu.edu*
• Jefferson, Joseph; PhD; Full Prof.; LPC, NCC; >81%;
• Newhouse, Geary; EdD; Assoc.; LPC; >81%;
• Broussard, Shanna; PhD; Assist.; CRC; >81%;
• Farenik, Kenneth; EdD; Assist.; LPC; >81%;
• Epps, Irvine; EdD; Assoc.; 41-60%;
• Venable, Riley H; PhD; Assoc.; LPC, NCC, RN; >81%; *RHVEA@aol.com*

Has CHI SIGMA IOTA (International Counseling Society) chapter.

TX: Texas Tech University

P.O. Box 41071-COE
Lubbock, TX 79409-1071
USA
Dean   Dean Gerald Skoog, COE
Administrator Loretta J. Bradley, Ph.D., Coordinator, Counselor Education
Department   College of Education-Counselor Education Program
                 (806) 742-1997 Ext. 263, fax (806) 742-2179, www.educ.ttu.edu/edce/

Key   See key for Data on Each Department (this section) on page 79.

Program
Accreditation   **CACREP:** Community Counseling, **CACREP:** Counselor Education and Supervision, **CACREP:** School Counseling

Uniqueness   Located in west Texas, this program provides academic preparation at the master's level for LPC licensure and school certification, and at the doctoral level, the emphasis is counselor education preparation. Faculty provide individual attention to students and students have the opportunity to learn to implement theory into practice. The programs are CACREP accredited at master's and doctoral levels. A member of the faculty is a past president of ACA and past president of ACES. Faculty members have been treasurer of ACA and treasurer of IAMFC.

Degrees   • Community Counseling: M.
                 • School Counseling: M.
                 • Counselor Education: EdD.

Contact   • Community Counseling: M = Bret Hendricks and Aretha Marbley.
                 • School Counseling: M = Jean Shen.
                 • Counselor Education: D = Loretta Bradley.

Admission and Graduation Data
Admission
Requirements   • Community Counseling(M): GPA 3.0+; GRE AVG; GRE V AVG; GRE Q AVG; GRE A AVG; MAT NR.
                 • School Counseling(M): GPA 3.0+; GRE AVG; GRE V AVG; GRE Q AVG; GRE A AVG; MAT NR.
                 • Counselor Education(D): Masters and GPA 3.0+; GRE prefer avg; GRE V prefer avg; GRE Q prefer avg; GRE A prefer avg; MAT not req.

Enrollment   • Community Counseling(M): 30 Admitted yearly; 20 Graduated yearly; 19 Female; 8 Male.
                 • School Counseling(M): 13 Admitted yearly; 10 Graduated yearly; 1 Male.
                 • Counselor Education(D): 6 Admitted yearly; 3 Graduated yearly; 3 Female; 3 Male.

Diversity   • African-American; Asian-American; Caucasian; Hispanic.

Graduation
Requirements   • Community Counseling(M): 48 Class hours; 100 Practicum hours; 600 Internship hours; Comprehensive exam; CPCE; Portfolio.
                 • School Counseling(M): 48 Class hours; 100 Practicum hours; 600 Internship hours; Comprehensive exam; CPCE; Portfolio.
                 • Counselor Education(D): 92 Class hours; 100 Practicum hours; 600 Internship hours; Comprehensive exam; Dissertation; Portfolio.

Postgraduation activity: Advanced education and employment setting percentages.
                 • Community Counseling(M): 5 Advanced education; 5 Managed care; 5 Private practice; 48 Agency practice; 8 Elementary school; 10 Middle school; 7 Secondary school; 2 Student affairs; 10 Other.
                 • School Counseling(M): 5 Advanced education; 2 Private practice; 10 Agency practice; 15 Elementary school; 20 Middle school; 40 Secondary school; 8 Other.
                 • Counselor Education(D): 10 Managed care; 15 Private practice; 40 Agency practice; 5 Elementary school; 5 Student affairs.

Planned Program Modifications
Courses   Drop   Add
                 • NP.   • Crisis/Violence Counseling.

Other   Decrease   Increase
                 • NP.   • NP.

Related Programs Clinical Social Workers
Marriage and Family Therapists
Psychology
Psychiatric Nurses
Psychiatrists
Communications
International Studies

Faculty

 Percent of faculty reported with NCC certification: 60%.

Percent in professional counseling practice: 60%.

Research interests The faculty research interests include: counselor supervision, group counseling, counseling diverse populations, developmental guidance, school counseling, play therapy, social justice advocacy, and ethics.

Diversity
• African-American; Asian-American; Caucasian.

Name, Degree, Rank, State/National Credentials, % time devoted to program, email
• Bradley, Loretta J; PhD; Full Prof.; LPC, NCC, TX LMFT; >81%; *Loretta.Bradley@ttu.edu*
• Hendricks, Bret C; EdD; Assist.; LPC; >81%; *Bret.Hendricks@ttu.edu*
• Marbley, Aretha F; PhD; Assist.; LPC, NCC; >81%; *Aretha.Marbley@ttu.edu*
• Parr, Gerald D; PhD; Full Prof.; LPC, NCC, Sch. psy; 22-40%; *Gerald.Parr@ttu.edu*
• Shen, Jean; EdD; Assist.; Play therapy; >81%; *Jean.Shen@ttu.edu*

Has CHI SIGMA IOTA (International Counseling Society) chapter.

TX: University of North Texas

PO Box 311337
Denton, TX 76203
USA

Dean Jean Keller
Administrator Michael Altekruse, Chair
Department Counseling, Development, & Higher Education
(940) 565-2910, fax (940) 565-2905, www.coe.unt.edu/cdhe/

Key See key for Data on Each Department (this section) on page 79.

Program

Accreditation Regional Accreditation, **CACREP:** College Counseling, **CACREP:** Community Counseling, **CACREP:** Counselor Education and Supervision, **CACREP:** School Counseling

Uniqueness • NP.

Degrees • Community Counseling: M.
• School Counseling: M.
• College Counseling: M.
• Counselor Education: PhD.

Contact • Community Counseling: M = Bob Berg.
• School Counseling: M = Doris Coy.
• College Counseling: M = Carolyn Kern.
• Counselor Education: D = Cynthia Chandler.

Admission and Graduation Data

Admission

Requirements • Community Counseling(M): GPA 3.00; GRE 710; GRE V 340; GRE Q 370; Interview.
• School Counseling(M): GPA 3.00; GRE 710; GRE V 340; GRE Q 370; Interview.
• College Counseling(M): GPA 3.00; GRE 710; GRE V 340; GRE Q 370; Interview.
• Counselor Education(D): Masters and GPA 3.50; GRE 710; GRE V 340; GRE Q 370; GRE A R.

Enrollment • Community Counseling(M): 70 Admitted yearly; 65 Graduated yearly; 64 Female; 5 Male.
• School Counseling(M): 75 Admitted yearly; 60 Graduated yearly; 69 Female; 4 Male.
• College Counseling(M): 5 Admitted yearly; 3 Graduated yearly; 2 Female; 1 Male.
• Counselor Education(D): 15 Admitted yearly; 9 Graduated yearly; 7 Female; 2 Male.

Diversity • African-American; Asian-American; Caucasian; Hispanic; Native American; Pacific Islander; Multiracial.

Graduation

Requirements • Community Counseling(M): 48 Class hours; 100 Practicum hours; 600 Internship hours.
• School Counseling(M): 48 Class hours; 100 Practicum hours; 600 Internship hours.
• College Counseling(M): 48 Class hours; 100 Practicum hours; 600 Internship hours.
• Counselor Education(D): 75 Class hours; 80 Practicum hours; 600 Internship hours; Dissertation.

Postgraduation activity: Advanced education and employment setting percentages.
• Community Counseling(M): 100 Agency practice.
• School Counseling(M): 50 Elementary school; 50 Secondary school.
• College Counseling(M): 100 Other.
• Counselor Education(D): 100 Student affairs.

Planned Program Modifications

Courses	Drop	Add
	• NP.	• NP.

Other	Decrease	Increase
	• NP.	• NP.

Related Programs

Faculty

Percent of faculty reported with NCC certification: 56%.

Percent in professional counseling practice: 23%.

Research interests Play Therapy, Group Therapy, Transpersonal Counseling, Dreamwork Counseling, Animal Assisted Therapy, Biofeedback, Multicultural Counseling

Diversity • African-American; Caucasian; Hispanic.

Name, Degree, Rank, State/National Credentials, % time devoted to program, email
• Altekruse, Michael K; EdD; Full Prof.; NCC; >81%; *altkrs@unt.edu*
• Berg, Robert C; EdD; Full Prof.; LPC; >81%; *Berg@coefs.coe.unt.edu*
• Bratton, Sue C; PhD; Assoc.; LPC; >81%; *Bratton@coefs.coe.unt.edu*
• Chandler, Cynthia K; EdD; Full Prof.; LPC; >81%; *Chandler@coefs.coe.unt.edu*
• Coy, Doris R; PhD; Assist.; LPC, NCC; >81%; *Coy@coefs.coe.unt.edu*
• Durodoye, Beth A; EdD; Assoc.; NCC; >81%; *Durodoye@coefs.coe.unt.edu*
• Engels, Dennis W; PhD; Full Prof.; NCC; >81%; *Engels@coefs.coe.unt.edu*
• Garza, Yvonne; MS; Lecturer; 22-40%; *Garza@coef.coe.unt.edu*
• Gieda, Martin J; PhD; Assist.; NCC; 22-40%; *Gieda@dsa.adm.unt.edu*
• Harris, Henry L; PhD; Assist.; LPC; >81%; *Hharris@coefs.coe.unt.edu*
• Holden, Janice M; EdD; Full Prof.; LPC; >81%; *Holden@unt.edu*
• Kern, Carolyn W; PhD; Assoc.; LPC, NCC; >81%; *Kern@coefs.coe.unt.edu*
• Landreth, Garry L; EdD; Full Prof.; LPC; >81%; *Landreth@coefs.coe.unt.edu*
• Norton, Earl D; PhD; Assoc.; LPC, NCC; >81%; *Norton@coefs.coe.unt.edu*
• Ray, Dee C; PhD; Assist.; LPC, NCC; >81%; *Ray@coefs.coe.unt.edu*
• Trevino, Lilia L; MA; Lecturer; 22-40%; *Trevino@coefs.coe.unt.edu*

Has CHI SIGMA IOTA (International Counseling Society) chapter.

TX: University of Texas at El Paso

	500 W. University
	El Paso, TX USA
	88005-7968
Dean	Dr. Josie Tinajero
Administrator	Don C. Combs, Ed.D., Counseling Program Coordinator
	Department Educational Psychology & Special Services
	(915) 747-7585, fax (915) 747-8410, N/A, www.utep.coe/edpsych

Key   See key for Data on Each Department (this section) on page 79.

Program
Accreditation   NP.

Uniqueness   We serve a border area multicultural region (Hispanic/Anglo).

Degrees   • Community Counseling: M.
• School Counseling: M.

Contact   • Community Counseling: M = Dr. Don C. Combs.
• School Counseling: M = Dr. Phillip Barbee.

Admission and Graduation Data
Admission
Requirements   • Community Counseling(M): GPA 3.00; GRE NR; Interview.
• School Counseling(M): GPA 3.00; GRE NR; Interview.

Enrollment   • Community Counseling(M): 15 Admitted yearly; 15 Graduated yearly; 27 Female; 13 Male.
• School Counseling(M): 25 Admitted yearly; 25 Graduated yearly.

Diversity   • African-American; Caucasian; Hispanic.

Graduation
Requirements   • Community Counseling(M): 48 Class hours; 100 Practicum hours; 600 Internship hours;
Comprehensive exam.
• School Counseling(M): 48 Class hours; 100 Practicum hours; 600 Internship hours;
Comprehensive exam.

Postgraduation activity: Advanced education and employment setting percentages.
• Community Counseling(M): 10 Advanced education; 20 Managed care; 60 Agency
practice; 33 Elementary school; 33 Middle school; 33 Secondary school.
• School Counseling(M): NP.

Planned Program Modifications

Courses	Drop	Add
	• Addictions	• NP.
	• Grief Counseling	
	• Legal/Ethical Issues	
	• Marriage and Family Counseling	
	• Research Methods	
	• School Counseling	
	• Supervision.	

Other	Decrease	Increase
	• NP.	• Admission Requirements
		• Clinical Supervision
		• National Accreditation
		• Number of Distance Education Courses
		• Number of On-Line Courses.

Related Programs Psychology
Psychiatric Nurses

Faculty

nbcc ❧   Percent of faculty reported with NCC certification: 25%.   **ncc** ❧

Percent in professional counseling practice: NP.

Research interests Grief and bereavement counseling, marriage and family counseling, career counseling, in-service learning models

Diversity   •   Caucasian; Hispanic.

Name, Degree, Rank, State/National Credentials, % time devoted to program, email
- Combs, Don C; EdD; Assoc.; LPC, NCC, CCMHC; >81%; *dcombs@utep.edu*
- Cortez-Gonzalez, Roberto; PhD; Assoc.; Lic Prof Psychologist; >81%; *rgonzale@utep.edu*
- Johnson, Steve W; PhD; Assoc.; LPC, LMFT; >81%; *stevej@utep.edu*
- Barbee, Phillip; PhD; Assist.; LPC; >81%; *pbarbee@utep.edu*

Has CHI SIGMA IOTA (International Counseling Society) chapter.

TX: University of Texas at Tyler

	3900 University Blvd
	Tyler, TX 75799
	USA
Dean	Mil Clark, Ph.D.
Administrator	Robert McClure, Ph.D., Psychology Graduate Coordinator
	Department Psychology
	(903) 566-7130, fax (903) 565-5656, rmcclure@uttyler.edu,
	www.uttyler.edu

Key   See key for Data on Each Department (this section) on page 79.

Program

Accreditation   Regional Accreditation

Uniqueness   This is an applied, practical program designed to turn out competent practicing counselors and therapists. There is no thesis, but rather many opportunities for applied counseling practice. School counselors receive training in assessment and testing. Marriage and family counseling program is an MA in counseling psychology.

Degrees
- School Counseling: M.
- Marriage and Family Counseling: M.

Contact
- School Counseling: M = Shirley Jones, Ed.D..
- Marriage and Family Counseling: M = Robert McClure, Ph.D.

Admission and Graduation Data

Admission

Requirements
- School Counseling(M): GPA 3.00; GRE 900.
- Marriage and Family Counseling(M): GPA 3.00; GRE 900.

Enrollment
- School Counseling(M): 10 Admitted yearly; 7 Graduated yearly; 20 Female; 5 Male.
- Marriage and Family Counseling(M): 8 Admitted yearly; 6 Graduated yearly; 16 Female; 4 Male.

Diversity
- African-American; Asian-American; Caucasian; Hispanic; Multiracial.

Graduation

Requirements
- School Counseling(M): 42 Class hours; 300 Practicum hours; Comprehensive exam; Oral exam.
- Marriage and Family Counseling(M): 60 Class hours; 300 Practicum hours; Oral exam.

Postgraduation activity: Advanced education and employment setting percentages.
- School Counseling(M): 35 Elementary school; 30 Middle school; 30 Secondary school; 5 Student affairs.
- Marriage and Family Counseling(M): 15 Advanced education; 40 Private practice; 40 Agency practice; 5 Other.

Planned Program Modifications

Courses	Drop		Add
	• NP.	• NP.	

Other	Decrease		Increase
	• NP.	• NP.	

Related Programs Psychology

Faculty

nbcc ❧   Percent of faculty reported with NCC certification: 14%.   ncc ❧

Percent in professional counseling practice: 71%.

Research interests Child sexual abuse and neglect, therapist theoretical orientations, assessment and testing, domestic abuse, school counseling and guidance, marriage and family, career counseling and assessment, special education, human growth and development (conception through gerontology).

Diversity
- Caucasian.

Name, Degree, Rank, State/National Credentials, % time devoted to program, email
- McClure, Robert F; PhD; Full Prof.; Psychologist; 61-80%; *rmcclure@uttyler.edu*
- Jones, Shirley M; EdD; Assoc.; NCC; >81%; *sjones@uttyler.edu*

- Lundberg-Love, Paula K; PhD; Full Prof.; LPC; 41-60%; *plundber@uttyler.edu*
- Livingston, Ronald B; PhD; Assoc.; Psychologist; 61-80%; *rlivings@uttyler.edu*
- Schreiber, Henry L; PhD; Assoc.; <21%; *hschreib@uttyler.edu*
- Mears, F G; PhD; Full Prof.; Psychologist; <21%; *gmears@uttyler.edu*
- Marmion, Shelly L; PhD; Assoc.; <21%; *smarmion@uttyler.edu*

TX: University of Texas of the Permian Basin

	4901 E. University
	Odessa, TX 79762
	USA
Dean	G. Peter Ienatsch, School of Education
Administrator	Cathleen Barrett-Kruse, EdD, NCC, Program Coordinator
	Department School of Education
	(915) 552-2140, fax (915) 552-2125, barrettkruse@utpb.edu

Key   See key for Data on Each Department (this section) on page 79.

Program

Accreditation   Regional Accreditation

Uniqueness   Adlerian and Developmental Counseling

Degrees   • Community Counseling: M.
              • School Counseling: M.

Contact   • Community Counseling: M = Cathleen Barrett-Kruse, EdD, NCC.
              • School Counseling: M = Cathleen Barrett-Kruse, EdD, NCC.

Admission and Graduation Data

Admission
Requirements   • Community Counseling(M): GPA 2.50; GRE 1200; GRE V 400; GRE Q 400; GRE A 400.
                   • School Counseling(M): GPA 2.50; GRE 1200; GRE V 400; GRE Q 400; GRE A 400.

Enrollment   • Community Counseling(M): 10 Admitted yearly; 3 Graduated yearly; 7 Female; 3 Male.
                 • School Counseling(M): 20 Admitted yearly; 6 Graduated yearly; 15 Female; 5 Male.

Diversity   • African-American; Caucasian; Hispanic.

Graduation
Requirements   • Community Counseling(M): 48 Class hours; 300 Practicum hours.
                   • School Counseling(M): 48 Class hours; 300 Practicum hours.

Postgraduation activity: Advanced education and employment setting percentages.
              • Community Counseling(M): 10 Private practice; 80 Agency practice; 10 Middle school.
              • School Counseling(M): 1 Advanced education; 35 Elementary school; 34 Middle school; 30
                Secondary school.

Planned Program Modifications

Courses	Drop	Add
	• NP.	• Abuse of Individual
		• Addictions.

Other	Decrease	Increase
	• NP.	• Diversity Recruiting of Faculty
		• Faculty FTE
		• National Accreditation
		• Number of Off-Campus Courses
		• Number of On-Line Courses.

Related Programs

Faculty

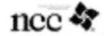

nbcc ❖   Percent of faculty reported with NCC certification: 67%.   ncc ❖

Percent in professional counseling practice: 0%.

Research interests Family resilience and family-school relations

Diversity   • Caucasian; Hispanic.

Name, Degree, Rank, State/National Credentials, % time devoted to program, email
• Barrett-Kruse, Cathleen M; EdD; Assoc.; NCC; 61-80%; *barrettkruse@utpb.edu*
• Jaramillo, Patricio T; PhD; Full Prof.; Psychologist; <21%; *jaramillo_p@utpb.edu*
• Milliren, Alan P; EdD; Assoc.; NCC; >81%; *milliren_a@utpb.edu*

UT: University of Phoenix

	5251 Green Street
	Salt Lake City, UT 84123
	USA
Dean	Patrick Romine, Ph.D. Phoenix Az.
Administrator	Don Beck, Associate Dean

Department   College of Social and Behavioral Sciences
(801) 905-4222, fax (801) 269-9766, Don.Beck@Phoenix.edu,
www.phoenix.edu

Key   See key for Data on Each Department (this section) on page 79.

Program

Accreditation   Regional Accreditation, **CACREP:** Mental Health Counseling

CACREP

Uniqueness   Program geared for working adults; employs adult learning models

Degrees
- Mental Health Counseling: M.
- School Counseling: S.

Contact
- Mental Health Counseling: M = Don Beck , Ph.D..
- School Counseling: S = NP.

Admission and Graduation Data

Admission

Requirements
- Mental Health Counseling(M): GPA 2.50; 3 Years work experience.
- School Counseling(S): GPA 2.50; 3 Years work experience.

Enrollment
- Mental Health Counseling(M): 60 Admitted yearly; 60% Female; 40% Male.
- School Counseling(S): 80 Admitted yearly; 35% Male.

Diversity
- African-American; Asian-American; Caucasian; Hispanic; Native American.

Graduation

Requirements
- Mental Health Counseling(M): 60 Class hours; 100 Practicum hours; 900 Internship hours; CPCE; Oral exam; Portfolio.
- School Counseling(S):

Postgraduation activity: Advanced education and employment setting percentages.
- Mental Health Counseling(M): 2 Advanced education; 5 Managed care; 5 Private practice; 75 Agency practice; 12 Other.
- School Counseling(S): 10 Elementary school; 45 Middle school; 40 Secondary school; 3 Student affairs.

Planned Program Modifications

Courses   Drop   Add
- NP.
                                           • Consultation
                                           • Marriage and Family Counseling.

Other   Decrease   Increase
- NP.
                                           • Course Offerings
                                           • Graduation Requirements
                                           • National Accreditation.

Related Programs

Faculty

nbcc   Percent of faculty reported with NCC certification: 0%.   ncc

Percent in professional counseling practice: 100%.

Research interests MMPI, Self-modeling, psychopharmocology, adult learning theory

Diversity
- Asian-American; Caucasian; Hispanic; Native American.

Name, Degree, Rank, State/National Credentials, % time devoted to program, email
- Alexander, Stephen; MS; Instructor; LPC, CSP; <21%; *steve.alexander@m.k-12.ut.us*
- Beck, Don; PhD; Instructor; Lic.Psych; >81%; *don.beck@phoenix.edu*
- Bircher, Del; MS; Instructor; LCSW; <21%; *delb@vmh.com*

- Brady, Susan; PhD; Instructor; <21%; *susan.brady@granite.k-12.ut.us*
- Brown, Art; PhD; Instructor; AAMFT; <21%; *abrown@sisna.com*
- Burnham, Lee; PhD; Instructor; Lic.Psych; >81%; *leeburnhjam@email.uophx.edu*
- Collihns-Jones, Teresa; PhD; Instructor; Lic.Psych; <21%; *dctjjones@aol.com*
- Dusoe, Michael; PhD; Instructor; LSAC; 22-40%; *mikey50@aol.com*
- Griffith, Sherry; MS; Instructor; LSSW; <21%; *sherryg@vmh.com*
- Hurd, Jeff; PhD; Instructor; Lic.Psych; <21%; *drhurd@earthlink.net*
- Jimenez, Carlie; MS; Instructor; LPC, LSAC; <21%; *artforms@networld.com*
- Jarreau-Wihongi, Lynn; MS; Instructor; LSAC, LCSW; >81%; *lymmjarreauwihongi@yahoo.com*
- Steven, Kay; PhD; Instructor; Lic.Psych; 41-60%; *steven@cornerstonesic.com*
- Korbanka, Juergen; PhD; Instructor; Lic.Psych; >81%; *juergen.korbanka@phoenix.edu*
- Macnamara, Susan; PhD; Instructor; Lic.Psych; >81%; *ldsmacna@ihc.com*
- Mendenhall, Marty; MS; Instructor; LPC, LPC; 22-40%; *rinpoche2@aol.com*
- Pankow, Shannon; PhD; Instructor; LMFT; 61-80%; *shannon_pankow@hotmail>com*
- Price, Donald; PhD; Instructor; AAMFT; <21%; *donprice@sisna.com*
- Shingleton, Richard; PhD; Instructor; Lic.Psych; <21%; *rshingleton@protocare.com*
- Simmons, Robert; PhD; Instructor; Lic.Psych; 61-80%; *robert.simmons@phoenix.com*
- Vandenaker, Pam; MS; Instructor; LPC, LMFT; *pjvamdemaker@aol.com*

Has CHI SIGMA IOTA (International Counseling Society) chapter.

VA: College of William and Mary

School of Education, PO Box 8795
Williamsburg, VA 23187-8795
USA

Dean Virginia McLaughlin, School of Education
Administrator Victoria Foster, Area Coordinator
Department School Psychology and Counselor Education
(757) 221-2321, fax (757) 221-2988, vafost@wm.edu,
http://www.wm.edu/education/index.html

Key See key for Data on Each Department (this section) on page 79.

Program
Accreditation Regional Accreditation, **CACREP:** Community Counseling, **CACREP:** Counselor Education and Supervision, **CACREP:** School Counseling

Uniqueness CACREP Accredited School, Community and Doctoral Programs. Specialties offered in Marriage and Family and in Addictions

Degrees
- Community Counseling: M.
- School Counseling: M.
- Addictions Counseling: M.
- Marriage and Family Counseling: M.
- Counselor Education: PhD.

Contact
- Community Counseling: M = Charles McAdams.
- School Counseling: M = Norma Day-Vines.
- Addictions Counseling: M = Charles Gressard.
- Marriage and Family Counseling: M = Charles McAdams.
- Counselor Education: D = Victoria Foster.

Admission and Graduation Data
Admission
Requirements
- Community Counseling(M): GPA 2.50; GRE 40%; GRE V 40%; GRE Q 40%.
- School Counseling(M): GPA 2.50; GRE 40%; GRE V 40%; GRE Q 40%.
- Addictions Counseling(M): GPA 2.50; GRE 40%; GRE V 40%; GRE Q 40%.
- Marriage and Family Counseling(M): GPA 2.50; GRE 40%; GRE V 40%; GRE Q 40%.
- Counselor Education(D): Masters and GPA 3.50; GRE 60%; GRE V 60%; GRE Q 60%; 2 Years work experience.

Enrollment
- Community Counseling(M): 10 Admitted yearly; 10 Graduated yearly; 8 Female; 2 Male.
- School Counseling(M): 10 Admitted yearly; 10 Graduated yearly; 8 Female; 2 Male.
- Addictions Counseling(M): 8 Admitted yearly; 6 Graduated yearly; 6 Female; 2 Male.
- Marriage and Family Counseling(M): 8 Admitted yearly; 6 Graduated yearly; 6 Female; 2 Male.
- Counselor Education(D): 10 Admitted yearly; 6 Graduated yearly; 8 Female; 2 Male.

Diversity
- African-American; Asian-American; Caucasian; Hispanic.

Graduation
Requirements
- Community Counseling(M): 51 Class hours; 100 Practicum hours; 600 Internship hours.
- School Counseling(M): 54 Class hours; 100 Practicum hours; 600 Internship hours.
- Addictions Counseling(M): 51 Class hours; 100 Practicum hours; 600 Internship hours.
- Marriage and Family Counseling(M): 63 Class hours; 100 Practicum hours; 600 Internship hours.
- Counselor Education(D): 63 Class hours; 100 Practicum hours; 600 Internship hours; Comprehensive exam; Oral exam; Dissertation.

Postgraduation activity: Advanced education and employment setting percentages.
- Community Counseling(M): 100 Agency practice.
- School Counseling(M): 34 Elementary school; 33 Middle school; 33 Secondary school.
- Addictions Counseling(M): 100 Agency practice.
- Marriage and Family Counseling(M): 100 Agency practice.
- Counselor Education(D): 80 Advanced education; 20 Private practice.

Planned Program Modifications
Courses	Drop	Add
	• NP.	• NP.

Other	Decrease	Increase
	• NP.	• NP.

Related Programs Psychology
                    International Studies

Faculty

nbcc 🔷   Percent of faculty reported with NCC certification: 75%.   **ncc** 🔷

Percent in professional counseling practice: 0%.

Research interests School Counseling, Addictions Counseling, Marriage and Family Counseling, Multicultural
                  Issues, Cognitive Development, Adolescent Development

Diversity   •   African-American; Caucasian.

Name, Degree, Rank, State/National Credentials, % time devoted to program, email
- Day-Vines, Norma; EdD; Assist.; >81%; *nldayv@wm.ede*
- Foster, Victoria; EdD; Assoc.; LPC, NCC, LMFT; >81%; *vafost@wm.edu*
- Gressard, Charles; PhD; Assoc.; LPC, NCC, MAC; >81%; *cfgres@wm.edu*
- McAdams, Charles; EdD; Assoc.; LPC, NCC, LMFT; >81%; *crmcad@wm.edu*

Has CHI SIGMA IOTA (International Counseling Society) chapter.

VA: George Mason University

MSN4B3, 4400 University Drive
Fairfax, VA 22030-4444
USA

Dean Jeffrey Gorrell
Administrator Fred Bemak, Professor and Program Coordinator
Department   Counseling and Development
(703) 993-3941, fax (703) 993-2013, fbemak@gmu.edu,
http://gse.gmu.edu/programs/counseling

Key   See key for Data on Each Department (this section) on page 79.

Program

Accreditation   Regional Accreditation

Uniqueness   This program, including Masters and Doctoral level work, has a unique mission statement that focuses on social justice, multiculturalism, advocacy, and leadership. Courses in the program reflect the mission with courses in social change, advocacy, an internship in multicultural counseling and an internship in social justice. The campus is located 15 miles from Washington D.C. and is one of the 10 most ethnically diverse universities in the U.S. while the surrounding community of Fairfax is one of the most diverse in the U.S.

Degrees
- Community Counseling: M, PhD.
- School Counseling: M, PhD.
- Counselor Education: PhD.

Contact
- Community Counseling: M = Dr. Regine Talleyrand.; D = Dr. Rita Chi-Ying Chung.
- School Counseling: M = Dr. Sally Murphy.; D = Dr. Carol Kaffenberger.
- Counselor Education: D = Dr. Fred Bemak.

Admission and Graduation Data

Admission

Requirements
- Community Counseling(M): GPA 3.00; Interview.
- Community Counseling(D): Masters and GPA 3.00; GRE 1000.
- School Counseling(M): GPA 3.00; Interview.
- School Counseling(D): Masters and GPA 3.00; GRE 1000.
- Counselor Education(D): Masters and GPA 3.00; GRE 1000.

Enrollment
- Community Counseling(M): 30 Admitted yearly; 10 Graduated yearly; 80% Female; 20% Male.
- Community Counseling(D): 3 Admitted yearly; 2 Graduated yearly; 50% Female; 50% Male.
- School Counseling(M): 40 Admitted yearly; 15 Graduated yearly; 80% Female; 20% Male.
- School Counseling(D): 3 Admitted yearly; 2 Graduated yearly; 50% Female; 50% Male.
- Counselor Education(D): 3 Admitted yearly; 2 Graduated yearly; 50% Female; 50% Male.

Diversity
- African-American; Asian-American; Caucasian; Hispanic; Multiracial.

Graduation

Requirements
- Community Counseling(M): 52 Class hours; 200 Practicum hours; 200 Internship hours.
- Community Counseling(D): 55-85 Class hours; 200 Practicum hours; 200 Internship hours; Comprehensive exam; CPCE; Oral exam.
- School Counseling(M): 45 Class hours; 200 Practicum hours; 200 Internship hours.
- School Counseling(D): 55-85 Class hours; 200 Practicum hours; 200 Internship hours; Dissertation; Portfolio.
- Counselor Education(D): 55-85 Class hours; 100 Internship hours; Dissertation; Portfolio.

Postgraduation activity: Advanced education and employment setting percentages.
- Community Counseling(M): 20 Advanced education; 20 Managed care; 5 Private practice; 30 Agency practice; 25 Other.
- Community Counseling(D): 20 Private practice; 60 Agency practice; 20 Other.
- School Counseling(M): 20 Advanced education; 20 Elementary school; 20 Middle school; 40 Secondary school.
- School Counseling(D): 10 Middle school; 10 Secondary school; 80 Student affairs.
- Counselor Education(D): 100 Other.

Planned Program Modifications

Courses	Drop	Add
	• NP.	Abuse of Individual
		Addictions
		Advocacy
		Computer and Related Technology
		Consultation
		Crisis/Violence Counseling
		Grief Counseling
		Group Work
		Human Sexuality
		Legal/Ethical Issues
		Play Therapy
		School Counseling
		Social Justice
		Supervision
		Testing, Appraisal, Assessment.

Other	Decrease	Increase
	• NP.	Diversity Recruiting of Faculty
		Diversity Recruiting of Students
		Faculty FTE
		Number of Off-Campus Courses.

Related Programs Psychology
International Studies

Faculty

nbcc ❖   Percent of faculty reported with NCC certification: 36%.   ncc ❖

Percent in professional counseling practice: NP.

Research interests Multicultural counseling, social justice, advocacy, leadership, at-risk youth and families, transforming school counseling, international cross-cultural counseling, racial identity development, inter-ethnic group relations, group counseling, refugee acculturation and mental health, bullying, wellness and health counseling.

Diversity   • African-American; Asian-American; Caucasian; Multiracial.

Name, Degree, Rank, State/National Credentials, % time devoted to program, email
• Bemak, Fred; EdD; Full Prof.; LPC, LCSW; >81%; *fbemak@gmu.edu*
• Chung, Rita Chi-Ying; PhD; Assoc.; >81%; *rchung@gmu.edu*
• Kaffenberger, Carol; PhD; Assist.; NCC, Licensed School Counselor; >81%; *ckaffenb@gmu.edu*
• Murphy, Sally; PhD; Assist.; NCC, Licensed School Counselor; >81%; *cmurphy@gmu.edu*
• Talleyrand, Regine; PhD; Assist.; Licensed Psychologist; >81%; *rtalleyr@gmu.edu*
• Gibb, Diana; PhD; Instructor; 41-60%; *dgibb@gmu.edu*
• Jackson, Morris; PhD; Adjunct; NCC; <21%; *mjacks@american.edu*
• Epp, Larry; PhD; Adjunct; <21%; *humortherapy@earthlink.net*
• Duval-Harvey, Jacqueline; PhD; Adjunct; <21%; *jduvalha@jhmi.edu*
• Crowley, Richard; MEd; Adjunct; Licensed School Counselor; <21%; *richcrowl@aol.com*
• Schumann, Mary; PhD; Adjunct; LPC; <21%; *mfschumann@aol.com*
• McCormick, Catherine; PhD; Adjunct; <21%; *Cmcormick27@yahoo.com*
• Seligman, Linda; PhD; Adjunct; LPC, NCC; <21%; *lseligma@gmu.edu*

Has CHI SIGMA IOTA (International Counseling Society) chapter.

VA: James Madison University

MSC 7401 James Madison University
Harrisonburg, VA 22807
USA
Dean   Jerry Benson, College of Integrated Science and Technology
Administrator Lennis G. Echterling, Director
                  Department   Counseling Psychology
                                 (540) 568-6522, fax (540) 568-3322, echterlg@jmu.edu,
                                 http://cep.jmu.edu/counselpsyc/

Key   See key for Data on Each Department (this section) on page 79.

Program
Accreditation   Regional Accreditation, **CACREP:** Community Counseling, **CACREP:** School Counseling

Uniqueness   Our philosophy of training is based on five principles.
- We learn by working together. Our program is a community of learners committed to support one another in the formidable enterprise of becoming a successful counselor.
- We learn by doing. In virtually every class period, faculty members involve students in some activity that requires them to practice the craft of counseling – the process of observing, gathering information, conceptualizing, and taking action.
- We learn throughout our lives. Counseling professionals have two simple options – to grow as persons and professionals by challenging ourselves, or to stagnate.
- We learn by example. The heart of a counselor education program is not the curriculum, but its people. Actions do speak louder than words, so it is vital that both faculty and students exemplify the values of the counseling profession.
- When we learn, we change. As students progress through this program, they do more than acquire knowledge and develop skills – they transform themselves professionally and personally.

Degrees
- Community Counseling: M.
- School Counseling: M.

Contact
- Community Counseling: M = Sue Rippy.
- School Counseling: M = Sue Rippy.

Admission and Graduation Data
Admission
Requirements
- Community Counseling(M): GRE required; Interview.
- School Counseling(M): GRE required; Interview.

Enrollment
- Community Counseling(M): 10 Admitted yearly; 10 Graduated yearly.
- School Counseling(M): 10 Admitted yearly; 10 Graduated yearly.

Diversity
- NP.

Graduation
Requirements
- Community Counseling(M): 60 Class hours; 100 Practicum hours; 900 Internship hours.
- School Counseling(M): 60 Class hours; 100 Practicum hours; 600 Internship hours.

Postgraduation activity: Advanced education and employment setting percentages.
- Community Counseling(M): NP.
- School Counseling(M): NP.

Planned Program Modifications
Courses   Drop   Add
- NP.   - NP.

Other   Decrease   Increase
- NP.   - NP.

Related Programs

Faculty

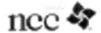 Percent of faculty reported with NCC certification: 38%.

Percent in professional counseling practice: 88%.

Research interests Michele Kielty Briggs – School counseling, spirituality, gender, self concept.Eric W. Cowan – Self psychology, eating disorders, counseling process. Recognized by the JMU Mortarboard for Outstanding Teaching.Lennis G. Echterling – Disasters and trauma, brief counseling, crisis intervention. Recipient of the national ACES Counseling Vision and Innovation Award and the Madison Distinguished Teacher Award.William Evans – Career development, spiritual issues in counseling, death and dying. Recipient of the JMU William Hall Student Service Award. J. Edson McKee – Counseling techniques, group dynamics, creativity and learning styles. Recipient of the national ACES Professional Service Award and the CISAT Distinguished Teaching Award.Jack H. Presbury – Creativity, artificial intelligence, brief therapy, cognitive psychology, history and systems. Recipient of the Madison Scholar Award.A. Renee Staton – Multicultural issues, community counseling, counselor supervision. President of the Virginia Association for Counselor Education and Supervision.

Diversity   • Caucasian; Multiracial.

Name, Degree, Rank, State/National Credentials, % time devoted to program, email
• Echterling, Lennis G; PhD; Full Prof.; >81%; *echterlg@jmu.edu*
• Evans, William; PhD; Assist.; LPC, NCC; 41-60%; *evansswf@jmu.edu*
• McKee, J.E.; EdD; Full Prof.; LPC; *mckeeje@jmu.edu*
• Presbury, Jack H; EdD; Full Prof.; LPC; 61-80%; *presubjh@jmu.edu*
• Stewart, Anne L; PhD; Full Prof.; 22-40%; *stewaral@jmu.edu*
• Briggs, Michele K; PhD; Assist.; LPC, NCC; >81%; *briggsmk@jmu.edu*
• Cowan, Eric; PsyD; Assist.; >81%; *cownawe@jmu.edu*
• Staton, Renee A; Assoc.; LPC, NCC; >81%; *statonar@jmu.edu*

Has CHI SIGMA IOTA (International Counseling Society) chapter.

VA: Old Dominion University

Education Building, Room 110
Norfolk, VA 23529-0157
USA
Dean William H. Graves
Administrator Dr. Alan Schwitzer, Counseling Graduate Program Director
Department   Educational Leadership and Counseling
(757) 683-3221, fax (757) 683-5756, delc@odu.edu,
http://web.odu.edu/webroot/orgs/Educ/ELC/elc.nsf/pages/home

Key See key for Data on Each Department (this section) on page 79.

Program

Accreditation   Regional Accreditation, **CACREP:** Community Counseling, **CACREP:** School Counseling, **CACREP:** Student Affairs - Counseling

Uniqueness Nationally-accredited by CACREP. Low faculty to student ratio.

Degrees
- Community Counseling: M.
- School Counseling: M.
- Other: S.
- Student Affairs: M.

Contact
- Community Counseling: M = Dr. Edward Neukrug.
- School Counseling: M = Dr. Radha Horton-Parker.
- Other: S = Dr. Alan Schwitzer.
- Student Affairs: M = Christopher Lovell.

Admission and Graduation Data

Admission

Requirements
- Community Counseling(M): GPA 3.00; GRE R; GRE V 400; GRE Q 400; GRE W 2.0.
- School Counseling(M): GPA 3.00; GRE R; GRE V 400; GRE Q 400; GRE W 2.0.
- Other(S):
- Student Affairs(M): GPA 3.00; GRE R; GRE V 400; GRE Q 400; GRE W 2.0.

Enrollment
- Community Counseling(M): 24 Admitted yearly; 19 Graduated yearly; 39 Female; 9 Male.
- School Counseling(M): 30 Admitted yearly; 24 Graduated yearly; 48 Female; 12 Male.
- Other(S): 2 Admitted yearly; 1 Graduated yearly; 4 Female; 1 Male.
- Student Affairs(M): 6 Admitted yearly; 4 Graduated yearly; 9 Female; 3 Male.

Diversity
- African-American; Asian-American; Caucasian; Hispanic; Native American; Pacific Islander; Multiracial.

Graduation

Requirements
- Community Counseling(M): 48 Class hours; 100 Practicum hours; 600 Internship hours; Comprehensive exam; CPCE.
- School Counseling(M): 48 Class hours; 100 Practicum hours; 600 Internship hours; Comprehensive exam; CPCE.
- Other(S): 30 Class hours; 100 Practicum hours; 300 Internship hours; Comprehensive exam.
- Student Affairs(M): 48 Class hours; 100 Practicum hours; 600 Internship hours; CPCE.

Postgraduation activity: Advanced education and employment setting percentages.
- Community Counseling(M): 5 Managed care; 10 Private practice; 85 Agency practice.
- School Counseling(M): 5 Advanced education; 35 Elementary school; 30 Middle school; 30 Secondary school.
- Other(S).
- Student Affairs(M): 20 Agency practice; 80 Other.

Planned Program Modifications

Courses	Drop	Add
	• NP.	• NP.

Other	Decrease	Increase
	• NP.	• NP.

Related Programs Psychology

Faculty

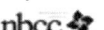 Percent of faculty reported with NCC certification: 40%.

Percent in professional counseling practice: 0%.

Research interests Counselor ethics, character disorders, counselor education and development, spirituality and values, skills, school counseling and federal/state mandates.

Diversity • African-American; Asian-American; Caucasian.

Name, Degree, Rank, State/National Credentials, % time devoted to program, email
• Neukrug, Edward; EdD; Full Prof.; LPC; *eneukrug@odu.edu*
• Brown, Nina; EdD; Full Prof.; LPC, NCC; *nbrown@odu.edu*
• Duggan, Molly; PhD; Lecturer; *mduggan@odu.edu*
• Horton-Parker, Radha; PhD; Assoc.; NCC; *rparker@odu.edu*
• Jurgens, Jill; EdD; Assist.; *jjurgens@odu.edu*
• Lovell, Christopher; PhD; Assoc.; NCC; *clovell@odu.edu*
• McAuliffe, Garrett; EdD; Assoc.; LPC; *gmacaulif@odu.edu*
• Parks-Savage, Agatha; EdD; Adjunct; LPC; *spsavage@odu.edu*
• Ripley, Vivian; EdD; Assist.; NCC; *vripley@odu.edu*
• Schwitzer, Alan; PhD; Assoc.; *aschwitz@odu.edu*

VA: Radford University

P.O. Box 6994
Radford, VA 24142
USA
Dean   Dr. Paul Sale, College of Education and Human Development
Administrator   Dr. Donald Anderson, Chairperson
                    Department   Dept of Counselor Education
                    (540) 831-5214, fax (540) 831-6755, danderso@radford.edu

Key   See key for Data on Each Department (this section) on page 79.

Program

Accreditation   Regional Accreditation, **CACREP:** Community Counseling, **CACREP:** School Counseling, **CACREP:** Student Affairs - Counseling

Uniqueness   The Dept. maintains an organizational culture that values academic excellence and promotes achievement of excellence through diversity of ideas and people. It provides a balanced curriculum blending knowledge in behavioral science with clinical or technical professions. Uniquely small academic community with strong clinical focus taught by experienced clinicians.

Degrees
- Community Counseling: M.
- School Counseling: M.
- Student Affairs: M.

Contact
- Community Counseling: M = Alan Forrest.
- School Counseling: M = James Gumaer.
- Student Affairs: M = Paul Harris.

Admission and Graduation Data

Admission

Requirements
- Community Counseling(M): GPA 2.75; GRE 900; GRE V 450; GRE Q 450; GRE A 0; MAT 45.
- School Counseling(M): GPA 2.75; GRE 900; GRE V 450; GRE Q 450; GRE A 0; MAT 45.
- Student Affairs(M): GPA 2.75; GRE 900; GRE V 450; GRE Q 450; GRE A 0; MAT 45.

Enrollment
- Community Counseling(M): 12 Admitted yearly; 12 Graduated yearly.
- School Counseling(M): 12 Admitted yearly; 12 Graduated yearly.
- Student Affairs(M): 12 Admitted yearly; 12 Graduated yearly.

Diversity
- African-American; Asian-American; Caucasian; Hispanic; Native American; Pacific Islander; Multiracial.

Graduation

Requirements
- Community Counseling(M): 48 Class hours; 100 Practicum hours; 600 Internship hours; Comprehensive exam.
- School Counseling(M): 48 Class hours; 100 Practicum hours; 600 Internship hours; Comprehensive exam.
- Student Affairs(M): 48 Class hours; 100 Practicum hours; 600 Internship hours.

Postgraduation activity: Advanced education and employment setting percentages.
- Community Counseling(M): 10 Advanced education; 90 Agency practice.
- School Counseling(M): 10 Advanced education; 5 Agency practice; 20 Elementary school; 32 Middle school; 33 Secondary school.
- Student Affairs(M): 10 Advanced education; 90 Other.

Planned Program Modifications

Courses   Drop   Add
- NP.   - Gender Issues in Counseling.

Other   Decrease   Increase
- NP.   - Diversity Recruiting of Faculty
                                          - Diversity Recruiting of Students
                                          - Faculty FTE
                                          - National Accreditation
                                          - Number of Degree Majors
                                          - Number of Off-Campus Courses.

Related Programs Clinical Social Workers
Psychology
Arts Therapists
Psychiatric Nurses

Faculty

nbcc 🔻   Percent of faculty reported with NCC certification: 80%.   ncc 🔻

Percent in professional counseling practice: 71%.

Research interests • NP.

Diversity   • African-American; Caucasian.

Name, Degree, Rank, State/National Credentials, % time devoted to program, email
- Anderson, Donald; EdD; Full Prof.; LPC, NCC, LMFT, NCMHC; >81%; *danderso@radford.edu*
- Forest, Alan; EdD; Full Prof.; LPC, NCC, LMFT; >81%; *aforrest@radford.edu*
- Gumaer, James; EdD; Full Prof.; LPC, LMFT; >81%; *dgumaer@radford.edu*
- Harris, Paul; EdD; Assoc.; >81%; *pharris@radford.edu*
- Scott, Wally W; PhD; Adjunct; LPC, NCC, LMFT; <21%; *wscott@radford.edu*
- Stanley, Paula H; PhD; Full Prof.; LPC, NCC, LMFT; 41-60%; *pstanley@radford.edu*
- Strosnider, J. Steve; MS; Adjunct; LPC, NCC, LMFT; <21%; *sstrosnider@lewisgaleclinic.com*
- Cutler, Heather; PhD; Assist.; NCC; >81%; *hcutler2@radford.edu*
- Steigerwald, Fran; PhD; Assist.; LPC, NCC; >81%; *fjsteiger@radford.edu*
- Murray, Lynda; PhD; Assist.; LPC, NCC; <21%; *lyndamurra@aol.com*

Has CHI SIGMA IOTA (International Counseling Society) chapter.

VA: Regent University

1000 Regent University Drive
Virginia Beach, VA 23464-9800
USA

Dean Dr. Rosemarie Scotti Hughes, Virginia Beach, VA
Administrator Dr. Rosemarie Hughes, Dean, School of Psychology & Counseling
Department School of Psychology & Counseling
(757) 226-4255, fax (757) 226-4263, psycoun@regent.edu,
www.regent.edu/psychology

Key See key for Data on Each Department (this section) on page 79.

Program

Accreditation Regional Accreditation, **CACREP:** Community Counseling, **CACREP:** School Counseling

Uniqueness CACREP accredited school and community programs on Virginia Beach campus. Alexandria, VA., CACS master's program beginning fall 2002. Diverse ethnically and by gender. Ability to take joint degree programs with other schools on campus. Programs founded on principles of integration of faith, spiritual values, and Judeo-Christian principles. Internships at over 100 sites

Degrees
- Community Counseling: M, S.
- School Counseling: M, S.
- Counselor Education: PhD.

Contact
- Community Counseling: M = Dr. Lee Underwood.; S = Dr. Kathleen Arveson.
- School Counseling: M = Dr. Robyn Rennie.; S = Dr. Kathleen Arveson.
- Counselor Education: D = Dr. Susan Scott.

Admission and Graduation Data

Admission

Requirements
- Community Counseling(M): GPA 2.75; GRE 1000; GRE V 500; GRE Q 500; MAT 50%; Interview.
- Community Counseling(S): GPA 2.75; GRE 1000; GRE V 500; GRE Q 500; MAT 50%; Interview.
- School Counseling(M): GPA 2.75; GRE 1000; GRE V 500; GRE Q 500; MAT 50%; Interview.
- School Counseling(S): GPA 2.75; GRE 1000; GRE V 500; GRE Q 500; MAT 50%; Interview.
- Counselor Education(D): GPA 3.50; GRE 1000; GRE V 500; GRE Q 500; MAT 50%.

Enrollment
- Community Counseling(M & S): 55 Admitted yearly; 38 Graduated yearly; 21 Female; 29 Male.
- School Counseling(M & S): 8 Admitted yearly; 8 Graduated yearly; 4 Female; 3 Male.
- Counselor Education(D): 15 Admitted yearly.

Diversity
- African-American; Asian-American; Caucasian; Hispanic; Native American; Multiracial; Other.

Graduation

Requirements
- Community Counseling(M): 51/60 Class hours; 100 Practicum hours; 600 Internship hours; CPCE.
- Community Counseling(S): 30 Class hours; 600 Practicum hours; 600 Internship hours.
- School Counseling(M): 51/60 Class hours; 100 Practicum hours; 600 Internship hours; CPCE.
- School Counseling(S): 30 Class hours; 100 Practicum hours; 600 Internship hours.
- Counselor Education(D): 60 Class hours; Dissertation.

Postgraduation activity: Advanced education and employment setting percentages.
- Community Counseling(M & S): 6 Advanced education; 7 Private practice; 50 Agency practice; 37 Other.
- School Counseling(M & S): 50 Elementary school; 20 Middle school; 19 Secondary school; 11 Other.
- Counselor Education(D):

Planned Program Modifications

Courses	Drop	Add
	• NP.	• Forensic Counseling.
		• Grief Counseling.

Other   Decrease   Increase
                        • Faculty FTE.   • Admission Requirements
                                                                    • Diversity Recruiting of Faculty
                                                                    • Financial Aid
                                                                    • Number of On-Line Courses.

Related Programs Psychology

Faculty

 nbcc   Percent of faculty reported with NCC certification: 32%.   ncc

Percent in professional counseling practice: 50%.

Research interests Research on Theophostic interventions, Marital Therapy, Juvenile Justice, Integrated
                  clinical faith interventions; Women's issues, ADHD, Play therapy, skills teaching of
                  counselors and sound counseling theory and practice..

Diversity   • African-American; Asian-American; Caucasian; Hispanic.

Name, Degree, Rank, State/National Credentials, % time devoted to program, email
• Arveson, Kathleen R; PhD; Assist.; LPC, NCC; >81%; *kathy@arveson.com*
• Garzon, Fernando L; PsyD; Assist.; LCP; >81%; *ferngar@regent.edu*
• Gatewood, Jacqueline J; PsyD; Assist.; LPC; >81%; *jacqgat@regent.edu*
• Hathaway, William L; PhD; Assoc.; LCP; <21%; *willhat@regent.edu*
• Hughes, Rosemarie S; PhD; Full Prof.; LPC, NCC; 41-60%; *rosehug@regent.edu*
• Hutchison, June W; PhD; Assist.; LPC, NCC; >81%; *junehut@regent.edu*
• Jefferson, George L; PhD; Assoc.; LPC; >81%; *georjef@regent.edu*
• Johnson, Judy L; PhD; Assoc.; LCP; <21%; *judyjoh@regent.edu*
• Maciak, Anna T; PsyD; Instructor; >81%; *annamac@regent.edu*
• Parker, Stephen E; PhD; Assoc.; LPC, NCC; >81%; *steppar@regent.edu*
• Rawles, Portia D; PsyD; Assist.; <21%; *portraw@regent.edu*
• Rennie, Robyn L; PhD; Assist.; LPC, NCC; >81%; *robyren@regent.edu*
• Ripley, Jennifer S; PhD; Assist.; LCP; <21%; *jennrip@regent.edu*
• Rondeau, Holiday; PsyD; Assoc.; LCP; <21%; *holiron@regent.edu*
• Sautter, Scott W; PhD; Assoc.; LCP; <21%; *scotsau@regent.edu*
• Scalise, Eric T; EdS; Assoc.; LPC, LMFT; MFCC; 61-80%; *ericsca@regent.edu*
• Scott, Susan W; PhD; Assist.; LPC, NCC; >81%; *susasco@regent.edu*
• Underwood, Lee A; PsyD; Assist.; LCP; PCC; >81%; *leeunde@regent.edu*
• Yarhouse, Mark A; PsyD; Assoc.; LCP; LMFT; <21%; *markyar@regent.edu*

VA: Virginia Tech

	308 East Eggleston Hall
	Blacksburg, VA 24061-0302
	United States
Dean	Dr. Jerry Niles, Blacksburg, VA
Administrator	Dr. David Alexander, Department Head
	Department Educational Leadership & Policy Studies
	(540) 231-5106, fax (540) 231-7845, vmeadows@vt.edu,
	http://filebox.vt.edu/users/thohen/index/

Key   See key for Data on Each Department (this section) on page 79.

Program

Accreditation   Regional Accreditation, **CACREP:** Community Counseling, **CACREP:** Counselor Education and Supervision, **CACREP:** School Counseling

Uniqueness   Students are first priority at both the master's and doctoral levels. Research and leadership are also highly valued. High tech instructional emphasis.

Degrees
- Community Counseling: M.
- School Counseling: M.
- Counselor Education: EdD, PhD.

Contact
- Community Counseling: M = NP.
- School Counseling: M = NP.
- Counselor Education: D = NP.

Admission and Graduation Data

Admission

Requirements
- Community Counseling(M): GPA 3.00; Interview.
- School Counseling(M): GPA 3.00; Interview.
- Counselor Education(D): Masters and GPA 3.00.

Enrollment
- Community Counseling(M): 20 Admitted yearly; 18 Graduated yearly; 15 Female; 5 Male.
- School Counseling(M): 20 Admitted yearly; 18 Graduated yearly; 15 Female; 5 Male.
- Counselor Education(D): 5-10 Admitted yearly; 5-8 Graduated yearly.

Diversity
- African-American; Asian-American; Caucasian; Hispanic; Native American; Multiracial.

Graduation

Requirements
- Community Counseling(M): 51 Class hours; 100 Practicum hours; 600 Internship hours; Comprehensive exam.
- School Counseling(M): 51 Class hours; 100 Practicum hours; 600 Internship hours; Comprehensive exam.
- Counselor Education(D): 100 Class hours; 600 Internship hours; Comprehensive exam; Oral exam; Dissertation.

Postgraduation activity: Advanced education and employment setting percentages.
- Community Counseling(M): 90 Agency practice; 10 Other.
- School Counseling(M): 30 Elementary school; 20 Middle school; 50 Secondary school.
- Counselor Education(D): 60 Advanced education; 15 Private practice; 10 Agency practice; 5 Middle school; 5 Secondary school; 5 Student affairs.

Planned Program Modifications

Courses	Drop	Add
	• NP.	• NP.

Other	Decrease	Increase
	• NP.	• NP.

Related Programs Marriage and Family Therapists
Psychology
Organizational Behaviorists
Communications
International Studies

Faculty

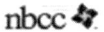   Percent of faculty reported with NCC certification: 43%.

Percent in professional counseling practice: 30%.

Research interests School counseling, community counseling, supervision, internet, career development, art therapy, international counseling

Diversity • African-American; Caucasian; Hispanic.

Name, Degree, Rank, State/National Credentials, % time devoted to program, email
- Bodenhorn, Nancy; PhD; Assist.; >81%; *pbrott@vt.edu*
- Brott, Pamelia; PhD; Assist.; LPC; >81%; *nanboden@vt.edu*
- Getz, Hildy; EdD; Assoc.; LPC, NCC, LMFT; >81%; *hgetz@vt.edu*
- Hohenshil, Thomas; PhD; Full Prof.; LPC, NCC; >81%; *thohen@vt.edu*
- Lawson, Gerard; PhD; Assist.; LPC, CAC; >81%;
- Madison-Colmore, Octavia; EdD; Assist.; LPC, NCC, CAC; >81%; *omadison@vt.edu*
- ter Maat, Mercedes; Assist.; LPC; >81%; *mtermaat@vt.edu*

Has CHI SIGMA IOTA (International Counseling Society) chapter.

WA: Central Washington University

400 E Eighth Avenue
Ellensburg, WA 98926-7575
USA

Dean
Administrator   Jeffrey Penick, Director
Department   Dept of Psychology
(509) 963-2381, fax (509) 963-2307, www.cwu.edu/~psych

Key   See key for Data on Each Department (this section) on page 79.

Program
Accreditation   • NP.

Uniqueness   The program includes five quarters of closely supervised practicum experience, followed by
an external internship. Certification in school counseling may also be obtained.

Degrees   • Mental Health Counseling: M.
• School Counseling: M.

Contact   • Mental Health Counseling: M = NP.
• School Counseling: M = NP.

Admission and Graduation Data
Admission
Requirements   • Mental Health Counseling(M): NP.
• School Counseling(M): NP.

Enrollment   • Mental Health Counseling(M): 12 Admitted yearly; 9 Graduated yearly.
• School Counseling(M): 2 Admitted yearly; 1 Graduated yearly.

Diversity   • NP.

Graduation
Requirements   • Mental Health Counseling(M): 90 Class hours; 325 Practicum hours; 600 Internship hours.
• School Counseling(M): 88 Class hours; 325 Practicum hours; 400 Internship hours.

Postgraduation activity: Advanced education and employment setting percentages.
• Mental Health Counseling(M): NP.
• School Counseling(M): NP.

Planned Program Modifications
Courses   <u>Drop</u>   <u>Add</u>
• NP.   • NP.

Other   <u>Decrease</u>   <u>Increase</u>
• NP.   • NP.

Related Programs

Faculty

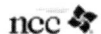

nbcc   Percent of faculty reported with NCC certification: 0%.   ncc

Percent in professional counseling practice: NP.

Research interests Counseling process research; Self-efficacy; ADHD; Developmental issues

Diversity   • Caucasian; Hispanic.

Name, Degree, Rank, State/National Credentials, % time devoted to program, email
• NP.

WA: City University

11900 NE First
Bellevue, WA 98005
USA

Dean   Elizabeth Fountain, MA
Administrator Theresa Wildt, MS, US Program Director and Arden Henley, MA, Canadian Program Director
                   Department   School of Human Services and Applied Behavioral Science
                   (425) 637-1010 Ext. 5459, fax (425) 709-5270, mjensen@cityu.edu, cityu.edu

Key   See key for Data on Each Department (this section) on page 79.

Program

Accreditation   • NP

Uniqueness   The Master of Arts in Counseling Psychology is a practitioner-based, theoretically diverse, cohort-model training program that emphasizes application of theory, ethical and legal obligations, diversity, and the self-awareness of the therapist.

Degrees   • Mental Health Counseling: M.

Contact   • Mental Health Counseling: M = Elizabeth Fountain, MA.

Admission and Graduation Data

Admission
Requirements   • Mental Health Counseling(M): GPA 2.75; Interview.

Enrollment   • Mental Health Counseling(M): 90 Admitted yearly; 25 Graduated yearly; 60 Female; 30 Male.

Diversity   • African-American; Asian-American; Caucasian; Hispanic; Native American; Pacific Islander; Multiracial.

Graduation
Requirements   • Mental Health Counseling(M): 250 Internship hours; Comprehensive exam; Oral exam; Thesis.

Postgraduation activity: Advanced education and employment setting percentages.
                    • Mental Health Counseling(M): 5 Advanced education; 5 Managed care; 5 Private practice; 85 Agency practice.

Planned Program Modifications

Courses   Drop   Add
                    • NP.   • Gerontological Counseling
                                                  • Marriage and Family Counseling.

Other   Decrease   Increase
                    • NP.   • Course Offerings
                                                  • Diversity Recruiting of Faculty
                                                  • Diversity Recruiting of Students
                                                  • Faculty FTE
                                                  • Number of Off-Campus Courses.

Related Programs Other

Faculty

nbcc   Percent of faculty reported with NCC certification: 20%.   ncc

Percent in professional counseling practice: 90%.

Research interests Marriage and family therapy, animal-assisted therapy, community-based approaches, narrative approaches.

Diversity   • Asian-American; Caucasian; Native American; Multiracial.

Name, Degree, Rank, State/National Credentials, % time devoted to program, email
• Fountain, Elizabeth A; MA; NCC, LMHC; 41-60%; *efountain@cityu.edu*
• Lilly, Karen F; MA; LMHC; 61-80%; *klilly@cityu.edu*
• Wildt, Theresa R; MA; LMFC; >81%; *twildt@cityu.edu*
• Henley, Arden; MA; RCC; >81%; *ahenley@cityu.edu*
• Chang, Jeff; MA; Counseling Psychology; 41-60%; *jchang@cityu.edu*

WA: Eastern Washington University

526 5th Street, MAR 213,
Cheney, WA 99004
USA
Dean   Dr. Fritz Erickson, College of Education and Human Development
Administrator   Dr. Val Appleton, Director
      Department   Counseling, Educational, and Developmental Psychology
      (509) 359-2827, fax (509) 359-4366, joanne.foster@mailserver.ewu.edu

Key   See key for Data on Each Department (this section) on page 79.

Program
Accreditation   Regional Accreditation, **CACREP:** Mental Health Counseling, **CACREP:** School Counseling

Uniqueness   CACREP accredited programs in School Counseling and Mental Health Counseling

Degrees
- Mental Health Counseling: M.
- School Counseling: M.

Contact
- Mental Health Counseling: M = Dr. Ken Engbresson.
- School Counseling: M = Dr. Sarah Leverett.

Admission and Graduation Data
Admission
Requirements
- Mental Health Counseling(M): NP.
- School Counseling(M): NP.

Enrollment
- Mental Health Counseling(M): 10 Admitted yearly.
- School Counseling(M): 10 Admitted yearly.

Diversity
- NP.

Graduation
Requirements
- Mental Health Counseling(M): NP.
- School Counseling(M): NP.

Postgraduation activity: Advanced education and employment setting percentages.
- Mental Health Counseling(M): NP.
- School Counseling(M): NP.

Planned Program Modifications
Courses   Drop   Add
- NP.   - NP.

Other   Decrease   Increase
- NP.   - NP.

Related Programs

Faculty

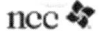
Percent of faculty reported with NCC certification: 0%.

Percent in professional counseling practice: NP.

Research interests Career, bilingual/multicultural, narrative, and family counseling

Diversity
- African-American; Caucasian; Hispanic; Native American; Other.

Name, Degree, Rank, State/National Credentials, % time devoted to program, email
- Engbresson, Ken
- Leverett, Sarah

Has CHI SIGMA IOTA (International Counseling Society) chapter.

WA: Seattle University

Broadway and Madison
Seattle, WA 98122
USA
Dean Sue Schmitt, School of Education, Seattle University
Administrator Hutch Haney, Chair
Department Department of Counseling and School Psychology
(206) 296-5750, fax (206) 296-1892, counsp@seattleu.edu,
www.seattleu.edu/soe/counseling

Key See key for Data on Each Department (this section) on page 79.

Program
Accreditation Regional Accreditation

Uniqueness Programs: school counseling, mental health counseling, post-secondary counseling, school psychology and post-master's certification in school counseling and school psychology. All programs designed for working students. All programs have a strong clinical sequence and courses in diversity and ethics.

Degrees
- Mental Health Counseling: M.
- School Counseling: M.
- College Counseling: M.

Contact
- Mental Health Counseling: M = Hutch Haney.
- School Counseling: M = Hutch Haney.
- College Counseling: M = Hutch Haney.

Admission and Graduation Data
Admission
Requirements
- Mental Health Counseling(M): GPA 3.00; 500hr Years work experience; Interview.
- School Counseling(M): GPA 3.00; 500hr Years work experience; Interview.
- College Counseling(M): GPA 3.00; 500hr Years work experience; Interview.

Enrollment
- Mental Health Counseling(M): 10 Admitted yearly; 10 Graduated yearly; 13 Female; 5 Male.
- School Counseling(M): 25 Admitted yearly; 25 Graduated yearly; 18 Female; 2 Male.
- College Counseling(M): 5 Admitted yearly; 5 Graduated yearly; 2 Female.

Diversity
- African-American; Asian-American; Caucasian; Hispanic; Multiracial.

Graduation
Requirements
- Mental Health Counseling(M): 80 Practicum hours; 520 Internship hours; Comprehensive exam.
- School Counseling(M): 80 Practicum hours; 520 Internship hours; Comprehensive exam; Portfolio.
- College Counseling(M): 80 Practicum hours; 520 Internship hours; Comprehensive exam.

Postgraduation activity: Advanced education and employment setting percentages.
- Mental Health Counseling(M): 5 Advanced education; 5 Managed care; 90 Agency practice.
- School Counseling(M): 6 Advanced education; 30 Elementary school; 40 Middle school; 30 Secondary school.
- College Counseling(M): 100 Other.

Planned Program Modifications

Courses	Drop	Add
	• NP.	• Social Justice.

Other	Decrease	Increase
	• NP.	• Diversity Recruiting of Faculty • Diversity Recruiting of Students.

Related Programs

Faculty

Percent of faculty reported with NCC certification: 50%.

Percent in professional counseling practice: NP.

Research interests School reform, spirituality, ethics and group counseling.

Diversity   •   Caucasian.

Name, Degree, Rank, State/National Credentials, % time devoted to program, email
- Owen, Yvonne J; PhD; Assoc.; NCC, State Lic Psych; >81%;
- Afanador, Josef C; EdD; Assoc.; NCC, CRCC/Stae Lic Psych; >81%;
- Haney, Hutch; MS; Assist.; CRCC; >81%;
- Jensen, Christine; EdD; Assist.; NCSC/ State Couns cert.; >81%;
- O'Connor, Michael; PhD; Assoc.; NCC; >81%;
- Leibsohn, Jackie; PhD; Assoc.; State Lic. Psych.; >81%;

WA: University of Puget Sound

1500 N. Warner CMB#1051
Tacoma, WA 98416-1051
USA

Dean Carol Merz
Administrator   Carol Merz, Dean
                      Department   Education
                      (253) 879-3375, fax (253) 879-3926, www.ups.edu/education/

Key   See key for Data on Each Department (this section) on page 79.

Program

Accreditation   Regional Accreditation

Uniqueness   Students study a wide range of counseling theories and learn to apply them in a variety of
               contexts.

Degrees   • Mental Health Counseling: M.
            • School Counseling: M.
            • Pastoral Counseling: M.

Contact   • Mental Health Counseling: M = Grace Kirchner.
            • School Counseling: M = Grace Kirchner.
            • Pastoral Counseling: M = Grace Kirchner.

Admission and Graduation Data
Admission
Requirements   • Mental Health Counseling(M): GPA 3.00; GRE 1500; Interview.
                 • School Counseling(M): GPA 3.00; GRE 1500; Interview.
                 • Pastoral Counseling(M): GPA 3.00; GRE 1500; Interview.

Enrollment   • Mental Health Counseling(M): 6 Admitted yearly; 6 Graduated yearly; 5 Female; 1 Male.
               • School Counseling(M): 6 Admitted yearly; 6 Graduated yearly; 5 Female; 1 Male.
               • Pastoral Counseling(M): 4 Admitted yearly; 2 Graduated yearly; 3 Female; 1 Male.

Diversity   • African-American; Asian-American; Caucasian; Pacific Islander.

Graduation
Requirements   • Mental Health Counseling(M): 48 Class hours; 32 Practicum hours; 400 Internship hours;
                   Comprehensive exam; Oral exam.
                 • School Counseling(M): 48 Class hours; 32 Practicum hours; 400 Internship hours;
                   Comprehensive exam; Oral exam.
                 • Pastoral Counseling(M): 48 Class hours; 100 Practicum hours; 500 Internship hours; Oral
                   exam.

Postgraduation activity: Advanced education and employment setting percentages.
               • Mental Health Counseling(M): 10 Advanced education; 40 Managed care; 50 Agency
                 practice.
               • School Counseling(M): 10 Elementary school; 30 Middle school; 30 Secondary school.
               • Pastoral Counseling(M): 100 Agency practice.

Planned Program Modifications
Courses   Drop   Add
                  • NP.   • NP.

Other   Decrease   Increase
                  • NP.   • NP.

Related Programs

Faculty

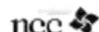 Percent of faculty reported with NCC certification: 25%.   ncc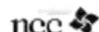

Percent in professional counseling practice: 50%.

Research interests Validity of admissions criteria to screen candidates for graduate study. Administrators'
                   perceptions of school counselors' roles.

Diversity   • Caucasian.

Name, Degree, Rank, State/National Credentials, % time devoted to program, email
• Kirchner, Grace L; PhD; Full Prof.; NCC; >81%; *kirchner@ups.edu*
• Gast, Joan E; MEd; Instructor; LPC; >81%; *bgast@ups.edu*
• Woodward, John; PhD; Full Prof.; <21%; *woodward@ups.edu*
• Setchfield, Margaret S; MEd; <21%; *msetchfield@ups.edu*

WA: Western Washington University

516 High Street
Bellingham, WA 98226-9089
USA
Dean Ronald Kleinknecht
Administrator Dale Dinnel, Chairperson
Department Psychology
(360) 650-3515, fax (360) 650-7305, www.ac.wwu.edu/~psych/

Key See key for Data on Each Department (this section) on page 79.

Program
Accreditation **CACREP:** Mental Health Counseling, **CACREP:** School Counseling

Uniqueness Highly selective, small, full-time programs in school and mental health counseling.

Degrees
- Mental Health Counseling: M.
- School Counseling: M.

Contact
- Mental Health Counseling: M = Davis Hayden.
- School Counseling: M = Arleen Lewis.

Admission and Graduation Data
Admission
Requirements
- Mental Health Counseling(M): GPA 3.00; GRE R; Interview.
- School Counseling(M): GPA 3.00; GRE R; Interview.

Enrollment
- Mental Health Counseling(M): 6 Admitted yearly; 6 Graduated yearly; 4 Female; 2 Male.
- School Counseling(M): 6 Admitted yearly; 6 Graduated yearly; 4 Female; 2 Male.

Diversity
- African-American; Asian-American; Caucasian; Native American.

Graduation
Requirements
- Mental Health Counseling(M): 100 Practicum hours; 900 Internship hours; Comprehensive exam.
- School Counseling(M): 100 Practicum hours; 600 Internship hours; Comprehensive exam.

Postgraduation activity: Advanced education and employment setting percentages.
- Mental Health Counseling(M): 100 Agency practice.
- School Counseling(M): 35 Elementary school; 30 Middle school; 35 Secondary school.

Planned Program Modifications
Courses | Drop | | Add
- NP. | | - NP.

Other | Decrease | | Increase
- NP. | | - NP.

Related Programs

Faculty

nbcc 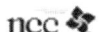 Percent of faculty reported with NCC certification: 0%. **ncc**

Percent in professional counseling practice: NP.

Research interests Suicide prevention, peer helping programs, women and anger expression, youth substance use, domestic violence, multicultural counseling.

Diversity
- Asian-American; Caucasian.

Name, Degree, Rank, State/National Credentials, % time devoted to program, email
- Byrne, Christina; PhD; Assoc.; Psychologist; 41-60%; *cbyrne@cc.wwu.edu*
- Forgays, Deborah K; PhD; Assoc.; Psychologist; 61-80%; *forgays@cc.wwu.edu*
- Hayes, Susanna; PhD; Assoc.; School Counseling; 61-80%; *hayes@cc.wwu.edu*
- Lewis, Arleen C; PhD; Full Prof.; psychologist; >81%; *Arleen.Lewis@wwu.edu*
- Hayden, Davis; PhD; Full Prof.; 61-80%; *hayden@cc.wwu.edu*
- David, Sue; PhD; Full Prof.; psychologist; 61-80%; *dsue@cc.wwu.edu*

WI: University of Wisconsin-La Crosse

	149 Graff Main Hall LaCrosse, WI 54601 USA
Dean	Garth Tymeson, College of Health, Physical Education and Teacher Education
Administrator	Larry J. Ringgenberg, Coordinator
	Department College Student Development & Administration
	(608) 785-8063, fax (608) 785-8933, ringgenb.larr@uwlax.edu,
	http://www.uwlax.edu/csda/

Key   See key for Data on Each Department (this section) on page 79.

Program
Accreditation   • NP.

Uniqueness   All faculty are practitioners. Therefore, we do an excellent job of connecting theory to practice.

Degrees   • Student Affairs: M.

Contact   • Student Affairs: M = Larry J. Ringgenberg, Ph.D..

Admission and Graduation Data
Admission
Requirements   • Student Affairs(M): GPA 2.85; GRE NR; Interview.

Enrollment   • Student Affairs(M): 15 Admitted yearly; 15 Graduated yearly; 10 Female; 5 Male.

Diversity   • Asian-American; Caucasian.

Graduation
Requirements   • Student Affairs(M): 38 Class hours; 140 Practicum hours; 210 Internship hours; Thesis.

Postgraduation activity: Advanced education and employment setting percentages.
• Student Affairs(M): 100 Other.

Planned Program Modifications
Courses	Drop	Add
	• NP.	• NP.

Other	Decrease	Increase
	• NP.	• Number of Distance Education Courses.

Related Programs

Faculty

    Percent of faculty reported with NCC certification: 0%.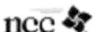

Percent in professional counseling practice: 25%.

Research interests   Student Development, college students and alcohol, Diversity.

Diversity   • Caucasian; Multiracial.

Name, Degree, Rank, State/National Credentials, % time devoted to program, email
• Goudie, Andrea K; PhD; Adjunct; <21%; *Goudie.Andr@uwlax.edu*
• Hageseth, Jon A; PhD; Adjunct; <21%; *Hageseth.Jon@uwlax.edu*
• Roter, Petra; PhD; Adjunct; <21%; *Roter.Petr@uwlax.edu*
• Bakkum, Chris S; PhD; Adjunct; <21%; *Bakkum.Chri@uwlax.edu*
• Miyamoto, Michael H; PhD; Adjunct; <21%; *Miyamoto.Mich@uwlax.edu*
• Nicklaus, Nick; EdD; Adjunct; <21%; *Nicklaus.Nick@uwlax.edu*
• Wagner, Jodie; PhD; Adjunct; <21%; *Wagner.Jodi@uwlax.edu*
• Ringgenberg, Larry J; PhD; Adjunct; <21%; *Ringgenb.larr@uwlax.edu*
• Vahala, Mary Beth; EdD; Adjunct; <21%; *Vahala.Mary@uwlax.edu*

WI: University of Wisconsin-Oshkosh

	800 Algoma Blvd. Oshkosh, WI 54901-8663 USA
Dean	Carmen Coballes-Vega, College of Education and Human Services
Administrator	Margaret Olson, Chairperson
	Department Department of Counselor Education (920) 424-1475, fax (920) 424-0858, olsonmj@uwosh.edu, http://www.coehs.uwosh.edu/departments/counselor_ed/

Key   See key for Data on Each Department (this section) on page 79.

Program

Accreditation   Regional Accreditation, **CACREP:** Community Counseling, **CACREP:** School Counseling, **CACREP:** Student Affairs - Counseling

Uniqueness   Program has a strong emphasis on personal growth and development of the counselor as a person.

Degrees
- Community Counseling: M.
- School Counseling: M.
- Student Affairs: M.

Contact
- Community Counseling: M = David Hargis.
- School Counseling: M = Robert Urofsky.
- Student Affairs: M = M. Alan Saginak.

Admission and Graduation Data

Admission

Requirements
- Community Counseling(M): GPA 3.00; 2 Years work experience; Interview.
- School Counseling(M): GPA 3.00; 2 Years work experience; Interview.
- Student Affairs(M): GPA 3.00; 2 Years work experience; Interview.

Enrollment
- Community Counseling(M): 20 Admitted yearly; 14 Graduated yearly; 39 Female; 10 Male.
- School Counseling(M): 30 Admitted yearly; 20 Graduated yearly; 63 Female; 11 Male.
- Student Affairs(M): 10 Admitted yearly; 6 Graduated yearly; 15 Female; 4 Male.

Diversity
- African-American; Asian-American; Caucasian; Hispanic; Native American; Multiracial.

Graduation

Requirements
- Community Counseling(M): 48 Class hours; 100 Practicum hours; 600 Internship hours; Portfolio.
- School Counseling(M): 48 Class hours; 100 Practicum hours; 600 Internship hours; Portfolio.
- Student Affairs(M): 48 Class hours; 100 Practicum hours; 600 Internship hours; Portfolio.

Postgraduation activity: Advanced education and employment setting percentages.
- Community Counseling(M): 2 Advanced education; 20 Managed care; 10 Private practice; 30 Agency practice; 38 Other.
- School Counseling(M): 1 Advanced education; 33 Elementary school; 33 Middle school; 33 Secondary school.
- Student Affairs(M): 1 Advanced education; 99 Other.

Planned Program Modifications

Courses	Drop	Add
	• NP.	• NP.

Other	Decrease	Increase
	• NP.	• Diversity Recruiting of Faculty • Diversity Recruiting of Students.

Related Programs Clinical Social Workers

Faculty

    Percent of faculty reported with NCC certification: 33%.   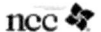

Percent in professional counseling practice: 0%.

Research interests Grief Counseling, Ethical Issues in Counseling, Gestalt Therapy and Counseling, Hypnosis and Pain Management, Media and Mental Health, Wellness, Spirituality and Counseling, College Students and Transition, Counselor Supervision

Diversity • Caucasian.

Name, Degree, Rank, State/National Credentials, % time devoted to program, email
- Barnes, Kristin; PhD; Assist.; NCC; >81%; *barnes@uwosh.edu*
- Hargis, David; PhD; Assist.; LPC; >81%; *hargis@uwosh.edu*
- Olson, Margaret; PhD; Assoc.; LPC, NCC, Sch. Couns; >81%; *olsonmj@uwosh.edu*
- Saginak, M. Alan; EdD; Assist.; >81%; *saginak@uwosh.edu*
- Urofsky, Robert; PhD; Assist.; >81%; *urofsky@uwosh.edu*
- Wilson, Nona; PhD; Assoc.; >81%; *wilsonn@uwosh.edu*

Has CHI SIGMA IOTA (International Counseling Society) chapter.

WI: University of Wisconsin-Whitewater

	6035 Winther Hall
	Whitewater, WI 53190-0296
	USA
Dean	Jeffrey Barnett, College of Education, University of Wis-Whitewater
Administrator	Aneneosa A. Okocha, Ph.D., NCC, Professor and Chairperson
	Department Dept of Counselor Education
	(262) 472-5426, fax (262) 472-2841, counslred@mail.uww.edu,
	http://academics.uww.edu/counseled

Key   See key for Data on Each Department (this section) on page 79.

Program

Accreditation   **CACREP:** Community Counseling, **CACREP:** School Counseling, **CACREP:** Student Affairs - Counseling, **CACREP:** Student Affairs - Professional Practice

Uniqueness   It is a 48-credit program with three major emphases: community, higher education and school. It is also a CACREP accredited program that emphasizes diversity/multiculturalism in its curriculum.

Degrees
- Community Counseling: M.
- School Counseling: M.
- Student Affairs: M.

Contact
- Community Counseling: M = NP.
- School Counseling: M = NP.
- Student Affairs: M = NP.

Admission and Graduation Data

Admission

Requirements
- Community Counseling(M): GPA 2.75; Interview.
- School Counseling(M): GPA 2.75; Interview.
- Student Affairs(M): GPA 2.75; Interview.

Enrollment
- Community Counseling(M): 27 Admitted yearly; 23 Graduated yearly.
- School Counseling(M): 23 Admitted yearly; 16 Graduated yearly.
- Student Affairs(M): 5 Admitted yearly; 3 Graduated yearly.

Diversity
- African-American; Asian-American; Caucasian; Hispanic.

Graduation

Requirements
- Community Counseling(M): 48 Class hours; 100 Practicum hours; 640 Internship hours.
- School Counseling(M): 48 Class hours; 100 Practicum hours; 640 Internship hours.
- Student Affairs(M): 48 Class hours; 100 Practicum hours; 640 Internship hours.

Postgraduation activity: Advanced education and employment setting percentages.
- Community Counseling(M): NP.
- School Counseling(M): NP.
- Student Affairs(M): NP.

Planned Program Modifications

Courses	Drop	Add
	• NP.	• NP.

Other	Decrease	Increase
	• NP.	• Diversity Recruiting of Students.

Related Programs

Faculty

nbcc ❧   Percent of faculty reported with NCC certification: 40%.   **ncc** ❧

Percent in professional counseling practice: NP.

Research interests • NP.

Diversity
- African-American; Caucasian.

Name, Degree, Rank, State/National Credentials, % time devoted to program, email
- Dollarhide, Colette; EdD; Assoc.; NCC; >81%; *dollarhc@mail.uww.edu*
- Norman, Donald; PhD; Assist.; >81%; *normand@mail.uww.edu*
- O'Beirne, Brenda; PhD; Assoc.; >81%; *obeirneb@mail.uww.edu*
- Okocha, Aneneosa; PhD; Full Prof.; NCC; >81%; *okochaa@mail.uww.edu*
- VanDoren, David; EdD; Assoc.; >81%; *vandored@mail.uww.edu*

Has CHI SIGMA IOTA (International Counseling Society) chapter.

WV: West Virginia University

502 Allen Hall, PO Box 6122
Morgantown, WV 26506-6122
USA

Dean Anne Nardi, Dean, 802 Allen Hall
Administrator Margaret Glenn, Interim Chair
Department Counseling, Rehab Counseling and Counseling Psychology
(304) 293-3807, fax (304) 293-4082, vicki.railing@mail.wvu.edu,
www.wvu.edu/~crc/couns/

Key   See key for Data on Each Department (this section) on page 79.

Program

Accreditation   Regional Accreditation, **CACREP:** Community Counseling, **CACREP:** School Counseling,
CORE: Rehabilitation Counseling

Uniqueness   Emphasis on rural service/needs,service-learning options for students,faculty/student
mentoring. Distance learning options.

Degrees
- Community Counseling: M.
- School Counseling: M.
- Other: PhD.
- Rehabilitation Counseling: M.

Contact
- Community Counseling: M = Ed Jacobs.
- School Counseling: M = Ed Jacobs.
- Other: D = NP.
- Rehabilitation Counseling: M = Margaret Glenn.

Admission and Graduation Data

Admission

Requirements
- Community Counseling(M): GPA 2.80; GRE 900; GRE V 450; GRE Q 450; Interview.
- School Counseling(M): GPA 2.80; GRE 900; GRE V 450; GRE Q 450; Interview.
- Other(D): Masters and GPA 3.25; GRE 1000; GRE V 500; GRE Q 500; GRE A NA; 1 Year work experience.
- Rehabilitation Counseling(M): GPA 2.80; GRE NA; Interview.

Enrollment
- Community Counseling(M): 22 Admitted yearly.
- School Counseling(M): 16 Admitted yearly.
- Other(D): 8 Admitted yearly; 6-8 Graduated yearly; 5 Female; 3 Male.
- Rehabilitation Counseling(M): 15 Admitted yearly.

Diversity
- African-American; Asian-American; Caucasian; Hispanic; Multiracial.

Graduation

Requirements
- Community Counseling(M): 51 Class hours; 100 Practicum hours; 600 Internship hours.
- School Counseling(M): 51 Class hours; 100 Practicum hours; 600 Internship hours.
- Other(D): 93 Class hours; 600 Practicum hours; 1200 Internship hours; Comprehensive exam; Dissertation.
- Rehabilitation Counseling(M): 51 Class hours; 100 Practicum hours; 600 Internship hours.

Postgraduation activity: Advanced education and employment setting percentages.
- Community Counseling(M): 25 Advanced education; 70 Agency practice; 5 Univ Other.
- School Counseling(M): 10 Advanced education; 90 Agency practice; 60 Elementary school; 10 Middle school; 30 Secondary school.
- Other(D): 10 Managed care; 30 Private practice; 30 Agency practice; 30 Univ Other.
- Rehabilitation Counseling(M): 10 Advanced education; 90 Agency practice.

Planned Program Modifications

Courses	Drop	Add
	• NP.	• Legal/Ethical Issues
		• Supervision.

Other	Decrease	Increase
	• NP.	• Course Offerings
		• Clinical Supervision
		• Graduation Requirements
		• Number of Distance Education Courses
		• Number of Off-Campus Courses
		• Number of On-Line Courses.

Related Programs Psychology
                      Communications

Faculty

                Percent of faculty reported with NCC certification: 30%.

Percent in professional counseling practice: NP.

Research interests Multicultural, rehabilitation service delivery, problem gambling, creative counseling
                   techniques, parent education for custody determination,career development/vocational
                   psychology, elementary guidance delivery/interventions, and play therapy.

Diversity   •   African-American; Caucasian; Multiracial.

Name, Degree, Rank, State/National Credentials, % time devoted to program, email
• Boyce, Justin; PhD; Assist.; 22-40%; *justin.boyce@mail.wvu.edu*
• Cormier, Sherry; PhD; Full Prof.; LPC; 41-60%; *sherry.cormier@mail.wvu.edu*
• Delo, James; PhD; Full Prof.; LPC; >81%; *jim.delo@mail.wvu.edu*
• Esposito, Judy; PhD; Assist.; LPC, NCC; >81%; *judy.esposito@mail.wvu.edu*
• Glenn, Margaret; PhD; Assoc.; LPC; <21%; *margaret.glenn@mail.wvu.edu*
• Jacobs, Ed; PhD; Full Prof.; LPC, NCC; >81%; *ed.jacobs@mail.wvu.edu*
• Marinelli, Robert; EdD; Full Prof.; <21%; *bob.marinelli@mail.wvu.edu*
• Srebalus, David; EdD; Full Prof.; LPC, NCC; >81%; *david.srebalus@mail.wvu.edu*
• Tunick, Roy; PhD; Full Prof.; 22-40%; *roy.tunick@mail.wvu.edu*
• Jones, Sharon; PhD; Assist.; 41-60%; *sharonb.jones@mail.wvu.edu*

Has CHI SIGMA IOTA (International Counseling Society) chapter.

WY: University of Wyoming

PO Box 3374, 16th and Gibbon
Laramie, WY 82071-3374
USA
Dean   Patricia McClurg, Education
Administrator   Mary Alice Bruce, Department Head
                    Department   Counselor Education
                    (307) 766-2366, fax (307) 766-6668, jleach@uwyo.edu,
                    http://ed.uwyo.edu/Departments/depcounsel/index.htm

Key   See key for Data on Each Department (this section) on page 79.

Program

Accreditation   Regional Accreditation, **CACREP:** Community Counseling, **CACREP:** Counselor Education and Supervision, **CACREP:** School Counseling, **CACREP:** Student Affairs - Counseling

Uniqueness   Small class environments, intensive class discussions, faculty focuses on encouraging and supporting self-examination and growth. Emphasis areas in Marriage & Family, Play Therapy, and Addictions

Degrees
- Community Counseling: M.
- School Counseling: M.
- Student Affairs: M.
- Counselor Education: PhD.

Contact
- Community Counseling: M = Michael D. Loos and Michael Morgan.
- School Counseling: M = Mary Alice Bruce and Michael Smith.
- Student Affairs: M = Deborah L. McGriff.
- Counselor Education: D = Kent W. Becker.

Admission and Graduation Data

Admission

Requirements
- Community Counseling(M): GPA 3.00; 2 Years work experience; Interview.
- School Counseling(M): GPA 3.00; 2 Years work experience; Interview.
- Student Affairs(M): GPA 3.00; 2 Years work experience; Interview.
- Counselor Education(D): Masters and GPA 3.00; 2 Years work experience.

Enrollment
- Community Counseling(M): 9 Admitted yearly; 5 Graduated yearly; 19 Female; 4 Male.
- School Counseling(M): 9 Admitted yearly; 5 Graduated yearly; 14 Female; 4 Male.
- Student Affairs(M): 2 Admitted yearly; 1 Graduated yearly; 1 Female.
- Counselor Education(D): 6 Admitted yearly; 4 Female; 2 Male.

Diversity
- African-American; Asian-American; Caucasian; Hispanic; Native American; Multiracial.

Graduation

Requirements
- Community Counseling(M): 48 Class hours; 100 Practicum hours; 600 Internship hours; Comprehensive exam.
- School Counseling(M): 48 Class hours; 100 Practicum hours; 600 Internship hours; Comprehensive exam.
- Student Affairs(M): 48 Class hours; 100 Practicum hours; 600 Internship hours.
- Counselor Education(D): 70+ Class hours; 600 Internship hours; Comprehensive exam; Oral exam; Dissertation.

Postgraduation activity: Advanced education and employment setting percentages.
- Community Counseling(M): 10 Advanced education; 90 Agency practice.
- School Counseling(M): 10 Advanced education; 30 Elementary school; 30 Middle school; 30 Secondary school.
- Student Affairs(M): 10 Advanced education; 90 Other.
- Counselor Education(D): 40 Advanced education; 10 Private practice; 40 Agency practice; 10 Student affairs.

Planned Program Modifications

Courses	Drop	Add
	• NP.	• Play Therapy.

Other	Decrease	Increase
	• Number of Degree Majors.	• Diversity Recruiting of Students
		• Number of On-Line Courses.

Related Programs Clinical Social Workers
Psychology
Psychiatric Nurses
Communications

Faculty

 Percent of faculty reported with NCC certification: 50%.

Percent in professional counseling practice: NP.

Research interests Marriage & Family, Addictions, Supervison, Spirituality, Treatment Outcome, Community Building, Play Therapy.

Diversity • African-American; Caucasian.

Name, Degree, Rank, State/National Credentials, % time devoted to program, email
• Bruce, Mary Alice; PhD; Assoc.; LPC, NCC; >81%; *mabruce@uwyo.edu*
• Becker, Kent W; EdD; Assist.; LPC, LMFT; >81%; *kwbecker@uwyo.edu*
• Loos, Michael D; PhD; Assist.; LPC, NCC, LAT; >81%; *mdloos@uwyo.edu*
• McGriff, Deborah L; PhD; Assist.; 41-60%; *mcgriff@uwyo.edu*
• Smith, Michael R; PhD; Assist.; NCC; >81%; *smithmr@uwyo.edu*
• Morgan, Michael; PhD; Assist.; LMFT; >81%

Has CHI SIGMA IOTA (International Counseling Society) chapter.

Part E

Data on
Program Areas

Key for Part E: Data on Program Areas

Admission Requirements:
Fin Aid - Financial Aid
GPA – Grade Point Average
GRE – Graduate Record Examinations
MAT – Miller Analogies Tests
Wrk Exp – Work Experience
Letters – Letters of Recommendation
Intervw – Interview
M – Master's

Graduation Requirements:
Hours C – Semester or quarter hours
Hours P – Practicum clock hours
Hours I – Internship clock hours
Comp – Comprehensive exam
CPCE – Counselor Preparation Comprehensive Exam
Oral – Oral comprehensive exam
Port. – Portfolio

Admissions and Enrollment:
Admit – Admitted yearly
Grad – Graduated yearly
F – Female
M – Male

Postgraduation Activity/Placement Percentages:
Adv Ed – Advanced Education
Mngd – Managed care
El – Elementary school counseling
Mddle – Middle school counseling
Sec – Secondary school counseling
Stu A – Higher Education/Student Affairs
Other – Other setting

Master's Degree Programs												
	Admission Requirements							Graduation Requirements				
Fin Aid	GPA	GRE	MAT	Wrk Exp	Letters	Intrvw	Hours C/P/I	Comp	CPCE	Oral	Thesis	Port.

Addictions Counseling
NC East Carolina University   Greenville   *Contact:* Lloyd Goodwin;

Y	~3.00		~35	0	0	Y	48/100/600			Y	Y	

Addictions Counseling
NJ The College of New Jersey   Ewing   *Contact:* Dr. Mark Woodford; woodford@tcnj.edu

Y	R				Y	Y	48/100/600					

Addictions Counseling
NV University of Nevada   Reno   *Contact:* Thomas Harrison; tch@unr.edu

Y	3.00	750		2	3		60/100/600	Y	Y			

Addictions Counseling
NY Queens College, City University of New York   Flushing

						//						

Addictions Counseling
RI Rhode Island College   Providence   *Contact:* MFinley

	3.00	900	45	2	3		36/90/					

Addictions Counseling
TX Houston Baptist University   Houston

Y		850					//					

Addictions Counseling
VA College of William and Mary   Williamsburg   *Contact:* Charles Gressard; cfgres@wm.edu

Y	2.50	40%		0	3		51/100/600					

Career Counseling
CA University of San Diego, School of Education   San Diego   *Contact:* Susan Zgliczynski

Y	2.75			1	3	Y	48/100/600	Y				

Career Counseling
CO University of Colorado at Denver Denver *Contact:* Andrew Helwig; Andrew_Helwig@ceo.cudenver.edu

Y	2.75	900	40	0	4	Y	60/150/600		Y	Y		

Career Counseling
MO University of Missouri - St. Louis   Saint Louis   *Contact:* Mark Pope, EdD; pope@umsl.edu

Y	3.00				3		48/150/600		Y			

Career Counseling
MO University of Missouri-Columbia Columbia *Contact:* Mary Heppner or Joe Johnson
HeppnerM@missouri.edu

	3.00	1000			3		48//					

Career Counseling
TX Houston Baptist University   Houston

	Y				3		450//					

College Counseling
CA San Jose University   San Jose

							//					

College Counseling
DE University of Delaware   Newark   *Contact:* John Bishop; John.Bishop@udel.edu

Y	2.50	1050			3	Y	48/210/420	Y				

Master's Degree Programs

College Counseling
LA Northwestern State University   Natchitoches   *Contact:* Robert Bowman; bowmanr@nsula.edu

Fin Aid	GPA	GRE	MAT	Wrk Exp	Letters	Intrvw	Hours C/P/I	Comp	CPCE	Oral	Thesis	Port.
Y	2.50	800		0	3	Y	48/100/600	Y				

College Counseling
LA Southeastern Louisiana University   Hammond   *Contact:* June Williams; jwilliams@selu.edu

Fin Aid	GPA	GRE	MAT	Wrk Exp	Letters	Intrvw	Hours C/P/I	Comp	CPCE	Oral	Thesis	Port.
Y				0	Y	Y	48/100/600	Y	Y			

College Counseling
LA University of New Orleans   New Orleans   *Contact:* Dr. Diana Hulse-Killacky; dhulseki@uno.edu

Fin Aid	GPA	GRE	MAT	Wrk Exp	Letters	Intrvw	Hours C/P/I	Comp	CPCE	Oral	Thesis	Port.
Y	2.50	R		0	0		60/100/600	Y	Y			

College Counseling
MI Eastern Michigan University   Ypsilanti   *Contact:* Yvonne Callaway; yvonne.callaway@emich.edu

Fin Aid	GPA	GRE	MAT	Wrk Exp	Letters	Intrvw	Hours C/P/I	Comp	CPCE	Oral	Thesis	Port.
Y	2.75				3	Y	48/100/600					Y

College Counseling
MS Mississippi State University   Mississippi State University   *Contact:* Dr. Mari Ann Callais; mcallais@colled.msstate.edu

Fin Aid	GPA	GRE	MAT	Wrk Exp	Letters	Intrvw	Hours C/P/I	Comp	CPCE	Oral	Thesis	Port.
Y	2.75	1200			3		48/100/600	Y	Y			

College Counseling
NY New York University   New York   *Contact:* Samuel Juni: sam.juni@nyu.edu

Fin Aid	GPA	GRE	MAT	Wrk Exp	Letters	Intrvw	Hours C/P/I	Comp	CPCE	Oral	Thesis	Port.
Y	3.00				2		48/84/84					

College Counseling
NY Plattsburgh State University   Plattsburgh   *Contact:* Dr. Beverly Burnell; beverly.burnell@plattsburgh.edu

Fin Aid	GPA	GRE	MAT	Wrk Exp	Letters	Intrvw	Hours C/P/I	Comp	CPCE	Oral	Thesis	Port.
Y	2.80	25th %tile	25th %tile	0	3	Y	48/115/600	Y	Y			

College Counseling
NY SUNY College of Brockport   Brockport   *Contact:* T. Hernandez

Fin Aid	GPA	GRE	MAT	Wrk Exp	Letters	Intrvw	Hours C/P/I	Comp	CPCE	Oral	Thesis	Port.
Y	2.50						48/100/600					

College Counseling
OR Oregon State University   Corvallis   *Contact:* Gene Eakin; gene.eakin@orst.edu

Fin Aid	GPA	GRE	MAT	Wrk Exp	Letters	Intrvw	Hours C/P/I	Comp	CPCE	Oral	Thesis	Port.
Y	3.00				3	Y	/100/600			Y		Y

College Counseling
PA Penn State University   University Park

Fin Aid	GPA	GRE	MAT	Wrk Exp	Letters	Intrvw	Hours C/P/I	Comp	CPCE	Oral	Thesis	Port.
							//					

College Counseling
PA Shippensburg University of PA   Shippensburg   *Contact:* Thomas Hozman; tlhozm@ship.edu

Fin Aid	GPA	GRE	MAT	Wrk Exp	Letters	Intrvw	Hours C/P/I	Comp	CPCE	Oral	Thesis	Port.
Y	2.75	800		1	3	Y	48/150/600					Y

College Counseling
SC Clemson University   Clemson

Fin Aid	GPA	GRE	MAT	Wrk Exp	Letters	Intrvw	Hours C/P/I	Comp	CPCE	Oral	Thesis	Port.
	3.00	1250			2		48/100/600	Y	Y			

College Counseling
TX University of North Texas   Denton   *Contact:* Carolyn Kern; Kern@coefs.coe.unt.edu

Fin Aid	GPA	GRE	MAT	Wrk Exp	Letters	Intrvw	Hours C/P/I	Comp	CPCE	Oral	Thesis	Port.
Y	3.00	710			3	Y	48/100/600					

College Counseling
WA Seattle University   Seattle   *Contact:* Hutch Haney

Fin Aid	GPA	GRE	MAT	Wrk Exp	Letters	Intrvw	Hours C/P/I	Comp	CPCE	Oral	Thesis	Port.
	3.00		500hr	2		Y	/80/520	Y				

Master's Degree Programs												
Admission Requirements							Graduation Requirements					
Fin Aid	GPA	GRE	MAT	Wrk Exp	Letters	Intrvw	Hours C/P/I	Examinations Comp	CPCE	Oral	Thesis	Port.

Community Counseling
AL Auburn University   Auburn   *Contact:* Irene Houston; houstis@auburn.edu

Fin Aid	GPA	GRE	MAT	Exp	Letters	Intrvw	C/P/I	Comp	CPCE	Oral	Thesis	Port.
Y	3.00	1000			3		48/100/600	Y	Y	Y		Y

Community Counseling
AL The University of Alabama   Tuscaloosa   *Contact:* S. Allen Wilcoxon, Ed.D.; awilcoxo@bamaed.ua.edu

Fin Aid	GPA	GRE	MAT	Exp	Letters	Intrvw	C/P/I	Comp	CPCE	Oral	Thesis	Port.
Y	3.00	1000 (V+Q)	50	0	3		60/100/600	Y				Y

Community Counseling
AL Troy State University   Troy   *Contact:* Jeane Wright

Fin Aid	GPA	GRE	MAT	Exp	Letters	Intrvw	C/P/I	Comp	CPCE	Oral	Thesis	Port.
	2.50	850	33		3	Y	48/100/600	Y				

Community Counseling
AL University of Montevallo   Montevallo   *Contact:* Debbie Grant; grantdd@montevallo.edu

Fin Aid	GPA	GRE	MAT	Exp	Letters	Intrvw	C/P/I	Comp	CPCE	Oral	Thesis	Port.
Y	2.50	850	35			Y	48/100/600	Y	Y			Y

Community Counseling
AL University of North Alabama   Florence   *Contact:* J. Paul Baird; pbaird@unanov.una.edu

Fin Aid	GPA	GRE	MAT	Exp	Letters	Intrvw	C/P/I	Comp	CPCE	Oral	Thesis	Port.
Y	3.00	900	40		3	Y	48/100/600	Y	Y			

Community Counseling
AL University of South Alabama   Mobile   *Contact:* Dr. Joseph G. Law, Jr.; jlaw@usouthal.edu

Fin Aid	GPA	GRE	MAT	Exp	Letters	Intrvw	C/P/I	Comp	CPCE	Oral	Thesis	Port.
Y	3.00						48/100/600	Y				

Community Counseling
AZ Arizona State University   Tempe   *Contact:* Terence Tracey; ttracey@asu.edu

Fin Aid	GPA	GRE	MAT	Exp	Letters	Intrvw	C/P/I	Comp	CPCE	Oral	Thesis	Port.
Y	no minima	R		0	3		60/100/600	Y	Y			

Community Counseling
CO Adams State College   Alamosa   *Contact:* Dr. Susan Varhely; scvarhel@adams.edu

Fin Aid	GPA	GRE	MAT	Exp	Letters	Intrvw	C/P/I	Comp	CPCE	Oral	Thesis	Port.
Y	2.75	1250	37	0	2		60/100/600	Y				

Community Counseling
CO Denver Seminary   Denver   *Contact:* James R. Beck; jim.beck@denverseminary.edu

Fin Aid	GPA	GRE	MAT	Exp	Letters	Intrvw	C/P/I	Comp	CPCE	Oral	Thesis	Port.
Y	3.00				3		62/125/600					

Community Counseling
CO University of Colorado - Colorado Springs   Colorado Springs   *Contact:* Beverly Snyder;
bsnyder@uccs.edu

Fin Aid	GPA	GRE	MAT	Exp	Letters	Intrvw	C/P/I	Comp	CPCE	Oral	Thesis	Port.
Y	2.50		3	4		Y	49/100/600	Y				Y

Community Counseling
CO University of Colorado at Denver   Denver   *Contact:* Andrew Helwig
Andrew_Helwig@ceo.cudenver.edu

Fin Aid	GPA	GRE	MAT	Exp	Letters	Intrvw	C/P/I	Comp	CPCE	Oral	Thesis	Port.
Y	2.75	900	40	0	4	Y	60/150/600	Y				

Community Counseling
CO University of Northern Colorado   Greeley   *Contact:* Basilia Softas-Nall; basilia.softas-nall@unco.edu

Fin Aid	GPA	GRE	MAT	Exp	Letters	Intrvw	C/P/I	Comp	CPCE	Oral	Thesis	Port.
Y	3.00				3	Y	60/340/600	Y				

Community Counseling
CO University of Phoenix   Colorado Springs   *Contact:* John West

Fin Aid	GPA	GRE	MAT	Exp	Letters	Intrvw	C/P/I	Comp	CPCE	Oral	Thesis	Port.
Y	2.50			3	3	Y	51/100/600					Y

Community Counseling
CT Saint Joseph College   West Hartford   *Contact:* Richard W. Halstead, Ph.D.; rhalstead@sjc.edu

Fin Aid	GPA	GRE	MAT	Exp	Letters	Intrvw	C/P/I	Comp	CPCE	Oral	Thesis	Port.
			R	0	2	Y	48/100/600	Y				Y

Master's Degree Programs												
	Admission Requirements						Graduation Requirements					
Fin				Wrk			Hours	Examinations				
Aid	GPA	GRE	MAT	Exp	Letters	Intrvw	C/P/I	Comp	CPCE	Oral	Thesis	Port.

Community Counseling
DC The George Washington University   Washington   *Contact:* Chris D. Erickson, Ph.D.; cerick@gwu.edu

Y	3.00	1000	50%		2	Y	48/100/600					

Community Counseling
GA Columbus State University   Columbus

	2.70	800	44		2	Y	48/100/600	Y				Y

Community Counseling
GA Georgia State University   Atlanta   *Contact:* Gary L. Arthur, Ed.D.; garthur@gsu.edu

Y	2.50	800	NA	6	3		48/100/600	Y				

Community Counseling
GA State University of West Georgia   Carrolton   *Contact:* Dr. Snow

Y	2.70	900		0	3	Y	48/150/600	Y	Y			

Community Counseling
IA The University of Iowa   IowaCity   *Contact:* Vilia M. Tarvydas; vilia-tarvydas@uiowa.edu

Y	3.00	1000		1	3	Y	60/300/600	Y				

Community Counseling
ID University of Idaho   Moscow   *Contact:* Dr. Dianne Phillips-Miller

	3.00				3	Y	60/150/850			Y		Y

Community Counseling
IL College of Arts and Sciences (CAS)   Wheaton   *Contact:* Susan Thorne-Devin; stdevin@nl.edu

Y	3.00				3	Y	48//600		Y			Y

Community Counseling
IL Concordia University   River Forest   *Contact:* Dr. Michael Smith

Y	3.00				3		48/100/600	Y		Y		

Community Counseling
IL Eastern Illinois University   Charleston   *Contact:* Dr. Roberts

Y	2.75			0	2	Y	48/100/600	Y				

Community Counseling
IL Lewis University   Romeoville   *Contact:* Edmund Kearney; kearneed@lewisu.edu

Y	3.00				2		48/100/600	Y				Y

Community Counseling
IL Southern Illinois University Carbondale   Carbondale   *Contact:* Dr. Kim Asner-Self

Y	2.70				3		48/100/600	Y				

Community Counseling
IL Western Illinois University   Moline   *Contact:* Melanie Rawlins

	2.50				2	Y	48/100/600					

Community Counseling
IN Ball State University   Muncie   *Contact:* Phyllis Gordon; pgordon@bsu.edu

Y	2.75				3		48/200/600	Y				

Community Counseling
IN Indiana University   Bloomington   *Contact:* Dr. Sue Whiston; swhiston@indiana.edu

Y	2.75	1300			3		48/100/600					

Community Counseling
IN Indiana Wesleyan University   Marion

Y	3.00	1000			3		48-60/100/ 600-900					Y

Master's Degree Programs

Fin Aid	Admission Requirements						Graduation Requirements					
	GPA	GRE	MAT	Wrk Exp	Letters	Intrvw	Hours C/P/I	Comp	CPCE	Oral	Thesis	Port.

Community Counseling
KS Pittsburg State University   Pittsburg   *Contact:* Donald Ward; dward@pittstate.edu

Fin Aid	GPA	GRE	MAT	Wrk Exp	Letters	Intrvw	Hours C/P/I	Comp	CPCE	Oral	Thesis	Port.
Y	3.00	1200			3		59/150/450					

Community Counseling
LA Louisiana State University   Baton Rouge   *Contact:* Laura G. Hensley, Ph.D.; lhensley@lsu.edu

Fin Aid	GPA	GRE	MAT	Wrk Exp	Letters	Intrvw	Hours C/P/I	Comp	CPCE	Oral	Thesis	Port.
Y	3.00	1000			3		48/100/600	Y				

Community Counseling
LA Louisiana State University in Shreveport   Shreveport   *Contact:* Meredith Nelson; nelson@pilot.lsus.edu

Fin Aid	GPA	GRE	MAT	Wrk Exp	Letters	Intrvw	Hours C/P/I	Comp	CPCE	Oral	Thesis	Port.
Y	2.75	800			3		48/100/600	Y	Y			Y

Community Counseling
LA Loyola University   New Orleans

Fin Aid	GPA	GRE	MAT	Wrk Exp	Letters	Intrvw	Hours C/P/I	Comp	CPCE	Oral	Thesis	Port.
Y	3.00	1600	45	0	3	Y	48/140/600	Y				

Community Counseling
LA Our Lady of Holy Cross   New Orleans   *Contact:* Dr. Judith Miranti

Fin Aid	GPA	GRE	MAT	Wrk Exp	Letters	Intrvw	Hours C/P/I	Comp	CPCE	Oral	Thesis	Port.
							51/100/600					

Community Counseling
LA Southeastern Louisiana University   Hammond   *Contact:* Hunter Alessi; halessi@selu.edu

Fin Aid	GPA	GRE	MAT	Wrk Exp	Letters	Intrvw	Hours C/P/I	Comp	CPCE	Oral	Thesis	Port.
Y				0	Y	Y	48/100/600	Y	Y			

Community Counseling
LA University of New Orleans   New Orleans   *Contact:* Dr. Diana Hulse-Killacky; dhulseki@uno.edu

Fin Aid	GPA	GRE	MAT	Wrk Exp	Letters	Intrvw	Hours C/P/I	Comp	CPCE	Oral	Thesis	Port.
Y	2.50	R		0	0		60/100/600	Y	Y			

Community Counseling
MA Lesley University   Cambridge   *Contact:* Yishiuan Chin (617) 349-8339; (800) 999-1959 ext. 8339

Fin Aid	GPA	GRE	MAT	Wrk Exp	Letters	Intrvw	Hours C/P/I	Comp	CPCE	Oral	Thesis	Port.
Y	3.00		40		3	Y	60/100/600/1200					

Community Counseling
MD Johns Hopkins University   Baltimore   *Contact:* Fred Hanna, Mary Guindon; fhanna@jhu.edu

Fin Aid	GPA	GRE	MAT	Wrk Exp	Letters	Intrvw	Hours C/P/I	Comp	CPCE	Oral	Thesis	Port.
Y	3.00				2	Y	48//500			Y		

Community Counseling
MD Loyola College in Maryland   Columbia   *Contact:* K. Elizabeth Oakes

Fin Aid	GPA	GRE	MAT	Wrk Exp	Letters	Intrvw	Hours C/P/I	Comp	CPCE	Oral	Thesis	Port.
Y	2.50			0	3	Y	52/250/750				Y	Y

Community Counseling
MD McDaniel College   Westminster   *Contact:* Dr. Simeon Schlossberg

Fin Aid	GPA	GRE	MAT	Wrk Exp	Letters	Intrvw	Hours C/P/I	Comp	CPCE	Oral	Thesis	Port.
Y	2.50				3	Y	39//200-500	Y				

Community Counseling
MI Andrews University   Berrien Springs   *Contact:* Elvin Gabriel; gabriel@andrews.edu

Fin Aid	GPA	GRE	MAT	Wrk Exp	Letters	Intrvw	Hours C/P/I	Comp	CPCE	Oral	Thesis	Port.
Y	2.70				2	Y	48/100/600	Y				

Community Counseling
MI Eastern Michigan University   Ypsilanti   *Contact:* Irene Ametrano; irene.ametrano@emich.edu

Fin Aid	GPA	GRE	MAT	Wrk Exp	Letters	Intrvw	Hours C/P/I	Comp	CPCE	Oral	Thesis	Port.
Y	2.75				3	Y	48/100/600					Y

Community Counseling
MI Oakland University   Rochester   *Contact:* ramey@oakland.edu

Fin Aid	GPA	GRE	MAT	Wrk Exp	Letters	Intrvw	Hours C/P/I	Comp	CPCE	Oral	Thesis	Port.
Y	3.00				2	Y	48/100/600					

Community Counseling
MI Siena Heights University   Adrian   *Contact:* Linda M. Brewster

Fin Aid	GPA	GRE	MAT	Wrk Exp	Letters	Intrvw	Hours C/P/I	Comp	CPCE	Oral	Thesis	Port.
	3.00			2	3	Y	48/100/600					

Master's Degree Programs

| | Admission Requirements | | | | | | Graduation Requirements | | | | | |
Fin Aid	GPA	GRE	MAT	Wrk Exp	Letters	Intrvw	Hours C/P/I	Comp	CPCE	Oral	Thesis	Port.

Community Counseling
MN Minnesota State University Moorhead   Moorhead   *Contact:* Wes Erwin

Y	3.00	R	R	0	3	Y	48/100/650	Y	Y	Y	Y	

Community Counseling
MN Minnesota State University, Mankato   Mankato   *Contact:* Diane Coursol & John Seymour; diane.coursol@mnsu.edu

Y	3.00	1350	44		3	Y	50/100/600	Y				Y

Community Counseling
MO Southeast Missouri State University   Cape Girardeau   *Contact:* Dr. Verl Pope; vpope@semo.edu

Y	3.00	1600		0	3	Y	48/100/600	Y	Y			Y

Community Counseling
MO Truman State University   Kirksville   *Contact:* Christopher J. Maglio, Ph.D.; cjmaglio@truman.edu

Y	3.00	50th%		0	3		48/150/600	Y			Y	

Community Counseling
MO University of Missouri - St. Louis   Saint Louis   *Contact:* Susan Kashubeck-West, PhD

Y	3.00				3		48/150/600	Y	Y			

Community Counseling
MO University of Missouri-Columbia   Columbia   *Contact:* Laurie Mintz; MintzL@missouri.edu

	3.00	1000			3		48//	Y				

Community Counseling
MS Mississippi State University   Mississippi State University   *Contact:* Dr. Joan Looby jlooby@colled.msstate.edu

Y	2.75	1200			3		60/100/600	Y	Y			

Community Counseling
MS William Carey College   Hattiesburg   *Contact:* Dr. Tommy King

Y	2.50	900			2		60/100/100					Y

Community Counseling
MT Montana Sate University-Northern   Havre   *Contact:* John Foley

Y	3.00	900	29	2	3		60/100/600	Y		Y		

Community Counseling
NC Appalachian State University   Boone   *Contact:* Diana Quealy-Berge

Y	R	R			3		60/100/600	Y	Y			

Community Counseling
NC Campbell University   Buies Creek   *Contact:* Wayne Hatcher; hatcher@mailcenter.cambell.edu

Y	3.00	850			3	Y	48/100/600	Y				

Community Counseling
NC North Carolina A&T State University   Greensboro   *Contact:* Dr. Wyatt D. Kirk

Y	R			0	3		48//	Y	Y			

Community Counseling
NC The University of North Carolina at Greensboro   Greensboro   *Contact:* For all programs in all tracks contact the Departmental admissions office at ced@uncg.edu or (336) 334-3434

Y	3.00	R			3		48/120+/600	Y				

Community Counseling
NC University of North Carolina at Charlotte   Charlotte   *Contact:* Phyllis Post; ppost@email.uncc.edu

Y	R	R	R	0	3	Y	60/150/600	Y				

| | | Admission Requirements | | | | | | Graduation Requirements | | | | |
Fin Aid	GPA	GRE	MAT	Wrk Exp	Letters	Intrvw	Hours C/P/I	Comp	CPCE	Oral	Thesis	Port.

Community Counseling
NC Wake Forest University   Winston-Salem   *Contact:* Laura Veach; veachlj@wfu.edu

| Y | 3.00 | 1000 | | | 3 | Y | 60/135/600 | | | | | |

Community Counseling
ND North Dakota State University   Fargo   *Contact:* Dr. Lee Covington Rush; Lee.Rush@ndsu.nodak.edu

| Y | 3.00 | | | | 3 | Y | 48/40/600/ 900 | Y | Y | | | |

Community Counseling
NE Chadron State College   Chadron   *Contact:* Linda Brockbank, PhD; lbrockbank@csc.edu

| | | | | | | | 48/40/600 | | | | | |

Community Counseling
NE University of Nebraska-Omaha   Omaha   *Contact:* Dept. Chair

| | 3.00 | | 35 | | 3 | Y | 48/170/130 | | | | | |

Community Counseling
NE Wayne State College   Wayne   *Contact:* Keith Willis; kewilli1@wsc.edu

| | | 1050 | | 0 | 2 | Y | 48/100/600 | | | | | Y |

Community Counseling
NJ The College of New Jersey   Ewing   *Contact:* Dr. Mark Woodford; woodford@tcnj.edu

| Y | R | | | | Y | Y | 48/100/600 | Y | | | | |

Community Counseling
NJ William Paterson University   Wayne   *Contact:* Paula R. Danzinger, Ph.D., LPC, CCMHC; danzingerp@wpunj.edu

| Y | 2.75 | | 42 | | 2 | Y | 48/100/600 | Y | | | Y | Y |

Community Counseling
NM University of Phoenix - Albuquerque, NM Campus   Albuquerque   *Contact:* Darren Adamson, Ph.D.; darren.adamson@phoenix.edu

| Y | 2.50 | | | 3 | 3 | Y | // | | | | | |

Community Counseling
NV University of Nevada   Reno   *Contact:* Thomas Harrison; tch@unr.edu

| Y | 3.00 | 750 | | 2 | 3 | | 60/100/600 | Y | | Y | | |

Community Counseling
NY Canisius College   Buffalo   *Contact:* David Farrugia; Farriguia@canisius.edu

| | 2.50 | 1300 | | | | Y | 42/160/340 | | | | | |

Community Counseling
NY College at Oswego SUNY   Oswego   *Contact:* Dr. Jodi Mullen

| Y | 3.00 | | | 2 | 3 | Y | 48/100/300 | Y | Y | | | |

Community Counseling
NY Marist College   Poughkeepsie   *Contact:* John Scileppi Ph.D.; John.Scileppi@Marist.edu

| Y | 3.00 | 1500 | | | 3 | Y | 45//360 | | | | | |

Community Counseling
NY New York University   New York   *Contact:* Samuel Juni; sam.juni@nyu.edu

| Y | 3.00 | | | | 2 | | 48/84/84 | | | | | |

Community Counseling
NY Plattsburgh State University   Plattsburgh   *Contact:* Dr. Stephen Saiz; stephen.saiz@plattsburgh.edu

| Y | 2.80 | 25th %tile | 25th %tile | 0 | 3 | Y | 48/115/600 | Y | Y | | | |

							Master's Degree Programs					
	Admission Requirements						Graduation Requirements					
Fin				Wrk			Hours		Examinations			
Aid	GPA	GRE	MAT	Exp	Letters	Intrvw	C/P/I	Comp	CPCE	Oral	Thesis	Port.

Community Counseling
NY SUNY College of Brockport   Brockport   *Contact:* S. R. Seem

Y	2.50			3		Y	48/100/600					

Community Counseling
NY Syracuse University   Syracuse   *Contact:* Janine Bernard; bernard@syr.edu

Y	3.00	NA		1	3	Y	48/100/600	Y	Y			Y

Community Counseling
NY University of Rochester   Rochester   *Contact:* Kathryn Douthit; duth@troi.cc.rochester.edu

Y		NR		0	2	Y	51/120/600				Y	

Community Counseling
OH Cleveland State University   Cleveland   *Contact:* Kathy MacCluskie

Y	2.75		R		2		60/100/600	Y				

Community Counseling
OH John Carroll University   Cleveland   *Contact:* Christopher M. Faiver, PhD; Faiver@JCU.EDU

Y	2.75	1000	50	0	3	Y	60/150/600	Y	Y			

Community Counseling
OH Kent State University   Kent   *Contact:* Dr. Jason McGlothlin; jmcgloth@kent.edu

Y	2.75			0	2	Y	60/100/600					

Community Counseling
OH Malone College   Canton   *Contact:* Dr. Dan Merz

	3.00			3		Y	48+12/ 100/600					

Community Counseling
OH Ohio University   Athens   *Contact:* Pat Beamish

Y	3.00	900			3		//					

Community Counseling
OH The University of Toledo   Toledo   *Contact:* Paula Dupuy; paula.dupuy@utoledo.edu

Y	3.00	800			3	Y	48/100/600					

Community Counseling
OH Xavier University   Cincinnati   *Contact:* Lon S. Kriner, PhD; kriner@xavier.edu

	2.7+		35	0	0	Y	60/100/600					

Community Counseling
OH Youngstown State University   Youngstown   *Contact:* Dr. Don Martin

Y	3.00	450	40	0	3	Y	60-64/200/ 600	Y				

Community Counseling
OR Oregon State University   Corvallis   *Contact:* Gene Eakin; gene.eakin@orst.edu

Y	3.00				3	Y	/100/600			Y		Y

Community Counseling
OR Portland State University   Portland   *Contact:* Capuzzi

Y	points as- signed	R	same	0	same	Y	/100/600	Y				

Community Counseling
PA Arcadia University   Glenside   *Contact:* Mrs. Carol Lyman

Y	3.00	R	R		3	Y	48-60/100/ 300-600					

Master's Degree Programs											
	Admission Requirements						Graduation Requirements				
Fin				Wrk			Hours	Examinations				
Aid	GPA	GRE	MAT	Exp	Letters	Intrvw	C/P/I	Comp	CPCE	Oral	Thesis	Port.

Community Counseling
PA California University of Pennsylvania   California   *Contact:* Gloria C. Brusoski, PhD; Brusoski@cup.edu

Fin Aid	GPA	GRE	MAT	Wrk Exp	Letters	Intrvw	Hours C/P/I	Comp	CPCE	Oral	Thesis	Port.
Y	3.00		45		3	Y	48/150/600	Y	Y			

Community Counseling
PA Duquesne University   Pittsburgh   *Contact:* Nicholas J. Hanna; Hannan@duq.edu

Fin Aid	GPA	GRE	MAT	Wrk Exp	Letters	Intrvw	Hours C/P/I	Comp	CPCE	Oral	Thesis	Port.
Y	3.00		40		2		60/125/600			Y		Y

Community Counseling
PA Indiana University of Pennsylvania   Indiana   *Contact:* Dr. Claire Dandeneau; cdanden@iup.edu

Fin Aid	GPA	GRE	MAT	Wrk Exp	Letters	Intrvw	Hours C/P/I	Comp	CPCE	Oral	Thesis	Port.
Y	2.80			0	2	Y	48/90/300-600					

Community Counseling
PA Kutztown University   Kutztown   *Contact:* Jo Cohen; cohen@kutztown.edu

Fin Aid	GPA	GRE	MAT	Wrk Exp	Letters	Intrvw	Hours C/P/I	Comp	CPCE	Oral	Thesis	Port.
	3.00	1200			3		60/100/700	Y				

Community Counseling
PA Shippensburg University of PA   Shippensburg   *Contact:* Thomas Hozman; tlhozm@ship.edu

Fin Aid	GPA	GRE	MAT	Wrk Exp	Letters	Intrvw	Hours C/P/I	Comp	CPCE	Oral	Thesis	Port.
Y	2.75	800		1	3	Y	48/150/600					Y

Community Counseling
PA West Chester University   West Chester

Fin Aid	GPA	GRE	MAT	Wrk Exp	Letters	Intrvw	Hours C/P/I	Comp	CPCE	Oral	Thesis	Port.
Y	3.00				3		48/360/	Y				Y

Community Counseling
SC Clemson University   Clemson

Fin Aid	GPA	GRE	MAT	Wrk Exp	Letters	Intrvw	Hours C/P/I	Comp	CPCE	Oral	Thesis	Port.
	3.00	1250			2		48/100/600	Y	Y			

Community Counseling
SC Winthrop University   Rock Hill   *Contact:* Dr. Johnny Sanders, Jr.; sandersj@winthrop.edu

Fin Aid	GPA	GRE	MAT	Wrk Exp	Letters	Intrvw	Hours C/P/I	Comp	CPCE	Oral	Thesis	Port.
Y	2.00	800	40	0	3	Y	51/100/600	Y				

Community Counseling
SD South Dakota State University   Brookings   *Contact:* Marla Muxen; Marla_Muxen@sdstate.edu

Fin Aid	GPA	GRE	MAT	Wrk Exp	Letters	Intrvw	Hours C/P/I	Comp	CPCE	Oral	Thesis	Port.
Y	3.00				2	Y	48/100/600	Y		Y		

Community Counseling
SD The University of South Dakota   Vermillion   *Contact:* Frank Main; fmain@usd.edu

Fin Aid	GPA	GRE	MAT	Wrk Exp	Letters	Intrvw	Hours C/P/I	Comp	CPCE	Oral	Thesis	Port.
	3.00	900	NA		3		51/45/600	Y				

Community Counseling
TN East Tennessee State University   Johnson City   *Contact:* Clifton Mitchell; Mitchelc@etsu.edu

Fin Aid	GPA	GRE	MAT	Wrk Exp	Letters	Intrvw	Hours C/P/I	Comp	CPCE	Oral	Thesis	Port.
Y		R			3	Y	48/100/600	Y				

Community Counseling
TN Peabody College, Vanderbilt University   Nashville   *Contact:* Gina Frieden; gina.frieden@vanderbilt.edu

Fin Aid	GPA	GRE	MAT	Wrk Exp	Letters	Intrvw	Hours C/P/I	Comp	CPCE	Oral	Thesis	Port.
Y	3.00	1000	50		3	Y	48/100/600	Y		Y		

Community Counseling
TX Lamar University   Beaumont

Fin Aid	GPA	GRE	MAT	Wrk Exp	Letters	Intrvw	Hours C/P/I	Comp	CPCE	Oral	Thesis	Port.
							45/300/					

Community Counseling
TX Southwest Texas State University   San Marcos   *Contact:* John Garcia; jg12@swt.edu

Fin Aid	GPA	GRE	MAT	Wrk Exp	Letters	Intrvw	Hours C/P/I	Comp	CPCE	Oral	Thesis	Port.
Y	see below						//					

		Master's Degree Programs										
	Admission Requirements						Graduation Requirements					
Fin Aid	GPA	GRE	MAT	Wrk Exp	Letters	Intrvw	Hours C/P/I	Comp	CPCE	Oral	Thesis	Port.

Community Counseling
TX Stephen F. Austin State University   Nacogdoches   *Contact:* Dr. Tom Caffery; tcaffery@sfasu.edu

Fin Aid	GPA	GRE	MAT	Wrk Exp	Letters	Intrvw	Hours C/P/I	Comp	CPCE	Oral	Thesis	Port.
Y					3	Y	48/150/600	Y		Y		

Community Counseling
TX Texas A & M University - Commerce   Commerce   *Contact:* Dr. Linda Ball; linda_ball@tamu-commerce.edu

Fin Aid	GPA	GRE	MAT	Wrk Exp	Letters	Intrvw	Hours C/P/I	Comp	CPCE	Oral	Thesis	Port.
Y					3		48/100/600	Y				

Community Counseling
TX Texas Southern University   Houston   *Contact:* Dr. Joyce K. Jones; Jones_JK@tsu.edu

Fin Aid	GPA	GRE	MAT	Wrk Exp	Letters	Intrvw	Hours C/P/I	Comp	CPCE	Oral	Thesis	Port.
	2.50	700			3		48/50/600	Y				

Community Counseling
TX Texas Tech University   Lubbock   *Contact:* Bret Hendricks and Aretha Marbley; Bret.Hendricks@ttu.edu

Fin Aid	GPA	GRE	MAT	Wrk Exp	Letters	Intrvw	Hours C/P/I	Comp	CPCE	Oral	Thesis	Port.
Y	3.0+	AVG	NR	0	3		48/100/600	Y	Y			Y

Community Counseling
TX University of North Texas   Denton   *Contact:* Bob Berg

Fin Aid	GPA	GRE	MAT	Wrk Exp	Letters	Intrvw	Hours C/P/I	Comp	CPCE	Oral	Thesis	Port.
Y	3.00	710			3	Y	48/100/600					

Community Counseling
TX University of Texas at El Paso   El Paso   *Contact:* Dr. Don C. Combs; dcombs@utep.edu

Fin Aid	GPA	GRE	MAT	Wrk Exp	Letters	Intrvw	Hours C/P/I	Comp	CPCE	Oral	Thesis	Port.
Y	3.00	NR		0	3	Y	48/100/600	Y				

Community Counseling
TX University of Texas of the Permian Basin   Odessa   *Contact:* Cathleen Barrett-Kruse, EdD, NCC; barrettkruse@utpb.edu

Fin Aid	GPA	GRE	MAT	Wrk Exp	Letters	Intrvw	Hours C/P/I	Comp	CPCE	Oral	Thesis	Port.
Y	2.50	1200		0	0		48/300/					

Community Counseling
VA College of William and Mary   Williamsburg   *Contact:* Charles McAdams; crmcad@wm.edu

Fin Aid	GPA	GRE	MAT	Wrk Exp	Letters	Intrvw	Hours C/P/I	Comp	CPCE	Oral	Thesis	Port.
Y	2.50	40%		0	3		51/100/600					

Community Counseling
VA George Mason University   Fairfax   *Contact:* Dr. Regine Talleyrand; rtalleyr@gmu.edu

Fin Aid	GPA	GRE	MAT	Wrk Exp	Letters	Intrvw	Hours C/P/I	Comp	CPCE	Oral	Thesis	Port.
Y	3.00			0	3	Y	52/200/200					

Community Counseling
VA James Madison University   Harrisonburg   *Contact:* Sue Rippy

Fin Aid	GPA	GRE	MAT	Wrk Exp	Letters	Intrvw	Hours C/P/I	Comp	CPCE	Oral	Thesis	Port.
							60/100/900					

Community Counseling
VA Old Dominion University   Norfolk   *Contact:* Dr. Edward Neukrug; eneukrug@odu.edu

Fin Aid	GPA	GRE	MAT	Wrk Exp	Letters	Intrvw	Hours C/P/I	Comp	CPCE	Oral	Thesis	Port.
Y	3.00	R			3		48/100/600	Y	Y			

Community Counseling
VA Radford University   Radford   *Contact:* Alan Forrest

Fin Aid	GPA	GRE	MAT	Wrk Exp	Letters	Intrvw	Hours C/P/I	Comp	CPCE	Oral	Thesis	Port.
	2.75	900	45		2		48/100/600	Y				

Community Counseling
VA Regent University   Virginia Beach   *Contact:* Dr. Lee Underwood; leeunde@regent.edu

Fin Aid	GPA	GRE	MAT	Wrk Exp	Letters	Intrvw	Hours C/P/I	Comp	CPCE	Oral	Thesis	Port.
Y	2.75	1000	50%	0	3	Y	51/60/100/ 600		Y			

Community Counseling
VA Virginia Tech   Blacksburg

Fin Aid	GPA	GRE	MAT	Wrk Exp	Letters	Intrvw	Hours C/P/I	Comp	CPCE	Oral	Thesis	Port.
Y	3.00				3	Y	51/100/600	Y				

		Master's Degree Programs										
	Admission Requirements						Graduation Requirements					
Fin Aid	GPA	GRE	MAT	Wrk Exp	Letters	Intrvw	Hours C/P/I	Examinations				
								Comp	CPCE	Oral	Thesis	Port.

Community Counseling
IL University of Wisconsin-Oshkosh   Oshkosh   *Contact:* David Hargis; hargis@uwosh.edu

Fin Aid	GPA	GRE	MAT	Wrk Exp	Letters	Intrvw	Hours C/P/I	Comp	CPCE	Oral	Thesis	Port.
Y	3.00			2	2	Y	48/100/600					Y

Community Counseling
WI University of Wisconsin-Whitewater   Whitewater

Fin Aid	GPA	GRE	MAT	Wrk Exp	Letters	Intrvw	Hours C/P/I	Comp	CPCE	Oral	Thesis	Port.
	2.75			2		Y	48/100/640					

Community Counseling
WV West Virginia University   Morgantown   *Contact:* Ed Jacobs; ed.jacobs@mail.wvu.edu

Fin Aid	GPA	GRE	MAT	Wrk Exp	Letters	Intrvw	Hours C/P/I	Comp	CPCE	Oral	Thesis	Port.
Y	2.80	900		0	3	Y	51/100/600					

Community Counseling
WY University of Wyoming   Laramie   *Contact:* Michael D. Loos and Michael Morgan; mdloos@uwyo.edu

Fin Aid	GPA	GRE	MAT	Wrk Exp	Letters	Intrvw	Hours C/P/I	Comp	CPCE	Oral	Thesis	Port.
Y	3.00			2	3	Y	48/100/600	Y				

Gerontological Counseling
IL College of Arts and Sciences (CAS)   Wheaton   *Contact:* Jim Ellor

Fin Aid	GPA	GRE	MAT	Wrk Exp	Letters	Intrvw	Hours C/P/I	Comp	CPCE	Oral	Thesis	Port.
Y	3.00				3	Y	48//600		Y			Y

Gerontological Counseling
MS William Carey College   Hattiesburg   *Contact:* Dr. Paul Cotten

Fin Aid	GPA	GRE	MAT	Wrk Exp	Letters	Intrvw	Hours C/P/I	Comp	CPCE	Oral	Thesis	Port.
Y	*	630+			2		54/100/100					Y

Gerontological Counseling
NC The University of North Carolina at Greensboro   Greensboro

Fin Aid	GPA	GRE	MAT	Wrk Exp	Letters	Intrvw	Hours C/P/I	Comp	CPCE	Oral	Thesis	Port.
Y	3.00	R			3		48//600					

Marriage and Family Counseling
AL University of Montevallo   Montevallo   *Contact:* Stephanie G. Puleo; puleos@montevallo.edu

Fin Aid	GPA	GRE	MAT	Wrk Exp	Letters	Intrvw	Hours C/P/I	Comp	CPCE	Oral	Thesis	Port.
Y	2.50	850	35			Y	60/100/900		Y			Y

Marriage and Family Counseling
AZ University of Phoenix   Phoenix   *Contact:* Paul Hagenburger, M.A.; hagenburger@cox.net

Fin Aid	GPA	GRE	MAT	Wrk Exp	Letters	Intrvw	Hours C/P/I	Comp	CPCE	Oral	Thesis	Port.
	2.50			2	3	Y	54/300/					Y

Marriage and Family Counseling
CA California State University-Fresno   Fresno   *Contact:* Sari H. Dworkin; sarid@csufresno.edu

Fin Aid	GPA	GRE	MAT	Wrk Exp	Letters	Intrvw	Hours C/P/I	Comp	CPCE	Oral	Thesis	Port.
Y	2.75				3	Y	60/80/600	·				

Marriage and Family Counseling
CO University of Colorado at Denver   Denver   *Contact:* Marsha Wiggins Frame;mframe@ceo.cudenver.edu

Fin Aid	GPA	GRE	MAT	Wrk Exp	Letters	Intrvw	Hours C/P/I	Comp	CPCE	Oral	Thesis	Port.
Y	2.75	900	40	0	4	Y	63/150/600					

Marriage and Family Counseling
CO University of Northern Colorado   Greeley   *Contact:* William Walsh; william.walsh@unco.edu

Fin Aid	GPA	GRE	MAT	Wrk Exp	Letters	Intrvw	Hours C/P/I	Comp	CPCE	Oral	Thesis	Port.
Y	3.00				3	Y	66/468/600					

Marriage and Family Counseling
FL Carlos Albizu University   Miami   *Contact:* Diana Barroso, M.S., LMHC

Fin Aid	GPA	GRE	MAT	Wrk Exp	Letters	Intrvw	Hours C/P/I	Comp	CPCE	Oral	Thesis	Port.
Y	3.00				3	Y	52/300/	Y				

Marriage and Family Counseling
FL University of Florida   Gainesville   *Contact:* M. Harry Daniels

Fin Aid	GPA	GRE	MAT	Wrk Exp	Letters	Intrvw	Hours C/P/I	Comp	CPCE	Oral	Thesis	Port.
	3.00	1000			3	Y	3/400/600			Y		

Marriage and Family Counseling
ID Idaho State University   Pocatello   *Contact:* Dr David Kleist; Kleidavi@isu.edu

Fin Aid	GPA	GRE	MAT	Wrk Exp	Letters	Intrvw	Hours C/P/I	Comp	CPCE	Oral	Thesis	Port.
Y	3.00		42		3	Y	64/150/850			Y		

Master's Degree Programs

	Admission Requirements						Graduation Requirements					
Fin Aid	GPA	GRE	MAT	Wrk Exp	Letters	Intrvw	Hours C/P/I	Comp	CPCE	Oral	Thesis	Port.

Marriage and Family Counseling
IL Southern Illinois University Carbondale   Carbondale   *Contact:* Dr. Jane Cox; janecox@siu.edu

Fin Aid	GPA	GRE	MAT	Wrk Exp	Letters	Intrvw	Hours C/P/I	Comp	CPCE	Oral	Thesis	Port.
Y	2.70			3			60/150/600					

Marriage and Family Counseling
IN Indiana State University   Terre Haute

Fin Aid	GPA	GRE	MAT	Wrk Exp	Letters	Intrvw	Hours C/P/I	Comp	CPCE	Oral	Thesis	Port.
Y	2.75	1455			3	Y	60/100/400					

Marriage and Family Counseling
IN Indiana Wesleyan University   Marion

Fin Aid	GPA	GRE	MAT	Wrk Exp	Letters	Intrvw	Hours C/P/I	Comp	CPCE	Oral	Thesis	Port.
Y	3.00	1000			3		60/100/900					Y

Marriage and Family Counseling
IN Indiana-Purdue University at Fort Wayne   Fort Wayne   *Contact:* Jim Burg

Fin Aid	GPA	GRE	MAT	Wrk Exp	Letters	Intrvw	Hours C/P/I	Comp	CPCE	Oral	Thesis	Port.
Y	3.20				3	Y	57/132/400					Y

Marriage and Family Counseling
KS Pittsburg State University   Pittsburg   *Contact:* Robert Sheverbush; rsheverb@pittstate.edu

Fin Aid	GPA	GRE	MAT	Wrk Exp	Letters	Intrvw	Hours C/P/I	Comp	CPCE	Oral	Thesis	Port.
Y	3.00	1200			3		32/450/150					

Marriage and Family Counseling
KY Western Kentucky University   Bowling Green

Fin Aid	GPA	GRE	MAT	Wrk Exp	Letters	Intrvw	Hours C/P/I	Comp	CPCE	Oral	Thesis	Port.
							60/100/600					

Marriage and Family Counseling
LA Our Lady of Holy Cross   New Orleans   *Contact:* Dr. Judith Miranti

Fin Aid	GPA	GRE	MAT	Wrk Exp	Letters	Intrvw	Hours C/P/I	Comp	CPCE	Oral	Thesis	Port.
							60/100/600					

Marriage and Family Counseling
LA Southeastern Louisiana University   Hammond   *Contact:* Peter Emerson; pemerson@selu.edu

Fin Aid	GPA	GRE	MAT	Wrk Exp	Letters	Intrvw	Hours C/P/I	Comp	CPCE	Oral	Thesis	Port.
Y						Y	63/100/600	Y	Y			

Marriage and Family Counseling
MA Fitchburg State College   Fitchburg   *Contact:* Michael Bloomfield

Fin Aid	GPA	GRE	MAT	Wrk Exp	Letters	Intrvw	Hours C/P/I	Comp	CPCE	Oral	Thesis	Port.
	2.80	1475	47		3		60/100/600					

Marriage and Family Counseling
MN Capella University   Minneapolis   *Contact:* Pamela Patrick

Fin Aid	GPA	GRE	MAT	Wrk Exp	Letters	Intrvw	Hours C/P/I	Comp	CPCE	Oral	Thesis	Port.
Y	2.70			0	2	Y	/100/900					Y

Marriage and Family Counseling
MS Mississippi College   Clinton   *Contact:* Bill Wheeler

Fin Aid	GPA	GRE	MAT	Wrk Exp	Letters	Intrvw	Hours C/P/I	Comp	CPCE	Oral	Thesis	Port.
Y	3.00	900		1	3	Y	60/100/600			Y		

Marriage and Family Counseling
MT Montana State University - Bozeman   Bozeman   *Contact:* Jill Thorngren; jillt@montana.edu

Fin Aid	GPA	GRE	MAT	Wrk Exp	Letters	Intrvw	Hours C/P/I	Comp	CPCE	Oral	Thesis	Port.
Y	3.00	900		1	3	Y	60/400/400	Y				

Marriage and Family Counseling
NC Appalachian State University   Boone   *Contact:* Jon Winek

Fin Aid	GPA	GRE	MAT	Wrk Exp	Letters	Intrvw	Hours C/P/I	Comp	CPCE	Oral	Thesis	Port.
Y	R	R			3	Y	48//500					

Marriage and Family Counseling
NM University of Phoenix - Albuquerque, NM Campus   Albuquerque   *Contact:* Darren Adamson, Ph.D.; darren.adamson@phoenix.edu

Fin Aid	GPA	GRE	MAT	Wrk Exp	Letters	Intrvw	Hours C/P/I	Comp	CPCE	Oral	Thesis	Port.
Y	2.50			3	3	Y	60//900					Y

Marriage and Family Counseling
OR George Fox University   Portland   *Contact:* Karin Jordan, Director

Fin Aid	GPA	GRE	MAT	Wrk Exp	Letters	Intrvw	Hours C/P/I	Comp	CPCE	Oral	Thesis	Port.
	2.70				3	Y	79//700					

Master's Degree Programs											
	Admission Requirements						Graduation Requirements				
Fin				Wrk			Hours	Examinations			
Aid	GPA	GRE	MAT	Exp	Letters	Intrvw	C/P/I	Comp	CPCE	Oral	Thesis	Port.

Marriage and Family Counseling
OR Portland State University   Portland   *Contact:* Halverson, Capuzzi

Y	points as-signed	R	same	0	same	Y	/100/600	Y			

Marriage and Family Counseling
PA Duquesne University   Pittsburgh   *Contact:* Paul M. Bernstein; BernsteinP@duq.edu

Y	3.00		40		2		60/125/600			Y		Y

Marriage and Family Counseling
PA Geneva College   Beaver Falls   *Contact:* Dr. Ronald Moslener; rwmoslener@geneva.edu

Y	3.00	1000			3		60/100/600	Y			

Marriage and Family Counseling
PA Kutztown University   Kutztown   *Contact:* Thomas Seay; seay@kutztown.edu

	3.00	1200			3	Y	60/100/700				

Marriage and Family Counseling
PR University of Phoenix, Puerto Rico Campus   Guaynabo   *Contact:* Ana M. Rodriguez, Ed.D.

	2.50			2	3	Y	60/100/900					Y

Marriage and Family Counseling
TN East Tennessee State University   Johnson City   *Contact:* Brent Morrow; MorrowB@etsu.edu

Y		R			3	Y	48//				

Marriage and Family Counseling
TN Travecca Nazarene University   Nashville   *Contact:* Don Harvey

Y	2.70	800	30		2		51/300/				

Marriage and Family Counseling
TX Houston Baptist University   Houston

Y		400				Y	//				

Marriage and Family Counseling
TX Our Lady of the Lake University   San Antonio   *Contact:* Joan Biever

Y	2.50	R	R		2	Y	60/500/				

Marriage and Family Counseling
TX Southwest Texas State University   San Marcos   *Contact:* Mike Carns; mc17@swt.edu

Y							//				

Marriage and Family Counseling
TX Tarleton State University   Stephenville   *Contact:* Bill LaBauve, Gary Mauldin; labauve@tarleton.edu

	3.00	850					48/9/500				

Marriage and Family Counseling
TX University of Texas at Tyler   Tyler   *Contact:* Robert McClure, Ph.D.; rmcclure@uttyler.edu

Y	3.00	900			3		60/300/				Y

Marriage and Family Counseling
VA College of William and Mary   Williamsburg   *Contact:* Charles McAdams; crmcad@wm.edu

Y	2.50	40%		0	3		63/100/600				

Mental Health Counseling
FL Carlos Albizu University   Miami   *Contact:* Diana Barroso, M.S., LMHC

Y	3.00				3	Y	61/1000/	Y			

Master's Degree Programs

| | Admission Requirements | | | | | | Graduation Requirements | | | | | |
Fin Aid	GPA	GRE	MAT	Wrk Exp	Letters	Intrvw	Hours C/P/I	Comp	CPCE	Oral	Thesis	Port.

Mental Health Counseling
FL Florida Atlantic University   Boca Raton   *Contact:* Dr. Alex Miranda; amiranda@fau.edu

Fin Aid	GPA	GRE	MAT	Wrk Exp	Letters	Intrvw	Hours C/P/I	Comp	CPCE	Oral	Thesis	Port.
Y	~3.00	~1000				Y	48/400/600					

Mental Health Counseling
FL Rollins College   Winter Park   *Contact:* Kathryn L. Norsworthy, Ph.D; Knorswor@rollins.edu

Fin Aid	GPA	GRE	MAT	Wrk Exp	Letters	Intrvw	Hours C/P/I	Comp	CPCE	Oral	Thesis	Port.
Y	3.00	1000	50	2	3		60/250/750					

Mental Health Counseling
FL University of Central Florida   Orlando   *Contact:* Mark Young; myoung@mail.ucf.edu

Fin Aid	GPA	GRE	MAT	Wrk Exp	Letters	Intrvw	Hours C/P/I	Comp	CPCE	Oral	Thesis	Port.
		1000			3	Y	63/200/1000		Y			Y

Mental Health Counseling
FL University of Florida   Gainesville   *Contact:* M. Harry Daniels

Fin Aid	GPA	GRE	MAT	Wrk Exp	Letters	Intrvw	Hours C/P/I	Comp	CPCE	Oral	Thesis	Port.
	3.00	1000			3	Y	3/400/600			Y		

Mental Health Counseling
FL University of North Florida   Jacksonville   *Contact:* Lynne Carroll; lcarroll@unf.edu

Fin Aid	GPA	GRE	MAT	Wrk Exp	Letters	Intrvw	Hours C/P/I	Comp	CPCE	Oral	Thesis	Port.
	3.00	1000		1	3	Y	60/100/900					

Mental Health Counseling
IA University of North Iowa   Cedar Falls   *Contact:* Dr. Ann Vernon; Ann.Vernon@uni.edu

Fin Aid	GPA	GRE	MAT	Wrk Exp	Letters	Intrvw	Hours C/P/I	Comp	CPCE	Oral	Thesis	Port.
Y	3.00	NR		0	3		62/100/900	Y			Y	

Mental Health Counseling
ID Idaho State University   Pocatello   *Contact:* Dr Nicole Hill; Hillnico@isu.edu

Fin Aid	GPA	GRE	MAT	Wrk Exp	Letters	Intrvw	Hours C/P/I	Comp	CPCE	Oral	Thesis	Port.
Y	3.00		42		3	Y	60/150/850	Y		Y		

Mental Health Counseling
IL Lewis University   Romeoville   *Contact:* Ann Barich; barichan@lewisu.edu

Fin Aid	GPA	GRE	MAT	Wrk Exp	Letters	Intrvw	Hours C/P/I	Comp	CPCE	Oral	Thesis	Port.
Y	3.00				2		48/100/600	Y				Y

Mental Health Counseling
IN Ball State University   Muncie   *Contact:* Phyllis Gordon; pgordon@bsu.edu

Fin Aid	GPA	GRE	MAT	Wrk Exp	Letters	Intrvw	Hours C/P/I	Comp	CPCE	Oral	Thesis	Port.
Y	2.75				3		60/200/900	Y				

Mental Health Counseling
IN Indiana State University   Terre Haute

Fin Aid	GPA	GRE	MAT	Wrk Exp	Letters	Intrvw	Hours C/P/I	Comp	CPCE	Oral	Thesis	Port.
Y	3.25	1455			3	Y	60/100/900	Y	Y	Y		

Mental Health Counseling
IN Purdue University   West Lafayette   *Contact:* M. Carole Pistole

Fin Aid	GPA	GRE	MAT	Wrk Exp	Letters	Intrvw	Hours C/P/I	Comp	CPCE	Oral	Thesis	Port.
	3.00	1000			3		60/100/900					

Mental Health Counseling
KS Emporia State University   Emporia   *Contact:* Dr. Wendy Enochs; enochswe@emporia.edu

Fin Aid	GPA	GRE	MAT	Wrk Exp	Letters	Intrvw	Hours C/P/I	Comp	CPCE	Oral	Thesis	Port.
Y	3.00	850	40	0	3	Y	60/100/900	Y				

Mental Health Counseling
KY Eastern Kentucky University   Richmond   *Contact:* Patricia Stevens; patricia.stevens@eku.edu

Fin Aid	GPA	GRE	MAT	Wrk Exp	Letters	Intrvw	Hours C/P/I	Comp	CPCE	Oral	Thesis	Port.
Y	3.00		30		3		60/100/900	Y	Y			

Mental Health Counseling
KY Western Kentucky University   Bowling Green   *Contact:* Fred Stickle

Fin Aid	GPA	GRE	MAT	Wrk Exp	Letters	Intrvw	Hours C/P/I	Comp	CPCE	Oral	Thesis	Port.
		1350			2		60/100/600					

Mental Health Counseling
LA McNeese State University   Lake Charles   *Contact:* M. Janelle Disney; mdisney@mail.mcneese.edu

Fin Aid	GPA	GRE	MAT	Wrk Exp	Letters	Intrvw	Hours C/P/I	Comp	CPCE	Oral	Thesis	Port.
Y	~3.00	~950				Y	60/100/900	Y				

Master's Degree Programs

Fin Aid	GPA	GRE	MAT	Wrk Exp	Letters	Intrvw	Hours C/P/I	Comp	CPCE	Oral	Thesis	Port.

Mental Health Counseling
MA Bridgewater State College   Bridgewater   *Contact:* Dr. Victoria L. Bacon; vbacon@bridgew.edu

| | 2.80 | 1000 | | 0 | 3 | Y | 60/100/900 | Y | | | | |

Mental Health Counseling
MA Fitchburg State College   Fitchburg   *Contact:* Richard J. Spencer

| | 2.80 | 1475 | 47 | | 3 | | 60/100/600 | | | | | |

Mental Health Counseling
MA Lesley University   Cambridge   *Contact:* Yishiuan Chin (617) 349-8339; (800) 999-1959 ext. 8339

| Y | 3.00 | | 40 | | 3 | Y | 60/100/600/ 1200 | | | | | |

Mental Health Counseling
MA Suffolk University   Boston   *Contact:* Dr. Glen Eskedal; gesekedal@suffolk.edu

| Y | 2.75 | R | R | | 3 | | 36/450/ | | | | | |

Mental Health Counseling
MD Frostburg State University   Frostburg   *Contact:* Ann R. Bristow; abristow@frostburg.edu

| Y | 3.00 | 1000 | 50 | 1 | 3 | Y | 49//450 | | | | | |

Mental Health Counseling
ME University of Southern Maine   Gorham   *Contact:* Reid D. Stevens, Ph.D.; stevens@usm.maine.edu

| Y | R | R | R | 0 | 3 | Y | 60/100/900 | Y | Y | | | |

Mental Health Counseling
MN Capella Uiversity   Minneapolis   *Contact:* Pamela Patrick

| Y | 2.70 | | | 0 | 2 | Y | /100/900 | | | | | Y |

Mental Health Counseling
MO Northwest Missouri State University   Maryville   *Contact:* Carla Ewdards

| Y | 3.00 | ~1500 | | 0 | Y | | 51/500/ | Y | | | Y | |

Mental Health Counseling
MS Mississippi College   Clinton   *Contact:* Katherine Jones

| Y | 3.00 | 900 | | 0 | 3 | Y | 60/100/900 | | | Y | | |

Mental Health Counseling
MT Montana State University - Bozeman   Bozeman   *Contact:* Patrick (Rick) Johnson; rjohnson@montana.edu

| Y | 3.00 | 900 | | 1 | 3 | Y | 60/400/400 | Y | | | | |

Mental Health Counseling
NC East Carolina University   Greenville   *Contact:* Lloyd Goodwin

| Y | ~3.00 | | ~35 | 0 | 0 | Y | 48/100/600 | | | Y | Y | |

Mental Health Counseling
NH Plymouth State College   Plymouth   *Contact:* Dr. Gail Mears; gmears@mail.plymouth.edu

| | 3.00 | | | | 3 | Y | 60/100/900 | | | | | |

Mental Health Counseling
NM University of Phoenix - Albuquerque, NM Campus   Albuquerque   *Contact:* Darren Adamson, Ph.D.; darren.adamson@phoenix.edu

| Y | 2.50 | | | 3 | 3 | Y | // | | | | | |

Mental Health Counseling
NY Niagara University   Niagara University   *Contact:* Dr.Shannon Hodges; sjp@niagara.edu

| Y | 2.75 | 880 | 40 | | 2 | Y | 60/100/900 | Y | | | | Y |

| | | Admission Requirements | | | | | Graduation Requirements | | | | | |
Fin Aid	GPA	GRE	MAT	Wrk Exp	Letters	Intrvw	Hours C/P/I	Comp	CPCE	Oral	Thesis	Port.

Master's Degree Programs

Mental Health Counseling
NY Queens College, City University of New York   Flushing   *Contact:* Dr. Lynn Howell

Fin Aid	GPA	GRE	MAT	Wrk Exp	Letters	Intrvw	Hours C/P/I	Comp	CPCE	Oral	Thesis	Port.
	3.00				3	Y	60/100/600	Y			Y	

Mental Health Counseling
OH University of Cincinnati   Cincinnati   *Contact:* F. Robert Wilson, Ph.D.

Fin Aid	GPA	GRE	MAT	Wrk Exp	Letters	Intrvw	Hours C/P/I	Comp	CPCE	Oral	Thesis	Port.
Y	2.80	1500			3	Y	/100/900	Y	Y			

Mental Health Counseling
OH Walsh University   North Canton   *Contact:* Linda L. Barclay Ph.D.; lbarclay@walsh.edu

Fin Aid	GPA	GRE	MAT	Wrk Exp	Letters	Intrvw	Hours C/P/I	Comp	CPCE	Oral	Thesis	Port.
	3.00	900	40		3	Y	60/100/600	Y	Y			

Mental Health Counseling
OR George Fox University   Portland   *Contact:* Karin Jordan, Director

Fin Aid	GPA	GRE	MAT	Wrk Exp	Letters	Intrvw	Hours C/P/I	Comp	CPCE	Oral	Thesis	Port.
	2.70				3	Y	64//600					

Mental Health Counseling
PA Geneva College   Beaver Falls   *Contact:* Dr. Joseph Peters; jepeters@geneva.edu

Fin Aid	GPA	GRE	MAT	Wrk Exp	Letters	Intrvw	Hours C/P/I	Comp	CPCE	Oral	Thesis	Port.
Y	3.00	1000			3		60/100/900	Y				

Mental Health Counseling
PA Shippensburg University of PA   Shippensburg   *Contact:* Thomas Hozman; tlhozm@ship.edu

Fin Aid	GPA	GRE	MAT	Wrk Exp	Letters	Intrvw	Hours C/P/I	Comp	CPCE	Oral	Thesis	Port.
Y	2.75	800		1	3	Y	60/150/900					Y

Mental Health Counseling
PR University of Phoenix, Puerto Rico Campus   Guaynabo   *Contact:* Ana M. Rodriguez, Ed.D.

Fin Aid	GPA	GRE	MAT	Wrk Exp	Letters	Intrvw	Hours C/P/I	Comp	CPCE	Oral	Thesis	Port.
	2.50			2	3	Y	60/100/900	Y				Y

Mental Health Counseling
RI Rhode Island College   Providence   *Contact:* M. Finely

Fin Aid	GPA	GRE	MAT	Wrk Exp	Letters	Intrvw	Hours C/P/I	Comp	CPCE	Oral	Thesis	Port.
	3.00	900	45	2	3		36/90/	Y				

Mental Health Counseling
TN Lee University   Cleveland   *Contact:* Doyle Goff, Ph.D.; drgoff@leeuniversity.edu

Fin Aid	GPA	GRE	MAT	Wrk Exp	Letters	Intrvw	Hours C/P/I	Comp	CPCE	Oral	Thesis	Port.
Y	3.00	~1000 V+Q		0	3	Y	60/150/500	Y	Y	Y		

Mental Health Counseling
TN The University of Tennessee at Knoxville   Knoxville   *Contact:* Dr. Charles Thompson; cthomps5@utk.edu

Fin Aid	GPA	GRE	MAT	Wrk Exp	Letters	Intrvw	Hours C/P/I	Comp	CPCE	Oral	Thesis	Port.
	3.00	1000			3		60/100/900	Y				

Mental Health Counseling
TN Trevecca Nazarene University   Nashville   *Contact:* Peter Wilson; pwilson@trevecca.edu

Fin Aid	GPA	GRE	MAT	Wrk Exp	Letters	Intrvw	Hours C/P/I	Comp	CPCE	Oral	Thesis	Port.
Y	2.70	800	30		2		48/300/200	Y				

Mental Health Counseling
TX Dallas Baptist University   Dallas   *Contact:* Mary Becerril

Fin Aid	GPA	GRE	MAT	Wrk Exp	Letters	Intrvw	Hours C/P/I	Comp	CPCE	Oral	Thesis	Port.
Y	3.00	850		0	3		48/300/					

Mental Health Counseling
TX Houston Baptist University   Houston

Fin Aid	GPA	GRE	MAT	Wrk Exp	Letters	Intrvw	Hours C/P/I	Comp	CPCE	Oral	Thesis	Port.
Y		850			3		48/450/					

Mental Health Counseling
TX Our Lady of the Lake University   San Antonio   *Contact:* Joan Biever

Fin Aid	GPA	GRE	MAT	Wrk Exp	Letters	Intrvw	Hours C/P/I	Comp	CPCE	Oral	Thesis	Port.
Y	2.50	R	R		2	Y	60/500/	Y				

Mental Health Counseling
TX Tarleton State University   Stephenville   *Contact:* All faculty

Fin Aid	GPA	GRE	MAT	Wrk Exp	Letters	Intrvw	Hours C/P/I	Comp	CPCE	Oral	Thesis	Port.
	3.00	850					48/6/300	Y				

Master's Degree Programs												
	Admission Requirements							Graduation Requirements				
Fin Aid	GPA	GRE	MAT	Wrk Exp	Letters	Intrvw	Hours C/P/I	Comp	CPCE	Oral	Thesis	Port.

Mental Health Counseling
UT University of Phoenix Salt Lake City *Contact:* Don Beck , Ph.D.; don.beck@phoenix.edu

Fin Aid	GPA	GRE	MAT	Wrk Exp	Letters	Intrvw	Hours C/P/I	Comp	CPCE	Oral	Thesis	Port.
Y	2.50			3	3		60/100/900		Y	Y		Y

Mental Health Counseling
WA Central Washington University Ellensburg

Fin Aid	GPA	GRE	MAT	Wrk Exp	Letters	Intrvw	Hours C/P/I	Comp	CPCE	Oral	Thesis	Port.
							90/325/600					

Mental Health Counseling
WA City University Bellevue *Contact:* Elizabeth Fountain, MA; efountain@cityu.edu

Fin Aid	GPA	GRE	MAT	Wrk Exp	Letters	Intrvw	Hours C/P/I	Comp	CPCE	Oral	Thesis	Port.
Y	2.75				3	Y	//250	Y		Y	Y	

Mental Health Counseling
WA Eastern Washington University Cheney *Contact:* Dr. Ken Engbresson

Fin Aid	GPA	GRE	MAT	Wrk Exp	Letters	Intrvw	Hours C/P/I	Comp	CPCE	Oral	Thesis	Port.
							//					

Mental Health Counseling
WA Seattle University Seattle *Contact:* Hutch Haney

Fin Aid	GPA	GRE	MAT	Wrk Exp	Letters	Intrvw	Hours C/P/I	Comp	CPCE	Oral	Thesis	Port.
	3.00			500hr	2	Y	/80/520	Y				

Mental Health Counseling
WA University of Puget Sound Tacoma *Contact:* Grace Kirchner; kirchner@ups.edu

Fin Aid	GPA	GRE	MAT	Wrk Exp	Letters	Intrvw	Hours C/P/I	Comp	CPCE	Oral	Thesis	Port.
	3.00	1500			2	Y	48/32/400	Y		Y		

Mental Health Counseling
WA Western Washington University Bellingham *Contact:* Davis Hayden; hayden@cc.wwu.edu

Fin Aid	GPA	GRE	MAT	Wrk Exp	Letters	Intrvw	Hours C/P/I	Comp	CPCE	Oral	Thesis	Port.
Y	3.00	R		0	3	Y	/100/900	Y				

Other
AL University of South Alabama Mobile *Contact:* Dr. Joe Law for psychometry

Fin Aid	GPA	GRE	MAT	Wrk Exp	Letters	Intrvw	Hours C/P/I	Comp	CPCE	Oral	Thesis	Port.
Y	3.00						39//300	Y				

Other
AZ Arizona State University Tempe

Fin Aid	GPA	GRE	MAT	Wrk Exp	Letters	Intrvw	Hours C/P/I	Comp	CPCE	Oral	Thesis	Port.
Y							//					

Other
CA University of San Diego, School of Education San Diego *Contact:* Ken Gonzalez - College

Fin Aid	GPA	GRE	MAT	Wrk Exp	Letters	Intrvw	Hours C/P/I	Comp	CPCE	Oral	Thesis	Port.
Y	2.75			1	3	Y	48/100/600	Y				

Other
CO Denver Seminary Denver

Fin Aid	GPA	GRE	MAT	Wrk Exp	Letters	Intrvw	Hours C/P/I	Comp	CPCE	Oral	Thesis	Port.
Y	2.50				3		62//400	Y				

Other – Leadership in Counseling
CO University of Colorado - Colorado Springs Colorado Springs *Contact:* David Ferrel

Fin Aid	GPA	GRE	MAT	Wrk Exp	Letters	Intrvw	Hours C/P/I	Comp	CPCE	Oral	Thesis	Port.
Y	2.75					Y	40//					

Other
IL College of Arts and Sciences (CAS) Wheaton *Contact:* Pat McGrath/Community Wellness
Janice Guerriero/Career Counseling; jguerriero@nl.edu

Fin Aid	GPA	GRE	MAT	Wrk Exp	Letters	Intrvw	Hours C/P/I	Comp	CPCE	Oral	Thesis	Port.
Y	3.00				3	Y	48//600		Y			Y

Other
KS Emporia State University Emporia *Contact:* Dr. Wendy Enochs; enochswe@emporia.edu

Fin Aid	GPA	GRE	MAT	Wrk Exp	Letters	Intrvw	Hours C/P/I	Comp	CPCE	Oral	Thesis	Port.
Y	3.00	850	40	0	3	Y	48/100/600	Y				

Master's Degree Programs

| | Admission Requirements | | | | | | | Graduation Requirements | | | | |
Fin Aid	GPA	GRE	MAT	Wrk Exp	Letters	Intrvw	Hours C/P/I	Comp	CPCE	Oral	Thesis	Port.

Other
KS University of Kansas   Lawrence

							/50/					

Other
MA Lesley University   Cambridge   *Contact:* Yishiuan Chin (617) 349-8339; (800) 999-1959 ext. 8339

Y	3.00		40		3	Y	48/60/100/ 600/1200					

Other
MA Suffolk University   Boston

Y	2.75	R	R		3		30/450/					

Other – Organizational Counseling
MD Johns Hopkins University   Baltimore   *Contact:* Organizationa Counseling -Mary Guindon; mguindon@jhu.edu

Y	3.00				3	Y	48//600			Y		

Other – Counseling Studies
MN Capella University   Minneapolis

Y	2.70					Y	//					

Other
MN Minnesota State University Moorhead   Moorhead   *Contact:* Bill Packwood

Y	3.00	R	R	0	3	Y	48/100/650	Y	Y	Y	Y	

Other
MO University of Missouri-Columbia   Columbia   *Contact:* Richard Cox; CoxRH@missouri.edu

	3.00	1000			3		48//					

Other
NC East Carolina University   Greenville   *Contact:* Steve Thomas

Y	~3.00		~30	0	0	Y	45/100/600			Y	Y	

Other
NC East Carolina University   Greenville

	2.50	1350	40		3	Y	48/90/225 minimum					

Other – School Psychology
TN Middle Tennessee State University   Murfreesboro   *Contact:* James O. Rust

Y	3.00	900		0	3		45/100/600	Y			Y	

Other
TN Travecca Nazarene University   Nashville   *Contact:* Peter Wilson; pwilson@trevecca.edu

Y	2.70	800	30		2		54/300/	Y			Y	

Other – Student Affairs
TX Southwest Texas State University   San Marcos   *Contact:* Jim Studer - Student Affairs

Y							//					

Pastoral Counseling
CO Denver Seminary   Denver

Y	2.50				3		92//400			Y		

Pastoral Counseling
MD Loyola College in Maryland   Columbia   *Contact:* K. Elizabeth Oakes

Y	same			0	same	Y	same/same/ same				Y	Y

Master's Degree Programs

| | | Admission Requirements | | | | | | Graduation Requirements | | | | |
| | | | | Wrk | | | Hours | | Examinations | | | |
Fin Aid	GPA	GRE	MAT	Exp	Letters	Intrvw	C/P/I	Comp	CPCE	Oral	Thesis	Port.

Pastoral Counseling
MS William Carey College Hattiesburg *Contact:* Dr. Tommy King

Fin Aid	GPA	GRE	MAT	Wrk Exp	Letters	Intrvw	C/P/I	Comp	CPCE	Oral	Thesis	Port.
Y	*	630+			2		60/100/100					Y

Pastoral Counseling
TX Houston Baptist University Houston

Fin Aid	GPA	GRE	MAT	Wrk Exp	Letters	Intrvw	C/P/I	Comp	CPCE	Oral	Thesis	Port.
Y							//					

Pastoral Counseling
WA University of Puget Sound Tacoma *Contact:* Grace Kirchner; kirchner@ups.edu

Fin Aid	GPA	GRE	MAT	Wrk Exp	Letters	Intrvw	C/P/I	Comp	CPCE	Oral	Thesis	Port.
	3.00	1500			2	Y	48/100/500			Y		

Rehabilitation Counseling
AL The University of Alabama Tuscaloosa *Contact:* Jamie F. Satcher, Ph.D.; jsatcher@bamaed.ua.edu

Fin Aid	GPA	GRE	MAT	Wrk Exp	Letters	Intrvw	C/P/I	Comp	CPCE	Oral	Thesis	Port.
Y	3.00	1000 (V+Q)	50	0	3		48/100/600	Y				Y

Rehabilitation Counseling
AL Troy State University Troy *Contact:* Linda Williams; lindaw@troyst.edu

Fin Aid	GPA	GRE	MAT	Wrk Exp	Letters	Intrvw	C/P/I	Comp	CPCE	Oral	Thesis	Port.
	2.50	850	33		3	Y	48/100/600	Y				

Rehabilitation Counseling
AL University of South Alabama Mobile *Contact:* Dr. Joseph G. Law, Jr.; jlaw@usouthal.edu

Fin Aid	GPA	GRE	MAT	Wrk Exp	Letters	Intrvw	C/P/I	Comp	CPCE	Oral	Thesis	Port.
Y	3.00						54/100/600	Y				

Rehabilitation Counseling
AR University of Arkansas at Little Rock Little Rock *Contact:* Larry R. Dickerson, PhD; lrdickerson@ualr.edu

Fin Aid	GPA	GRE	MAT	Wrk Exp	Letters	Intrvw	C/P/I	Comp	CPCE	Oral	Thesis	Port.
Y	2.75			0	NA	Y	54/100/600					

Rehabilitation Counseling
CA California State University-Fresno Fresno *Contact:* Charles Arokiasamy; charles@csufresno.edu

Fin Aid	GPA	GRE	MAT	Wrk Exp	Letters	Intrvw	C/P/I	Comp	CPCE	Oral	Thesis	Port.
Y	2.75				3		60//					

Rehabilitation Counseling
CA San Diego State University San Diego *Contact:* Fred McFarlane; fmfarla@mail.sdsu.edu

Fin Aid	GPA	GRE	MAT	Wrk Exp	Letters	Intrvw	C/P/I	Comp	CPCE	Oral	Thesis	Port.
	2.75	950			3	Y	60/9/600					

Rehabilitation Counseling
DC The George Washington University Washington *Contact:* Jorge Garcia, Rh.D.; Garcia@gwu.edu

Fin Aid	GPA	GRE	MAT	Wrk Exp	Letters	Intrvw	C/P/I	Comp	CPCE	Oral	Thesis	Port.
Y	3.00	1000	50%		2	Y	48/100/600					

Rehabilitation Counseling
FL Florida Atlantic University Boca Raton *Contact:* Dr. Larry Kontosh

Fin Aid	GPA	GRE	MAT	Wrk Exp	Letters	Intrvw	C/P/I	Comp	CPCE	Oral	Thesis	Port.
Y	~3.00	~1000				Y	60/150/600					

Rehabilitation Counseling
IA The University of Iowa Iowa City *Contact:* Vilia Tarvydas; vilia-tarvydas@uiowa.edu

Fin Aid	GPA	GRE	MAT	Wrk Exp	Letters	Intrvw	C/P/I	Comp	CPCE	Oral	Thesis	Port.
Y	3.00	1000		1	3	Y	60/350/600	Y				

Rehabilitation Counseling
ID University of Idaho Moscow *Contact:* Dr. Jerry Fischer; jfischer@uidaho.edu

Fin Aid	GPA	GRE	MAT	Wrk Exp	Letters	Intrvw	C/P/I	Comp	CPCE	Oral	Thesis	Port.
	3.00				3	Y	60/150/850					

Rehabilitation Counseling
IL Illinois Institute of Technology Chicago *Contact:* Dr. Chow S. Lam; Lam@iit.edu

Fin Aid	GPA	GRE	MAT	Wrk Exp	Letters	Intrvw	C/P/I	Comp	CPCE	Oral	Thesis	Port.
Y	3.00				3	Y	60/200/600				Y	

Master's Degree Programs												
	Admission Requirements						Graduation Requirements					
Fin				Wrk			Hours	Examinations				
Aid	GPA	GRE	MAT	Exp	Letters	Intrvw	C/P/I	Comp	CPCE	Oral	Thesis	Port.

Rehabilitation Counseling
IN Ball State University   Muncie   *Contact:* Phyllis Gordon; pgordon@bsu.edu

Y	2.75			3			48/100/600	Y				

Rehabilitation Counseling
KS Emporia State University   Emporia   *Contact:* Dr. Marvin Kuehn; kuehnmar@emporia.edu

Y	3.00	850	40	0	3	Y	60/100/600	Y				

Rehabilitation Counseling
KY University of Kentucky   Lexington   *Contact:* Ralph M. Crystal; crystal@uky.edu

Y	2.75	1200		0	3	Y	55-60/300/600	Y		Y		

Rehabilitation Counseling
ME University of Southern Maine   Gorham   *Contact:* Stephen T. Murphy, Ph.D.; smurphy@usm.maine.edu

Y		R	R	0	3	Y	48/100/600	Y	Y			

Rehabilitation Counseling
MO University of Missouri-Columbia   Columbia   *Contact:* David Roberts

	3.00	1000			3		48//	Y				

Rehabilitation Counseling
MS Mississippi State University   Mississippi State University   *Contact:* Dr. Glen Hendren; glen@ra.msstate.edu

Y	2.75	1200			3		48/100/600	Y	Y			

Rehabilitation Counseling
MT Montana State University - Billings   Billings   *Contact:* Alan Davis; adavis@msubillings.edu

Y	3.00	1371			3	Y	60//600	Y				

Rehabilitation Counseling
NC East Carolina University   Greenville   *Contact:* Mark Stebnicki; stebnickim@mail.ecu.edu

Y	~3.00		~35	0	0	Y	48/100/600			Y	Y	

Rehabilitation Counseling
NY New York University   New York   *Contact:* David Peterson; david.peterson@nyu.edu

Y	2.50			2		Y	54/100/600	Y				

Rehabilitation Counseling
NY SUNY University at Buffalo   Buffalo   *Contact:* Dr. Tim Janikowski

				3		Y	48/300/300				Y	

Rehabilitation Counseling
NY Syracuse University   Syracuse   *Contact:* Dennis Gilbride; ddgilbri@syr.edu

Y	3.00	NA		1	3	Y	48/100/600	Y				

Rehabilitation Counseling
OH Ohio University   Athens   *Contact:* Jerry Olsheski; olsheski@ohio.edu

Y	3.00	900			3		//					

Rehabilitation Counseling
OR Portland State University   Portland   *Contact:* Livneh

Y	points assigned	R	same	0	same	Y	/100/600	Y				

Rehabilitation Counseling
PA Penn State University   University Park

							//					

	Master's Degree Programs											
Fin Aid	Admission Requirements						Graduation Requirements					
	GPA	GRE	MAT	Wrk Exp	Letters	Intrvw	Hours C/P/I	Examinations				
								Comp	CPCE	Oral	Thesis	Port.

Rehabilitation Counseling
TN The University of Tennessee at Knoxville   Knoxville

	GPA	GRE	MAT	Wrk Exp	Letters	Intrvw	Hours C/P/I	Comp	CPCE	Oral	Thesis	Port.
	2.70	1000			3	Y	54/150/600	Y				

Rehabilitation Counseling
TX Stephen F. Austin State University   Nacogdoches   *Contact:* Dr. Robert Choate; rchoate@sfasu.edu

	GPA	GRE	MAT	Wrk Exp	Letters	Intrvw	Hours C/P/I	Comp	CPCE	Oral	Thesis	Port.
Y					3	Y	48/150/600	Y		Y		

Rehabilitation Counseling
WV West Virginia University   Morgantown   *Contact:* Margaret Glenn; margaret.glenn@mail.wvu.edu

	GPA	GRE	MAT	Wrk Exp	Letters	Intrvw	Hours C/P/I	Comp	CPCE	Oral	Thesis	Port.
Y	2.80	NA		0	3	Y	51/100/600					

School Counseling
AL Auburn University   Auburn   *Contact:* Debra Cobia; cobiadc@mail.auburn.edu

	GPA	GRE	MAT	Wrk Exp	Letters	Intrvw	Hours C/P/I	Comp	CPCE	Oral	Thesis	Port.
Y	3.00	1000			3		48-51/100/600	Y	Y	Y		Y

School Counseling
AL The University of Alabama   Tuscaloosa   *Contact:* Karla D. Carmichael, Ph.D.; kcarmich@bamaed.ua.edu

	GPA	GRE	MAT	Wrk Exp	Letters	Intrvw	Hours C/P/I	Comp	CPCE	Oral	Thesis	Port.
Y	3.00	1000 (V+Q)	50	0	3		48/100/600	Y				Y

School Counseling
AL Troy State University   Troy   *Contact:* Dianne Gossett; dgossett@troyst.edu

	GPA	GRE	MAT	Wrk Exp	Letters	Intrvw	Hours C/P/I	Comp	CPCE	Oral	Thesis	Port.
	2.50	850	33		3		48/100/600	Y				

School Counseling
AL University of Montevallo   Montevallo   *Contact:* Charlotte Daughhetee; daughh@montevallo.edu

	GPA	GRE	MAT	Wrk Exp	Letters	Intrvw	Hours C/P/I	Comp	CPCE	Oral	Thesis	Port.
Y	2.50	850	35			Y	48/100/600	Y	Y			Y

School Counseling
AL University of North Alabama   Florence   *Contact:* J. Paul Baird; pbaird@unanov.una.edu

	GPA	GRE	MAT	Wrk Exp	Letters	Intrvw	Hours C/P/I	Comp	CPCE	Oral	Thesis	Port.
Y	3.00	900	40		3	Y	48/100/600	Y	Y			

School Counseling
AL University of South Alabama   Mobile   *Contact:* Dr. Jean Clark; jclark@usouthal.edu

	GPA	GRE	MAT	Wrk Exp	Letters	Intrvw	Hours C/P/I	Comp	CPCE	Oral	Thesis	Port.
Y	3.00						39/100/300	Y				

School Counseling
AZ Arizona State University   Tempe   *Contact:* Andrea DixonRayle; andrea_dixon.rayle@asu.edu

	GPA	GRE	MAT	Wrk Exp	Letters	Intrvw	Hours C/P/I	Comp	CPCE	Oral	Thesis	Port.
Y		R	R	0	3		60/100/600	Y	Y			

School Counseling
CA California Lutheran University   Thousand Oaks

	GPA	GRE	MAT	Wrk Exp	Letters	Intrvw	Hours C/P/I	Comp	CPCE	Oral	Thesis	Port.
	3.00	900			3	Y	48/100/600	Y				Y

School Counseling
CA California State University-Fresno   Fresno   *Contact:* Sarah Lam; renees@csufresno.edu

	GPA	GRE	MAT	Wrk Exp	Letters	Intrvw	Hours C/P/I	Comp	CPCE	Oral	Thesis	Port.
Y	2.75				3	Y	48/600/					

School Counseling
CA La Sierra University   Riverside   *Contact:* Lennard A. Jorgensen; ljorgens@lasierra.edu

	GPA	GRE	MAT	Wrk Exp	Letters	Intrvw	Hours C/P/I	Comp	CPCE	Oral	Thesis	Port.
Y	3.0	1000			3	Y	/450/	Y				Y

School Counseling
CA San Jose University   San Jose

	GPA	GRE	MAT	Wrk Exp	Letters	Intrvw	Hours C/P/I	Comp	CPCE	Oral	Thesis	Port.
							48//600	Y			Y	

Master's Degree Programs

Fin Aid	GPA	GRE	MAT	Wrk Exp	Letters	Intrvw	Hours C/P/I	Comp	CPCE	Oral	Thesis	Port.

Header spans: Admission Requirements (GPA, GRE, MAT, Wrk Exp, Letters, Intrvw) | Graduation Requirements (Hours C/P/I, Examinations: Comp, CPCE, Oral, Thesis, Port.)

School Counseling
CA University of San Diego, School of Education   San Diego   *Contact:* Lonnie Rowell

Fin Aid	GPA	GRE	MAT	Wrk Exp	Letters	Intrvw	Hours C/P/I	Comp	CPCE	Oral	Thesis	Port.
Y	2.75			1	3	Y	48/100/600	Y				

School Counseling
CO Adams State College   Alamosa   *Contact:* Dr. Susan Varhely; scvarhel@adams.edu

Fin Aid	GPA	GRE	MAT	Wrk Exp	Letters	Intrvw	Hours C/P/I	Comp	CPCE	Oral	Thesis	Port.
Y	2.75	1250	37	0	2		60/100/600	Y				

School Counseling
CO University of Colorado - Colorado Springs   Colorado Springs   *Contact:* Donna Kelsch; dkelsch@uccs.edu

Fin Aid	GPA	GRE	MAT	Wrk Exp	Letters	Intrvw	Hours C/P/I	Comp	CPCE	Oral	Thesis	Port.
Y	2.75					Y	49/100/600	Y				Y

School Counseling
CO University of Colorado at Denver   Denver   *Contact:* Joseph Lasky; Joe_Lasky@ceo.cudenver.edu

Fin Aid	GPA	GRE	MAT	Wrk Exp	Letters	Intrvw	Hours C/P/I	Comp	CPCE	Oral	Thesis	Port.
Y	2.75	900	40	0	4	Y	60/150/600	Y				

School Counseling
CO University of Northern Colorado   Greeley   *Contact:* Linda Black; linda.black@unco.edu

Fin Aid	GPA	GRE	MAT	Wrk Exp	Letters	Intrvw	Hours C/P/I	Comp	CPCE	Oral	Thesis	Port.
Y	3.00				3	Y	57/340/600	Y				

School Counseling
CO University of Phoenix   Colorado Springs   *Contact:* John West

Fin Aid	GPA	GRE	MAT	Wrk Exp	Letters	Intrvw	Hours C/P/I	Comp	CPCE	Oral	Thesis	Port.
Y	2.50			3		Y	49//600					Y

School Counseling
DC The George Washington University   Washington, D.C.   *Contact:* Pat Schwallie-Giddis, Ph.D.

Fin Aid	GPA	GRE	MAT	Wrk Exp	Letters	Intrvw	Hours C/P/I	Comp	CPCE	Oral	Thesis	Port.
Y	3.00	1000	50%		2	Y	48/100/600					

School Counseling
FL Carlos Albizu University   Miami   *Contact:* Diana Barroso, M.S., LMHC

Fin Aid	GPA	GRE	MAT	Wrk Exp	Letters	Intrvw	Hours C/P/I	Comp	CPCE	Oral	Thesis	Port.
Y	3.00				3	Y	49/240/	Y				

School Counseling
FL Florida Atlantic University   Boca Raton   *Contact:* Dr. Greg Brigman; gbrigman@fau.edu

Fin Aid	GPA	GRE	MAT	Wrk Exp	Letters	Intrvw	Hours C/P/I	Comp	CPCE	Oral	Thesis	Port.
Y	~3.00	~1000				Y	60/150/600					Y

School Counseling
FL Rollins College   Winter Park   *Contact:* Kathryn L. Norsworthy, Ph.D.; Knorswor@rollins.edu

Fin Aid	GPA	GRE	MAT	Wrk Exp	Letters	Intrvw	Hours C/P/I	Comp	CPCE	Oral	Thesis	Port.
Y	3.00	1000	50	2	3		48/100/600					

School Counseling
FL University of Central Florida   Orlando   *Contact:* B. Grant Hayes; ghayes@mail.ucf.edu

Fin Aid	GPA	GRE	MAT	Wrk Exp	Letters	Intrvw	Hours C/P/I	Comp	CPCE	Oral	Thesis	Port.
		1000			3	Y	51/60/ 150/600		Y			Y

School Counseling
FL University of Florida   Gainesville   *Contact:* M. Harry Daniels

Fin Aid	GPA	GRE	MAT	Wrk Exp	Letters	Intrvw	Hours C/P/I	Comp	CPCE	Oral	Thesis	Port.
	3.00	1000			3	Y	3/300/600			Y		

School Counseling
FL University of North Florida   Jacksonville   *Contact:* Carolyn Stone; Cstone@uaf.edu

Fin Aid	GPA	GRE	MAT	Wrk Exp	Letters	Intrvw	Hours C/P/I	Comp	CPCE	Oral	Thesis	Port.
	3.00	1000		1	3	Y	51/100/600					

School Counseling
GA Columbus State University   Columbus

Fin Aid	GPA	GRE	MAT	Wrk Exp	Letters	Intrvw	Hours C/P/I	Comp	CPCE	Oral	Thesis	Port.
	2.70	800	44	2	2	Y	48/100/600	Y				Y

School Counseling
GA Georgia State University   Atlanta   *Contact:* Fran Mullis, Ph.D.

Fin Aid	GPA	GRE	MAT	Wrk Exp	Letters	Intrvw	Hours C/P/I	Comp	CPCE	Oral	Thesis	Port.
Y	2.50	800	NA	1	3		48/100/600	Y				

Master's Degree Programs												
	Admission Requirements							Graduation Requirements				
Fin				Wrk			Hours		Examinations			
Aid	GPA	GRE	MAT	Exp	Letters	Intrvw	C/P/I	Comp	CPCE	Oral	Thesis	Port.

School Counseling
GA State University of West Georgia Carrolton *Contact:* Dr. Snow

Y	2.70	900		0	3	Y	48/100/600	Y	Y			

School Counseling
IA Iowa State University Ames *Contact:* John M. Littrell; jlittrel@iastate.edu

Y	3.20			2	3	Y	36-42/100 /400			Y		Y

School Counseling
IA The University of Iowa Iowa City *Contact:* David A. Jepsen; david-jepsen-@uiowa.edu

Y	3.00	1000		0	3	Y	48-61/100 /600	Y				Y

School Counseling
IA University of North Iowa Cedar Falls *Contact:* Dr. Ann Vernon; Ann.Vernon@uni.edu

Y	3.00	NR		0	3		56 or 62 for nonteaching majors /150/600	Y			Y	

School Counseling
ID Boise State University Boise *Contact:* Dr. Bobbie Birdsall; bbirdsa@boisestate.edu

Y					3	Y	60/100/700	Y				Y

School Counseling
ID Idaho State University Pocatello *Contact:* Dr. Virginia Allen; Allevirg@isu.edu

Y	3.00		42		3	Y	48/150/600	Y		Y		

School Counseling
ID Northwest Nazarene University Nampa *Contact:* Brenda Freeman; bjfreeman@nnu.edu

Y	3.00				2	Y	53/200/600	Y				Y

School Counseling
ID University of Idaho Moscow *Contact:* Dr. Tom Trotter

	3.00				3	Y	60/150/850					

School Counseling
IL Concordia University River Forest *Contact:* Dr. Dale J. Septeowski; crfsepteodj@curf.edu

Y	3.00				3		48/100/600			Y		Y

School Counseling
IL Eastern Illinois University Charleston *Contact:* Dr. Roberts

Y	2.75			0	2	Y	48/100/600	Y				

School Counseling
IL Lewis University Romeoville *Contact:* Richard Guerra; guerrari@lewisu.edu

Y	3.00				2		40/100/300	Y				

School Counseling
IL Southern Illinois University Carbondale Carbondale *Contact:* Dr. David Duys; duys@siu.edu

Y	2.70				3		48/100/600	Y				

School Counseling
IL Western Illinois University Moline *Contact:* Melanie Rawlins

	2.50				2	Y	48/100/600					

School Counseling
IN Ball State University Muncie *Contact:* Charlene Alexander; calexander@bsu.edu

Y	2.75				3		48/200/600	Y				Y

	Master's Degree Programs											
Fin Aid	Admission Requirements						Graduation Requirements					
	GPA	GRE	MAT	Wrk Exp	Letters	Intrvw	Hours C/P/I	Examinations				
								Comp	CPCE	Oral	Thesis	Port.

School Counseling
IN Butler University Indianapolis *Contact:* Dr.Ron Goodman

Y	3.00	875	40		2	Y	48/100/600		Y			Y

School Counseling
IN Indiana State University Terre Haute

Y	2.50				3	Y	52/100/600			Y		Y

School Counseling
IN Indiana University Bloomington *Contact:* Dr. Sue Whiston; swhiston@indiana.edu

Y	2.75	1300			3		48/100/600					

School Counseling
IN Indiana-Purdue University at Fort Wayne Fort Wayne *Contact:* William E. Utesch; utesch@ipfw.edu

Y	3.20				3	Y	51/100/9mo	Y				Y

School Counseling
IN Purdue University West Lafayette *Contact:* Jean Peterson; jeanp@purdue.edu

	3.00	1000			3		48/100/600					

School Counseling
KS Emporia State University Emporia *Contact:* Dr. Dennis Pelsma; pelsmade@emporia.edu

Y	3.00	850	40	0	3	Y	48/100/	Y				

School Counseling
KS Kansas State University Manhattan *Contact:* Dr. Judith Hughey; jhughey@ksu.edu

Y	3.00	970	50	1	3		48/100/600	Y				

School Counseling
KS Pittsburg State University Pittsburg *Contact:* Becky Brannock; rbrannoc@pittstate.edu

Y	3.00	1200			3		48/150/300					

School Counseling
KS University of Kansas Lawrence

							/50/					

School Counseling
KY Eastern Kentucky University Richmond *Contact:* Patricia Stevens; patricia.stevens@eku.edu

Y	3.00		30		3		48/100/600	Y	Y			

School Counseling
LA Louisiana State University Baton Rouge *Contact:* David A. Spruill, Ph.D.; dspruill@lsu.edu

Y	3.00	1000			3		48/100/600	Y				

School Counseling
LA McNeese State University Lake Charles *Contact:* M. Janelle Disney; mdisney@mail.mcneese.edu

Y	~2.70	~895				Y	48/100/600	Y				

School Counseling
LA Our Lady of Holy Cross New Orleans *Contact:* Dr. Judith Miranti

							54/100/600					

School Counseling
LA Southeastern Louisiana University Hammond *Contact:* Mary Ballard; mballard2@selu.edu

Y				0	Y	Y	48/100/600	Y	Y			

School Counseling
LA University of New Orleans New Orleans *Contact:* Dr. Diana Hulse-Killacky; dhulseki@uno.edu

Y	2.50	R		0	0		60/100/600	Y	Y			

		Master's Degree Programs										
	Admission Requirements						Graduation Requirements					
Fin Aid	GPA	GRE	MAT	Wrk Exp	Letters	Intrvw	Hours C/P/I	Comp	CPCE	Oral	Thesis	Port.

School Counseling
MA Bridgewater State College   Bridgewater   *Contact:* Dr. Maxine Rawlins; mrawlins@bridgew.edu

	GPA	GRE	MAT	Wrk Exp	Letters	Intrvw	Hours C/P/I	Comp	CPCE	Oral	Thesis	Port.
	2.80	1000		0	3	Y	48/100/600	Y				

School Counseling
MA Fitchburg State College   Fitchburg   *Contact:* Carol Globiano

	GPA	GRE	MAT	Wrk Exp	Letters	Intrvw	Hours C/P/I	Comp	CPCE	Oral	Thesis	Port.
	2.80	1475	47		3		51/100/450					

School Counseling
MA Lesley University   Cambridge   *Contact:* Yishiuan Chin (617) 349-8339; (800) 999-1959 ext. 8339

	GPA	GRE	MAT	Wrk Exp	Letters	Intrvw	Hours C/P/I	Comp	CPCE	Oral	Thesis	Port.
Y	3.00		40		3	Y	48/60/100/600/1200					

School Counseling
MA Suffolk University   Boston   *Contact:* Dr. R. Arthur Winters

	GPA	GRE	MAT	Wrk Exp	Letters	Intrvw	Hours C/P/I	Comp	CPCE	Oral	Thesis	Port.
Y	2.75	R	R		3		36/450/					Y

School Counseling
MD Johns Hopkins University   Baltimore   *Contact:* Alan Green, Susan Keys; keys@jhu.edu

	GPA	GRE	MAT	Wrk Exp	Letters	Intrvw	Hours C/P/I	Comp	CPCE	Oral	Thesis	Port.
Y	3.00			2	Y		48//200			Y		

School Counseling
MD McDaniel College   Westminster   *Contact:* Dr. Julia Orza; jorza@mcdaniel.edu

	GPA	GRE	MAT	Wrk Exp	Letters	Intrvw	Hours C/P/I	Comp	CPCE	Oral	Thesis	Port.
Y	2.50			3	Y		45//200-500	Y				

School Counseling
ME University of Southern Maine   Gorham   *Contact:* Marijane Fall, Ed.D.; mjfall@usm.maine.edu

	GPA	GRE	MAT	Wrk Exp	Letters	Intrvw	Hours C/P/I	Comp	CPCE	Oral	Thesis	Port.
Y	R	R	R	0	3	Y	54/100/600	Y	Y			Y

School Counseling
MI Andrews University   Berrien Springs   *Contact:* Frederick Kosinski, Jr.; kosinskf@andrews.edu

	GPA	GRE	MAT	Wrk Exp	Letters	Intrvw	Hours C/P/I	Comp	CPCE	Oral	Thesis	Port.
Y	2.70			2	Y		48/100/600	Y				

School Counseling
MI Eastern Michigan University   Ypsilanti   *Contact:* Sue Stickel; sue.stickel@emich.edu

	GPA	GRE	MAT	Wrk Exp	Letters	Intrvw	Hours C/P/I	Comp	CPCE	Oral	Thesis	Port.
Y	2.75			3	Y		48/100/600					Y

School Counseling
MI Oakland University   Rochester   *Contact:* parfitt@oakland.edu

	GPA	GRE	MAT	Wrk Exp	Letters	Intrvw	Hours C/P/I	Comp	CPCE	Oral	Thesis	Port.
Y	3.00			2	Y		48/100/600					

School Counseling
MI Siena Heights University   Adrian   *Contact:* Linda M. Brewster

	GPA	GRE	MAT	Wrk Exp	Letters	Intrvw	Hours C/P/I	Comp	CPCE	Oral	Thesis	Port.
	3.00			1	3	Y	48/100/600					

School Counseling
MN Minnesota State University Moorhead   Moorhead

	GPA	GRE	MAT	Wrk Exp	Letters	Intrvw	Hours C/P/I	Comp	CPCE	Oral	Thesis	Port.
Y	3.00	R	R	0	3	Y	48/100/650	Y	Y	Y	Y	

School Counseling
MN Minnesota State University, Mankato   Mankato   *Contact:* Walter Roberts & Richard Auger; walter.roberts@mnsu.edu

	GPA	GRE	MAT	Wrk Exp	Letters	Intrvw	Hours C/P/I	Comp	CPCE	Oral	Thesis	Port.
Y	3.00	1350	44		3	Y	50/100/700	Y				Y

School Counseling
MO Northwest Missouri State University   Maryville   *Contact:* Rochelle Hiatt

	GPA	GRE	MAT	Wrk Exp	Letters	Intrvw	Hours C/P/I	Comp	CPCE	Oral	Thesis	Port.
Y	2.50	~1400		0	Y		44/150/	Y				Y

School Counseling
MO Southeast Missouri State University   Cape Girardeau   *Contact:* Dr. Doris Skelton; dskelton@semo.edu

	GPA	GRE	MAT	Wrk Exp	Letters	Intrvw	Hours C/P/I	Comp	CPCE	Oral	Thesis	Port.
Y	3.00	1600		0	3	Y	48/100/600	Y	Y			Y

Master's Degree Programs

Fin Aid	GPA	GRE	MAT	Wrk Exp	Letters	Intrvw	Hours C/P/I	Comp	CPCE	Oral	Thesis	Port.

School Counseling
MO Truman State University   Kirksville   *Contact:* Tricia K. Brown, Ph.D.; tbrown@truman.edu

Fin Aid	GPA	GRE	MAT	Wrk Exp	Letters	Intrvw	Hours C/P/I	Comp	CPCE	Oral	Thesis	Port.
Y	3.00	50th%		0	3		48/150/600	Y			Y	Y

School Counseling
MO University of Missouri - St. Louis   Saint Louis   *Contact:* Therese Cristiani, EdD; cristiani@umsl.edu

Fin Aid	GPA	GRE	MAT	Wrk Exp	Letters	Intrvw	Hours C/P/I	Comp	CPCE	Oral	Thesis	Port.
Y	3.00				3		48/150/600	Y	Y			Y

School Counseling
MO University of Missouri-Columbia   Columbia   *Contact:* Norman Gysbers or Richard Lapan; GysbersN@missouri.edu

Fin Aid	GPA	GRE	MAT	Wrk Exp	Letters	Intrvw	Hours C/P/I	Comp	CPCE	Oral	Thesis	Port.
	3.00	1000			3		48//			Y		Y

School Counseling
MS Mississippi College   Clinton   *Contact:* Edith Carlisle; carlisle@mc.edu

Fin Aid	GPA	GRE	MAT	Wrk Exp	Letters	Intrvw	Hours C/P/I	Comp	CPCE	Oral	Thesis	Port.
Y	2.50	Praxis		1	3	Y	48/100/600			Y		

School Counseling
MS Mississippi State University   Mississippi State University   *Contact:* Dr. Joe Ray Underwood; joeray@colled.msstate.edu

Fin Aid	GPA	GRE	MAT	Wrk Exp	Letters	Intrvw	Hours C/P/I	Comp	CPCE	Oral	Thesis	Port.
Y	2.75	1200			3		48/100/600	Y	Y			

School Counseling
MS William Carey College   Hattiesburg   *Contact:* Dr. Tommy King

Fin Aid	GPA	GRE	MAT	Wrk Exp	Letters	Intrvw	Hours C/P/I	Comp	CPCE	Oral	Thesis	Port.
Y	2.50	850			2		48/100/100					Y

School Counseling
MT Montana State University-Northern   Havre   *Contact:* John Foley

Fin Aid	GPA	GRE	MAT	Wrk Exp	Letters	Intrvw	Hours C/P/I	Comp	CPCE	Oral	Thesis	Port.
Y	3.00	900	29	3	3		50/100/600					Y

School Counseling
MT Montana State University - Billings   Billings   *Contact:* James Nowlin; jnowlin@msubillings.edu

Fin Aid	GPA	GRE	MAT	Wrk Exp	Letters	Intrvw	Hours C/P/I	Comp	CPCE	Oral	Thesis	Port.
Y	3.00	1350					40-60/100/600					Y

School Counseling
MT Montana State University - Bozeman   Bozeman   *Contact:* Mark Nelson; markn@montana.edu

Fin Aid	GPA	GRE	MAT	Wrk Exp	Letters	Intrvw	Hours C/P/I	Comp	CPCE	Oral	Thesis	Port.
Y	3.00	900		1	3	Y	48/200/600	Y				

School Counseling
NC Appalachian State University   Boone   *Contact:* Laurie Williamson

Fin Aid	GPA	GRE	MAT	Wrk Exp	Letters	Intrvw	Hours C/P/I	Comp	CPCE	Oral	Thesis	Port.
Y	R	R			3	Y	48/100/600	Y	Y			

School Counseling
NC Campbell University   Buies Creek   *Contact:* Harriet Enzor

Fin Aid	GPA	GRE	MAT	Wrk Exp	Letters	Intrvw	Hours C/P/I	Comp	CPCE	Oral	Thesis	Port.
Y	3.00	850			3	Y	48/100/600	Y				

School Counseling
NC North Carolina A&T State University   Greensboro   *Contact:* Dr. Wyatt D. Kirk

Fin Aid	GPA	GRE	MAT	Wrk Exp	Letters	Intrvw	Hours C/P/I	Comp	CPCE	Oral	Thesis	Port.
Y	R			0	3		60//	Y	Y			

School Counseling
NC The University of North Carolina at Chapel Hill   Chapel Hill   *Contact:* John P. Galassi; jgalassi@email.unc.edu

Fin Aid	GPA	GRE	MAT	Wrk Exp	Letters	Intrvw	Hours C/P/I	Comp	CPCE	Oral	Thesis	Port.
Y	3.00				3	Y	60/100/600 min.	Y				

School Counseling
NC The University of North Carolina at Greensboro   Greensboro

Fin Aid	GPA	GRE	MAT	Wrk Exp	Letters	Intrvw	Hours C/P/I	Comp	CPCE	Oral	Thesis	Port.
Y	3.00	R			3		48/120+/600	Y				

Master's Degree Programs												
	Admission Requirements							Graduation Requirements				
Fin Aid	GPA	GRE	MAT	Wrk Exp	Letters	Intrvw	Hours C/P/I	Comp	CPCE	Oral	Thesis	Port.

School Counseling
NC University of North Carolina at Charlotte   Charlotte   *Contact:* Phyllis Post; ppost@email.uncc.edu

Fin Aid	GPA	GRE	MAT	Wrk Exp	Letters	Intrvw	Hours C/P/I	Comp	CPCE	Oral	Thesis	Port.
Y	R	R	R	0			60/150/600	Y				

School Counseling
NC Wake Forest University   Winston-Salem   *Contact:* Donna Henderson; henderda@wfu.edu

Fin Aid	GPA	GRE	MAT	Wrk Exp	Letters	Intrvw	Hours C/P/I	Comp	CPCE	Oral	Thesis	Port.
Y	3.00	1000			3	Y	60/135/600					

School Counseling
ND North Dakota State University   Fargo

Fin Aid	GPA	GRE	MAT	Wrk Exp	Letters	Intrvw	Hours C/P/I	Comp	CPCE	Oral	Thesis	Port.
Y	3.00				3	Y	48/40/600/ 900	Y	Y			

School Counseling
NE Chadron State College   Chadron   *Contact:* Laura Gaudet, PhD; lgaudet@csc.edu

Fin Aid	GPA	GRE	MAT	Wrk Exp	Letters	Intrvw	Hours C/P/I	Comp	CPCE	Oral	Thesis	Port.
							39/20/300					

School Counseling
NE University of Nebraska-Omaha   Omaha   *Contact:* Dept. Chair

Fin Aid	GPA	GRE	MAT	Wrk Exp	Letters	Intrvw	Hours C/P/I	Comp	CPCE	Oral	Thesis	Port.
	3.00		35	2		Y	51/100/500					

School Counseling
NE Wayne State College   Wayne

Fin Aid	GPA	GRE	MAT	Wrk Exp	Letters	Intrvw	Hours C/P/I	Comp	CPCE	Oral	Thesis	Port.
		1050		0	2	Y	48/100/450					Y

School Counseling
NH Plymouth State College   Plymouth   *Contact:* Dr. Gary Goodnough; ggoodno@mail.plymouth.edu

Fin Aid	GPA	GRE	MAT	Wrk Exp	Letters	Intrvw	Hours C/P/I	Comp	CPCE	Oral	Thesis	Port.
	3.00				3	Y	48/100/600					

School Counseling
NJ The College of New Jersey   Ewing   *Contact:* Dr. MaryLou Ramsey; ramsey@tcnj.edu

Fin Aid	GPA	GRE	MAT	Wrk Exp	Letters	Intrvw	Hours C/P/I	Comp	CPCE	Oral	Thesis	Port.
Y	R				Y	Y	48/100/600	Y				

School Counseling
NJ William Paterson University   Wayne   *Contact:* Mathilda Catarina, Ph.D., LPC; catarinam@wpunj.ed

Fin Aid	GPA	GRE	MAT	Wrk Exp	Letters	Intrvw	Hours C/P/I	Comp	CPCE	Oral	Thesis	Port.
Y	2.75		42		2	Y	48/100/600	Y			Y	Y

School Counseling
NV University of Nevada   Reno   *Contact:* Jill Packman; packman@unr.edu

Fin Aid	GPA	GRE	MAT	Wrk Exp	Letters	Intrvw	Hours C/P/I	Comp	CPCE	Oral	Thesis	Port.
Y	3.00	750		2	3		60/100/600	Y	Y			

School Counseling
NY Canisius College   Buffalo   *Contact:* David Farrugia; Farriguia@canisius.edu

Fin Aid	GPA	GRE	MAT	Wrk Exp	Letters	Intrvw	Hours C/P/I	Comp	CPCE	Oral	Thesis	Port.
	2.50	1300				Y	42/160/340					

School Counseling
NY College at Oswego SUNY   Oswego   *Contact:* Dr. Jean Casey; casey@oswego.edu

Fin Aid	GPA	GRE	MAT	Wrk Exp	Letters	Intrvw	Hours C/P/I	Comp	CPCE	Oral	Thesis	Port.
Y	3.00	1000			3	Y	48/100/300	Y	Y			

School Counseling
NY Lehman College of the City University of New York   Bronx   *Contact:* Stuart Chen-Hayes; stuartc@lehman.cuny.edu

Fin Aid	GPA	GRE	MAT	Wrk Exp	Letters	Intrvw	Hours C/P/I	Comp	CPCE	Oral	Thesis	Port.
Y	3.00	R		0	3	Y	48/100/600					Y

School Counseling
NY Marist College   Poughkeepsie   *Contact:* Paul Egan Ph.D.

Fin Aid	GPA	GRE	MAT	Wrk Exp	Letters	Intrvw	Hours C/P/I	Comp	CPCE	Oral	Thesis	Port.
Y	3.00	1500			3	Y	62/100/600					

School Counseling
NY New York University   New York   *Contact:* Samuel Juni; sam.juni@nyu.edu

Fin Aid	GPA	GRE	MAT	Wrk Exp	Letters	Intrvw	Hours C/P/I	Comp	CPCE	Oral	Thesis	Port.
Y	3.00				2		48/84/84					

		Master's Degree Programs									
	Admission Requirements						Graduation Requirements				
Fin Aid	GPA	GRE	MAT	Wrk Exp	Letters	Intrvw	Hours C/P/I	Examinations				
								Comp	CPCE	Oral	Thesis	Port.

School Counseling
NY Niagara University   Niagara University   *Contact:* Dr. Morgan Brocks Conway; mcc@niagara.edu

Fin Aid	GPA	GRE	MAT	Wrk Exp	Letters	Intrvw	Hours C/P/I	Comp	CPCE	Oral	Thesis	Port.
Y	2.75	880	40		2	Y	36/100/100	Y				Y

School Counseling
NY Plattsburgh State University   Plattsburgh   *Contact:* Dr. Rachelle Perusse; rachelle.perusse@plattsburgh.edu

Fin Aid	GPA	GRE	MAT	Wrk Exp	Letters	Intrvw	Hours C/P/I	Comp	CPCE	Oral	Thesis	Port.
Y	2.80	25th %tile	25th %tile	0	3	Y	60/115/600	Y	Y			

School Counseling
NY Queens College, City University of New York   Flushing   *Contact:* Dr. John Pellitteri; Jpellitter@aol.com

Fin Aid	GPA	GRE	MAT	Wrk Exp	Letters	Intrvw	Hours C/P/I	Comp	CPCE	Oral	Thesis	Port.
	3.00				3	Y	60/100/600	Y			Y	

School Counseling
NY State University of New York at Oneonta   Oneonta   *Contact:* Emily Phillips; phillie@oneonta.edu

Fin Aid	GPA	GRE	MAT	Wrk Exp	Letters	Intrvw	Hours C/P/I	Comp	CPCE	Oral	Thesis	Port.
	2.80				2	Y	33/will be 60 by 2005/ 180/600	Y				Y

School Counseling
NY SUNY College of Brockport   Brockport   *Contact:* J. Cochran

Fin Aid	GPA	GRE	MAT	Wrk Exp	Letters	Intrvw	Hours C/P/I	Comp	CPCE	Oral	Thesis	Port.
Y	2.50				3	Y	48/100/600					

School Counseling
NY SUNY University at Buffalo   Buffalo   *Contact:* Dr. Janis DeLucia Waack

Fin Aid	GPA	GRE	MAT	Wrk Exp	Letters	Intrvw	Hours C/P/I	Comp	CPCE	Oral	Thesis	Port.
					3	Y	36/150/	Y				

School Counseling
NY Syracuse University   Syracuse   *Contact:* Janna Scarborough; scarboro@syr.edu

Fin Aid	GPA	GRE	MAT	Wrk Exp	Letters	Intrvw	Hours C/P/I	Comp	CPCE	Oral	Thesis	Port.
Y	3.00	NA		1	3	Y	48/100/600	Y	Y			Y

School Counseling
NY University of Rochester   Rochester   *Contact:* Howard Kirschenbaum; Howard.Kirschenbaum@rochester.edu

Fin Aid	GPA	GRE	MAT	Wrk Exp	Letters	Intrvw	Hours C/P/I	Comp	CPCE	Oral	Thesis	Port.
Y		NR		0	2	Y	48/120/600				Y	

School Counseling
OH Cleveland State University   Cleveland   *Contact:* Elliott Ingersoll; r.ingersoll@csuohio.edu

Fin Aid	GPA	GRE	MAT	Wrk Exp	Letters	Intrvw	Hours C/P/I	Comp	CPCE	Oral	Thesis	Port.
Y	2.75		R		2		48/100/600	Y				

School Counseling
OH John Carroll University   Cleveland   *Contact:* David C. Helsel, PhD; DHelsel@JCU.EDU

Fin Aid	GPA	GRE	MAT	Wrk Exp	Letters	Intrvw	Hours C/P/I	Comp	CPCE	Oral	Thesis	Port.
Y	2.75	1000	50	2	2	Y	48/150/600	Y				

School Counseling
OH Kent State University   Kent   *Contact:* Dr. Jason McGlothlin; jmcgloth@kent.edu

Fin Aid	GPA	GRE	MAT	Wrk Exp	Letters	Intrvw	Hours C/P/I	Comp	CPCE	Oral	Thesis	Port.
Y	2.75				2	Y	49/100/600					

School Counseling
OH Malone College   Canton   *Contact:* Dr. Ken McCurdy

Fin Aid	GPA	GRE	MAT	Wrk Exp	Letters	Intrvw	Hours C/P/I	Comp	CPCE	Oral	Thesis	Port.
	3.00				3	Y	48/100/600					

School Counseling
OH Ohio University   Athens   *Contact:* Tracy Leinbaugh; leinbaug@ohio.edu

Fin Aid	GPA	GRE	MAT	Wrk Exp	Letters	Intrvw	Hours C/P/I	Comp	CPCE	Oral	Thesis	Port.
Y	3.00	900			3		//					

School Counseling
OH The University of Toledo   Toledo   *Contact:* Martin Ritchie; martin.ritchie@utoledo.edu

Fin Aid	GPA	GRE	MAT	Wrk Exp	Letters	Intrvw	Hours C/P/I	Comp	CPCE	Oral	Thesis	Port.
Y	3.00	800			3	Y	48/100/600					

Master's Degree Programs												
	Admission Requirements							Graduation Requirements				
Fin Aid	GPA	GRE	MAT	Wrk Exp	Letters	Intrvw	Hours C/P/I	Comp	CPCE	Oral	Thesis	Port.

School Counseling
OH University of Cincinnati Cincinnati *Contact:* Mei Tang, Ph.D.; mei.tang@uc.edu

Fin Aid	GPA	GRE	MAT	Wrk Exp	Letters	Intrvw	Hours C/P/I	Comp	CPCE	Oral	Thesis	Port.
Y	2.80	1500			3	Y	/100/600	Y	Y			

School Counseling
OH Walsh University North Canton *Contact:* Judy Green Ph.D.; jgreen@walsh.edu

Fin Aid	GPA	GRE	MAT	Wrk Exp	Letters	Intrvw	Hours C/P/I	Comp	CPCE	Oral	Thesis	Port.
	3.00	900	40		3	Y	48/100/600	Y	Y			

School Counseling
OH Xavier University Cincinnati *Contact:* Lon S. Kriner, PhD; kriner@xavier.edu

Fin Aid	GPA	GRE	MAT	Wrk Exp	Letters	Intrvw	Hours C/P/I	Comp	CPCE	Oral	Thesis	Port.
	2.7+		35	0	0	Y	48/100/600					

School Counseling
OH Youngstown State University Youngstown

Fin Aid	GPA	GRE	MAT	Wrk Exp	Letters	Intrvw	Hours C/P/I	Comp	CPCE	Oral	Thesis	Port.
Y		same				Y	51/200/600	Y				

School Counseling
OR George Fox University Portland *Contact:* Karin Jordan, Director

Fin Aid	GPA	GRE	MAT	Wrk Exp	Letters	Intrvw	Hours C/P/I	Comp	CPCE	Oral	Thesis	Port.
	2.70				3	Y	60/200/600					

School Counseling
OR Oregon State University Corvallis *Contact:* Gene Eakin; gene.eakin@orst.edu

Fin Aid	GPA	GRE	MAT	Wrk Exp	Letters	Intrvw	Hours C/P/I	Comp	CPCE	Oral	Thesis	Port.
Y	3.00				3	Y	/100/600			Y		Y

School Counseling
OR Portland State University Portland *Contact:* Lewis, Halverson

Fin Aid	GPA	GRE	MAT	Wrk Exp	Letters	Intrvw	Hours C/P/I	Comp	CPCE	Oral	Thesis	Port.
Y	points as-signed	R	same	0	same	Y	/100/600	Y				Y

School Counseling
PA Arcadia University Glenside *Contact:* Mrs. Carol Lyman

Fin Aid	GPA	GRE	MAT	Wrk Exp	Letters	Intrvw	Hours C/P/I	Comp	CPCE	Oral	Thesis	Port.
Y	3.00	R	R		3	Y	54-57/100/300-600					

School Counseling
PA California University of Pennsylvania California *Contact:* Gloria C. Brusoski, PhD; Brusoski@cup.edu

Fin Aid	GPA	GRE	MAT	Wrk Exp	Letters	Intrvw	Hours C/P/I	Comp	CPCE	Oral	Thesis	Port.
Y	3.00		45		3	Y	48/300/	Y	Y			

School Counseling
PA Duquesne University Pittsburgh *Contact:* William J. Casile; Casile@duq.edu

Fin Aid	GPA	GRE	MAT	Wrk Exp	Letters	Intrvw	Hours C/P/I	Comp	CPCE	Oral	Thesis	Port.
Y	3.00		40		2		60/125/600			Y		Y

School Counseling
PA Geneva College Beaver Falls *Contact:* Dr. David Harvey; dharvey@geneva.edu

Fin Aid	GPA	GRE	MAT	Wrk Exp	Letters	Intrvw	Hours C/P/I	Comp	CPCE	Oral	Thesis	Port.
Y	3.00	1000			3		51/100/600	Y				

School Counseling
PA Indiana University of Pennsylvania Indiana *Contact:* Dr. Claire Dandeneau; cdanden@iup.edu

Fin Aid	GPA	GRE	MAT	Wrk Exp	Letters	Intrvw	Hours C/P/I	Comp	CPCE	Oral	Thesis	Port.
Y	3.00			0	2	Y	48/90/300					

School Counseling
PA Kutztown University Kutztown *Contact:* Deborah Barlieb, Sandra McSwain; barlieb@kutztown.edu

Fin Aid	GPA	GRE	MAT	Wrk Exp	Letters	Intrvw	Hours C/P/I	Comp	CPCE	Oral	Thesis	Port.
	3.00	1200			3	Y	51/100/700	Y				

School Counseling
PA Penn State University University Park

Fin Aid	GPA	GRE	MAT	Wrk Exp	Letters	Intrvw	Hours C/P/I	Comp	CPCE	Oral	Thesis	Port.
						//						

Master's Degree Programs

		Admission Requirements					Graduation Requirements					
Fin Aid	GPA	GRE	MAT	Wrk Exp	Letters	Intrvw	Hours C/P/I	Comp	CPCE	Oral	Thesis	Port.

School Counseling

PA Shippensburg University of PA Shippensburg *Contact:* Thomas Hozman; tlhozm@ship.edu

Fin Aid	GPA	GRE	MAT	Wrk Exp	Letters	Intrvw	Hours C/P/I	Comp	CPCE	Oral	Thesis	Port.
Y	3.00	800		1	3	Y	48/150/600					Y

School Counseling

PA West Chester University West Chester *Contact:* Dr. Angelo Gadaleto; Agadaleto@wcupa.edu

Fin Aid	GPA	GRE	MAT	Wrk Exp	Letters	Intrvw	Hours C/P/I	Comp	CPCE	Oral	Thesis	Port.
Y	3.00				3		48/360/	Y				Y

School Counseling

PA Westminster College New Wilmington *Contact:* William J. Evans Ph.D.b; evanswj@westminster.edu

Fin Aid	GPA	GRE	MAT	Wrk Exp	Letters	Intrvw	Hours C/P/I	Comp	CPCE	Oral	Thesis	Port.
Y	3.00				2		30/100/ 300/600	Y				

School Counseling

RI Rhode Island College Providence *Contact:* M. Finley

Fin Aid	GPA	GRE	MAT	Wrk Exp	Letters	Intrvw	Hours C/P/I	Comp	CPCE	Oral	Thesis	Port.
	3.00	900	45	2	3		36/90/600	Y				

School Counseling

SC Clemson University Clemson

Fin Aid	GPA	GRE	MAT	Wrk Exp	Letters	Intrvw	Hours C/P/I	Comp	CPCE	Oral	Thesis	Port.
	3.00	1250			2		51/100/600	Y	Y			

School Counseling

SC Winthrop University Rock Hill *Contact:* Dr. Johnny Sanders, Jr.; sandersj@winthrop.edu

Fin Aid	GPA	GRE	MAT	Wrk Exp	Letters	Intrvw	Hours C/P/I	Comp	CPCE	Oral	Thesis	Port.
Y	2.00	800	40	0	3	Y	51/100/600	Y				

School Counseling

SD South Dakota State University Brookings *Contact:* Jay Trenhaile

Fin Aid	GPA	GRE	MAT	Wrk Exp	Letters	Intrvw	Hours C/P/I	Comp	CPCE	Oral	Thesis	Port.
Y	3.00				2	Y	48/100/600	Y		Y		

School Counseling

SD The University of South Dakota Vermillion *Contact:* Frank Main; fmain@usd.edu

Fin Aid	GPA	GRE	MAT	Wrk Exp	Letters	Intrvw	Hours C/P/I	Comp	CPCE	Oral	Thesis	Port.
	3.00	900			3		51/45/600	Y				

School Counseling

TN East Tennessee State University Johnson City *Contact:* Patricia Robertson; RobertPE@etsu.edu

Fin Aid	GPA	GRE	MAT	Wrk Exp	Letters	Intrvw	Hours C/P/I	Comp	CPCE	Oral	Thesis	Port.
Y		R			3	Y	48/100/600	Y				

School Counseling

TN Lee University Cleveland *Contact:* Susan Carter, Ph.D.; scarter@leeuniversity.edu

Fin Aid	GPA	GRE	MAT	Wrk Exp	Letters	Intrvw	Hours C/P/I	Comp	CPCE	Oral	Thesis	Port.
Y	3.00	~1000 V+Q			0	3	Y	48/150/600	Y				

School Counseling

TN Middle Tennessee State University Murfreesboro *Contact:* Virginia S. Dansby; vdansby@mtsu.edu

Fin Aid	GPA	GRE	MAT	Wrk Exp	Letters	Intrvw	Hours C/P/I	Comp	CPCE	Oral	Thesis	Port.
Y	3.00	900			0	3	Y	49/100/600	Y				

School Counseling

TN Peabody College, Vanderbilt University Nashville *Contact:* H. Lori Schnieders; lori.schnieders@vanderbilt.edu

Fin Aid	GPA	GRE	MAT	Wrk Exp	Letters	Intrvw	Hours C/P/I	Comp	CPCE	Oral	Thesis	Port.
Y	3.00	1000	50		3	Y	48/100/600	Y		Y		Y

School Counseling

TN The University of Tennessee at Knoxville Knoxville *Contact:* Dr. William Poppen; poppen@utk.edu

Fin Aid	GPA	GRE	MAT	Wrk Exp	Letters	Intrvw	Hours C/P/I	Comp	CPCE	Oral	Thesis	Port.
	2.70	1000			3		48/100/600	Y				

School Counseling

TX Houston Baptist University Houston

Fin Aid	GPA	GRE	MAT	Wrk Exp	Letters	Intrvw	Hours C/P/I	Comp	CPCE	Oral	Thesis	Port.
Y							//					

Master's Degree Programs

Fin Aid	GPA	GRE	MAT	Wrk Exp	Letters	Intrvw	Hours C/P/I	Comp	CPCE	Oral	Thesis	Port.

School Counseling
TX Lamar University   Beaumont

Fin Aid	GPA	GRE	MAT	Wrk Exp	Letters	Intrvw	Hours C/P/I	Comp	CPCE	Oral	Thesis	Port.
						45/300/						

School Counseling
TX Our Lady of the Lake University   San Antonio   *Contact:* Nadene Peterson

Fin Aid	GPA	GRE	MAT	Wrk Exp	Letters	Intrvw	Hours C/P/I	Comp	CPCE	Oral	Thesis	Port.
Y	2.75	R	R		2	Y	48/300/	Y				

School Counseling
TX Southwest Texas State University   San Marcos   *Contact:* JoLynne Reynolds; jr36@swt.edu

Fin Aid	GPA	GRE	MAT	Wrk Exp	Letters	Intrvw	Hours C/P/I	Comp	CPCE	Oral	Thesis	Port.
Y							//					

School Counseling
TX Stephen F. Austin State University   Nacogdoches   *Contact:* Dr. Jan Stalling; jstalling@sfasu.edu

Fin Aid	GPA	GRE	MAT	Wrk Exp	Letters	Intrvw	Hours C/P/I	Comp	CPCE	Oral	Thesis	Port.
Y					3	Y	48/150/600	Y		Y		

School Counseling
TX Tarleton State University   Stephenville   *Contact:* Albrecht, Duncan, Weissenberger;

Fin Aid	GPA	GRE	MAT	Wrk Exp	Letters	Intrvw	Hours C/P/I	Comp	CPCE	Oral	Thesis	Port.
	3.00	850					48/6/300	Y				

School Counseling
TX Texas A & M University - Commerce   Commerce   *Contact:* Dr. Richard Lampe; Richard_lampe@tamu-commerce.edu

Fin Aid	GPA	GRE	MAT	Wrk Exp	Letters	Intrvw	Hours C/P/I	Comp	CPCE	Oral	Thesis	Port.
Y					3		48/100/600	Y				

School Counseling
TX Texas Southern University   Houston   *Contact:* Dr. Joyce K. Jones; Jones_JK@tsu.edu

Fin Aid	GPA	GRE	MAT	Wrk Exp	Letters	Intrvw	Hours C/P/I	Comp	CPCE	Oral	Thesis	Port.
	2.50	700			3		48/50/600	Y				

School Counseling
TX Texas Tech University   Lubbock   *Contact:* Jean Shen; Jean.Shen@ttu.edu

Fin Aid	GPA	GRE	MAT	Wrk Exp	Letters	Intrvw	Hours C/P/I	Comp	CPCE	Oral	Thesis	Port.
Y	3.0+	AVG	NR	0	3		48/100/600	Y	Y			Y

School Counseling
TX University of North Texas   Denton   *Contact:* Doris Coy; Coy@coefs.coe.unt.edu

Fin Aid	GPA	GRE	MAT	Wrk Exp	Letters	Intrvw	Hours C/P/I	Comp	CPCE	Oral	Thesis	Port.
Y	3.00	710			3	Y	48/100/600					

School Counseling
TX University of Texas at El Paso   El Paso   *Contact:* Dr. Phillip Barbee; pbarbee@utep.edu

Fin Aid	GPA	GRE	MAT	Wrk Exp	Letters	Intrvw	Hours C/P/I	Comp	CPCE	Oral	Thesis	Port.
Y	3.00	NR		0	3	Y	48/100/600	Y				

School Counseling
TX University of Texas at Tyler   Tyler   *Contact:* Shirley Jones, Ed.D.; sjones@uttyler.edu

Fin Aid	GPA	GRE	MAT	Wrk Exp	Letters	Intrvw	Hours C/P/I	Comp	CPCE	Oral	Thesis	Port.
Y	3.00	900			3		42/300/	Y		Y		

School Counseling
TX University of Texas of the Permian Basin   Odessa   *Contact:* Cathleen Barrett-Kruse, EdD, NCC; barrettkruse@utpb.edu

Fin Aid	GPA	GRE	MAT	Wrk Exp	Letters	Intrvw	Hours C/P/I	Comp	CPCE	Oral	Thesis	Port.
Y	2.50	1200		0	0		48/300/					

School Counseling
VA College of William and Mary   Williamsburg   *Contact:* Norma Day-Vines; nldayv@wm.ede

Fin Aid	GPA	GRE	MAT	Wrk Exp	Letters	Intrvw	Hours C/P/I	Comp	CPCE	Oral	Thesis	Port.
Y	2.50	40%		0	3		54/100/600					

School Counseling
VA George Mason University   Fairfax   *Contact:* Dr. Sally Murphy; cmurphy@gmu.edu

Fin Aid	GPA	GRE	MAT	Wrk Exp	Letters	Intrvw	Hours C/P/I	Comp	CPCE	Oral	Thesis	Port.
Y	3.00			0	3	Y	45/200/200					

School Counseling
VA James Madison University   Harrisonburg   *Contact:* Sue Rippy

Fin Aid	GPA	GRE	MAT	Wrk Exp	Letters	Intrvw	Hours C/P/I	Comp	CPCE	Oral	Thesis	Port.
							60/100/600					

Master's Degree Programs												
	Admission Requirements						Graduation Requirements					
Fin Aid	GPA	GRE	MAT	Wrk Exp	Letters	Intrvw	Hours C/P/I	Comp	CPCE	Oral	Thesis	Port.

School Counseling
VA Old Dominion University Norfolk *Contact:* Dr. Radha Horton-Parker; rparker@odu.edu

Fin Aid	GPA	GRE	MAT	Wrk Exp	Letters	Intrvw	Hours C/P/I	Comp	CPCE	Oral	Thesis	Port.
Y	3.00	R			3		48/100/600	Y	Y			

School Counseling
VA Radford University Radford *Contact:* James Gumaer; dgumaer@radford.edu

Fin Aid	GPA	GRE	MAT	Wrk Exp	Letters	Intrvw	Hours C/P/I	Comp	CPCE	Oral	Thesis	Port.
	2.75	900	45		2		48/100/600	Y				

School Counseling
VA Regent University Virginia Beach *Contact:* Dr. Robyn Rennie; robyren@regent.edu

Fin Aid	GPA	GRE	MAT	Wrk Exp	Letters	Intrvw	Hours C/P/I	Comp	CPCE	Oral	Thesis	Port.
Y	2.75	1000	50%	0	3	Y	51/60/100/600		Y			

School Counseling
VA Virginia Tech Blacksburg

Fin Aid	GPA	GRE	MAT	Wrk Exp	Letters	Intrvw	Hours C/P/I	Comp	CPCE	Oral	Thesis	Port.
Y	3.00				3	Y	51/100/600	Y				

School Counseling
WA Central Washington University Ellensburg

Fin Aid	GPA	GRE	MAT	Wrk Exp	Letters	Intrvw	Hours C/P/I	Comp	CPCE	Oral	Thesis	Port.
							88/325/400					

School Counseling
WA Eastern Washington University Cheney *Contact:* Dr. Sarah Leverett

Fin Aid	GPA	GRE	MAT	Wrk Exp	Letters	Intrvw	Hours C/P/I	Comp	CPCE	Oral	Thesis	Port.
							//					

School Counseling
WA Seattle University Seattle *Contact:* Hutch Haney

Fin Aid	GPA	GRE	MAT	Wrk Exp	Letters	Intrvw	Hours C/P/I	Comp	CPCE	Oral	Thesis	Port.
	3.00			500hr	2	Y	/80/520	Y				Y

School Counseling
WA University of Puget Sound Tacoma *Contact:* Grace Kirchner; kirchner@ups.edu

Fin Aid	GPA	GRE	MAT	Wrk Exp	Letters	Intrvw	Hours C/P/I	Comp	CPCE	Oral	Thesis	Port.
	3.00	1500			2	Y	48/32/400	Y		Y		

School Counseling
WA Western Washington University Bellingham *Contact:* Arleen Lewis; Arleen.Lewis@wwu.edu

Fin Aid	GPA	GRE	MAT	Wrk Exp	Letters	Intrvw	Hours C/P/I	Comp	CPCE	Oral	Thesis	Port.
Y	3.00	R		0	3	Y	/100/600	Y				

School Counseling
WI University of Wisconsin-Oshkosh Oshkosh *Contact:* Robert Urofsky; urofsky@uwosh.edu

Fin Aid	GPA	GRE	MAT	Wrk Exp	Letters	Intrvw	Hours C/P/I	Comp	CPCE	Oral	Thesis	Port.
Y	3.00			2	2	Y	48/100/600					Y

School Counseling
WI University of Wisconsin-Whitewater Whitewater

Fin Aid	GPA	GRE	MAT	Wrk Exp	Letters	Intrvw	Hours C/P/I	Comp	CPCE	Oral	Thesis	Port.
	2.75				2	Y	48/100/640					

School Counseling
WV West Virginia University Morgantown *Contact:* Ed Jacobs; ed.jacobs@mail.wvu.edu

Fin Aid	GPA	GRE	MAT	Wrk Exp	Letters	Intrvw	Hours C/P/I	Comp	CPCE	Oral	Thesis	Port.
Y	2.80	900		0	3	Y	51/100/600					

School Counseling
WY University of Wyoming Laramie *Contact:* Mary Alice Bruce and Michael Smith; mabruce@uwyo.edu

Fin Aid	GPA	GRE	MAT	Wrk Exp	Letters	Intrvw	Hours C/P/I	Comp	CPCE	Oral	Thesis	Port.
Y	3.00			2	3	Y	48/100/600	Y				

Student Affairs
CA California Lutheran University Thousand Oaks

Fin Aid	GPA	GRE	MAT	Wrk Exp	Letters	Intrvw	Hours C/P/I	Comp	CPCE	Oral	Thesis	Port.
	3.00	900			3	Y	38/150/150					

Student Affairs
CA California State University-Fresno Fresno *Contact:* Sarah Lam; renees@csufresno.edu

Fin Aid	GPA	GRE	MAT	Wrk Exp	Letters	Intrvw	Hours C/P/I	Comp	CPCE	Oral	Thesis	Port.
Y	2.75						//					

Master's Degree Programs

| | Admission Requirements | | | | | | Graduation Requirements | | | | | |
| | GPA | GRE | MAT | Wrk Exp | Letters | Intrvw | Hours C/P/I | Comp | CPCE | Oral | Thesis | Port. |
Fin Aid												

Student Affairs
CA San Jose University San Jose

| | | | | | | | 48//400 | | | | Y | |

Student Affairs
CO University of Colorado - Colorado Springs Colorado Springs *Contact:* Beverly Snyder; bsnyder@uccs.edu

| Y | 2.75 | | | | | Y | 49/100/600 | Y | | | | Y |

Student Affairs
DE University of Delaware Newark *Contact:* John Bishop; John.Bishop@udel.edu

| Y | 2.50 | 1050 | | | 3 | Y | 48/210/420 | | | | | |

Student Affairs
IA The University of Iowa Iowa City *Contact:* Elizabeth Whitt; elizabeth-whitt@uiowa.edu

| Y | 3.00 | 1000 | | 1 | 3 | Y | 48/100/600 | | | | | |

Student Affairs
ID Idaho State University Pocatello *Contact:* Dr Don Paulson; Pauldona@isu.edu

| Y | 3.00 | | 42 | | 3 | Y | 48/150/600 | | | Y | | |

Student Affairs
IN Indiana State University Terre Haute

| Y | 2.50 | 1455 | | | 3 | Y | 48/100/600 | | | | | |

Student Affairs
IN Purdue University West Lafayette *Contact:* Deborah J. Taub; dtaub@purdue.edu

| | 3.00 | 1000 | | | 3 | | 42/100/200 | | | | | |

Student Affairs
KS Kansas State University Manhattan *Contact:* Dr. Adrienne Leslie-Toogood-; atoogood@ksu.edu

| Y | 3.00 | 1000 | 50 | | 3 | | 39/50/160 | | | | | |

Student Affairs
KY Western Kentucky University Bowling Green *Contact:* Aaron Hughey

| | 2.75 | | | | 2 | | 48/100/600 | | | | | |

Student Affairs
LA Northwestern State University Natchitoches *Contact:* Robert Bowman; bowmanr@nsula.edu

| Y | 2.50 | 800 | | 0 | 3 | Y | 48/100/600 | | | | | |

Student Affairs
MA Bridgewater State College Bridgewater *Contact:* Dr. Michael Kocet; mkocet@bridgew.edu

| | 2.80 | 1000 | | 0 | 3 | Y | 48/100/600 | Y | | | | |

Student Affairs
MN Minnesota State University, Mankato Mankato *Contact:* Anne Blackhurst & Jacqueline Lewis; anne.blackhurst@mnsu.edu

| Y | 3.00 | 1350 | | | 3 | Y | 50/100/600 | | | | | Y |

Student Affairs
MO Truman State University Kirksville *Contact:* Michael Mann, Ph.D.; mmann@truman.edu

| Y | 3.00 | 50th% | | 0 | 3 | | 48/150/600 | | | Y | | |

Student Affairs
MO University of Missouri-Columbia Columbia *Contact:* Glenn Good; GoodG@missouri.edu

| | 3.00 | 1000 | | | 3 | | 48// | | | | | |

Master's Degree Programs

| | Admission Requirements | | | | | | Graduation Requirements | | | | | |
Fin Aid	GPA	GRE	MAT	Wrk Exp	Letters	Intrvw	Hours C/P/I	Comp	CPCE	Oral	Thesis	Port.

Student Affairs
MS Mississippi State University   Mississippi State University   *Contact:* Dr. Mari Ann Callais; mcallais@colled.msstate.edu

Fin Aid	GPA	GRE	MAT	Wrk Exp	Letters	Intrvw	Hours C/P/I	Comp	CPCE	Oral	Thesis	Port.
Y	2.75	1200			3		48/100/600		Y			

Student Affairs
NC Appalachian State University   Boone   *Contact:* Cathy Clark

Fin Aid	GPA	GRE	MAT	Wrk Exp	Letters	Intrvw	Hours C/P/I	Comp	CPCE	Oral	Thesis	Port.
Y	R	R			3		48/100/600					

Student Affairs
NC The University of North Carolina at Greensboro   Greensboro

Fin Aid	GPA	GRE	MAT	Wrk Exp	Letters	Intrvw	Hours C/P/I	Comp	CPCE	Oral	Thesis	Port.
Y	3.00	R			3		48/120+/600	Y				

Student Affairs
NE University of Nebraska-Omaha   Omaha   *Contact:* Dept. Chair

Fin Aid	GPA	GRE	MAT	Wrk Exp	Letters	Intrvw	Hours C/P/I	Comp	CPCE	Oral	Thesis	Port.
	3.00		35		3	Y	48//600					

Student Affairs
NE Wayne State College   Wayne   *Contact:* Keith Willis; kewilli1@wsc.edu

Fin Aid	GPA	GRE	MAT	Wrk Exp	Letters	Intrvw	Hours C/P/I	Comp	CPCE	Oral	Thesis	Port.
		1050		0	2	Y	36/100/600					Y

Student Affairs
NV University of Nevada   Reno   *Contact:* Mary Maples; maples@unr.edu

Fin Aid	GPA	GRE	MAT	Wrk Exp	Letters	Intrvw	Hours C/P/I	Comp	CPCE	Oral	Thesis	Port.
Y	3.00	750		2	3		60/100/600		Y			

Student Affairs
NY Canisius College   Buffalo   *Contact:* Sandra Estanek

Fin Aid	GPA	GRE	MAT	Wrk Exp	Letters	Intrvw	Hours C/P/I	Comp	CPCE	Oral	Thesis	Port.
	2.50	1300				Y	36//500					

Student Affairs
NY Syracuse University   Syracuse   *Contact:* Janine Bernard; bernard@syr.edu

Fin Aid	GPA	GRE	MAT	Wrk Exp	Letters	Intrvw	Hours C/P/I	Comp	CPCE	Oral	Thesis	Port.
Y	3.00	NA		1	3	Y	48/100/600		Y			Y

Student Affairs
OH Youngstown State University   Youngstown

Fin Aid	GPA	GRE	MAT	Wrk Exp	Letters	Intrvw	Hours C/P/I	Comp	CPCE	Oral	Thesis	Port.
Y		same				Y	36/200/600					

Student Affairs
PA Kutztown University   Kutztown   *Contact:* Kelley Kenney; kenney@kutztown.edu

Fin Aid	GPA	GRE	MAT	Wrk Exp	Letters	Intrvw	Hours C/P/I	Comp	CPCE	Oral	Thesis	Port.
	3.00	1200			3	Y	48//500					

Student Affairs
PA Shippensburg University of PA   Shippensburg   *Contact:* Thomas Hozman; tlhozm@ship.edu

Fin Aid	GPA	GRE	MAT	Wrk Exp	Letters	Intrvw	Hours C/P/I	Comp	CPCE	Oral	Thesis	Port.
Y	2.75	800		1	3	Y	48/150/600					Y

Student Affairs
PA West Chester University   West Chester   *Contact:* Dr. Angelo Gadaleto; Agadaleto@wcupa.edu

Fin Aid	GPA	GRE	MAT	Wrk Exp	Letters	Intrvw	Hours C/P/I	Comp	CPCE	Oral	Thesis	Port.
Y	3.00				3		48/360/					Y

Student Affairs
SC Clemson University   Clemson

Fin Aid	GPA	GRE	MAT	Wrk Exp	Letters	Intrvw	Hours C/P/I	Comp	CPCE	Oral	Thesis	Port.
	3.00	1250			2		48/100/600		Y			

Student Affairs
SD South Dakota State University   Brookings   *Contact:* Ruth Harper; Ruth_Harper@sdstate.edu

Fin Aid	GPA	GRE	MAT	Wrk Exp	Letters	Intrvw	Hours C/P/I	Comp	CPCE	Oral	Thesis	Port.
Y	3.00				2	Y	48/100/600			Y		

Student Affairs
SD The University of South Dakota   Vermillion   *Contact:* Frank Main; fmain@usd.edu

Fin Aid	GPA	GRE	MAT	Wrk Exp	Letters	Intrvw	Hours C/P/I	Comp	CPCE	Oral	Thesis	Port.
	3.00	900			3		51/45/600	Y				

Master's Degree Programs												
	Admission Requirements						Graduation Requirements					
Fin				Wrk			Hours	Examinations				
Aid	GPA	GRE	MAT	Exp	Letters	Intrvw	C/P/I	Comp	CPCE	Oral	Thesis	Port.

Student Affairs
　　TX Texas A & M University - Commerce   Commerce   *Contact:* Dr. Chester Robinson;
　　Chester_Robinson@tamu-commerce.edu

Y					3		48/100/600					

Student Affairs
　　VA Old Dominion University   Norfolk   *Contact:* Christopher Lovell; clovell@odu.edu

Y	3.00	R			3		48/100/600		Y			

Student Affairs
　　VA Radford University   Radford   *Contact:* Paul Harris; pharris@radford.edu

	2.75	900	45		2		48/100/600					

Student Affairs
　　WI University of Wisconsin-La Crosse   LaCrosse   *Contact:* Larry J. Ringgenberg, Ph.D.;
　　　　Ringgenb.larr@uwlax.edu

Y	2.85	NR		0	3	Y	38/140/210				Y	

Student Affairs
　　WI University of Wisconsin-Oshkosh   Oshkosh   *Contact:* M. Alan Saginak; saginak@uwosh.edu

Y	3.00			2	2	Y	48/100/600					Y

Student Affairs
　　WI University of Wisconsin-Whitewater   Whitewater

	2.75				2	Y	48/100/640					

Student Affairs
　　WY University of Wyoming   Laramie   *Contact:* Deborah L. McGriff; mcgriff@uwyo.edu

Y	3.00			2	3	Y	48/100/600					

				Specialist Degree Programs								
	Admission Requirements						Graduation Requirements					
Fin				Wrk			Hours		Examinations			
Aid	GPA	GRE	MAT	Exp	Letters	Intrvw	C/P/I	Comp	CPCE	Oral	Thesis	Port.

Career Counseling
MO University of Missouri-Columbia   Columbia

		1000					30/same/	Y				

College Counseling
MS Mississippi State University   Mississippi State University   *Contact:* Dr. Mari Ann Callais;
mcallais@colled.msstate.edu

Y	3.3	1400					78/100/600	Y				

College Counseling
NY New York University   New York   *Contact:* Samuel Juni; sam.juni@nyu.edu

Y							30//					Y

Community Counseling
AL The University of Alabama   Tuscaloosa   *Contact:* S. Allen Wilcoxon, Ed.D.; awilcoxo@bamaed.ua.edu

Y		1000 (V+Q)					30//300					Y

Community Counseling
GA Georgia State University   Atlanta   *Contact:* Gary L. Arthur, Ed.D.; garthur@gsu.edu

Y		900					30/300/NA					Y

Community Counseling
GA State University of West Georgia   Carrolton   *Contact:* Dr. Snow

Y		900					27//VAR			Y		

Community Counseling
ID University of Idaho   Moscow   *Contact:* Dr. Dianne Phillips-Miller

							72/100/500			Y		Y

Community Counseling
KS Pittsburg State University   Pittsburg   *Contact:* Donald Ward; dward@pittstate.edu

Y		1200					30//					

Community Counseling
LA Louisiana State University   Baton Rouge   *Contact:* Gary G. Gintner, Ph.D.; gintner@lsu.edu

Y		1000					60//300	Y				

Community Counseling
MA Lesley University   Cambridge   *Contact:* Yishiuan Chin (617) 349-8339; (800) 999-1959 ext. 8339

Y							36//600					

Community Counseling
MD Johns Hopkins University   Baltimore   *Contact:* Fred Hanna; fhanna@jhu.edu

Y							30//300					

Community Counseling
MO University of Missouri-Columbia   Columbia

		1000					30/one practicum course: hours in consultation with advisor/	Y				

Community Counseling
MS Mississippi State University   Mississippi State University   *Contact:* Dr. Joan Looby;
jlooby@colled.msstate.edu

Y	3.3	1400					90/100/600	Y				

Specialist Degree Programs

Fin Aid	GPA	GRE	MAT	Wrk Exp	Letters	Intrvw	Hours C/P/I	Comp	CPCE	Oral	Thesis	Port.

Community Counseling
NC The University of North Carolina at Greensboro   Greensboro   *Contact:* For all programs in all tracks contact the Departmental admissions office at ced@uncg.edu or (336) 334-3434

| Y | 3.0 | R | | | 3 | | 66/120+/600 | Y | | | | |

Community Counseling
NV University of Nevada   Reno   *Contact:* Thomas Harrison; tch@unr.edu

| Y | | 750 | | | | | MA+35//600 | Y | Y | | Y | |

Community Counseling
NY New York University   New York   *Contact:* Samuel Juni; sam.juni@nyu.edu

| Y | | | | | | | 30// | | | | | Y |

Community Counseling
NY Syracuse University   Syracuse   *Contact:* Janine Bernard; bernard@syr.edu

| Y | | NA | | | | | 60 to include M.A.// | | | | | |

Community Counseling
NY University of Rochester   Rochester

| Y | | NR | | | | | at least 12// | | | | | |

Community Counseling
PA Arcadia University   Glenside   *Contact:* Mrs. Carol Lyman

| Y | | R | | | | | 12// | | | | | |

Community Counseling
PA Duquesne University   Pittsburgh   *Contact:* Nicholas J. Hanna; Hannan@duq.edu

| Y | | | | | | | 78/125/600 | | | Y | | Y |

Community Counseling
VA Regent University   Virginia Beach   *Contact:* Dr. Kathleen Arveson; kathy@arveson.com

| Y | | 1000 | | | | | 30/600/600 | | | | | |

Gerontologicial Counseling
NC The University of North Carolina at Greensboro   Greensboro

| Y | | R | | | | | 66/120+/600 | Y | | | | |

Marriage and Family Counseling
KS Pittsburg State University   Pittsburg   *Contact:* Robert Sheverbush; rsheverb@pittstate.edu

| Y | | 1200 | | | | | 30// | | | | | |

Marriage and Family Counseling
PA Duquesne University   Pittsburgh   *Contact:* Paul M. Bernstein; BernsteinP@duq.edu

| Y | | | | | | | 78/125/600 | | | Y | | Y |

Mental Health Counseling
FL Florida Atlantic University   Boca Raton   *Contact:* Dr. Alex Miranda; amiranda@fau.edu

| Y | 3.5 | 1000 | | | | Y | 33/33+/ | | | | | |

Mental Health Counseling
FL University of Florida   Gainesville   *Contact:* M. Harry Daniels

| | | 1000 | | | | | 72/400/600 | | | Y | | |

Mental Health Counseling
IN Indiana University   Bloomington   *Contact:* Dr. Sue Whiston; swhiston@indiana.edu

| Y | | 1300 | | | | | 65/100/900 | Y | | | | |

	Specialist Degree Programs											
	Admission Requirements							Graduation Requirements				
Fin Aid	GPA	GRE	MAT	Wrk Exp	Letters	Intrvw	Hours C/P/I	Comp	CPCE	Oral	Thesis	Port.

Mental Health Counseling
MA Bridgewater State College Bridgewater

		1000					//					

Mental Health Counseling
MA Lesley University Cambridge *Contact:* Yishiuan Chin (617) 349-8339; (800) 999-1959 ext. 8339

Y							36//600					

Mental Health Counseling
MA Suffolk University Boston *Contact:* Dr. Glen Eskedal; gesekedal@suffolk.edu

Y		R					30//600					

Mental Health Counseling
NC The University of North Carolina at Greensboro Greensboro

Y	3.0	R			3		66/120+/600	Y				

Mental Health Counseling
RI Rhode Island College Providence *Contact:* M. Finley

		900					36/225/600				Y	

Other
MA Lesley University Cambridge *Contact:* Yishiuan Chin (617) 349-8339; (800) 999-1959 ext. 8339

Y							//					

Other
MO University of Missouri-Columbia Columbia

		1000					30/same/	Y				

Other
NC East Carolina University Greenville

		1350					30//	Y				

Other – School Psychology
TN Middle Tennessee State University Murfreesboro *Contact:* James O. Rust

Y		900					30/100/1200	Y			Y	

Pastoral Counseling
MD Loyola College in Maryland Columbia

Y							same/same/same					

Rehabilitation Counseling
AL The University of Alabama Tuscaloosa *Contact:* Jamie F. Satcher, Ph.D.; jsatcher@bamaed.ua.edu

Y		1000 (V+Q)					30//300					Y

Rehabilitation Counseling
ID University of Idaho Moscow, ID

							72//	Y				

Rehabilitation Counseling
MO University of Missouri-Columbia Columbia

		1000					30/same/	Y				

Rehabilitation Counseling
MS Mississippi State University Mississippi State University *Contact:* Dr. Glen Hendren; glen@ra.msstate.edu

Y	3.3	1400					78/100/600	Y				

Specialist Degree Programs												
	Admission Requirements							Graduation Requirements				
Fin Aid	GPA	GRE	MAT	Wrk Exp	Letters	Intrvw	Hours C/P/I	Comp	CPCE	Oral	Thesis	Port.

School Counseling

AL The University of Alabama   Tuscaloosa   *Contact:* Karla D. Carmichael, Ph.D.; kcarmich@bamaed.ua.edu

Fin Aid	GPA	GRE	MAT	Wrk Exp	Letters	Intrvw	Hours C/P/I	Comp	CPCE	Oral	Thesis	Port.
Y		1000 (V+Q)					30//300					Y

School Counseling

AL University of South Alabama   Mobile

Fin Aid	GPA	GRE	MAT	Wrk Exp	Letters	Intrvw	Hours C/P/I	Comp	CPCE	Oral	Thesis	Port.
Y							//					

School Counseling

CA La Sierra University   Riverside   *Contact:* Lennard A. Jorgensen; ljorgens@lasierra.edu

Fin Aid	GPA	GRE	MAT	Wrk Exp	Letters	Intrvw	Hours C/P/I	Comp	CPCE	Oral	Thesis	Port.
Y		1000					/500/1200	Y				Y

School Counseling

FL Florida Atlantic University   Boca Raton   *Contact:* Dr. Greg Brigman; gbrigman@fau.edu

Fin Aid	GPA	GRE	MAT	Wrk Exp	Letters	Intrvw	Hours C/P/I	Comp	CPCE	Oral	Thesis	Port.
Y	3.5	1000					33/33+/					Y

School Counseling

FL University of Central Florida   Orlando   *Contact:* B. Grant Hayes; ghayes@mail.ucf.edu

Fin Aid	GPA	GRE	MAT	Wrk Exp	Letters	Intrvw	Hours C/P/I	Comp	CPCE	Oral	Thesis	Port.
		1000					48/150/600		Y			Y

School Counseling

FL University of Florida   Gainesville   *Contact:* M. Harry Daniels

Fin Aid	GPA	GRE	MAT	Wrk Exp	Letters	Intrvw	Hours C/P/I	Comp	CPCE	Oral	Thesis	Port.
		1000					72/300/600			Y		

School Counseling

GA Columbus State University   Columbus

Fin Aid	GPA	GRE	MAT	Wrk Exp	Letters	Intrvw	Hours C/P/I	Comp	CPCE	Oral	Thesis	Port.
		800					30//VAR					

School Counseling

GA Georgia State University   Atlanta   *Contact:* Fran Mullis, Ph.D.

Fin Aid	GPA	GRE	MAT	Wrk Exp	Letters	Intrvw	Hours C/P/I	Comp	CPCE	Oral	Thesis	Port.
Y		900					30/300/NA					Y

School Counseling

GA State University of West Georgia   Carrolton   *Contact:* Dr. Snow

Fin Aid	GPA	GRE	MAT	Wrk Exp	Letters	Intrvw	Hours C/P/I	Comp	CPCE	Oral	Thesis	Port.
Y		900					27//VAR			Y		

School Counseling

ID University of Idaho   Moscow, ID

Fin Aid	GPA	GRE	MAT	Wrk Exp	Letters	Intrvw	Hours C/P/I	Comp	CPCE	Oral	Thesis	Port.
							72//	Y				

School Counseling

KS Pittsburg State University   Pittsburg   *Contact:* Becky Brannock; rbrannoc@pittstate.edu

Fin Aid	GPA	GRE	MAT	Wrk Exp	Letters	Intrvw	Hours C/P/I	Comp	CPCE	Oral	Thesis	Port.
Y		1200					30//					

School Counseling

LA Louisiana State University   Baton Rouge   *Contact:* David A. Spruill, Ph.D.; dspruill@lsu.edu

Fin Aid	GPA	GRE	MAT	Wrk Exp	Letters	Intrvw	Hours C/P/I	Comp	CPCE	Oral	Thesis	Port.
Y		1000					60//300	Y				

School Counseling

MA Lesley University   Cambridge   *Contact:* Yishiuan Chin (617) 349-8339; (800) 999-1959 ext. 8339

Fin Aid	GPA	GRE	MAT	Wrk Exp	Letters	Intrvw	Hours C/P/I	Comp	CPCE	Oral	Thesis	Port.
Y							indiv./ 100/600					

School Counseling

MA Suffolk University   Boston

Fin Aid	GPA	GRE	MAT	Wrk Exp	Letters	Intrvw	Hours C/P/I	Comp	CPCE	Oral	Thesis	Port.
Y		R					30//600					Y

	Specialist Degree Programs											
	Admission Requirements							Graduation Requirements				
Fin Aid	GPA	GRE	MAT	Wrk Exp	Letters	Intrvw	Hours C/P/I	Comp	Examinations CPCE	Oral	Thesis	Port.

School Counseling
MO University of Missouri-Columbia   Columbia

		1000					30/same/	Y				

School Counseling
MS Mississippi College   Clinton   *Contact:* Edith Carlisle; carlisle@mc.edu

Y		Praxis					36/100/300			Y		

School Counseling
MS Mississippi State University   Mississippi State University   *Contact:* Dr. Joe Ray Underwood
joeray@colled.msstate.edu

Y	3.3	1400					78/100/600	Y				

School Counseling
NC The University of North Carolina at Greensboro   Greensboro

Y	3.0	R		3			66/120+/600	Y				

School Counseling
NV University of Nevada   Reno   *Contact:* Jill Packman; packman@unr.edu

Y		750					MA+35/ /600	Y	Y		Y	

School Counseling
NY College at Oswego SUNY   Oswego   *Contact:* Dr. Jean Casey; casey@oswego.edu

Y		1000					60/200/300	Y	Y		Y	

School Counseling
NY New York University   New York   *Contact:* Samuel Juni; sam.juni@nyu.edu

Y							30//					Y

School Counseling
NY Plattsburgh State University   Plattsburgh   *Contact:* Dr. Rachelle Perusse;
rachelle.perusse@plattsburgh.edu

Y		25th %tile					60/115/600	Y	Y			

School Counseling
NY State University of New York at Oneonta   Oneonta   *Contact:* Emily Phillips; phillie@oneonta.edu

							27//600					

School Counseling
NY Syracuse University   Syracuse   *Contact:* Janna Scarborough; scarboro@syr.edu

Y		NA					60//					

School Counseling
NY University of Rochester   Rochester

Y		NR					at least 12//					

School Counseling
PA Duquesne University   Pittsburgh   *Contact:* William J. Casile; Casile@duq.edu

Y							78/125/600			Y		Y

School Counseling
RI Rhode Island College   Providence   *Contact:* M. Finley

		900					36/225/600			Y		

School Counseling
TN The University of Tennessee at Knoxville   Knoxville

		1000					70//					

Specialist Degree Programs

Fin Aid	GPA	GRE	MAT	Wrk Exp	Letters	Intrvw	Hours C/P/I	Comp	CPCE	Oral	Thesis	Port.
	Admission Requirements							Graduation Requirements				
								Examinations				

School Counseling

VA Regent University   Virginia Beach   *Contact:* Dr. Kathleen Arveson; kathy@arveson.com

Fin Aid	GPA	GRE	MAT	Wrk Exp	Letters	Intrvw	Hours C/P/I	Comp	CPCE	Oral	Thesis	Port.
Y		1000					30/100/600					

Student Affairs

MO University of Missouri-Columbia   Columbia

Fin Aid	GPA	GRE	MAT	Wrk Exp	Letters	Intrvw	Hours C/P/I	Comp	CPCE	Oral	Thesis	Port.
		1000					30/same/	Y				

Student Affairs

MS Mississippi State University   Mississippi State University   *Contact:* Dr. Mari Ann Callais; mcallais@colled.msstate.edu

Fin Aid	GPA	GRE	MAT	Wrk Exp	Letters	Intrvw	Hours C/P/I	Comp	CPCE	Oral	Thesis	Port.
Y	3.3	1400					78/100/600	Y				

Student Affairs

NC The University of North Carolina at Greensboro   Greensboro

Fin Aid	GPA	GRE	MAT	Wrk Exp	Letters	Intrvw	Hours C/P/I	Comp	CPCE	Oral	Thesis	Port.
Y	3.0	R		3			66/120+/600	Y				

Student Affairs

NV University of Nevada   Reno   *Contact:* Mary Maples; maples@unr.edu

Fin Aid	GPA	GRE	MAT	Wrk Exp	Letters	Intrvw	Hours C/P/I	Comp	CPCE	Oral	Thesis	Port.
Y		750					MA+35//600	Y	Y		Y	

Student Affairs

NY Syracuse University   Syracuse   *Contact:* Janine Bernard; bernard@syr.edu

Fin Aid	GPA	GRE	MAT	Wrk Exp	Letters	Intrvw	Hours C/P/I	Comp	CPCE	Oral	Thesis	Port.
Y		NA					60//					

Doctoral Degree Programs												
	Admission Requirements						Graduation Requirements					
Fin Aid	GPA	GRE	MAT	Wrk Exp	Letters	Intrvw	Hours C/P/I	Comp	CPCE	Oral	Thesis	Port.

Addictions Counseling
NV University of Nevada Reno *Contact:* Thomas Harrison; tch@unr.edu

Fin Aid	GPA	GRE	MAT	Wrk Exp	Letters	Intrvw	Hours C/P/I	Comp	CPCE	Oral	Thesis	Port.
Y	M3.50	1000		2	3	1	100//600	Y	Y	Y	Y	

Career Counseling
MI Oakland University Rochester *Contact:* blume@oakland.edu

Fin Aid	GPA	GRE	MAT	Wrk Exp	Letters	Intrvw	Hours C/P/I	Comp	CPCE	Oral	Thesis	Port.
Y	M3.60	R		2	1		82/100/600	Y			Y	

Community Counseling
MI Oakland University Rochester *Contact:* blume@oakland.edu

Fin Aid	GPA	GRE	MAT	Wrk Exp	Letters	Intrvw	Hours C/P/I	Comp	CPCE	Oral	Thesis	Port.
Y	M3.60	R		2	1		82/100/600	Y			Y	

Community Counseling
NC University of North Carolina at Charlotte Charlotte *Contact:* Robert Barret; rlbarret@email.uncc.edu

Fin Aid	GPA	GRE	MAT	Wrk Exp	Letters	Intrvw	Hours C/P/I	Comp	CPCE	Oral	Thesis	Port.
Y	MR	R	yes	0	3	1	57/150/600	Y		Y	Y	

Community Counseling
NV University of Nevada Reno *Contact:* Thomas Harrison; tch@unr.edu

Fin Aid	GPA	GRE	MAT	Wrk Exp	Letters	Intrvw	Hours C/P/I	Comp	CPCE	Oral	Thesis	Port.
Y	M3.50	1000		2	3	1	100//600	Y	Y	Y	Y	

Community Counseling
OH The University of Toledo Toledo *Contact:* Nick Piazza; nick.piazza@utoledo.edu

Fin Aid	GPA	GRE	MAT	Wrk Exp	Letters	Intrvw	Hours C/P/I	Comp	CPCE	Oral	Thesis	Port.
Y	M3.00	1040		2	3	1	96/100/600	Y			Y	Y

Community Counseling
VA George Mason University Fairfax *Contact:* Dr. Rita Chi-Ying Chung; rchung@gmu.edu

Fin Aid	GPA	GRE	MAT	Wrk Exp	Letters	Intrvw	Hours C/P/I	Comp	CPCE	Oral	Thesis	Port.
Y	M3.00	1000			3	1	55-85/ 200/200	Y	Y	Y		

Counselor Education
AL Auburn University Auburn *Contact:* Jamie Carney; carneyjs@auburn.edu

Fin Aid	GPA	GRE	MAT	Wrk Exp	Letters	Intrvw	Hours C/P/I	Comp	CPCE	Oral	Thesis	Port.
Y	M	1000		0	3	1	50 Post-master's/ 100/600			Y	Y	Y

Counselor Education
AL The University of Alabama Tuscaloosa *Contact:* S. Allen Wilcoxon, Ed.D.; awilcoxo@bamaed.ua.edu

Fin Aid	GPA	GRE	MAT	Wrk Exp	Letters	Intrvw	Hours C/P/I	Comp	CPCE	Oral	Thesis	Port.
Y	M3.00	1000	50	1	3	1	72/300/600	Y			Y	

Counselor Education
CO University of Northern Colorado Greeley *Contact:* Tracy Baldo; tracy.baldo@unco.edu

Fin Aid	GPA	GRE	MAT	Wrk Exp	Letters	Intrvw	Hours C/P/I	Comp	CPCE	Oral	Thesis	Port.
Y	M3.25	1000			3	1	89/1270+/ 1200	Y			Y	Y

Counselor Education
DC The George Washington University Washington, D. C. *Contact:* Richard Lanthier, Ph.D.; lanthier@gwu.edu

Fin Aid	GPA	GRE	MAT	Wrk Exp	Letters	Intrvw	Hours C/P/I	Comp	CPCE	Oral	Thesis	Port.
Y	M3.50	1000		2	3	1	69/300/600	Y			Y	Y

Counselor Education
FL University of Central Florida Orlando *Contact:* E.H. Mike Robinson, III

Fin Aid	GPA	GRE	MAT	Wrk Exp	Letters	Intrvw	Hours C/P/I	Comp	CPCE	Oral	Thesis	Port.
	M3.00	1000		0	3	1	84/300/900	Y			Y	Y

Counselor Education
GA Georgia State University Atlanta *Contact:* Roy M. Kern, Ed.D.; rkern@gsu.edu

Fin Aid	GPA	GRE	MAT	Wrk Exp	Letters	Intrvw	Hours C/P/I	Comp	CPCE	Oral	Thesis	Port.
Y	M3.25	1000	NA	1	3	1	97/360/600	Y			Y	Y

Doctoral Degree Programs

Fin Aid	Admission Requirements: GPA	GRE	MAT	Wrk Exp	Letters	Intrvw	Graduation Requirements: Hours C/P/I	Examinations: Comp	CPCE	Oral	Thesis	Port.
Counselor Education — IA The University of Iowa Iowa City *Contact:* David A.Jepsen; david-jepsen-@uiowa.edu												
Y	M3.00	1100			3	1	96/180/600	Y		Y	Y	
Counselor Education — ID Idaho State University Pocatello *Contact:* Dr Stephen Feit; Feitstep@isu.edu												
Y			42		3	1	96/150/1000	Y			Y	
Counselor Education — ID University of Idaho Moscow, ID *Contact:* Dr. Tom Trotter												
	M3.50	1100			3	1	124/100/500		Y		Y	
Counselor Education — IL Southern Illinois University Carbondale Carbondale *Contact:* Dr. Karen Prichard; prichard@siu.edu												
Y					3	1	80/180/600	Y			Y	
Counselor Education — KS Kansas State University Manhattan *Contact:* Dr. Fred Bradley; fbradley@ksu.edu												
Y	M3.00	1000		2	3		120/100/600	Y			Y	
Counselor Education — LA University of New Orleans New Orleans *Contact:* Dr. Diana Hulse-Killacky; dhulseki@uno.edu												
Y	M3.00	R		0	3	1	112/200/ 1200	Y	Y	Y	Y	
Counselor Education — MI Oakland University Rochester *Contact:* blume@oakland.edu												
Y	M3.60	R			2	1	82/100/600	Y			Y	
Counselor Education — MO University of Missouri - St. Louis Saint Louis *Contact:* R. Rocco Cottone, PhD; cottone@umsl.edu												
Y	M3.00	1000			3	1	110/150/600	Y		Y	Y	
Counselor Education — MS Mississippi State University Mississippi State University *Contact:* Dr. Joan Looby; jlooby@colled.msstate.edu												
Y							98//1200			Y	Y	
Counselor Education — NC The University of North Carolina at Greensboro Greensboro												
Y	M3.00	R		0	3	1	60 min/ 100/600	Y		Y	Y	
Counselor Education — NC University of North Carolina at Charlotte Charlotte *Contact:* Robert Barret; rlbarret@email.uncc.edu												
Y	MR	R	yes	0	3	1	57/150/600	Y		Y	Y	
Counselor Education — ND North Dakota State University Fargo *Contact:* Dr. Robert Nielsen; Robert.Nielsen@ndsu.nodak.edu												
Y					3	1	71+ Masters// 600	Y		Y	Y	
Counselor Education — NV University of Nevada Reno *Contact:* Marlowe Smaby; smaby@unr.edu												
Y							100//600	Y	Y	Y	Y	
Counselor Education — NY SUNY University at Buffalo Buffalo *Contact:* Dr. T.T. Frantz												
	M			1	3	1	90/500/	Y			Y	

Doctoral Degree Programs

Fin Aid	GPA	GRE	MAT	Wrk Exp	Letters	Intrvw	Hours C/P/I	Comp	CPCE	Oral	Thesis	Port.

Counselor Education
NY Syracuse University   Syracuse   *Contact:* Harold (Dick) Hackney; hackney@syr.edu

Fin Aid	GPA	GRE	MAT	Wrk Exp	Letters	Intrvw	Hours C/P/I	Comp	CPCE	Oral	Thesis	Port.
Y	M3.50			1	3	1	102/100/600	Y		Y	Y	

Counselor Education
NY University of Rochester   Rochester   *Contact:* Howard Kirschenbaum; Howard.Kirschenbaum@rochester.edu

Fin Aid	GPA	GRE	MAT	Wrk Exp	Letters	Intrvw	Hours C/P/I	Comp	CPCE	Oral	Thesis	Port.
Y	Mno spec.	NR	not req.	2	3 video tape interview possible	1	96/100/600	Y			Y	

Counselor Education
OH Kent State University   Kent   *Contact:* Dr. John West; jwest@kent.edu

Fin Aid	GPA	GRE	MAT	Wrk Exp	Letters	Intrvw	Hours C/P/I	Comp	CPCE	Oral	Thesis	Port.
Y	M3.50			0	3	1	110//600	Y		Y	Y	

Counselor Education
OH Ohio University   Athens   *Contact:* Tom Davis

Fin Aid	GPA	GRE	MAT	Wrk Exp	Letters	Intrvw	Hours C/P/I	Comp	CPCE	Oral	Thesis	Port.
Y	M	1000			3	1	//720	Y			Y	

Counselor Education
OH University of Cincinnati   Cincinnati   *Contact:* Ellen Cook; ellen.cook@uc.edu

Fin Aid	GPA	GRE	MAT	Wrk Exp	Letters	Intrvw	Hours C/P/I	Comp	CPCE	Oral	Thesis	Port.
Y	M3.20	1500		1	3	1	/1000/600	Y		Y	Y	Y

Counselor Education
OR Oregon State University   Corvallis   *Contact:* Cass Dykeman

Fin Aid	GPA	GRE	MAT	Wrk Exp	Letters	Intrvw	Hours C/P/I	Comp	CPCE	Oral	Thesis	Port.
Y	M3.00			0	3	1	//600	Y		Y	Y	

Counselor Education
PA Duquesne University   Pittsburgh   *Contact:* Joseph F. Maola; maola@duq.edu

Fin Aid	GPA	GRE	MAT	Wrk Exp	Letters	Intrvw	Hours C/P/I	Comp	CPCE	Oral	Thesis	Port.
Y	M3.25	1800		2	3	1	67/150/600	Y		Y	Y	

Counselor Education
PA Penn State University   University Park

Fin Aid	GPA	GRE	MAT	Wrk Exp	Letters	Intrvw	Hours C/P/I	Comp	CPCE	Oral	Thesis	Port.
							//					

Counselor Education
SC University of South Carolina   Columbia   *Contact:* Josh Gold, PhD

Fin Aid	GPA	GRE	MAT	Wrk Exp	Letters	Intrvw	Hours C/P/I	Comp	CPCE	Oral	Thesis	Port.
Y	M3.00	800		2	2	1	96/300/900			Y	Y	

Counselor Education
SD The University of South Dakota   Vermillion   *Contact:* Frank Main, Chair CPE; fmain@usd.edu

Fin Aid	GPA	GRE	MAT	Wrk Exp	Letters	Intrvw	Hours C/P/I	Comp	CPCE	Oral	Thesis	Port.
	M3.40	1500			5	1	/90/600	Y		Y	Y	

Counselor Education
TN The University of Tennessee at Knoxville   Knoxville

Fin Aid	GPA	GRE	MAT	Wrk Exp	Letters	Intrvw	Hours C/P/I	Comp	CPCE	Oral	Thesis	Port.
	M3.50	1100		2	3		110//					

Counselor Education
TX Texas A & M University - Commerce   Commerce   *Contact:* Dr. Richard Lampe; Richard_lampe@tamu-commerce.edu

Fin Aid	GPA	GRE	MAT	Wrk Exp	Letters	Intrvw	Hours C/P/I	Comp	CPCE	Oral	Thesis	Port.
Y	M3.50				3	1	69/300/600	Y		Y	Y	

Counselor Education
TX Texas Southern University   Houston   *Contact:* Dr. Joyce Jones; Jones_JK@tsu.edu

Fin Aid	GPA	GRE	MAT	Wrk Exp	Letters	Intrvw	Hours C/P/I	Comp	CPCE	Oral	Thesis	Port.
	M3.25	750				1	60/100/600	Y		Y	Y	

Counselor Education
TX Texas Tech University   Lubbock   *Contact:* Loretta Bradley; Loretta.Bradley@ttu.edu

Fin Aid	GPA	GRE	MAT	Wrk Exp	Letters	Intrvw	Hours C/P/I	Comp	CPCE	Oral	Thesis	Port.
Y	M3.0+	prefer avg	not req	0	3		92/100/600	Y			Y	Y

Doctoral Degree Programs

Fin Aid	GPA	GRE	MAT	Wrk Exp	Letters	Intrvw	Hours C/P/I	Comp	CPCE	Oral	Thesis	Port.

Counselor Education
TX University of North Texas   Denton   *Contact:* Cynthia Chandler; Chandler@coefs.coe.unt.edu

Fin Aid	GPA	GRE	MAT	Wrk Exp	Letters	Intrvw	Hours C/P/I	Comp	CPCE	Oral	Thesis	Port.
Y	M3.50	710			3	1	75/80/600				Y	

Counselor Education
VA College of William and Mary   Williamsburg   *Contact:* Victoria Foster; vafost@wm.edu

Fin Aid	GPA	GRE	MAT	Wrk Exp	Letters	Intrvw	Hours C/P/I	Comp	CPCE	Oral	Thesis	Port.
Y	M3.50	60%		2	3	1	63/100/600	Y		Y	Y	

Counselor Education
VA George Mason University   Fairfax   *Contact:* Dr. Fred Bemak; fbemak@gmu.edu

Fin Aid	GPA	GRE	MAT	Wrk Exp	Letters	Intrvw	Hours C/P/I	Comp	CPCE	Oral	Thesis	Port.
Y	M3.00	1000			3	1	55-85//100				Y	Y

Counselor Education
VA Regent University   Virginia Beach   *Contact:* Dr. Susan Scott; susasco@regent.edu

Fin Aid	GPA	GRE	MAT	Wrk Exp	Letters	Intrvw	Hours C/P/I	Comp	CPCE	Oral	Thesis	Port.
Y	3.50	1000	50%	0	3	1	60//				Y	

Counselor Education
VA Virginia Tech   Blacksburg

Fin Aid	GPA	GRE	MAT	Wrk Exp	Letters	Intrvw	Hours C/P/I	Comp	CPCE	Oral	Thesis	Port.
Y	M3.00			0	3	1	100//600	Y		Y	Y	

Counselor Education
WY University of Wyoming   Laramie   *Contact:* Kent W. Becker; kwbecker@uwyo.edu

Fin Aid	GPA	GRE	MAT	Wrk Exp	Letters	Intrvw	Hours C/P/I	Comp	CPCE	Oral	Thesis	Port.
Y	M3.00			2	3	1	70+//600	Y		Y	Y	

Marriage and Family Counseling
CO Denver Seminary   Denver

Fin Aid	GPA	GRE	MAT	Wrk Exp	Letters	Intrvw	Hours C/P/I	Comp	CPCE	Oral	Thesis	Port.
Y							//					

Marriage and Family Counseling
FL University of Florida   Gainesville   *Contact:* M. Harry Daniels

Fin Aid	GPA	GRE	MAT	Wrk Exp	Letters	Intrvw	Hours C/P/I	Comp	CPCE	Oral	Thesis	Port.
	M3.20	1100		0	3	1	120//1200	Y		Y	Y	

Marriage and Family Counseling
MI Oakland University   Rochester   *Contact:* blume@oakland.edu

Fin Aid	GPA	GRE	MAT	Wrk Exp	Letters	Intrvw	Hours C/P/I	Comp	CPCE	Oral	Thesis	Port.
Y	M3.60	R			2	1	82/100/600	Y			Y	

Mental Health Counseling
FL University of Florida   Gainesville   *Contact:* M. Harry Daniels

Fin Aid	GPA	GRE	MAT	Wrk Exp	Letters	Intrvw	Hours C/P/I	Comp	CPCE	Oral	Thesis	Port.
	M3.20	1100		0	3	1	120//1200	Y		Y	Y	

Mental Health Counseling
IN Indiana University   Bloomington   *Contact:* Dr. Chalmer Thompson; chathomp@indiana.edu

Fin Aid	GPA	GRE	MAT	Wrk Exp	Letters	Intrvw	Hours C/P/I	Comp	CPCE	Oral	Thesis	Port.
Y	3.00						96/150-500/2000	Y		Y	Y	

Mental Health Counseling
MI Andrews University   Berrien Springs

Fin Aid	GPA	GRE	MAT	Wrk Exp	Letters	Intrvw	Hours C/P/I	Comp	CPCE	Oral	Thesis	Port.
Y							//					

Mental Health Counseling
MI Oakland University   Rochester   *Contact:* blume@oakland.edu

Fin Aid	GPA	GRE	MAT	Wrk Exp	Letters	Intrvw	Hours C/P/I	Comp	CPCE	Oral	Thesis	Port.
Y	M3.60	R			2	1	82/100/600	Y			Y	

Other
AL Auburn University   Auburn

Fin Aid	GPA	GRE	MAT	Wrk Exp	Letters	Intrvw	Hours C/P/I	Comp	CPCE	Oral	Thesis	Port.
Y							//					

Doctoral Degree Programs												
	Admission Requirements						Graduation Requirements					
Fin Aid	GPA	GRE	MAT	Wrk Exp	Letters	Intrvw	Hours C/P/I	Comp	CPCE	Oral	Thesis	Port.

Other
IN Ball State University   Muncie   *Contact:* Lawrence Gerstein; rangzen@aol.com

Fin Aid	GPA	GRE	MAT	Wrk Exp	Letters	Intrvw	Hours C/P/I	Comp	CPCE	Oral	Thesis	Port.
Y	3.20	1000					97/400/1500	Y		Y	Y	Y

Other
MI Oakland University   Rochester

Fin Aid	GPA	GRE	MAT	Wrk Exp	Letters	Intrvw	Hours C/P/I	Comp	CPCE	Oral	Thesis	Port.
Y							//					

Other
MN Capella Uiversity   Minneapolis   *Contact:* Pamela Patrick

Fin Aid	GPA	GRE	MAT	Wrk Exp	Letters	Intrvw	Hours C/P/I	Comp	CPCE	Oral	Thesis	Port.
Y	M3.00			0			//			Y	Y	

Other
MO University of Missouri-Columbia   Columbia   *Contact:* Laurie Mintz; MintzL@missouri.edu

Fin Aid	GPA	GRE	MAT	Wrk Exp	Letters	Intrvw	Hours C/P/I	Comp	CPCE	Oral	Thesis	Port.
	M3.00	1200			3		82/400/2000			Y	Y	Y

Other
NY New York University   New York   *Contact:* Lisa Suzuki; las1@nyu.edu

Fin Aid	GPA	GRE	MAT	Wrk Exp	Letters	Intrvw	Hours C/P/I	Comp	CPCE	Oral	Thesis	Port.
Y	M	800			3	1	96//			Y	Y	

Other – Counseling Psychology
NY SUNY University at Buffalo   Buffalo   *Contact:* Dr. Scott Meier; stmeier@acsu.buffalo.edu

Fin Aid	GPA	GRE	MAT	Wrk Exp	Letters	Intrvw	Hours C/P/I	Comp	CPCE	Oral	Thesis	Port.
					3	1	90/1000/2000	Y			Y	

Other
WV West Virginia University   Morgantown

Fin Aid	GPA	GRE	MAT	Wrk Exp	Letters	Intrvw	Hours C/P/I	Comp	CPCE	Oral	Thesis	Port.
Y	M3.25	1000		1	3	1	93/600/1200	Y			Y	

Pastoral Counseling
MD Loyola College in Maryland   Columbia   *Contact:* Ralph Piedmont; RPiedmont@Loyola.edu

Fin Aid	GPA	GRE	MAT	Wrk Exp	Letters	Intrvw	Hours C/P/I	Comp	CPCE	Oral	Thesis	Port.
Y	M			2	5	1	60//1500	Y			Y	

Rehabilitation Counseling
IA The University of Iowa   Iowa City   *Contact:* Vilia Tarvydas; vilia-tarvydas@uiowa.edu

Fin Aid	GPA	GRE	MAT	Wrk Exp	Letters	Intrvw	Hours C/P/I	Comp	CPCE	Oral	Thesis	Port.
Y	M3.00	1100		1	3	1	96/180/					

Rehabilitation Counseling
IL Illinois Institute of Technology   Chicago   *Contact:* Dr. Chow S. Lam; Lam@iit.edu

Fin Aid	GPA	GRE	MAT	Wrk Exp	Letters	Intrvw	Hours C/P/I	Comp	CPCE	Oral	Thesis	Port.
Y	M3.50	1000			3	1	110/900/2000			Y	Y	

School Counseling
FL University of Florida   Gainesville   *Contact:* M. Harry Daniels

Fin Aid	GPA	GRE	MAT	Wrk Exp	Letters	Intrvw	Hours C/P/I	Comp	CPCE	Oral	Thesis	Port.
	M3.20	1100		0	3	1	120//1200			Y	Y	

School Counseling
KS Kansas State University   Manhattan   *Contact:* Dr. Ken Hughey

Fin Aid	GPA	GRE	MAT	Wrk Exp	Letters	Intrvw	Hours C/P/I	Comp	CPCE	Oral	Thesis	Port.
Y	M3.00	1000		2	3		94//300				Y	

School Counseling
MI Oakland University   Rochester   *Contact:* blume@oakland.edu

Fin Aid	GPA	GRE	MAT	Wrk Exp	Letters	Intrvw	Hours C/P/I	Comp	CPCE	Oral	Thesis	Port.
Y	M3.60	R			2	1	82/100/600				Y	

School Counseling
MS Mississippi State University   Mississippi State University   *Contact:* Dr. Joe Ray Underwood; joeray@colled.msstate.edu

Fin Aid	GPA	GRE	MAT	Wrk Exp	Letters	Intrvw	Hours C/P/I	Comp	CPCE	Oral	Thesis	Port.
Y	M3.50	1500		2	3	1	98//1200			Y	Y	

	Doctoral Degree Programs											
	Admission Requirements							Graduation Requirements				
Fin Aid	GPA	GRE	MAT	Wrk Exp	Letters	Intrvw	Hours C/P/I		Examinations			
								Comp	CPCE	Oral	Thesis	Port.

School Counseling
NC University of North Carolina at Charlotte   Charlotte   *Contact:* Robert Barret; rlbarret@email.uncc.edu

Fin Aid	GPA	GRE	MAT	Wrk Exp	Letters	Intrvw	Hours C/P/I	Comp	CPCE	Oral	Thesis	Port.
Y	MR	R	yes	0	3	1	57/150/600			Y	Y	

School Counseling
NV University of Nevada   Reno   *Contact:* Marlowe Smaby; smaby@unr.edu

Fin Aid	GPA	GRE	MAT	Wrk Exp	Letters	Intrvw	Hours C/P/I	Comp	CPCE	Oral	Thesis	Port.
Y	M3.50	1000		2	3	1	100//600	Y		Y	Y	

School Counseling
OH The University of Toledo   Toledo   *Contact:* Nick Piazza; nick.piazza@utoledo.edu

Fin Aid	GPA	GRE	MAT	Wrk Exp	Letters	Intrvw	Hours C/P/I	Comp	CPCE	Oral	Thesis	Port.
Y	M3.00	1040		2	3	1	96/100/600			Y	Y	

School Counseling
VA George Mason University   Fairfax   *Contact:* Dr. Carol Kaffenberger; ckaffenb@gmu.edu

Fin Aid	GPA	GRE	MAT	Wrk Exp	Letters	Intrvw	Hours C/P/I	Comp	CPCE	Oral	Thesis	Port.
Y	M3.00	1000			3	1	55-85/200/200				Y	Y

Student Affairs
IA The University of Iowa   Iowa City   *Contact:* Elizabeth Whitt; elizabeth-whitt@uiowa.edu

Fin Aid	GPA	GRE	MAT	Wrk Exp	Letters	Intrvw	Hours C/P/I	Comp	CPCE	Oral	Thesis	Port.
Y	M3.00	1100			3	1	96/180/600					

Student Affairs
KS Kansas State University   Manhattan   *Contact:* Dr. Doris Wright-Carroll

Fin Aid	GPA	GRE	MAT	Wrk Exp	Letters	Intrvw	Hours C/P/I	Comp	CPCE	Oral	Thesis	Port.
Y	M3.00	1000			3		120/50/160	Y			Y	

Master's and Specialist Degree Programs												
Admission and Enrollment				Postgraduation Activity/Placement Percentages								
2002				Adv	Mngd	Private	Agency	School and Student Affairs				
Admit	Grad	F	M	Ed	Care	Practice		EI	Mddle	Sec	Stu A	Other

Addictions Counseling
NC East Carolina University Greenville

Admit	Grad	F	M	Adv Ed	Mngd Care	Private Practice	Agency Practice	EI	Mddle	Sec	Stu A	Other
15	15	10	5				95					5

Addictions Counseling
NJ The College of New Jersey Ewing

Admit	Grad	F	M	Adv Ed	Mngd Care	Private Practice	Agency Practice	EI	Mddle	Sec	Stu A	Other
10	10			5			50					45

Addictions Counseling
NV University of Nevada Reno

Admit	Grad	F	M	Adv Ed	Mngd Care	Private Practice	Agency Practice	EI	Mddle	Sec	Stu A	Other
5	3	8	2	20	30	20	30					

Addictions Counseling
NY Queens College, City University of New York Flushing

Admit	Grad	F	M	Adv Ed	Mngd Care	Private Practice	Agency Practice	EI	Mddle	Sec	Stu A	Other

Addictions Counseling
RI Rhode Island College Providence

Admit	Grad	F	M	Adv Ed	Mngd Care	Private Practice	Agency Practice	EI	Mddle	Sec	Stu A	Other
10	5	6	5	0	65	0	35		0	0	0	0

Addictions Counseling
TX Houston Baptist University Houston

Admit	Grad	F	M	Adv Ed	Mngd Care	Private Practice	Agency Practice	EI	Mddle	Sec	Stu A	Other

Addictions Counseling
VA College of William and Mary Williamsburg

Admit	Grad	F	M	Adv Ed	Mngd Care	Private Practice	Agency Practice	EI	Mddle	Sec	Stu A	Other
8	6	6	2				100					

Career Counseling
CA San Jose University San Jose

Admit	Grad	F	M	Adv Ed	Mngd Care	Private Practice	Agency Practice	EI	Mddle	Sec	Stu A	Other

Career Counseling
CA University of San Diego, School of Education San Diego

Admit	Grad	F	M	Adv Ed	Mngd Care	Private Practice	Agency Practice	EI	Mddle	Sec	Stu A	Other
15	10	16	2	10		10	20				30	30 Business

Career Counseling
CO University of Colorado at Denver Denver

Admit	Grad	F	M	Adv Ed	Mngd Care	Private Practice	Agency Practice	EI	Mddle	Sec	Stu A	Other
5	0											

Career Counseling
MO University of Missouri - St. Louis Saint Louis

Admit	Grad	F	M	Adv Ed	Mngd Care	Private Practice	Agency Practice	EI	Mddle	Sec	Stu A	Other
10	8	24	8									

Career Counseling
MO University of Missouri-Columbia Columbia

Admit	Grad	F	M	Adv Ed	Mngd Care	Private Practice	Agency Practice	EI	Mddle	Sec	Stu A	Other
6	6	7	6	25	0	0	25		0	0	0	50

Career Counseling
TX Houston Baptist University Houston

Admit	Grad	F	M	Adv Ed	Mngd Care	Private Practice	Agency Practice	EI	Mddle	Sec	Stu A	Other

College Counseling
CA San Jose University San Jose

Admit	Grad	F	M	Adv Ed	Mngd Care	Private Practice	Agency Practice	EI	Mddle	Sec	Stu A	Other
			20									

Master's and Specialist Degree Programs												
Admission and Enrollment 2002				Postgraduation Activity/Placement Percentages								
Admit	Grad	F	M	Adv Ed	Mngd Care	Private Practice	Agency	EI	Mddle	Sec	Stu A	Other

College Counseling
DE University of Delaware   Newark

Admit	Grad	F	M	Adv Ed	Mngd Care	Private	Agency	EI	Mddle	Sec	Stu A	Other
6	6	10	2	10								90

College Counseling
LA Northwestern State University   Natchitoches

Admit	Grad	F	M	Adv Ed	Mngd Care	Private	Agency	EI	Mddle	Sec	Stu A	Other
20	15			15	0	10	10					65

College Counseling
LA Southeastern Louisiana University   Hammond

Admit	Grad	F	M	Adv Ed	Mngd Care	Private	Agency	EI	Mddle	Sec	Stu A	Other

College Counseling
LA University of New Orleans   New Orleans

Admit	Grad	F	M	Adv Ed	Mngd Care	Private	Agency	EI	Mddle	Sec	Stu A	Other
10	10	20	10	5							95	

College Counseling
MI Eastern Michigan University   Ypsilanti

Admit	Grad	F	M	Adv Ed	Mngd Care	Private	Agency	EI	Mddle	Sec	Stu A	Other
10	3	2	1	10	0	0	2		0	0	0	88

College Counseling
MS Mississippi State University   Mississippi State University

Admit	Grad	F	M	Adv Ed	Mngd Care	Private	Agency	EI	Mddle	Sec	Stu A	Other
10	8	16	2									100

College Counseling
NY New York University   New York

Admit	Grad	F	M	Adv Ed	Mngd Care	Private	Agency	EI	Mddle	Sec	Stu A	Other
				20		26.7	30.7				8	14.7

College Counseling
NY Plattsburgh State University   Plattsburgh

Admit	Grad	F	M	Adv Ed	Mngd Care	Private	Agency	EI	Mddle	Sec	Stu A	Other
2	2	1	1	5	0	0	0				90	5

College Counseling
NY SUNY College of Brockport   Brockport

Admit	Grad	F	M	Adv Ed	Mngd Care	Private	Agency	EI	Mddle	Sec	Stu A	Other
5	5	4	1	0	0	0	0					0

College Counseling
OR Oregon State University   Corvallis

Admit	Grad	F	M	Adv Ed	Mngd Care	Private	Agency	EI	Mddle	Sec	Stu A	Other
3	3	2	1									100

College Counseling
PA Penn State University   University Park

Admit	Grad	F	M	Adv Ed	Mngd Care	Private	Agency	EI	Mddle	Sec	Stu A	Other

College Counseling
PA Shippensburg University of PA   Shippensburg

Admit	Grad	F	M	Adv Ed	Mngd Care	Private	Agency	EI	Mddle	Sec	Stu A	Other
1	1	1	3	15	5	0	0					80

College Counseling
SC Clemson University   Clemson

Admit	Grad	F	M	Adv Ed	Mngd Care	Private	Agency	EI	Mddle	Sec	Stu A	Other
5	2	4	1	0	0	0	0		0	0	0	0

College Counseling
TX University of North Texas   Denton

Admit	Grad	F	M	Adv Ed	Mngd Care	Private	Agency	EI	Mddle	Sec	Stu A	Other
5	3	2	1									100

College Counseling
WA Seattle University   Seattle

Admit	Grad	F	M	Adv Ed	Mngd Care	Private	Agency	EI	Mddle	Sec	Stu A	Other
5	5	2		0	0	0						100

Master's and Specialist Degree Programs												
Admission and Enrollment				Postgraduation Activity/Placement Percentages								
2002				Adv	Mngd	Private	Agency	School and Student Affairs				
Admit	Grad	F	M	Ed	Care	Practice		El	Mddle	Sec	Stu A	Other

Community Counseling
AL Auburn University Auburn

Admit	Grad	F	M	Adv Ed	Mngd Care	Private	Agency	El	Mddle	Sec	Stu A	Other
15-20	15-20	22	5	5	0	0	90		0	0		5

Community Counseling
AL The University of Alabama Tuscaloosa

Admit	Grad	F	M	Adv Ed	Mngd Care	Private	Agency	El	Mddle	Sec	Stu A	Other
14	9	28	8	25	5	5	70					

Community Counseling
AL Troy State University Troy

Admit	Grad	F	M	Adv Ed	Mngd Care	Private	Agency	El	Mddle	Sec	Stu A	Other
40	45											

Community Counseling
AL University of Montevallo Montevallo

Admit	Grad	F	M	Adv Ed	Mngd Care	Private	Agency	El	Mddle	Sec	Stu A	Other
20	18	35	5	2		3	87					3

Community Counseling
AL University of North Alabama Florence

Admit	Grad	F	M	Adv Ed	Mngd Care	Private	Agency	El	Mddle	Sec	Stu A	Other
15	12	33	7		30	20	35			5	5	

Community Counseling
AL University of South Alabama Mobile

Admit	Grad	F	M	Adv Ed	Mngd Care	Private	Agency	El	Mddle	Sec	Stu A	Other
23	10											

Community Counseling
AZ Arizona State University Tempe

Admit	Grad	F	M	Adv Ed	Mngd Care	Private	Agency	El	Mddle	Sec	Stu A	Other
50	45	105	38	15	25	10	40					10

Community Counseling
CO Adams State College Alamosa

Admit	Grad	F	M	Adv Ed	Mngd Care	Private	Agency	El	Mddle	Sec	Stu A	Other
60	58	58	24				66	5	5	10		10

Community Counseling
CO Denver Seminary Denver

Admit	Grad	F	M	Adv Ed	Mngd Care	Private	Agency	El	Mddle	Sec	Stu A	Other
75	50	60%	40%		0	50	40					5

Community Counseling
CO University of Colorado - Colorado Springs Colorado Springs

Admit	Grad	F	M	Adv Ed	Mngd Care	Private	Agency	El	Mddle	Sec	Stu A	Other
20	15	10	5									

Community Counseling
CO University of Colorado at Denver Denver

Admit	Grad	F	M	Adv Ed	Mngd Care	Private	Agency	El	Mddle	Sec	Stu A	Other
25	25	160	40									

Community Counseling
CO University of Northern Colorado Greeley

Admit	Grad	F	M	Adv Ed	Mngd Care	Private	Agency	El	Mddle	Sec	Stu A	Other
50	48	38	12	20	10	15	50					5

Community Counseling
CO University of Phoenix Colorado Springs

Admit	Grad	F	M	Adv Ed	Mngd Care	Private	Agency	El	Mddle	Sec	Stu A	Other
30		30	15									

Community Counseling
CT Saint Joseph College West Hartford

Admit	Grad	F	M	Adv Ed	Mngd Care	Private	Agency	El	Mddle	Sec	Stu A	Other
24	18	90	10		10	5	84					

Community Counseling
DC The George Washington University Washington, D.C.

Admit	Grad	F	M	Adv Ed	Mngd Care	Private	Agency	El	Mddle	Sec	Stu A	Other
15	10	12	3	20	4	10	33					33

Master's and Specialist Degree Programs												
Admission and Enrollment						Postgraduation Activity/Placement Percentages						
2002				Adv Ed	Mngd Care	Private Practice	Agency	School and Student Affairs				
Admit	Grad	F	M					EI	Mddle	Sec	Stu A	Other

Community Counseling
GA Columbus State University   Columbus

Admit	Grad	F	M	Adv Ed	Mngd Care	Private	Agency	EI	Mddle	Sec	Stu A	Other
60	30	20	10	15	20	5	60		0	0	0	0

Community Counseling
GA Georgia State University   Atlanta

Admit	Grad	F	M	Adv Ed	Mngd Care	Private	Agency	EI	Mddle	Sec	Stu A	Other
150	115	245	52	16	3	1	76		0	0	0	4

Community Counseling
GA State University of West Georgia   Carrolton

Admit	Grad	F	M	Adv Ed	Mngd Care	Private	Agency	EI	Mddle	Sec	Stu A	Other
15	15	10	5	20	0	5	75		0	0	0	0

Community Counseling
IA The University of Iowa   Iowa City

Admit	Grad	F	M	Adv Ed	Mngd Care	Private	Agency	EI	Mddle	Sec	Stu A	Other
15	15			10	10	10	70		0	0	0	0

Community Counseling
ID University of Idaho   Moscow

Admit	Grad	F	M	Adv Ed	Mngd Care	Private	Agency	EI	Mddle	Sec	Stu A	Other
15				5	5	10	70		0	0	0	0

Community Counseling
IL College of Arts and Sciences (CAS)   Wheaton

Admit	Grad	F	M	Adv Ed	Mngd Care	Private	Agency	EI	Mddle	Sec	Stu A	Other
120	60	100	20	10	10	5	65	10				

Community Counseling
IL Concordia University   River Forest

Admit	Grad	F	M	Adv Ed	Mngd Care	Private	Agency	EI	Mddle	Sec	Stu A	Other
15	7			10			90					

Community Counseling
IL Eastern Illinois University   Charleston

Admit	Grad	F	M	Adv Ed	Mngd Care	Private	Agency	EI	Mddle	Sec	Stu A	Other
20	20			5	0		90		0	0	0	5

Community Counseling
IL Lewis University   Romeoville

Admit	Grad	F	M	Adv Ed	Mngd Care	Private	Agency	EI	Mddle	Sec	Stu A	Other
15	7	90%	10%	5		10	50				5	30

Community Counseling
IL Southern Illinois University Carbondale   Carbondale

Admit	Grad	F	M	Adv Ed	Mngd Care	Private	Agency	EI	Mddle	Sec	Stu A	Other
15	13	12	3	20		10	50					10

Community Counseling
IL Western Illinois University   Moline

Admit	Grad	F	M	Adv Ed	Mngd Care	Private	Agency	EI	Mddle	Sec	Stu A	Other
				30	0		70		0	0	0	0

Community Counseling
IN Ball State University   Muncie

Admit	Grad	F	M	Adv Ed	Mngd Care	Private	Agency	EI	Mddle	Sec	Stu A	Other
10	10			25	10	15	50		0	0	0	0

Community Counseling
IN Indiana University   Bloomington

Admit	Grad	F	M	Adv Ed	Mngd Care	Private	Agency	EI	Mddle	Sec	Stu A	Other
25	22			30			60					10

Community Counseling
IN Indiana Wesleyan University   Marion

Admit	Grad	F	M	Adv Ed	Mngd Care	Private	Agency	EI	Mddle	Sec	Stu A	Other

Community Counseling
KS Pittsburg State University   Pittsburg

Admit	Grad	F	M	Adv Ed	Mngd Care	Private	Agency	EI	Mddle	Sec	Stu A	Other
20	20			5			95					

Master's and Specialist Degree Programs												
Admission and Enrollment				Postgraduation Activity/Placement Percentages								
2002				Adv Ed	Mngd Care	Private | Agency Practice		School and Student Affairs				Other
Admit	Grad	F	M			Private	Agency	EI	Mddle	Sec	Stu A	
Community Counseling — LA Louisiana State University Baton Rouge												
10	9	22	1	10			70					20
Community Counseling — LA Louisiana State University in Shreveport Shreveport												
20	15	65%	35%	15	30	20	20				5	10
Community Counseling — LA Loyola University New Orleans												
20	10	85%	15%	20	0	0	40		10	10	10	10
Community Counseling — LA Our Lady of Holy Cross New Orleans												
10	5											
Community Counseling — LA Southeastern Louisiana University Hammond												
Community Counseling — LA University of New Orleans New Orleans												
30	30	70	20		5		90					
Community Counseling — MA Lesley University Cambridge												
Community Counseling — MD Johns Hopkins University Baltimore												
56	42											
Community Counseling — MD Loyola College in Maryland Columbia												
120	80	250	150			10	50	1	1	3	10	10
Community Counseling — MD McDaniel College Westminster												
15	5			5		5	40					50
Community Counseling — MI Andrews University Berrien Springs												
15	12	8	7			20	60					
Community Counseling — MI Eastern Michigan University Ypsilanti												
15	8	6	2	5	0	0	90		0	0	0	5
Community Counseling — MI Oakland University Rochester												
85	70	61	9		10	10	45					20
Community Counseling — MI Siena Heights University Adrian												
30	20			10		20	60		0	0	0	0
Community Counseling — MN Minnesota State University Moorhead Moorhead												
7		4	1		10	10	80					

Master's and Specialist Degree Programs												
Admission and Enrollment				Postgraduation Activity/Placement Percentages								
2002				Adv	Mngd	Private	Agency	School and Student Affairs				
Admit	Grad	F	M	Ed	Care	Practice		El	Mddle	Sec	Stu A	Other

Community Counseling
MN Minnesota State University, Mankato   Mankato

Admit	Grad	F	M	Adv Ed	Mngd Care	Private Practice	Agency	El	Mddle	Sec	Stu A	Other
15	15	11	4	2			98					

Community Counseling
MO Southeast Missouri State University   Cape Girardeau

Admit	Grad	F	M	Adv Ed	Mngd Care	Private Practice	Agency	El	Mddle	Sec	Stu A	Other
15	12			20			80					

Community Counseling
MO Truman State University   Kirksville

Admit	Grad	F	M	Adv Ed	Mngd Care	Private Practice	Agency	El	Mddle	Sec	Stu A	Other
7	7	4	3	30			70					

Community Counseling
MO University of Missouri - St. Louis   Saint Louis

Admit	Grad	F	M	Adv Ed	Mngd Care	Private Practice	Agency	El	Mddle	Sec	Stu A	Other
40	30	96	24									

Community Counseling
MO University of Missouri-Columbia   Columbia

Admit	Grad	F	M	Adv Ed	Mngd Care	Private Practice	Agency	El	Mddle	Sec	Stu A	Other
6-10	6-10	15	10	30		30	40					

Community Counseling
MS Mississippi State University   Mississippi State University

Admit	Grad	F	M	Adv Ed	Mngd Care	Private Practice	Agency	El	Mddle	Sec	Stu A	Other
16	15	27	4	10	5	5	65		5			10

Community Counseling
MS William Carey College   Hattiesburg

Admit	Grad	F	M	Adv Ed	Mngd Care	Private Practice	Agency	El	Mddle	Sec	Stu A	Other
10	10	8	12				80					

Community Counseling
MT Montana Sate University Northern   Havre

Admit	Grad	F	M	Adv Ed	Mngd Care	Private Practice	Agency	El	Mddle	Sec	Stu A	Other
5	5											

Community Counseling
NC Appalachian State University   Boone

Admit	Grad	F	M	Adv Ed	Mngd Care	Private Practice	Agency	El	Mddle	Sec	Stu A	Other
25	20			5	0	5	80		0	0	0	10

Community Counseling
NC Campbell University   Buies Creek

Admit	Grad	F	M	Adv Ed	Mngd Care	Private Practice	Agency	El	Mddle	Sec	Stu A	Other
10	8-10	20	10	5	0	5	85		0	0	0	5

Community Counseling
NC North Carolina A&T State University   Greensboro

Admit	Grad	F	M	Adv Ed	Mngd Care	Private Practice	Agency	El	Mddle	Sec	Stu A	Other

Community Counseling
NC The University of North Carolina at Greensboro   Greensboro

Admit	Grad	F	M	Adv Ed	Mngd Care	Private Practice	Agency	El	Mddle	Sec	Stu A	Other
12	12	18	6	10	5	30	45					10

Community Counseling
NC University of North Carolina at Charlotte   Charlotte

Admit	Grad	F	M	Adv Ed	Mngd Care	Private Practice	Agency	El	Mddle	Sec	Stu A	Other

Community Counseling
NC Wake Forest University   Winston-Salem

Admit	Grad	F	M	Adv Ed	Mngd Care	Private Practice	Agency	El	Mddle	Sec	Stu A	Other
8	8	6	2	12.5	25	12.5	37.5					12.5

Community Counseling
ND North Dakota State University   Fargo

Admit	Grad	F	M	Adv Ed	Mngd Care	Private Practice	Agency	El	Mddle	Sec	Stu A	Other
7	4	27	3	3	0	1	70		0	0	0	23

Master's and Specialist Degree Programs

| | Admission and Enrollment 2002 | | | Postgraduation Activity/Placement Percentages | | | | | | | | |
| | Admit | Grad | F | M | Adv Ed | Mngd Care | Private | Agency Practice | El | Mddle | Sec | Stu A | Other |

Community Counseling
NE Chadron State College   Chadron

Admit	Grad	F	M	Adv Ed	Mngd Care	Private	Agency Practice	El	Mddle	Sec	Stu A	Other
15	10											

Community Counseling
NE University of Nebraska-Omaha   Omaha

Admit	Grad	F	M	Adv Ed	Mngd Care	Private	Agency Practice	El	Mddle	Sec	Stu A	Other
40	38			5	30	5	60		0	0	0	0

Community Counseling
NE Wayne State College   Wayne

Admit	Grad	F	M	Adv Ed	Mngd Care	Private	Agency Practice	El	Mddle	Sec	Stu A	Other
12	8					10	90					

Community Counseling
NJ The College of New Jersey   Ewing

Admit	Grad	F	M	Adv Ed	Mngd Care	Private	Agency Practice	El	Mddle	Sec	Stu A	Other
20	20			5			40					35

Community Counseling
NJ William Paterson University   Wayne

Admit	Grad	F	M	Adv Ed	Mngd Care	Private	Agency Practice	El	Mddle	Sec	Stu A	Other
6	5	12	3				85					15

Community Counseling
NM University of Phoenix - Albuquerque, NM Campus   Albuquerque

Admit	Grad	F	M	Adv Ed	Mngd Care	Private	Agency Practice	El	Mddle	Sec	Stu A	Other

Community Counseling
NV University of Nevada   Reno

Admit	Grad	F	M	Adv Ed	Mngd Care	Private	Agency Practice	El	Mddle	Sec	Stu A	Other
15	12	35	20	20			80					

Community Counseling
NY Canisius College   Buffalo

Admit	Grad	F	M	Adv Ed	Mngd Care	Private	Agency Practice	El	Mddle	Sec	Stu A	Other
10	10			10	10	10	50		0	0	0	10

Community Counseling
NY College at Oswego SUNY   Oswego

Admit	Grad	F	M	Adv Ed	Mngd Care	Private	Agency Practice	El	Mddle	Sec	Stu A	Other
30	25	60	20	2		2	85					9

Community Counseling
NY Marist College   Poughkeepsie

Admit	Grad	F	M	Adv Ed	Mngd Care	Private	Agency Practice	El	Mddle	Sec	Stu A	Other
46	41	65	27	10			70					10

Community Counseling
NY New York University   New York

Admit	Grad	F	M	Adv Ed	Mngd Care	Private	Agency Practice	El	Mddle	Sec	Stu A	Other
				20			26.7	30.7			8	14.7

Community Counseling
NY Plattsburgh State University   Plattsburgh

Admit	Grad	F	M	Adv Ed	Mngd Care	Private	Agency Practice	El	Mddle	Sec	Stu A	Other
12	11	6	5		5	0	70					20

Community Counseling
NY SUNY College of Brockport   Brockport

Admit	Grad	F	M	Adv Ed	Mngd Care	Private	Agency Practice	El	Mddle	Sec	Stu A	Other
10	10	3	7	0	0	5	95		0	0	0	0

Community Counseling
NY Syracuse University   Syracuse

Admit	Grad	F	M	Adv Ed	Mngd Care	Private	Agency Practice	El	Mddle	Sec	Stu A	Other
10	8	8	2				New program					

Community Counseling
NY University of Rochester   Rochester

Admit	Grad	F	M	Adv Ed	Mngd Care	Private	Agency Practice	El	Mddle	Sec	Stu A	Other
8	6	11	3		25		75					

Master's and Specialist Degree Programs

All programs below are **Community Counseling**.

Institution (City)	Admit	Grad	F	M	Adv Ed	Mngd Care	Private Practice	Agency	El	Mddle	Sec	Stu A	Other
OH Cleveland State University — Cleveland	30	26											
OH John Carroll University — Cleveland	35	35	75	25		10	10	75	0	0	0	0	0
OH Kent State University — Kent	40	34	90	30	12	5		75					8
OH Malone College — Canton	15-20	10-15	90%	10%	5	0	0	85		0	0	0	10
OH Ohio University — Athens	30	25	20	10									
OH The University of Toledo — Toledo	20	18	13	7	5	20	5	70					
OH Xavier University — Cincinnati	75	30	70%	30%	10	10	5	70		0	0	0	5
OH Youngstown State University — Youngstown	50	25	70	20	5			95		30	40	40	100
OR Oregon State University — Corvallis	3	3	3	0				50					50
OR Portland State University — Portland	14	14-28	75%	25%	10	10	10	70					
PA Arcadia University — Glenside	14 (2001)	13 (2001)	30	5	10	10		80					
PA California University of Pennsylvania — California	15	15	38	9	2	0	0	80		0	0	0	18
PA Duquesne University — Pittsburgh	25	16			10	0	5	75		0	0	0	10
PA Indiana University of Pennsylvania — Indiana	50												
PA Kutztown University — Kutztown	20	10			2	10	2	86		0	0	0	

Master's and Specialist Degree Programs												
Admission and Enrollment				Postgraduation Activity/Placement Percentages								
2002				Adv Ed	Mngd Care	Private	Agency	School and Student Affairs				
Admit	Grad	F	M			Practice		El	Mddle	Sec	Stu A	Other

Community Counseling
PA Shippensburg University of PA   Shippensburg

Admit	Grad	F	M	Adv Ed	Mngd Care	Private	Agency	El	Mddle	Sec	Stu A	Other
15	8	13	4	10	10	5	75		0	0	0	0

Community Counseling
PA West Chester University   West Chester

Admit	Grad	F	M	Adv Ed	Mngd Care	Private	Agency	El	Mddle	Sec	Stu A	Other
10	5											

Community Counseling
SC Clemson University   Clemson

Admit	Grad	F	M	Adv Ed	Mngd Care	Private	Agency	El	Mddle	Sec	Stu A	Other
60	30	50	10	10	0	20	70		0	0	0	0

Community Counseling
SC Winthrop University   Rock Hill

Admit	Grad	F	M	Adv Ed	Mngd Care	Private	Agency	El	Mddle	Sec	Stu A	Other
12	10	10	2	1			80	19%				

Community Counseling
SD South Dakota State University   Brookings

Admit	Grad	F	M	Adv Ed	Mngd Care	Private	Agency	El	Mddle	Sec	Stu A	Other
25	25											

Community Counseling
SD The University of South Dakota   Vermillion

Admit	Grad	F	M	Adv Ed	Mngd Care	Private	Agency	El	Mddle	Sec	Stu A	Other
12		75%	25%	100	25	25	50					

Community Counseling
TN East Tennessee State University   Johnson City

Admit	Grad	F	M	Adv Ed	Mngd Care	Private	Agency	El	Mddle	Sec	Stu A	Other
10	9			2	0	5	85		0	0	0	8

Community Counseling
TN Peabody College, Vanderbilt University   Nashville

Admit	Grad	F	M	Adv Ed	Mngd Care	Private	Agency	El	Mddle	Sec	Stu A	Other
12	12	90%	10%	10	10	15	45				2	18

Community Counseling
TX Lamar University   Beaumont

Admit	Grad	F	M	Adv Ed	Mngd Care	Private	Agency	El	Mddle	Sec	Stu A	Other
	15											

Community Counseling
TX Southwest Texas State University   San Marcos

Admit	Grad	F	M	Adv Ed	Mngd Care	Private	Agency	El	Mddle	Sec	Stu A	Other

Community Counseling
TX Stephen F. Austin State University   Nacogdoches

Admit	Grad	F	M	Adv Ed	Mngd Care	Private	Agency	El	Mddle	Sec	Stu A	Other
15	15	13	2	10	10	10	70					

Community Counseling
TX Texas A & M University - Commerce   Commerce

Admit	Grad	F	M	Adv Ed	Mngd Care	Private	Agency	El	Mddle	Sec	Stu A	Other
37	34			10	40	10	40		0	0	0	0

Community Counseling
TX Texas Southern University   Houston

Admit	Grad	F	M	Adv Ed	Mngd Care	Private	Agency	El	Mddle	Sec	Stu A	Other
35	20	75	30		10	10	75	0	0	0	0	

Community Counseling
TX Texas Tech University   Lubbock

Admit	Grad	F	M	Adv Ed	Mngd Care	Private	Agency	El	Mddle	Sec	Stu A	Other
30	20	19	8	5	5	5	48	8	10	7	2	10 state

Community Counseling
TX University of North Texas   Denton

Admit	Grad	F	M	Adv Ed	Mngd Care	Private	Agency	El	Mddle	Sec	Stu A	Other
70	65	64	5				100					

Master's and Specialist Degree Programs

Admit	Grad	F	M	Adv Ed	Mngd Care	Private Practice	Agency	EI	Mddle	Sec	Stu A	Other
		2002				Postgraduation Activity/Placement Percentages			School and Student Affairs			

Community Counseling
TX University of Texas at El Paso   El Paso

Admit	Grad	F	M	Adv Ed	Mngd Care	Private Practice	Agency	EI	Mddle	Sec	Stu A	Other
15	15	27	13	10	20		60	33	33	33		

Community Counseling
TX University of Texas of the Permian Basin   Odessa

Admit	Grad	F	M	Adv Ed	Mngd Care	Private Practice	Agency	EI	Mddle	Sec	Stu A	Other
10	3	7	3	0	0	10	80		10			

Community Counseling
VA College of William and Mary   Williamsburg

Admit	Grad	F	M	Adv Ed	Mngd Care	Private Practice	Agency	EI	Mddle	Sec	Stu A	Other
10	10	8	2				100					

Community Counseling
VA George Mason University   Fairfax

Admit	Grad	F	M	Adv Ed	Mngd Care	Private Practice	Agency	EI	Mddle	Sec	Stu A	Other
30	10	80%	20%	20	20	5	30					25

Community Counseling
VA James Madison University   Harrisonburg

Admit	Grad	F	M	Adv Ed	Mngd Care	Private Practice	Agency	EI	Mddle	Sec	Stu A	Other
10	10											

Community Counseling
VA Old Dominion University   Norfolk

Admit	Grad	F	M	Adv Ed	Mngd Care	Private Practice	Agency	EI	Mddle	Sec	Stu A	Other
24	19	39	9		5	10	85					

Community Counseling
VA Radford University   Radford

Admit	Grad	F	M	Adv Ed	Mngd Care	Private Practice	Agency	EI	Mddle	Sec	Stu A	Other
12	12			10	0	0	90		0	0	0	0

Community Counseling
VA Regent University   Virginia Beach

Admit	Grad	F	M	Adv Ed	Mngd Care	Private Practice	Agency	EI	Mddle	Sec	Stu A	Other
55	38	121	29	6		7	50					37

Community Counseling
VA Virginia Tech   Blacksburg

Admit	Grad	F	M	Adv Ed	Mngd Care	Private Practice	Agency	EI	Mddle	Sec	Stu A	Other
20	18	15	5				90					10

Community Counseling
WI University of Wisconsin-Oshkosh   Oshkosh

Admit	Grad	F	M	Adv Ed	Mngd Care	Private Practice	Agency	EI	Mddle	Sec	Stu A	Other
20	14	39	10	2	20	10	30					38

Community Counseling
WI University of Wisconsin-Whitewater   Whitewater

Admit	Grad	F	M	Adv Ed	Mngd Care	Private Practice	Agency	EI	Mddle	Sec	Stu A	Other
27	23											

Community Counseling
WV West Virginia University   Morgantown

Admit	Grad	F	M	Adv Ed	Mngd Care	Private Practice	Agency	EI	Mddle	Sec	Stu A	Other
22				25			70					5 Univ

Community Counseling
WY University of Wyoming   Laramie

Admit	Grad	F	M	Adv Ed	Mngd Care	Private Practice	Agency	EI	Mddle	Sec	Stu A	Other
9	5	19	4	10	0	0	90					

Gerontological Counseling
IL College of Arts and Sciences (CAS)   Wheaton

Admit	Grad	F	M	Adv Ed	Mngd Care	Private Practice	Agency	EI	Mddle	Sec	Stu A	Other
10	5	10	0	5	15	5	75	5				

Gerontological Counseling
MS William Carey College   Hattiesburg

Admit	Grad	F	M	Adv Ed	Mngd Care	Private Practice	Agency	EI	Mddle	Sec	Stu A	Other
10	10	12	8									

Master's and Specialist Degree Programs												
Admission and Enrollment 2002				Postgraduation Activity/Placement Percentages								
				Adv Ed	Mngd Care	Private Practice	Agency Practice	School and Student Affairs				
Admit	Grad	F	M					El	Mddle	Sec	Stu A	Other

Gerontological Counseling
NC The University of North Carolina at Greensboro   Greensboro

Admit	Grad	F	M	Adv Ed	Mngd Care	Private	Agency	El	Mddle	Sec	Stu A	Other
2	2	2	0				30					70

Marriage and Family Counseling
AL University of Montevallo   Montevallo

Admit	Grad	F	M	Adv Ed	Mngd Care	Private	Agency	El	Mddle	Sec	Stu A	Other
10	9	20	4									

Marriage and Family Counseling
AZ University of Phoenix   Phoenix

Admit	Grad	F	M	Adv Ed	Mngd Care	Private	Agency	El	Mddle	Sec	Stu A	Other
40	35	110	70	25	20	15	40					

Marriage and Family Counseling
CA California State University-Fresno   Fresno

Admit	Grad	F	M	Adv Ed	Mngd Care	Private	Agency	El	Mddle	Sec	Stu A	Other
40	30			10	10	20	50	0	0	0		10

Marriage and Family Counseling
CO University of Colorado at Denver   Denver

Admit	Grad	F	M	Adv Ed	Mngd Care	Private	Agency	El	Mddle	Sec	Stu A	Other
50	40											

Marriage and Family Counseling
CO University of Northern Colorado   Greeley

Admit	Grad	F	M	Adv Ed	Mngd Care	Private	Agency	El	Mddle	Sec	Stu A	Other
25	23	17	8	25	10	20	45					

Marriage and Family Counseling
FL Carlos Albizu University   Miami

Admit	Grad	F	M	Adv Ed	Mngd Care	Private	Agency	El	Mddle	Sec	Stu A	Other
13	11	23	8									

Marriage and Family Counseling
FL University of Florida   Gainesville

Admit	Grad	F	M	Adv Ed	Mngd Care	Private	Agency	El	Mddle	Sec	Stu A	Other
16	11			25	10	15	50					

Marriage and Family Counseling
ID Idaho State University   Pocatello

Admit	Grad	F	M	Adv Ed	Mngd Care	Private	Agency	El	Mddle	Sec	Stu A	Other
10	10	14	6	10			90					

Marriage and Family Counseling
IL Southern Illinois University Carbondale   Carbondale

Admit	Grad	F	M	Adv Ed	Mngd Care	Private	Agency	El	Mddle	Sec	Stu A	Other
12	6	10	2	20		10	70					

Marriage and Family Counseling
IN Indiana State University   Terre Haute

Admit	Grad	F	M	Adv Ed	Mngd Care	Private	Agency	El	Mddle	Sec	Stu A	Other
8	7	8	2	10	10	10	70					

Marriage and Family Counseling
IN Indiana Wesleyan University   Marion

Admit	Grad	F	M	Adv Ed	Mngd Care	Private	Agency	El	Mddle	Sec	Stu A	Other

Marriage and Family Counseling
IN Indiana-Purdue University at Fort Wayne   Fort Wayne

Admit	Grad	F	M	Adv Ed	Mngd Care	Private	Agency	El	Mddle	Sec	Stu A	Other
14	12	32	22	2	13	5	80					

Marriage and Family Counseling
KS Pittsburg State University   Pittsburg

Admit	Grad	F	M	Adv Ed	Mngd Care	Private	Agency	El	Mddle	Sec	Stu A	Other
10	10			5		25	70					

Marriage and Family Counseling
KY Western Kentucky University   Bowling Green

Admit	Grad	F	M	Adv Ed	Mngd Care	Private	Agency	El	Mddle	Sec	Stu A	Other
15	10											

Master's and Specialist Degree Programs

Admission and Enrollment 2002				Postgraduation Activity/Placement Percentages								
				Adv Ed	Mngd Care	Private Practice	Agency	School and Student Affairs				
Admit	Grad	F	M	Ed	Care	Practice		EI	Mddle	Sec	Stu A	Other

Marriage and Family Counseling
LA Our Lady of Holy Cross New Orleans

Admit	Grad	F	M	Adv Ed	Mngd Care	Private Practice	Agency	EI	Mddle	Sec	Stu A	Other
25	25											

Marriage and Family Counseling
LA Southeastern Louisiana University Hammond

Admit	Grad	F	M	Adv Ed	Mngd Care	Private Practice	Agency	EI	Mddle	Sec	Stu A	Other

Marriage and Family Counseling
MA Fitchburg State College Fitchburg

Admit	Grad	F	M	Adv Ed	Mngd Care	Private Practice	Agency	EI	Mddle	Sec	Stu A	Other
1	1	6	0				100					

Marriage and Family Counseling
MN Capella Uiversity Minneapolis

Admit	Grad	F	M	Adv Ed	Mngd Care	Private Practice	Agency	EI	Mddle	Sec	Stu A	Other
20		19	1									

Marriage and Family Counseling
MS Mississippi College Clinton

Admit	Grad	F	M	Adv Ed	Mngd Care	Private Practice	Agency	EI	Mddle	Sec	Stu A	Other
15	5				10		10	20				60

Marriage and Family Counseling
MT Montana State University - Bozeman Bozeman

Admit	Grad	F	M	Adv Ed	Mngd Care	Private Practice	Agency	EI	Mddle	Sec	Stu A	Other
8-96	6-8	6	2	10	10	30	50					

Marriage and Family Counseling
NC Appalachian State University Boone

Admit	Grad	F	M	Adv Ed	Mngd Care	Private Practice	Agency	EI	Mddle	Sec	Stu A	Other
12	11			3	25	25	25		0	0	0	22

Marriage and Family Counseling
NC University of North Carolina at Greensboro Greensboro

Admit	Grad	F	M	Adv Ed	Mngd Care	Private Practice	Agency	EI	Mddle	Sec	Stu A	Other
8	8	4	4	10	5	35	50					

Marriage and Family Counseling
NM University of Phoenix - Albuquerque, NM Campus Albuquerque

Admit	Grad	F	M	Adv Ed	Mngd Care	Private Practice	Agency	EI	Mddle	Sec	Stu A	Other
20	18	36	6	14	4	21	39		4	4		14

Marriage and Family Counseling
OR George Fox University Portland

Admit	Grad	F	M	Adv Ed	Mngd Care	Private Practice	Agency	EI	Mddle	Sec	Stu A	Other
40	25	73	22	1	0	20	75	0	2	2		0

Marriage and Family Counseling
OR Portland State University Portland

Admit	Grad	F	M	Adv Ed	Mngd Care	Private Practice	Agency	EI	Mddle	Sec	Stu A	Other
14				10	10	10	70					

Marriage and Family Counseling
PA Duquesne University Pittsburgh

Admit	Grad	F	M	Adv Ed	Mngd Care	Private Practice	Agency	EI	Mddle	Sec	Stu A	Other
10	4			10	15	5	70					

Marriage and Family Counseling
PA Geneva College Beaver Falls

Admit	Grad	F	M	Adv Ed	Mngd Care	Private Practice	Agency	EI	Mddle	Sec	Stu A	Other
7	6											

Marriage and Family Counseling
PA Kutztown University Kutztown

Admit	Grad	F	M	Adv Ed	Mngd Care	Private Practice	Agency	EI	Mddle	Sec	Stu A	Other
14	7			5	10	5	80		0	0	0	0

Marriage and Family Counseling
PR University of Phoenix, Puerto Rico Campus Guaynabo

Admit	Grad	F	M	Adv Ed	Mngd Care	Private Practice	Agency	EI	Mddle	Sec	Stu A	Other
50	50	37	13	5	15	5	65					10

Master's and Specialist Degree Programs												
Admission and Enrollment				Postgraduation Activity/Placement Percentages								
2002				Adv	Mngd	Private	Agency	School and Student Affairs				
Admit	Grad	F	M	Ed	Care	Practice		EI	Mddle	Sec	Stu A	Other

Marriage and Family Counseling
TN East Tennessee State University   Johnson City

10	9			2	0	5	85		0	0	0	8

Marriage and Family Counseling
TN Travecca Nazarene University   Nashville

Marriage and Family Counseling
TX Houston Baptist University   Houston

Marriage and Family Counseling
TX Our Lady of the Lake University   San Antonio

10	10			10		10	70					10

Marriage and Family Counseling
TX Southwest Texas State University   San Marcos

Marriage and Family Counseling
TX Tarleton State University   Stephenville

30	30			10			90					

Marriage and Family Counseling
TX University of Texas at Tyler   Tyler

8	6	16	4	15		40	40					5

Marriage and Family Counseling
VA College of William and Mary   Williamsburg

8	6	6	2				100					

Mental Health Counseling
FL Carlos Albizu University   Miami

38	7	39	19									

Mental Health Counseling
FL Florida Atlantic University   Boca Raton

50	20	20	10	5	30	05	60					

Mental Health Counseling
FL Rollins College   Winter Park

30	20	85	5	10	5	0	70					15

Mental Health Counseling
FL University of Central Florida   Orlando

25/30	22	54	8	15	10	05	65					10

Mental Health Counseling
FL University of Florida   Gainesville

18	12			25	10	15	50					

Mental Health Counseling
FL University of North Florida   Jacksonville

25	25			5	5	0	90					0

Mental Health Counseling
IA University of North Iowa   Cedar Falls

30-40	10-15	40	30	2	3	5	80		0	0	0	10

Master's and Specialist Degree Programs

	Admission and Enrollment 2002						Postgraduation Activity/Placement Percentages						
					Adv Ed	Mngd Care	Private Practice	Agency	School and Student Affairs				
	Admit	Grad	F	M					El	Mddle	Sec	Stu A	Other

Mental Health Counseling
ID Idaho State University Pocatello

Admit	Grad	F	M	Adv Ed	Mngd Care	Private Practice	Agency	El	Mddle	Sec	Stu A	Other
10	10	14	6	10			90					

Mental Health Counseling
IL Lewis University Romeoville

Admit	Grad	F	M	Adv Ed	Mngd Care	Private Practice	Agency	El	Mddle	Sec	Stu A	Other
15	7	90%	10%	5		10	50				5	30

Mental Health Counseling
IN Ball State University Muncie

Admit	Grad	F	M	Adv Ed	Mngd Care	Private Practice	Agency	El	Mddle	Sec	Stu A	Other
20	15											

Mental Health Counseling
IN Indiana State University Terre Haute

Admit	Grad	F	M	Adv Ed	Mngd Care	Private Practice	Agency	El	Mddle	Sec	Stu A	Other
20	20	35	4	30	10	10	50					

Mental Health Counseling
IN Indiana University Bloomington

Admit	Grad	F	M	Adv Ed	Mngd Care	Private Practice	Agency	El	Mddle	Sec	Stu A	Other
10	10			5	15	10	60					5

Mental Health Counseling
IN Purdue University West Lafayette

Admit	Grad	F	M	Adv Ed	Mngd Care	Private Practice	Agency	El	Mddle	Sec	Stu A	Other
10	7-8	10	5									

Mental Health Counseling
KS Emporia State University Emporia

Admit	Grad	F	M	Adv Ed	Mngd Care	Private Practice	Agency	El	Mddle	Sec	Stu A	Other
7-12	7-12	4-8	3-4	10			90					

Mental Health Counseling
KY Eastern Kentucky University Richmond

Admit	Grad	F	M	Adv Ed	Mngd Care	Private Practice	Agency	El	Mddle	Sec	Stu A	Other
14				5	5	5	80					5

Mental Health Counseling
KY Western Kentucky University Bowling Green

Admit	Grad	F	M	Adv Ed	Mngd Care	Private Practice	Agency	El	Mddle	Sec	Stu A	Other
30	10			5	50	15	25		0	0	0	5

Mental Health Counseling
LA McNeese State University Lake Charles

Admit	Grad	F	M	Adv Ed	Mngd Care	Private Practice	Agency	El	Mddle	Sec	Stu A	Other
5	4	4	1	1	5		94					

Mental Health Counseling
MA Bridgewater State College Bridgewater

Admit	Grad	F	M	Adv Ed	Mngd Care	Private Practice	Agency	El	Mddle	Sec	Stu A	Other
30	15	50	40	2	90							

Mental Health Counseling
MA Fitchburg State College Fitchburg

Admit	Grad	F	M	Adv Ed	Mngd Care	Private Practice	Agency	El	Mddle	Sec	Stu A	Other
10	8	28	2		5	20	75					

Mental Health Counseling
MA Lesley University Cambridge

Admit	Grad	F	M	Adv Ed	Mngd Care	Private Practice	Agency	El	Mddle	Sec	Stu A	Other

Mental Health Counseling
MA Suffolk University Boston

Admit	Grad	F	M	Adv Ed	Mngd Care	Private Practice	Agency	El	Mddle	Sec	Stu A	Other
25	15	20	5	5	60	5	20					10

Mental Health Counseling
MD Frostburg State University Frostburg

Admit	Grad	F	M	Adv Ed	Mngd Care	Private Practice	Agency	El	Mddle	Sec	Stu A	Other
15	12	25	7	10		10	70					10

Master's and Specialist Degree Programs												
Admission and Enrollment				Postgraduation Activity/Placement Percentages								
2002				Adv	Mngd	Private	Agency	School and Student Affairs				
Admit	Grad	F	M	Ed	Care	Practice		EI	Mddle	Sec	Stu A	Other

Mental Health Counseling
ME University of Southern Maine   Gorham

Admit	Grad	F	M	Adv Ed	Mngd Care	Private	Agency	EI	Mddle	Sec	Stu A	Other
15	15	11	4	5	5	10	80					

Mental Health Counseling
MN Capella University   Minneapolis

Admit	Grad	F	M	Adv Ed	Mngd Care	Private	Agency	EI	Mddle	Sec	Stu A	Other
40		35	5									

Mental Health Counseling
MO Northwest Missouri State University   Maryville

Admit	Grad	F	M	Adv Ed	Mngd Care	Private	Agency	EI	Mddle	Sec	Stu A	Other
12	10			5			95					

Mental Health Counseling
MS Mississippi College   Clinton

Admit	Grad	F	M	Adv Ed	Mngd Care	Private	Agency	EI	Mddle	Sec	Stu A	Other
15	8			10		10	50					30

Mental Health Counseling
MT Montana State University - Bozeman   Bozeman

Admit	Grad	F	M	Adv Ed	Mngd Care	Private	Agency	EI	Mddle	Sec	Stu A	Other
8-9	6-8	6	2	10	20	20	50					

Mental Health Counseling
NC East Carolina University   Greenville

Admit	Grad	F	M	Adv Ed	Mngd Care	Private	Agency	EI	Mddle	Sec	Stu A	Other
15	15	10	5				95					5

Mental Health Counseling
NH Plymouth State College   Plymouth

Admit	Grad	F	M	Adv Ed	Mngd Care	Private	Agency	EI	Mddle	Sec	Stu A	Other
10	8	4	4		25		75					

Mental Health Counseling
NM University of Phoenix - Albuquerque, NM Campus   Albuquerque

Admit	Grad	F	M	Adv Ed	Mngd Care	Private	Agency	EI	Mddle	Sec	Stu A	Other

Mental Health Counseling
NY Niagara University   Niagara University

Admit	Grad	F	M	Adv Ed	Mngd Care	Private	Agency	EI	Mddle	Sec	Stu A	Other
5	5			0	0	0	100		0	0	0	0

Mental Health Counseling
NY Queens College, City University of New York   Flushing

Admit	Grad	F	M	Adv Ed	Mngd Care	Private	Agency	EI	Mddle	Sec	Stu A	Other

Mental Health Counseling
OH University of Cincinnati   Cincinnati

Admit	Grad	F	M	Adv Ed	Mngd Care	Private	Agency	EI	Mddle	Sec	Stu A	Other
20	15	40	5	25	5	5	55					10

Mental Health Counseling
OH Walsh University   North Canton

Admit	Grad	F	M	Adv Ed	Mngd Care	Private	Agency	EI	Mddle	Sec	Stu A	Other
10-15	8-10			10	5	5	80		0	0	0	0

Mental Health Counseling
OR George Fox University   Portland

Admit	Grad	F	M	Adv Ed	Mngd Care	Private	Agency	EI	Mddle	Sec	Stu A	Other
47	25	99	24	1	0	20	75	21				2

Mental Health Counseling
PA Geneva College   Beaver Falls

Admit	Grad	F	M	Adv Ed	Mngd Care	Private	Agency	EI	Mddle	Sec	Stu A	Other
7	6											

Mental Health Counseling
PA Shippensburg University of PA   Shippensburg

Admit	Grad	F	M	Adv Ed	Mngd Care	Private	Agency	EI	Mddle	Sec	Stu A	Other
4	3	31	5	10	10	5	75		0	0	0	0

Master's and Specialist Degree Programs

	Admission and Enrollment 2002				Postgraduation Activity/Placement Percentages								
					Adv Ed	Mngd Care	Private Practice	Agency	EI	Mddle	Sec	Stu A	Other
	Admit	Grad	F	M									

Mental Health Counseling
PR University of Phoenix, Puerto Rico Campus Guaynabo

Admit	Grad	F	M	Adv Ed	Mngd Care	Private Practice	Agency	EI	Mddle	Sec	Stu A	Other
50	50	35	15	10	15	5	60					10

Mental Health Counseling
RI Rhode Island College Providence

Admit	Grad	F	M	Adv Ed	Mngd Care	Private Practice	Agency	EI	Mddle	Sec	Stu A	Other
42	22	65	15	50	50	25	25		0	0	0	0

Mental Health Counseling
TN Lee University Cleveland

Admit	Grad	F	M	Adv Ed	Mngd Care	Private Practice	Agency	EI	Mddle	Sec	Stu A	Other
18	15	40	11	12		35	48					5

Mental Health Counseling
TN The University of Tennessee at Knoxville Knoxville

Admit	Grad	F	M	Adv Ed	Mngd Care	Private Practice	Agency	EI	Mddle	Sec	Stu A	Other
20	20			25	0	20	55		0	0	0	0

Mental Health Counseling
TN Travecca Nazarene University Nashville

Admit	Grad	F	M	Adv Ed	Mngd Care	Private Practice	Agency	EI	Mddle	Sec	Stu A	Other

Mental Health Counseling
TX Dallas Baptist University Dallas

Admit	Grad	F	M	Adv Ed	Mngd Care	Private Practice	Agency	EI	Mddle	Sec	Stu A	Other
95	30	75	22									

Mental Health Counseling
TX Houston Baptist University Houston

Admit	Grad	F	M	Adv Ed	Mngd Care	Private Practice	Agency	EI	Mddle	Sec	Stu A	Other
	17											

Mental Health Counseling
TX Our Lady of the Lake University San Antonio

Admit	Grad	F	M	Adv Ed	Mngd Care	Private Practice	Agency	EI	Mddle	Sec	Stu A	Other
10	10			10		10	70					10

Mental Health Counseling
TX Tarleton State University Stephenville

Admit	Grad	F	M	Adv Ed	Mngd Care	Private Practice	Agency	EI	Mddle	Sec	Stu A	Other
20	20			10	0	0	90		0	0	0	0

Mental Health Counseling
UT University of Phoenix Salt Lake City

Admit	Grad	F	M	Adv Ed	Mngd Care	Private Practice	Agency	EI	Mddle	Sec	Stu A	Other
60		60%	40%	2	5	5	75					12

Mental Health Counseling
WA Central Washington University Ellensburg

Admit	Grad	F	M	Adv Ed	Mngd Care	Private Practice	Agency	EI	Mddle	Sec	Stu A	Other
12	9											

Mental Health Counseling
WA City University Bellevue

Admit	Grad	F	M	Adv Ed	Mngd Care	Private Practice	Agency	EI	Mddle	Sec	Stu A	Other
90	25	60	30	5	5	5	85					

Mental Health Counseling
WA Eastern Washington University Cheney

Admit	Grad	F	M	Adv Ed	Mngd Care	Private Practice	Agency	EI	Mddle	Sec	Stu A	Other

Mental Health Counseling
WA Seattle University Seattle

Admit	Grad	F	M	Adv Ed	Mngd Care	Private Practice	Agency	EI	Mddle	Sec	Stu A	Other
10	10	13	5	5	5	0	90					

Mental Health Counseling
WA University of Puget Sound Tacoma

Admit	Grad	F	M	Adv Ed	Mngd Care	Private Practice	Agency	EI	Mddle	Sec	Stu A	Other
6	6	5	1	10	40		50					

Master's and Specialist Degree Programs

Admission and Enrollment 2002				Postgraduation Activity/Placement Percentages								
Admit	Grad	F	M	Adv Ed	Mngd Care	Private	Agency Practice	EI	Mddle	Sec	Stu A	Other

Mental Health Counseling

WA Western Washington University   Bellingham

Admit	Grad	F	M	Adv Ed	Mngd Care	Private	Agency	EI	Mddle	Sec	Stu A	Other
6	6	4	2				100					

Other

AL University of South Alabama   Mobile

Admit	Grad	F	M	Adv Ed	Mngd Care	Private	Agency	EI	Mddle	Sec	Stu A	Other
12	8											

Other

AZ Arizona State University   Tempe

Admit	Grad	F	M	Adv Ed	Mngd Care	Private	Agency	EI	Mddle	Sec	Stu A	Other

Other

CA University of San Diego, School of Education   San Diego

Admit	Grad	F	M	Adv Ed	Mngd Care	Private	Agency	EI	Mddle	Sec	Stu A	Other
15	12	15	5	10			20				70	

Other

CO Denver Seminary   Denver

Admit	Grad	F	M	Adv Ed	Mngd Care	Private	Agency	EI	Mddle	Sec	Stu A	Other
15	10	60%	40%	0	0	50	0					50

Other

CO University of Colorado - Colorado Springs   Colorado Springs

Admit	Grad	F	M	Adv Ed	Mngd Care	Private	Agency	EI	Mddle	Sec	Stu A	Other
20	20											

Other

ID University of Idaho   Moscow

Admit	Grad	F	M	Adv Ed	Mngd Care	Private	Agency	EI	Mddle	Sec	Stu A	Other
12				100					30	30	30	

Other

IL College of Arts and Sciences (CAS)   Wheaton

Admit	Grad	F	M	Adv Ed	Mngd Care	Private	Agency	EI	Mddle	Sec	Stu A	Other
10	5	10	0	5	10	0	80	5				

Other

KS Emporia State University   Emporia

Admit	Grad	F	M	Adv Ed	Mngd Care	Private	Agency	EI	Mddle	Sec	Stu A	Other
7-12	7-12	4-6	3-6	10							90	

Other

KS University of Kansas   Lawrence

Admit	Grad	F	M	Adv Ed	Mngd Care	Private	Agency	EI	Mddle	Sec	Stu A	Other
15	15											

Other

MA Lesley University   Cambridge

Admit	Grad	F	M	Adv Ed	Mngd Care	Private	Agency	EI	Mddle	Sec	Stu A	Other

Other

MA Suffolk University   Boston

Admit	Grad	F	M	Adv Ed	Mngd Care	Private	Agency	EI	Mddle	Sec	Stu A	Other
10	6	9	1	2		5	75					18

Other

MD Johns Hopkins University   Baltimore

Admit	Grad	F	M	Adv Ed	Mngd Care	Private	Agency	EI	Mddle	Sec	Stu A	Other
49	15											

Other

MN Capella University   Minneapolis

Admit	Grad	F	M	Adv Ed	Mngd Care	Private	Agency	EI	Mddle	Sec	Stu A	Other
20		19	1									

Other

MN Minnesota State University Moorhead   Moorhead

Admit	Grad	F	M	Adv Ed	Mngd Care	Private	Agency	EI	Mddle	Sec	Stu A	Other
7	4										100	

Master's and Specialist Degree Programs

Admission and Enrollment 2002				Postgraduation Activity/Placement Percentages								
Admit	Grad	F	M	Adv Ed	Mngd Care	Private Practice	Agency	El	Mddle	Sec	Stu A	Other

Other
MO University of Missouri-Columbia   Columbia

Admit	Grad	F	M	Adv Ed	Mngd Care	Private Practice	Agency	El	Mddle	Sec	Stu A	Other
3	3	3	1									100

Other
NC East Carolina University   Greenville

Admit	Grad	F	M	Adv Ed	Mngd Care	Private Practice	Agency	El	Mddle	Sec	Stu A	Other
10	10	7	3				95					5

Other
NC East Carolina University   Greenville

Admit	Grad	F	M	Adv Ed	Mngd Care	Private Practice	Agency	El	Mddle	Sec	Stu A	Other
40	28	80%	20%	5			5		40	20	15	15

Other
TN Middle Tennessee State University   Murfreesboro

Admit	Grad	F	M	Adv Ed	Mngd Care	Private Practice	Agency	El	Mddle	Sec	Stu A	Other
20	16	12	8	10			90					

Other
TN Travecca Nazarene University   Nashville

Admit	Grad	F	M	Adv Ed	Mngd Care	Private Practice	Agency	El	Mddle	Sec	Stu A	Other

Other
TX Southwest Texas State University   San Marcos

Admit	Grad	F	M	Adv Ed	Mngd Care	Private Practice	Agency	El	Mddle	Sec	Stu A	Other

Pastoral Counseling
CO Denver Seminary   Denver

Admit	Grad	F	M	Adv Ed	Mngd Care	Private Practice	Agency	El	Mddle	Sec	Stu A	Other
10	5	0%	100%	5	0	0	0					95

Pastoral Counseling
MD Loyola College in Maryland   Columbia

Admit	Grad	F	M	Adv Ed	Mngd Care	Private Practice	Agency	El	Mddle	Sec	Stu A	Other
same	same	same	same	15		10	50	1	1	3	10	10

Pastoral Counseling
MS William Carey College   Hattiesburg

Admit	Grad	F	M	Adv Ed	Mngd Care	Private Practice	Agency	El	Mddle	Sec	Stu A	Other
10	10	4	16									

Pastoral Counseling
TX Houston Baptist University   Houston

Admit	Grad	F	M	Adv Ed	Mngd Care	Private Practice	Agency	El	Mddle	Sec	Stu A	Other
6												

Pastoral Counseling
WA University of Puget Sound   Tacoma

Admit	Grad	F	M	Adv Ed	Mngd Care	Private Practice	Agency	El	Mddle	Sec	Stu A	Other
4	2	3	1				100					

Rehabilitation Counseling
AL The University of Alabama   Tuscaloosa

Admit	Grad	F	M	Adv Ed	Mngd Care	Private Practice	Agency	El	Mddle	Sec	Stu A	Other
14	12	17	6	5	10	0	85					

Rehabilitation Counseling
AL Troy State University   Troy

Admit	Grad	F	M	Adv Ed	Mngd Care	Private Practice	Agency	El	Mddle	Sec	Stu A	Other
5 new program												

Rehabilitation Counseling
AL University of South Alabama   Mobile

Admit	Grad	F	M	Adv Ed	Mngd Care	Private Practice	Agency	El	Mddle	Sec	Stu A	Other
12	8											

Master's and Specialist Degree Programs												
Admission and Enrollment				Postgraduation Activity/Placement Percentages								
2002				Adv Ed	Mngd Care	Private	Agency	School and Student Affairs				Other
Admit	Grad	F	M			Practice		El	Mddle	Sec	Stu A	
Rehabilitation Counseling AR University of Arkansas at Little Rock Little Rock												
138	15	97	41	10		10	80					
Rehabilitation Counseling CA California State University-Fresno Fresno												
15	10			0	0	30	70	0	0	0		0
Rehabilitation Counseling CA San Diego State University San Diego												
25	12			5	10	25	25	0	0		5	20
Rehabilitation Counseling DC The George Washington University Washington, D.C.												
10	10	7	3	20			40					40
Rehabilitation Counseling FL Florida Atlantic University Boca Raton												
10	5	7	3	0		20	70					
Rehabilitation Counseling IA The University of Iowa Iowa City												
15	15	28	2	10	10	40	40	0	0	0		0
Rehabilitation Counseling ID University of Idaho Moscow												
15				0	0	10	90	0	0	0		0
Rehabilitation Counseling IL Illinois Institute of Technology Chicago												
15	12	12	3				100					
Rehabilitation Counseling IN Ball State University Muncie												
12	11			10	5	20	60	0	0	0		5
Rehabilitation Counseling KS Emporia State University Emporia												
7-12	7-12	4-6	3-6	10			10					80
Rehabilitation Counseling KY University of Kentucky Lexington												
20	20	15	5	10		10	80					
Rehabilitation Counseling ME University of Southern Maine Gorham												
10	5	9	1		2	1	96					1
Rehabilitation Counseling MO University of Missouri-Columbia Columbia												
6	5	5	7	20	0	0	80	0	0	0		0
Rehabilitation Counseling MS Mississippi State University Mississippi State University												
16	15	27	4	10	5	15	70					
Rehabilitation Counseling MT Montana State University - Billings Billings												
				5		5	90					

Master's and Specialist Degree Programs												
Admission and Enrollment 2002				Adv Ed	Mngd Care	Postgraduation Activity/Placement Percentages		School and Student Affairs				
						Private Agency Practice						
Admit	Grad	F	M			Private	Agency	El	Mddle	Sec	Stu A	Other

Rehabilitation Counseling
NC East Carolina University   Greenville

Admit	Grad	F	M	Adv Ed	Mngd Care	Private	Agency	El	Mddle	Sec	Stu A	Other
25	25	17	8				95					5

Rehabilitation Counseling
NY New York University   New York

Admit	Grad	F	M	Adv Ed	Mngd Care	Private	Agency	El	Mddle	Sec	Stu A	Other
				1	2	3	84					10

Rehabilitation Counseling
NY SUNY University at Buffalo   Buffalo

Admit	Grad	F	M	Adv Ed	Mngd Care	Private	Agency	El	Mddle	Sec	Stu A	Other
10	10	6	4	20	0	10	70		0	0	0	0

Rehabilitation Counseling
NY Syracuse University   Syracuse

Admit	Grad	F	M	Adv Ed	Mngd Care	Private	Agency	El	Mddle	Sec	Stu A	Other
10	8	15	8	10			90					

Rehabilitation Counseling
OH Ohio University   Athens

Admit	Grad	F	M	Adv Ed	Mngd Care	Private	Agency	El	Mddle	Sec	Stu A	Other
7	7											

Rehabilitation Counseling
OR Portland State University   Portland

Admit	Grad	F	M	Adv Ed	Mngd Care	Private	Agency	El	Mddle	Sec	Stu A	Other
14				10	10	10	70					

Rehabilitation Counseling
PA Penn State University   University Park

Admit	Grad	F	M	Adv Ed	Mngd Care	Private	Agency	El	Mddle	Sec	Stu A	Other

Rehabilitation Counseling
TN The University of Tennessee at Knoxville   Knoxville

Admit	Grad	F	M	Adv Ed	Mngd Care	Private	Agency	El	Mddle	Sec	Stu A	Other
15	11			10	5	10	75		0	0	0	0

Rehabilitation Counseling
TX Stephen F. Austin State University   Nacogdoches

Admit	Grad	F	M	Adv Ed	Mngd Care	Private	Agency	El	Mddle	Sec	Stu A	Other
8	6	4	4	10			60					

Rehabilitation Counseling
WV West Virginia University   Morgantown

Admit	Grad	F	M	Adv Ed	Mngd Care	Private	Agency	El	Mddle	Sec	Stu A	Other
15				10			90					

School Counseling
AL Auburn University   Auburn

Admit	Grad	F	M	Adv Ed	Mngd Care	Private	Agency	El	Mddle	Sec	Stu A	Other
5-10	5-10	8	2	0	0	0	0					0

School Counseling
AL The University of Alabama   Tuscaloosa

Admit	Grad	F	M	Adv Ed	Mngd Care	Private	Agency	El	Mddle	Sec	Stu A	Other
6	3	11	0	15	0	0	0	40	10	35		

School Counseling
AL Troy State University   Troy

Admit	Grad	F	M	Adv Ed	Mngd Care	Private	Agency	El	Mddle	Sec	Stu A	Other
15	5											

School Counseling
AL University of Montevallo   Montevallo

Admit	Grad	F	M	Adv Ed	Mngd Care	Private	Agency	El	Mddle	Sec	Stu A	Other
10	9	15	1	2				30	34	34		

School Counseling
AL University of North Alabama   Florence

Admit	Grad	F	M	Adv Ed	Mngd Care	Private	Agency	El	Mddle	Sec	Stu A	Other
15	12		5	5				40	20	35		

Master's and Specialist Degree Programs												
Admission and Enrollment				Postgraduation Activity/Placement Percentages								
2002				Adv	Mngd	Private	Agency	School and Student Affairs				
Admit	Grad	F	M	Ed	Care	Practice		El	Mddle	Sec	Stu A	Other

School Counseling
AL University of South Alabama Mobile

Admit	Grad	F	M	Adv Ed	Mngd Care	Private/Agency Practice		El	Mddle	Sec	Stu A	Other
16	9											

School Counseling
AZ Arizona State University Tempe

Admit	Grad	F	M	Adv Ed	Mngd Care	Private/Agency Practice		El	Mddle	Sec	Stu A	Other
15								10	20	40		20

School Counseling
CA California Lutheran University Thousand Oaks

Admit	Grad	F	M	Adv Ed	Mngd Care	Private/Agency Practice		El	Mddle	Sec	Stu A	Other
				98	0	0	0	10	25	65		0

School Counseling
CA California State University-Fresno Fresno

Admit	Grad	F	M	Adv Ed	Mngd Care	Private/Agency Practice		El	Mddle	Sec	Stu A	Other
30	20			0	0	0	0	10	20	70		0

School Counseling
CA La Sierra University Riverside

Admit	Grad	F	M	Adv Ed	Mngd Care	Private/Agency Practice		El	Mddle	Sec	Stu A	Other
20	10		5					33.3	33.3	33.3		

School Counseling
CA San Jose University San Jose

Admit	Grad	F	M	Adv Ed	Mngd Care	Private/Agency Practice		El	Mddle	Sec	Stu A	Other
60	50			60				15	15	30		40

School Counseling
CA University of San Diego, School of Education San Diego

Admit	Grad	F	M	Adv Ed	Mngd Care	Private/Agency Practice		El	Mddle	Sec	Stu A	Other
25	25		10				10	25	25	40		

School Counseling
CO Adams State College Alamosa

Admit	Grad	F	M	Adv Ed	Mngd Care	Private/Agency Practice		El	Mddle	Sec	Stu A	Other
60	58		7									

School Counseling
CO Univiversity of Colorado - Colorado Springs Colorado Springs

Admit	Grad	F	M	Adv Ed	Mngd Care	Private/Agency Practice		El	Mddle	Sec	Stu A	Other
40	35		10									

School Counseling
CO University of Colorado at Denver Denver

Admit	Grad	F	M	Adv Ed	Mngd Care	Private/Agency Practice		El	Mddle	Sec	Stu A	Other
45	40											

School Counseling
CO University of Northern Colorado Greeley

Admit	Grad	F	M	Adv Ed	Mngd Care	Private/Agency Practice		El	Mddle	Sec	Stu A	Other
25	22	17	8	15				15	30	40		

School Counseling
CO University of Phoenix Colorado Springs

Admit	Grad	F	M	Adv Ed	Mngd Care	Private/Agency Practice		El	Mddle	Sec	Stu A	Other

School Counseling
DC The George Washington University Washington, D. C.

Admit	Grad	F	M	Adv Ed	Mngd Care	Private/Agency Practice		El	Mddle	Sec	Stu A	Other
15	10	12	3	10				33	10	27		

School Counseling
FL Carlos Albizu University Miami

Admit	Grad	F	M	Adv Ed	Mngd Care	Private/Agency Practice		El	Mddle	Sec	Stu A	Other
11	11	20	1									

School Counseling
FL Florida Atlantic University Boca Raton

Admit	Grad	F	M	Adv Ed	Mngd Care	Private/Agency Practice		El	Mddle	Sec	Stu A	Other
50	20		10	5				30	30	40		

Master's and Specialist Degree Programs												
Admission and Enrollment				Postgraduation Activity/Placement Percentages								
2002				Adv	Mngd	Private	Agency	School and Student Affairs				
Admit	Grad	F	M	Ed	Care	Practice		EI	Mddle	Sec	Stu A	Other

School Counseling
FL Rollins College   Winter Park

Admit	Grad	F	M	Adv Ed	Mngd Care	Private	Agency	EI	Mddle	Sec	Stu A	Other
5	5	4	1	5	0	0		45	10	30		10

School Counseling
FL University of Central Florida   Orlando

Admit	Grad	F	M	Adv Ed	Mngd Care	Private	Agency	EI	Mddle	Sec	Stu A	Other
25/30	23	52	7	10				15	25	40		10

School Counseling
FL University of Florida   Gainesville

Admit	Grad	F	M	Adv Ed	Mngd Care	Private	Agency	EI	Mddle	Sec	Stu A	Other
18	16			10				30	30	30		

School Counseling
FL University of North Florida   Jacksonville

Admit	Grad	F	M	Adv Ed	Mngd Care	Private	Agency	EI	Mddle	Sec	Stu A	Other
30	30			0	0	0	0	50	25	25		0

School Counseling
GA Columbus State University   Columbus

Admit	Grad	F	M	Adv Ed	Mngd Care	Private	Agency	EI	Mddle	Sec	Stu A	Other
40	15	10	5	0	0	0	0	40	20	40		0

School Counseling
GA Georgia State University   Atlanta

Admit	Grad	F	M	Adv Ed	Mngd Care	Private	Agency	EI	Mddle	Sec	Stu A	Other
28	23	63	2	5	0	0	0	60	15	20		0

School Counseling
GA State University of West Georgia   Carrolton

Admit	Grad	F	M	Adv Ed	Mngd Care	Private	Agency	EI	Mddle	Sec	Stu A	Other
70	45	40	5	10	0	0	0	30	30	30		0

School Counseling
IA Iowa State University   Ames

Admit	Grad	F	M	Adv Ed	Mngd Care	Private	Agency	EI	Mddle	Sec	Stu A	Other
12-15	12-15	20	10					30	20	50		

School Counseling
IA The University of Iowa   Iowa City

Admit	Grad	F	M	Adv Ed	Mngd Care	Private	Agency	EI	Mddle	Sec	Stu A	Other
20	20	25	5	5	0	0	0	60	5	30		0

School Counseling
IA University of North Iowa   Cedar Falls

Admit	Grad	F	M	Adv Ed	Mngd Care	Private	Agency	EI	Mddle	Sec	Stu A	Other
30-40	10-15	60	15	0	0	0	0	40	30	30		0

School Counseling
ID Boise State University   Boise

Admit	Grad	F	M	Adv Ed	Mngd Care	Private	Agency	EI	Mddle	Sec	Stu A	Other
15-18	15-16	32	19			10	15	20	30	15		10

School Counseling
ID Idaho State University   Pocatello

Admit	Grad	F	M	Adv Ed	Mngd Care	Private	Agency	EI	Mddle	Sec	Stu A	Other
10	10	14	6	10				40	40	20		

School Counseling
ID Northwest Nazarene University   Nampa

Admit	Grad	F	M	Adv Ed	Mngd Care	Private	Agency	EI	Mddle	Sec	Stu A	Other
13	10		10					40	35	18		7

School Counseling
ID University of Idaho   Moscow

Admit	Grad	F	M	Adv Ed	Mngd Care	Private	Agency	EI	Mddle	Sec	Stu A	Other
15				0	0	0	0	40	30	30		0

School Counseling
IL Concordia University   River Forest

Admit	Grad	F	M	Adv Ed	Mngd Care	Private	Agency	EI	Mddle	Sec	Stu A	Other
7	3							10	10	80		

Master's and Specialist Degree Programs											
Admission and Enrollment				Postgraduation Activity/Placement Percentages							
2002				Adv	Mngd	Private	Agency	School and Student Affairs			
Admit	Grad	F	M	Ed	Care	\ Practice /		El	Mddle	Sec	Stu A	Other

School Counseling
IL Eastern Illinois University   Charleston

Admit	Grad	F	M	Adv Ed	Mngd Care	Private/Agency Practice		El	Mddle	Sec	Stu A	Other
20	20			0	0		0	10	15	70		

School Counseling
IL Lewis University   Romeoville

Admit	Grad	F	M	Adv Ed	Mngd Care	Private/Agency Practice		El	Mddle	Sec	Stu A	Other
40	20	75%	25%	0				5	5	90		

School Counseling
IL Southern Illinois University Carbondale   Carbondale

Admit	Grad	F	M	Adv Ed	Mngd Care	Private/Agency Practice		El	Mddle	Sec	Stu A	Other
20	18	19	1	10								5

School Counseling
IL Western Illinois University   Moline

Admit	Grad	F	M	Adv Ed	Mngd Care	Private/Agency Practice		El	Mddle	Sec	Stu A	Other
				0	0	0	0	15	20	65		0

School Counseling
IN Ball State University   Muncie

Admit	Grad	F	M	Adv Ed	Mngd Care	Private/Agency Practice		El	Mddle	Sec	Stu A	Other
12	10			5	0	0	0	30	20	40		5

School Counseling
IN Butler University   Indianapolis

Admit	Grad	F	M	Adv Ed	Mngd Care	Private/Agency Practice		El	Mddle	Sec	Stu A	Other
24	20	55	15		0	0	10	30	20	40		0

School Counseling
IN Indiana State University   Terre Haute

Admit	Grad	F	M	Adv Ed	Mngd Care	Private/Agency Practice		El	Mddle	Sec	Stu A	Other
20	17	32	8				5	30	30	30		

School Counseling
IN Indiana University   Bloomington

Admit	Grad	F	M	Adv Ed	Mngd Care	Private/Agency Practice		El	Mddle	Sec	Stu A	Other
25	22			10				20	35	35		

School Counseling
IN Indiana-Purdue University at Fort Wayne   Fort Wayne

Admit	Grad	F	M	Adv Ed	Mngd Care	Private/Agency Practice		El	Mddle	Sec	Stu A	Other
14	12	34	18					35	40	25		

School Counseling
IN Purdue University   West Lafayette

Admit	Grad	F	M	Adv Ed	Mngd Care	Private/Agency Practice		El	Mddle	Sec	Stu A	Other
10	8-10	19	1									

School Counseling
KS Emporia State University   Emporia

Admit	Grad	F	M	Adv Ed	Mngd Care	Private/Agency Practice		El	Mddle	Sec	Stu A	Other
10-20	10-20		3-6					25	15	60		

School Counseling
KS Kansas State University   Manhattan

Admit	Grad	F	M	Adv Ed	Mngd Care	Private/Agency Practice		El	Mddle	Sec	Stu A	Other
25	15	40	8	0	0	0	0	35	20	45		0

School Counseling
KS Pittsburg State University   Pittsburg

Admit	Grad	F	M	Adv Ed	Mngd Care	Private/Agency Practice		El	Mddle	Sec	Stu A	Other
20	20							25	15	60		

School Counseling
KS University of Kansas   Lawrence

Admit	Grad	F	M	Adv Ed	Mngd Care	Private/Agency Practice		El	Mddle	Sec	Stu A	Other
15	15											

School Counseling
KY Eastern Kentucky University   Richmond

Admit	Grad	F	M	Adv Ed	Mngd Care	Private/Agency Practice		El	Mddle	Sec	Stu A	Other
30				2	0	0	0	32.6	32.6	32.6		

Master's and Specialist Degree Programs

Admit	Grad	F	M	Adv Ed	Mngd Care	Private Practice	Agency	El	Mddle	Sec	Stu A	Other

Admission and Enrollment 2002 — Admit, Grad, F, M; **Postgraduation Activity/Placement Percentages** — Adv Ed, Mngd Care, Private | Agency Practice, School and Student Affairs (El, Mddle, Sec, Stu A, Other)

School Counseling
LA Louisiana State University Baton Rouge

Admit	Grad	F	M	Adv Ed	Mngd Care	Private	Agency	El	Mddle	Sec	Stu A	Other
5	5	10						40	20	40		

School Counseling
LA McNeese State University Lake Charles

Admit	Grad	F	M	Adv Ed	Mngd Care	Private	Agency	El	Mddle	Sec	Stu A	Other
4	4		0					50		50		

School Counseling
LA Our Lady of Holy Cross New Orleans

Admit	Grad	F	M	Adv Ed	Mngd Care	Private	Agency	El	Mddle	Sec	Stu A	Other
10	10											

School Counseling
LA Southeastern Louisiana University Hammond

Admit	Grad	F	M	Adv Ed	Mngd Care	Private	Agency	El	Mddle	Sec	Stu A	Other

School Counseling
LA University of New Orleans New Orleans

Admit	Grad	F	M	Adv Ed	Mngd Care	Private	Agency	El	Mddle	Sec	Stu A	Other
20	20		15	5				10	40	50		

School Counseling
MA Bridgewater State College Bridgewater

Admit	Grad	F	M	Adv Ed	Mngd Care	Private	Agency	El	Mddle	Sec	Stu A	Other
15	8		10	0				5	25	70		

School Counseling
MA Fitchburg State College Fitchburg

Admit	Grad	F	M	Adv Ed	Mngd Care	Private	Agency	El	Mddle	Sec	Stu A	Other
16	18		7					15	10	75		

School Counseling
MA Lesley University Cambridge

Admit	Grad	F	M	Adv Ed	Mngd Care	Private	Agency	El	Mddle	Sec	Stu A	Other

School Counseling
MA Suffolk University Boston

Admit	Grad	F	M	Adv Ed	Mngd Care	Private	Agency	El	Mddle	Sec	Stu A	Other
12	8	10	2	2					10	84		5

School Counseling
MD Johns Hopkins University Baltimore

Admit	Grad	F	M	Adv Ed	Mngd Care	Private	Agency	El	Mddle	Sec	Stu A	Other
50	43											

School Counseling
MD McDaniel College Westminster

Admit	Grad	F	M	Adv Ed	Mngd Care	Private	Agency	El	Mddle	Sec	Stu A	Other
60	25							30	30	40		

School Counseling
ME University of Southern Maine Gorham

Admit	Grad	F	M	Adv Ed	Mngd Care	Private	Agency	El	Mddle	Sec	Stu A	Other
15	15	11	4	5				35	30	35		

School Counseling
MI Andrews University Berrien Springs

Admit	Grad	F	M	Adv Ed	Mngd Care	Private	Agency	El	Mddle	Sec	Stu A	Other
5	4		2	10				30	30	30		

School Counseling
MI Eastern Michigan University Ypsilanti

Admit	Grad	F	M	Adv Ed	Mngd Care	Private	Agency	El	Mddle	Sec	Stu A	Other
35	29	20	9	0	0	0	0	20	40	40		0

School Counseling
MI Oakland University Rochester

Admit	Grad	F	M	Adv Ed	Mngd Care	Private	Agency	El	Mddle	Sec	Stu A	Other
75	60		8					10	40	40	10	

Master's and Specialist Degree Programs												
Admission and Enrollment				Postgraduation Activity/Placement Percentages								
2002				Adv	Mngd	Private	Agency	School and Student Affairs				
Admit	Grad	F	M	Ed	Care	Practice		El	Mddle	Sec	Stu A	Other

School Counseling
MI Siena Heights University   Adrian

Admit	Grad	F	M	Adv Ed	Mngd Care	Private	Agency	El	Mddle	Sec	Stu A	Other
7	5			0	0	0	0	10	20	60	10	0

School Counseling
MN Minnesota State University Moorhead   Moorhead

Admit	Grad	F	M	Adv Ed	Mngd Care	Private	Agency	El	Mddle	Sec	Stu A	Other
7	4											

School Counseling
MN Minnesota State University, Mankato   Mankato

Admit	Grad	F	M	Adv Ed	Mngd Care	Private	Agency	El	Mddle	Sec	Stu A	Other
15	15	10	5					20	20	60		

School Counseling
MO Northwest Missouri State University   Maryville

Admit	Grad	F	M	Adv Ed	Mngd Care	Private	Agency	El	Mddle	Sec	Stu A	Other
12	12							30	20	50		

School Counseling
MO Southeast Missouri State University   Cape Girardeau

Admit	Grad	F	M	Adv Ed	Mngd Care	Private	Agency	El	Mddle	Sec	Stu A	Other
20	18			5				35	20	30	10	

School Counseling
MO Truman State University   Kirksville

Admit	Grad	F	M	Adv Ed	Mngd Care	Private	Agency	El	Mddle	Sec	Stu A	Other
5	5	4	1	10				50	0	40		

School Counseling
MO University of Missouri - St. Louis   Saint Louis

Admit	Grad	F	M	Adv Ed	Mngd Care	Private	Agency	El	Mddle	Sec	Stu A	Other
50	40	120	30									

School Counseling
MO University of Missouri-Columbia   Columbia

Admit	Grad	F	M	Adv Ed	Mngd Care	Private	Agency	El	Mddle	Sec	Stu A	Other
6-8	6-8	15	2	0	0	0	0	50	25	25		0

School Counseling
MS Mississippi College   Clinton

Admit	Grad	F	M	Adv Ed	Mngd Care	Private	Agency	El	Mddle	Sec	Stu A	Other
10	3			10				20	30	40		

School Counseling
MS Mississippi State University   Mississippi State University

Admit	Grad	F	M	Adv Ed	Mngd Care	Private	Agency	El	Mddle	Sec	Stu A	Other
20	18	34	4	5			10	15	35	35		

School Counseling
MS William Carey College   Hattiesburg

Admit	Grad	F	M	Adv Ed	Mngd Care	Private	Agency	El	Mddle	Sec	Stu A	Other
10	10		8				100	20	20	60		

School Counseling
MT Montana Sate University-Northern   Havre

Admit	Grad	F	M	Adv Ed	Mngd Care	Private	Agency	El	Mddle	Sec	Stu A	Other
15	15	20	10									

School Counseling
MT Montana State University - Billings   Billings

Admit	Grad	F	M	Adv Ed	Mngd Care	Private	Agency	El	Mddle	Sec	Stu A	Other
15-25	10-20	75%	25%	5			15%	26	26	26		2

School Counseling
MT Montana State University - Bozeman   Bozeman

Admit	Grad	F	M	Adv Ed	Mngd Care	Private	Agency	El	Mddle	Sec	Stu A	Other
8-9	6-8	6	2	10				10	40	40		

School Counseling
NC Appalachian State University   Boone

Admit	Grad	F	M	Adv Ed	Mngd Care	Private	Agency	El	Mddle	Sec	Stu A	Other
20	17			5	0	0	0	55	20	20		0

Master's and Specialist Degree Programs

Admit	Grad	F	M	Adv Ed	Mngd Care	Private Practice	Agency	El	Mddle	Sec	Stu A	Other
Admission and Enrollment 2002				Postgraduation Activity/Placement Percentages				School and Student Affairs				

School Counseling
NC Campbell University Buies Creek

Admit	Grad	F	M	Adv Ed	Mngd Care	Private Practice	Agency	El	Mddle	Sec	Stu A	Other
15	13-15	60	10	0	0	0	0	40	40	20		0

School Counseling
NC North Carolina A&T State University Greensboro

Admit	Grad	F	M	Adv Ed	Mngd Care	Private Practice	Agency	El	Mddle	Sec	Stu A	Other

School Counseling
NC The University of North Carolina at Chapel Hill Chapel Hill

Admit	Grad	F	M	Adv Ed	Mngd Care	Private Practice	Agency	El	Mddle	Sec	Stu A	Other
15-20	15-20							40	20	40		

School Counseling
NC The University of North Carolina at Greensboro Greensboro

Admit	Grad	F	M	Adv Ed	Mngd Care	Private Practice	Agency	El	Mddle	Sec	Stu A	Other
12	12	21	3	10				30	30	25		5

School Counseling
NC University of North Carolina at Charlotte Charlotte

Admit	Grad	F	M	Adv Ed	Mngd Care	Private Practice	Agency	El	Mddle	Sec	Stu A	Other

School Counseling
NC Wake Forest University Winston-Salem

Admit	Grad	F	M	Adv Ed	Mngd Care	Private Practice	Agency	El	Mddle	Sec	Stu A	Other
7	7	6	1	16				28	28	28		

School Counseling
ND North Dakota State University Fargo

Admit	Grad	F	M	Adv Ed	Mngd Care	Private Practice	Agency	El	Mddle	Sec	Stu A	Other
19	11	34	6	5	0	0	0	25	15	40		15

School Counseling
NE Chadron State College Chadron

Admit	Grad	F	M	Adv Ed	Mngd Care	Private Practice	Agency	El	Mddle	Sec	Stu A	Other
7	5											

School Counseling
NE University of Nebraska-Omaha Omaha

Admit	Grad	F	M	Adv Ed	Mngd Care	Private Practice	Agency	El	Mddle	Sec	Stu A	Other
10	9			0	0	0	0	0	0	90		0

School Counseling
NE Wayne State College Wayne

Admit	Grad	F	M	Adv Ed	Mngd Care	Private Practice	Agency	El	Mddle	Sec	Stu A	Other
15	10							50	50	50		

School Counseling
NH Plymouth State College Plymouth

Admit	Grad	F	M	Adv Ed	Mngd Care	Private Practice	Agency	El	Mddle	Sec	Stu A	Other
25	15	9	6	2				38	30	30		

School Counseling
NJ The College of New Jersey Ewing

Admit	Grad	F	M	Adv Ed	Mngd Care	Private Practice	Agency	El	Mddle	Sec	Stu A	Other
20	20			5					33	33		

School Counseling
NJ William Paterson University Wayne

Admit	Grad	F	M	Adv Ed	Mngd Care	Private Practice	Agency	El	Mddle	Sec	Stu A	Other
24	15		10					32	32	32		3

School Counseling
NV University of Nevada Reno

Admit	Grad	F	M	Adv Ed	Mngd Care	Private Practice	Agency	El	Mddle	Sec	Stu A	Other
15	12	35	20	20				40	40	20	20	

School Counseling
NY Canisius College Buffalo

Admit	Grad	F	M	Adv Ed	Mngd Care	Private Practice	Agency	El	Mddle	Sec	Stu A	Other
50	50			10	0	0	0	20	20	30		20

Master's and Specialist Degree Programs												
Admission and Enrollment				Postgraduation Activity/Placement Percentages								
2002				Adv	Mngd	Private	Agency	School and Student Affairs				
Admit	Grad	F	M	Ed	Care	Practice		El	Mddle	Sec	Stu A	Other
School Counseling NY College at Oswego SUNY Oswego												
20	25	75	10	10	0	0	10	10	30	40		0
School Counseling NY Lehman College of the City University of New York Bronx												
30	25		20				10	10	10	60	10	
School Counseling NY Marist College Poughkeepsie												
30	23	30	22	10				30	30	30		
School Counseling NY New York University New York												
			0			13.8	9.9	33	33		8.6	
School Counseling NY Niagara University Niagara University												
25	25			0	0	0	0	10	45	45		0
School Counseling NY Plattsburgh State University Plattsburgh												
20	16		4	5	0	0	0	30	30	30		5
School Counseling NY Queens College, City University of New York Flushing												
35	30 - 40	85	10	1				14	30	50		5
School Counseling NY State University of New York at Oneonta Oneonta												
30	30				0	0	0	35	30	35		2.5
School Counseling NY SUNY College of Brockport Brockport												
30	30	20	10	0	0	0	0	30	30	40		0
School Counseling NY SUNY University at Buffalo Buffalo												
30	27	24	6	15			5			80		
School Counseling NY Syracuse University Syracuse												
20	20	50	10	10				10	30	30		
School Counseling NY University of Rochester Rochester												
25	23	36	10				5	15	30	45		5
School Counseling OH Cleveland State University Cleveland												
30	26											
School Counseling OH John Carroll University Cleveland												
20	15		5	0	0	0	0	20	20	60	0	0
School Counseling OH Kent State University Kent												
32	25	52	5					35	25	40		

Master's and Specialist Degree Programs												
Admission and Enrollment 2002				Postgraduation Activity/Placement Percentages								
				Adv Ed	Mngd Care	Private Practice	Agency	School and Student Affairs				
Admit	Grad	F	M					El	Mddle	Sec	Stu A	Other
School Counseling OH Malone College Canton												
15-20	10-15	80%	20%	10	0	0	0	25	25	40		0
School Counseling OH Ohio University Athens												
8	8											
School Counseling OH The University of Toledo Toledo												
20	18		8	2				40	18	40		
School Counseling OH University of Cincinnati Cincinnati												
20	8	14	4					33	33	33		
School Counseling OH Walsh University North Canton												
12	10-12			0	0	0	0	20	20	60		0
School Counseling OH Xavier University Cincinnati												
75	30	70%	30%	10	0	0	0	20	20	25		20
School Counseling OH Youngstown State University Youngstown												
20	10			5				95				
School Counseling OR George Fox University Portland												
25	new pgm		7									
School Counseling OR Oregon State University Corvallis												
20	20	15	5					30	20	50		
School Counseling OR Portland State University Portland												
14				0	0	0	0	20	20	60		
School Counseling PA Arcadia University Glenside												
17 (2001)	1 (2001)		5					60		40		
School Counseling PA California University of Pennsylvania California												
18	13	31	8	0	0	0	25	20	10	20		20
School Counseling PA Duquesne University Pittsburgh												
25	15			6	0	0	0	38	23	33		0
School Counseling PA Geneva College Beaver Falls												
7	6											
School Counseling PA Indiana University of Pennsylvania Indiana												
45												

Master's and Specialist Degree Programs

Admit	Grad	F	M	Adv Ed	Mngd Care	Private Practice	Agency	El	Mddle	Sec	Stu A	Other

School Counseling
PA Kutztown University   Kutztown

Admit	Grad	F	M	Adv Ed	Mngd Care	Private Practice	Agency	El	Mddle	Sec	Stu A	Other
29	18			5	0	0	5	17	18	55		0

School Counseling
PA Penn State University   University Park

Admit	Grad	F	M	Adv Ed	Mngd Care	Private Practice	Agency	El	Mddle	Sec	Stu A	Other

School Counseling
PA Shippensburg University of PA   Shippensburg

Admit	Grad	F	M	Adv Ed	Mngd Care	Private Practice	Agency	El	Mddle	Sec	Stu A	Other
29	20	83	15	2	2	0	1	30	30	35		0

School Counseling
PA West Chester University   West Chester

Admit	Grad	F	M	Adv Ed	Mngd Care	Private Practice	Agency	El	Mddle	Sec	Stu A	Other
80	40			0	0	0	0	30	20	50		0

School Counseling
PA Westminster College   New Wilmington

Admit	Grad	F	M	Adv Ed	Mngd Care	Private Practice	Agency	El	Mddle	Sec	Stu A	Other
30	30	70	30					15	70	70		

School Counseling
RI Rhode Island College   Providence

Admit	Grad	F	M	Adv Ed	Mngd Care	Private Practice	Agency	El	Mddle	Sec	Stu A	Other
25	15	30	10	0	0	0	0	40	30	30		0

School Counseling
SC Clemson University   Clemson

Admit	Grad	F	M	Adv Ed	Mngd Care	Private Practice	Agency	El	Mddle	Sec	Stu A	Other
60	30	50	10	0	0	0	0	50	0	50		0

School Counseling
SC Winthrop University   Rock Hill

Admit	Grad	F	M	Adv Ed	Mngd Care	Private Practice	Agency	El	Mddle	Sec	Stu A	Other
12	14	22	3	0				40	30	30		

School Counseling
SD South Dakota State University   Brookings

Admit	Grad	F	M	Adv Ed	Mngd Care	Private Practice	Agency	El	Mddle	Sec	Stu A	Other
25	25											

School Counseling
SD The University of South Dakota   Vermillion

Admit	Grad	F	M	Adv Ed	Mngd Care	Private Practice	Agency	El	Mddle	Sec	Stu A	Other
12		75%	25%	100				25	25	50		

School Counseling
TN East Tennessee State University   Johnson City

Admit	Grad	F	M	Adv Ed	Mngd Care	Private Practice	Agency	El	Mddle	Sec	Stu A	Other
10	9			2	0	0	0	30	30	30		8

School Counseling
TN Lee University   Cleveland

Admit	Grad	F	M	Adv Ed	Mngd Care	Private Practice	Agency	El	Mddle	Sec	Stu A	Other
15	0 (new)		New					0 - New	0 - New	0 - New		

School Counseling
TN Middle Tennessee State University   Murfreesboro

Admit	Grad	F	M	Adv Ed	Mngd Care	Private Practice	Agency	El	Mddle	Sec	Stu A	Other
20	16		2					60	10	30		

School Counseling
TN Peabody College, Vanderbilt University   Nashville

Admit	Grad	F	M	Adv Ed	Mngd Care	Private Practice	Agency	El	Mddle	Sec	Stu A	Other
12	12	90%	10%	5				25	30	30		10

School Counseling
TN The University of Tennessee at Knoxville   Knoxville

Admit	Grad	F	M	Adv Ed	Mngd Care	Private Practice	Agency	El	Mddle	Sec	Stu A	Other
13	11			10	0	0	0	40	20	30		0

Master's and Specialist Degree Programs

Admission and Enrollment				Postgraduation Activity/Placement Percentages								
2002				Adv Ed	Mngd Care	Private Practice	Agency	School and Student Affairs				
Admit	Grad	F	M					El	Mddle	Sec	Stu A	Other
School Counseling TX Houston Baptist University Houston												
School Counseling TX Lamar University Beaumont												
	25											
School Counseling TX Our Lady of the Lake University San Antonio												
7	7							30	40	40		
School Counseling TX Southwest Texas State University San Marcos												
School Counseling TX Stephen F. Austin State University Nacogdoches												
10	10		1					50	30	20		
School Counseling TX Tarleton State University Stephenville												
40	40			0	0	0	0	73	15	15		0
School Counseling TX Texas A & M University - Commerce Commerce												
43	40			5	0	0	0	45	15	35		0
School Counseling TX Texas Southern University Houston												
20	10		15	5	0	0	0	20	35	39	1	0
School Counseling TX Texas Tech University Lubbock												
13	10		1	5	0	2	10	15	20	40	0	8
School Counseling TX University of North Texas Denton												
75	60	69	4					50		50		
School Counseling TX University of Texas at El Paso El Paso												
25	25											
School Counseling TX University of Texas at Tyler Tyler												
10	7	20	5					35	30	30	5	
School Counseling TX University of Texas of the Permian Basin Odessa												
20	6	15	5	1	0	0	0	35	34	30		
School Counseling VA College of William and Mary Williamsburg												
10	10	8	2					34	33	33		
School Counseling VA George Mason University Fairfax												
40	15	80%	20%	20				20	20	40		

Master's and Specialist Degree Programs												
Admission and Enrollment 2002				Postgraduation Activity/Placement Percentages								
Admit	Grad	F	M	Adv Ed	Mngd Care	Private Practice	Agency Practice	El	Mddle	Sec	Stu A	Other

School Counseling
VA James Madison University Harrisonburg

Admit	Grad	F	M	Adv Ed	Mngd Care	Private	Agency	El	Mddle	Sec	Stu A	Other
10	10											

School Counseling
VA Old Dominion University Norfolk

Admit	Grad	F	M	Adv Ed	Mngd Care	Private	Agency	El	Mddle	Sec	Stu A	Other
30	24	48	12	5				35	30	30		

School Counseling
VA Radford University Radford

Admit	Grad	F	M	Adv Ed	Mngd Care	Private	Agency	El	Mddle	Sec	Stu A	Other
12	12			10	0	0	5	20	32	33		0

School Counseling
VA Regent University Virginia Beach

Admit	Grad	F	M	Adv Ed	Mngd Care	Private	Agency	El	Mddle	Sec	Stu A	Other
8	8	4	3					50	20	19		11

School Counseling
VA Virginia Tech Blacksburg

Admit	Grad	F	M	Adv Ed	Mngd Care	Private	Agency	El	Mddle	Sec	Stu A	Other
20	18	15	5					30	20	50		

School Counseling
WA Central Washington University Ellensburg

Admit	Grad	F	M	Adv Ed	Mngd Care	Private	Agency	El	Mddle	Sec	Stu A	Other
2	1											

School Counseling
WA Eastern Washington University Cheney

Admit	Grad	F	M	Adv Ed	Mngd Care	Private	Agency	El	Mddle	Sec	Stu A	Other

School Counseling
WA Seattle University Seattle

Admit	Grad	F	M	Adv Ed	Mngd Care	Private	Agency	El	Mddle	Sec	Stu A	Other
25	25	18	2	6	0	0		30	40	30		

School Counseling
WA University of Puget Sound Tacoma

Admit	Grad	F	M	Adv Ed	Mngd Care	Private	Agency	El	Mddle	Sec	Stu A	Other
6	6	5	1					10	30	30		

School Counseling
WA Western Washington University Bellingham

Admit	Grad	F	M	Adv Ed	Mngd Care	Private	Agency	El	Mddle	Sec	Stu A	Other
6	6	4	2					35	30	35		

School Counseling
WI University of Wisconsin-Oshkosh Oshkosh

Admit	Grad	F	M	Adv Ed	Mngd Care	Private	Agency	El	Mddle	Sec	Stu A	Other
30	20	63	11	1				33	33	33		

School Counseling
WI University of Wisconsin-Whitewater Whitewater

Admit	Grad	F	M	Adv Ed	Mngd Care	Private	Agency	El	Mddle	Sec	Stu A	Other
23	16											

School Counseling
WV West Virginia University Morgantown

Admit	Grad	F	M	Adv Ed	Mngd Care	Private	Agency	El	Mddle	Sec	Stu A	Other
16				10			90	60	10	30		

School Counseling
WY University of Wyoming Laramie

Admit	Grad	F	M	Adv Ed	Mngd Care	Private	Agency	El	Mddle	Sec	Stu A	Other
9	5	14	4	10	0	0		30	30	30		

Student Affairs
CA California Lutheran University Thousand Oaks

Admit	Grad	F	M	Adv Ed	Mngd Care	Private	Agency	El	Mddle	Sec	Stu A	Other
				80	0	0	0		0	0	0	100

Master's and Specialist Degree Programs												
Admission and Enrollment 2002				Postgraduation Activity/Placement Percentages								
				Adv Ed	Mngd Care	Private Practice	Agency	School and Student Affairs				Other
Admit	Grad	F	M			Private	Agency	El	Mddle	Sec	Stu A	

Student Affairs
CA California State University-Fresno   Fresno

Admit	Grad	F	M	Adv Ed	Mngd Care	Private	Agency	El	Mddle	Sec	Stu A	Other
20	14			0	0	0	0		0	0	0	100

Student Affairs
CA San Jose University   San Jose

Admit	Grad	F	M	Adv Ed	Mngd Care	Private	Agency	El	Mddle	Sec	Stu A	Other
30	20			20								

Student Affairs
CO University of Colorado - Colorado Springs   Colorado Springs

Admit	Grad	F	M	Adv Ed	Mngd Care	Private	Agency	El	Mddle	Sec	Stu A	Other
5	5	3	2									

Student Affairs
DE University of Delaware   Newark

Admit	Grad	F	M	Adv Ed	Mngd Care	Private	Agency	El	Mddle	Sec	Stu A	Other
6	6	8	4	10								90

Student Affairs
IA The University of Iowa   Iowa City

Admit	Grad	F	M	Adv Ed	Mngd Care	Private	Agency	El	Mddle	Sec	Stu A	Other
15	15	12	3	25	0	0	0		0	0	0	75

Student Affairs
ID Idaho State University   Pocatello

Admit	Grad	F	M	Adv Ed	Mngd Care	Private	Agency	El	Mddle	Sec	Stu A	Other
3	3	1	2									100

Student Affairs
IN Indiana State University   Terre Haute

Admit	Grad	F	M	Adv Ed	Mngd Care	Private	Agency	El	Mddle	Sec	Stu A	Other
20	15	20	15									100

Student Affairs
IN Purdue University   West Lafayette

Admit	Grad	F	M	Adv Ed	Mngd Care	Private	Agency	El	Mddle	Sec	Stu A	Other
10	8	11	5									100

Student Affairs
KS Kansas State University   Manhattan

Admit	Grad	F	M	Adv Ed	Mngd Care	Private	Agency	El	Mddle	Sec	Stu A	Other
20	10	20	20	10	0	0	0		0	0	0	90

Student Affairs
KY Eastern Kentucky University   Richmond

Admit	Grad	F	M	Adv Ed	Mngd Care	Private	Agency	El	Mddle	Sec	Stu A	Other
				8	0	0	2					90

Student Affairs
KY Western Kentucky University   Bowling Green

Admit	Grad	F	M	Adv Ed	Mngd Care	Private	Agency	El	Mddle	Sec	Stu A	Other
15	13			4	0	0	0		0	0	0	96

Student Affairs
LA Northwestern State University   Natchitoches

Admit	Grad	F	M	Adv Ed	Mngd Care	Private	Agency	El	Mddle	Sec	Stu A	Other
20	15			15	0	0	10		0	0	0	75

Student Affairs
MA Bridgewater State College   Bridgewater

Admit	Grad	F	M	Adv Ed	Mngd Care	Private	Agency	El	Mddle	Sec	Stu A	Other
15	8	15	12	2							100	

Student Affairs
MN Minnesota State University, Mankato   Mankato

Admit	Grad	F	M	Adv Ed	Mngd Care	Private	Agency	El	Mddle	Sec	Stu A	Other
15	15	12	3	1							99	

Student Affairs
MO Truman State University   Kirksville

Admit	Grad	F	M	Adv Ed	Mngd Care	Private	Agency	El	Mddle	Sec	Stu A	Other
3	3	1	2	10			10					80

Master's and Specialist Degree Programs

| Admission and Enrollment 2002 | | | | Postgraduation Activity/Placement Percentages | | | | | | | | |
Admit	Grad	F	M	Adv Ed	Mngd Care	Private Practice	Agency Practice	EI	Mddle	Sec	Stu A	Other

Student Affairs
MO University of Missouri-Columbia Columbia

Admit	Grad	F	M	Adv Ed	Mngd Care	Private	Agency	EI	Mddle	Sec	Stu A	Other
1-2	1-2	2	2	50	0	0	0		0	0	0	50

Student Affairs
MS Mississippi State University Mississippi State University

Admit	Grad	F	M	Adv Ed	Mngd Care	Private	Agency	EI	Mddle	Sec	Stu A	Other
16	10	23	3									100

Student Affairs
NC Appalachian State University Boone

Admit	Grad	F	M	Adv Ed	Mngd Care	Private	Agency	EI	Mddle	Sec	Stu A	Other
15	13			4	0	0	0		0	0	75	21

Student Affairs
NC The University of North Carolina at Greensboro Greensboro

Admit	Grad	F	M	Adv Ed	Mngd Care	Private	Agency	EI	Mddle	Sec	Stu A	Other
5	5	7	3									100

Student Affairs
NE University of Nebraska-Omaha Omaha

Admit	Grad	F	M	Adv Ed	Mngd Care	Private	Agency	EI	Mddle	Sec	Stu A	Other
5	4			0	0	0	0		0	0	0	100

Student Affairs
NE Wayne State College Wayne

Admit	Grad	F	M	Adv Ed	Mngd Care	Private	Agency	EI	Mddle	Sec	Stu A	Other
1	1											100

Student Affairs
NV University of Nevada Reno

Admit	Grad	F	M	Adv Ed	Mngd Care	Private	Agency	EI	Mddle	Sec	Stu A	Other
5	3	8	2	20								80

Student Affairs
NY Canisius College Buffalo

Admit	Grad	F	M	Adv Ed	Mngd Care	Private	Agency	EI	Mddle	Sec	Stu A	Other
25	25			10	0	0			0	0	30	20

Student Affairs
NY Syracuse University Syracuse

Admit	Grad	F	M	Adv Ed	Mngd Care	Private	Agency	EI	Mddle	Sec	Stu A	Other
5	5	5	5	10							90	

Student Affairs
OH Youngstown State University Youngstown

Admit	Grad	F	M	Adv Ed	Mngd Care	Private	Agency	EI	Mddle	Sec	Stu A	Other
			5					95				

Student Affairs
PA Kutztown University Kutztown

Admit	Grad	F	M	Adv Ed	Mngd Care	Private	Agency	EI	Mddle	Sec	Stu A	Other
7	7			5	0	0	0	0	0	0	0	95

Student Affairs
PA Shippensburg University of PA Shippensburg

Admit	Grad	F	M	Adv Ed	Mngd Care	Private	Agency	EI	Mddle	Sec	Stu A	Other
10	7	24	9	10	0	0	0		0	0	0	90

Student Affairs
PA West Chester University West Chester

Admit	Grad	F	M	Adv Ed	Mngd Care	Private	Agency	EI	Mddle	Sec	Stu A	Other
40	20			20	10	0	0		0	10	10	50

Student Affairs
SC Clemson University Clemson

Admit	Grad	F	M	Adv Ed	Mngd Care	Private	Agency	EI	Mddle	Sec	Stu A	Other
30	20	20	10	10	0	0	0		0	0	0	90

Student Affairs
SD South Dakota State University Brookings

Admit	Grad	F	M	Adv Ed	Mngd Care	Private	Agency	EI	Mddle	Sec	Stu A	Other
10	10											

	Master's and Specialist Degree Programs										
Admission and Enrollment				Postgraduation Activity/Placement Percentages							
2002				Adv Ed	Mngd Care	Private | Agency Practice		School and Student Affairs				Other
Admit	Grad	F	M					EI	Mddle	Sec	Stu A	

Student Affairs
SD The University of South Dakota   Vermillion

Admit	Grad	F	M	Adv Ed	Mngd Care	Private	Agency	EI	Mddle	Sec	Stu A	Other
5		75%	25%	100								

Student Affairs
TX Texas A & M University - Commerce   Commerce

Admit	Grad	F	M	Adv Ed	Mngd Care	Private	Agency	EI	Mddle	Sec	Stu A	Other
5	2			10	0	0	0		0	0	0	90

Student Affairs
VA Old Dominion University   Norfolk

Admit	Grad	F	M	Adv Ed	Mngd Care	Private	Agency	EI	Mddle	Sec	Stu A	Other
6	4	9	3				20					80

Student Affairs
VA Radford University   Radford

Admit	Grad	F	M	Adv Ed	Mngd Care	Private	Agency	EI	Mddle	Sec	Stu A	Other
12	12			10	0	0	0		0	0	0	90

Student Affairs
WI University of Wisconsin-La Crosse   LaCrosse

Admit	Grad	F	M	Adv Ed	Mngd Care	Private	Agency	EI	Mddle	Sec	Stu A	Other
15	15	10	5									100

Student Affairs
WI University of Wisconsin-Oshkosh   Oshkosh

Admit	Grad	F	M	Adv Ed	Mngd Care	Private	Agency	EI	Mddle	Sec	Stu A	Other
10	6	15	4	1								99

Student Affairs
WI University of Wisconsin-Whitewater   Whitewater

Admit	Grad	F	M	Adv Ed	Mngd Care	Private	Agency	EI	Mddle	Sec	Stu A	Other
5	3											

Student Affairs
WY University of Wyoming   Laramie

Admit	Grad	F	M	Adv Ed	Mngd Care	Private	Agency	EI	Mddle	Sec	Stu A	Other
2	1	1	0	10	0	0						90

Doctoral Degree Programs

| Admission and Enrollment 2002 | | | | Postgraduation Activity/Placement Percentages | | | | | | | | |
Admit	Grad	F	M	Adv Ed	Mngd Care	Private Practice	Agency Practice	EI	Mddle	Sec	Stu A	Other
Addictions Counseling — NV University of Nevada Reno												
1	1	4	1	20	30	20	30					
Career Counseling — MI Oakland University Rochester												
1												
Community Counseling — MI Oakland University Rochester												
1												
Community Counseling — NC University of North Carolina at Charlotte Charlotte												
Community Counseling — NV University of Nevada Reno												
2	1	12	2	20	30	20	30					
Community Counseling — OH The University of Toledo Toledo												
10	8	5	5		10	70	20					
Community Counseling — VA George Mason University Fairfax												
3	2	50%	50%			20	60					20
Counselor Education — AL Auburn University Auburn												
1-2	3-6	12	1	80			5		5	5	5	
Counselor Education — AL The University of Alabama Tuscaloosa												
9	4	13	6	5	25	25				15	10	20
Counselor Education — CO University of Northern Colorado Greeley												
6	6	13	5			30						70
Counselor Education — DC The George Washington University Washington, D.C.												
10	~5	40	10	40								60
Counselor Education — FL University of Central Florida Orlando												
6	6	12	7				16.7	16.7			66.6	
Counselor Education — GA Georgia State University Atlanta												
4-6	2-4	12	4	0	10	10	20	20	10	10	20	
Counselor Education — IA The University of Iowa Iowa City												
3	3	8	7	0	0	20	15		0	0	65	0

Doctoral Degree Programs

| Admission and Enrollment 2002 | | | | Postgraduation Activity/Placement Percentages | | | | | | | | |
Admit	Grad	F	M	Adv Ed	Mngd Care	Private Practice	Agency	EI	Mddle	Sec	Stu A	Other

Counselor Education
ID Idaho State University   Pocatello

Admit	Grad	F	M	Adv Ed	Mngd Care	Private Practice	Agency	EI	Mddle	Sec	Stu A	Other
4	4	7	3	90		10						

Counselor Education
ID University of Idaho   Moscow

Admit	Grad	F	M	Adv Ed	Mngd Care	Private Practice	Agency	EI	Mddle	Sec	Stu A	Other

Counselor Education
IL Southern Illinois University Carbondale   Carbondale

Admit	Grad	F	M	Adv Ed	Mngd Care	Private Practice	Agency	EI	Mddle	Sec	Stu A	Other
10	8	15	3	75		5	10					10

Counselor Education
KS Kansas State University   Manhattan

Admit	Grad	F	M	Adv Ed	Mngd Care	Private Practice	Agency	EI	Mddle	Sec	Stu A	Other
5	2	14	5	0	0	0	10		5	0	5	90

Counselor Education
LA University of New Orleans   New Orleans

Admit	Grad	F	M	Adv Ed	Mngd Care	Private Practice	Agency	EI	Mddle	Sec	Stu A	Other
15	15	30	18		5	20	50			5	20	

Counselor Education
MI Oakland University   Rochester

Admit	Grad	F	M	Adv Ed	Mngd Care	Private Practice	Agency	EI	Mddle	Sec	Stu A	Other
3	3											

Counselor Education
MO University of Missouri - St. Louis   Saint Louis

Admit	Grad	F	M	Adv Ed	Mngd Care	Private Practice	Agency	EI	Mddle	Sec	Stu A	Other

Counselor Education
MS Mississippi State University   Mississippi State University

Admit	Grad	F	M	Adv Ed	Mngd Care	Private Practice	Agency	EI	Mddle	Sec	Stu A	Other
						10					90	

Counselor Education
NC University of North Carolina at Charlotte   Charlotte

Admit	Grad	F	M	Adv Ed	Mngd Care	Private Practice	Agency	EI	Mddle	Sec	Stu A	Other

Counselor Education
NC University of North Carolina at Greensboro   Greensboro

Admit	Grad	F	M	Adv Ed	Mngd Care	Private Practice	Agency	EI	Mddle	Sec	Stu A	Other
8	8	15	15	There no place to put placement of doctoral graduates for UNCG	teaching /counsel or education 60	agency 10	private practice 10					student affairs administration

Counselor Education
ND North Dakota State University   Fargo

Admit	Grad	F	M	Adv Ed	Mngd Care	Private Practice	Agency	EI	Mddle	Sec	Stu A	Other
8	New Program	5	3	0	5	10	10		0	0	0	75

Counselor Education
NV University of Nevada   Reno

Admit	Grad	F	M	Adv Ed	Mngd Care	Private Practice	Agency	EI	Mddle	Sec	Stu A	Other
				10								90

Counselor Education
NY SUNY University at Buffalo   Buffalo

Admit	Grad	F	M	Adv Ed	Mngd Care	Private Practice	Agency	EI	Mddle	Sec	Stu A	Other
6	5	3	3	0	0	0	35	0	0	0	60	5

Doctoral Degree Programs												
Admission and Enrollment 2002				Adv Ed	Mngd Care	Private | Agency Practice		School and Student Affairs				Other
Admit	Grad	F	M			Private	Agency	El	Mddle	Sec	Stu A	

Counselor Education
NY Syracuse University Syracuse

Admit	Grad	F	M	Adv Ed	Mngd Care	Private	Agency	El	Mddle	Sec	Stu A	Other
4-6	4-6	13	8			10	20					70

Counselor Education
NY University of Rochester Rochester

Admit	Grad	F	M	Adv Ed	Mngd Care	Private	Agency	El	Mddle	Sec	Stu A	Other
5 re-cently	2 in past	13	11	40	15	15	15		5	5	5	

Counselor Education
OH Kent State University Kent

Admit	Grad	F	M	Adv Ed	Mngd Care	Private	Agency	El	Mddle	Sec	Stu A	Other
14	10	62	18		4	10	35	2	2	2	45	

Counselor Education
OH Ohio University Athens

Admit	Grad	F	M	Adv Ed	Mngd Care	Private	Agency	El	Mddle	Sec	Stu A	Other
12	12											

Counselor Education
OH University of Cincinnati Cincinnati

Admit	Grad	F	M	Adv Ed	Mngd Care	Private	Agency	El	Mddle	Sec	Stu A	Other
8	3	19	10	0	10	25	40				25	

Counselor Education
OR Oregon State University Corvallis

Admit	Grad	F	M	Adv Ed	Mngd Care	Private	Agency	El	Mddle	Sec	Stu A	Other
4	4	12				50					50	

Counselor Education
PA Duquesne University Pittsburgh

Admit	Grad	F	M	Adv Ed	Mngd Care	Private	Agency	El	Mddle	Sec	Stu A	Other
11	4	15	15		10	20	25		5	5	5	30

Counselor Education
PA Penn State University University Park

Admit	Grad	F	M	Adv Ed	Mngd Care	Private	Agency	El	Mddle	Sec	Stu A	Other

Counselor Education
SC University of South Carolina Columbia

Admit	Grad	F	M	Adv Ed	Mngd Care	Private	Agency	El	Mddle	Sec	Stu A	Other
9	3	16	7	0	0	0	0	0	0	0	100	0

Counselor Education
SD The University of South Dakota Vermillion

Admit	Grad	F	M	Adv Ed	Mngd Care	Private	Agency	El	Mddle	Sec	Stu A	Other
8	3	50%	50%	75	12	12						

Counselor Education
TN The University of Tennessee at Knoxville Knoxville

Admit	Grad	F	M	Adv Ed	Mngd Care	Private	Agency	El	Mddle	Sec	Stu A	Other
5		3	2									

Counselor Education
TX Texas A & M University - Commerce Commerce

Admit	Grad	F	M	Adv Ed	Mngd Care	Private	Agency	El	Mddle	Sec	Stu A	Other
11	8			0	10	10	10	2	1	2		65

Counselor Education
TX Texas Southern University Houston

Admit	Grad	F	M	Adv Ed	Mngd Care	Private	Agency	El	Mddle	Sec	Stu A	Other
15	10	30	30	0	5	5	10	10	20	20	15	15

Counselor Education
TX Texas Tech University Lubbock

Admit	Grad	F	M	Adv Ed	Mngd Care	Private	Agency	El	Mddle	Sec	Stu A	Other
6	3	3	3	0	10	15	40	5	0	0	5	univ 25

Counselor Education
TX University of North Texas Denton

Admit	Grad	F	M	Adv Ed	Mngd Care	Private	Agency	El	Mddle	Sec	Stu A	Other
15	9	7	2								100	

Doctoral Degree Programs												
Admission and Enrollment				Postgraduation Activity/Placement Percentages								
2002				Adv Ed	Mngd Care	Private Practice	Agency	School and Student Affairs				
Admit	Grad	F	M					EI	Mddle	Sec	Stu A	Other
Counselor Education VA College of William and Mary Williamsburg												
10	6	8	2	80		20						
Counselor Education VA George Mason University Fairfax												
3	2	50%	50%	0								100
Counselor Education VA Regent University Virginia Beach												
15	0											
Counselor Education VA Virginia Tech Blacksburg												
5-10	5-8			60		15	10		5	5	5	
Counselor Education WY University of Wyoming Laramie												
6		4	2	40		10	40				10	
Marriage and Family Counseling CO Denver Seminary Denver												
Marriage and Family Counseling FL University of Florida Gainesville												
3	5											
Marriage and Family Counseling MI Oakland University Rochester												
1	1											
Mental Health Counseling FL University of Florida Gainesville												
7	5											
Mental Health Counseling IN Indiana University Bloomington												
5-8	5-8	22	20				40				40	20
Mental Health Counseling MI Andrews University Berrien Springs												
Mental Health Counseling MI Oakland University Rochester												
2	2											
Other AL Auburn University Auburn												
5	5	25	5									
Other IN Ball State University Muncie												
10	7	31	11		20	25	25				20	10
Other MI Oakland University Rochester												
		18	5									

525

Doctoral Degree Programs												
Admission and Enrollment				Postgraduation Activity/Placement Percentages								
2002				Adv Ed	Mngd Care	Private | Agency		School and Student Affairs				
Admit	Grad	F	M			Practice		EI	Mddle	Sec	Stu A	Other

Other
MN Capella University Minneapolis

Admit	Grad	F	M	Adv Ed	Mngd Care	Private	Agency	EI	Mddle	Sec	Stu A	Other
20		17	3									

Other
MO University of Missouri-Columbia Columbia

Admit	Grad	F	M	Adv Ed	Mngd Care	Private	Agency	EI	Mddle	Sec	Stu A	Other
8	6	44	23	0	1	1	49	0	0	0	33	16

Other
NY New York University New York

Admit	Grad	F	M	Adv Ed	Mngd Care	Private	Agency	EI	Mddle	Sec	Stu A	Other
4												

Other
NY SUNY University at Buffalo Buffalo

Admit	Grad	F	M	Adv Ed	Mngd Care	Private	Agency	EI	Mddle	Sec	Stu A	Other
10	10	7	3	0	60	30	10		0	0	0	0

Other
WV West Virginia University Morgantown

Admit	Grad	F	M	Adv Ed	Mngd Care	Private	Agency	EI	Mddle	Sec	Stu A	Other
8	6-8	5	3		10	30	30					30 Univ

Pastoral Counseling
MD Loyola College in Maryland Columbia

Admit	Grad	F	M	Adv Ed	Mngd Care	Private	Agency	EI	Mddle	Sec	Stu A	Other
12	6-10	25	15	25		35	15			2	3	20

Rehabilitation Counseling
IA The University of Iowa Iowa City

Admit	Grad	F	M	Adv Ed	Mngd Care	Private	Agency	EI	Mddle	Sec	Stu A	Other
3	3	6	3	0	10	10	20		0	0	60	0

Rehabilitation Counseling
IL Illinois Institute of Technology Chicago

Admit	Grad	F	M	Adv Ed	Mngd Care	Private	Agency	EI	Mddle	Sec	Stu A	Other
3	2	2	1									

School Counseling
FL University of Florida Gainesville

Admit	Grad	F	M	Adv Ed	Mngd Care	Private	Agency	EI	Mddle	Sec	Stu A	Other
3	2											

School Counseling
KS Kansas State University Manhattan

Admit	Grad	F	M	Adv Ed	Mngd Care	Private	Agency	EI	Mddle	Sec	Stu A	Other
2	0	2	1	0	0	0	0		40		40	20

School Counseling
MI Oakland University Rochester

Admit	Grad	F	M	Adv Ed	Mngd Care	Private	Agency	EI	Mddle	Sec	Stu A	Other

School Counseling
MS Mississippi State University Mississippi State University

Admit	Grad	F	M	Adv Ed	Mngd Care	Private	Agency	EI	Mddle	Sec	Stu A	Other
						10						90

School Counseling
NC University of North Carolina at Charlotte Charlotte

Admit	Grad	F	M	Adv Ed	Mngd Care	Private	Agency	EI	Mddle	Sec	Stu A	Other

School Counseling
NV University of Nevada Reno

Admit	Grad	F	M	Adv Ed	Mngd Care	Private	Agency	EI	Mddle	Sec	Stu A	Other
2	1	12	2	20					40	20	20	

Doctoral Degree Programs												
Admission and Enrollment				Postgraduation Activity/Placement Percentages								
2002				Adv Ed	Mngd Care	Private Practice	Agency	School and Student Affairs				Other
Admit	Grad	F	M					El	Mddle	Sec	Stu A	

School Counseling
OH The University of Toledo   Toledo

Admit	Grad	F	M	Adv Ed	Mngd Care	Private Practice	Agency	El	Mddle	Sec	Stu A	Other
4	3	3	1			20	80					

School Counseling
VA George Mason University   Fairfax

Admit	Grad	F	M	Adv Ed	Mngd Care	Private Practice	Agency	El	Mddle	Sec	Stu A	Other
3	2	50%	50%						10	10	80	

Student Affairs
IA The University of Iowa   Iowa City

Admit	Grad	F	M	Adv Ed	Mngd Care	Private Practice	Agency	El	Mddle	Sec	Stu A	Other
4		7	1	0	0	10	0		0	0	55	35

Student Affairs
KS Kansas State University   Manhattan

Admit	Grad	F	M	Adv Ed	Mngd Care	Private Practice	Agency	El	Mddle	Sec	Stu A	Other
3	1	3	1	0	0	0	0	0	0	0	100	0

Student Affairs
NV University of Nevada   Reno

Admit	Grad	F	M	Adv Ed	Mngd Care	Private Practice	Agency	El	Mddle	Sec	Stu A	Other
1	1	4	1	20								80

Faculty Index